3402984395

Health Care

ersity of
rdshire

7

D1426469

Prevention and Treatment of Ischemic Stroke

Blue Books of Practical Neurology

(Volumes 1-14 published as BIMR Neurology)

1. **Clinical Neurophysiology**
   Eric Stalberg and Robert R. Young

2. **Movement Disorders**
   C. David Marsden and
   Stanley Fahn

3. **Cerebral Vascular Disease**
   Michael J.G. Harrison and
   Mark L. Dyken

4. **Peripheral Nerve Disorders**
   Arthur K. Asbury and R.W. Gilliatt

5. **The Epilepsies**
   Roger J. Porter and
   Paolo I. Morselli

6. **Multiple Sclerosis**
   W. Ian McDonald and
   Donald H. Silberberg

7. **Movement Disorders 2**
   C. David Marsden and
   Stanley Fahn

8. **Infections of the Nervous System**
   Peter G.E. Kennedy and
   Richard T. Johnson

9. **The Molecular Biology of
   Neurological Disease**
   Roger N. Rosenberg and
   Anita E. Harding

10. **Pain Syndromes in Neurology**
    Howard L. Fields

11. **Principles and Practice of
    Restorative Neurology**
    Robert R. Young and
    Paul J. Delwaide

12. **Stroke: Populations, Cohorts, and
    Clinical Trials**
    Jack P. Whisnant

13. **Movement Disorders 3**
    C. David Marsden and
    Stanley Fahn

14. **Mitochondrial Disorders in
    Neurology**
    A.H.V. Schapira and
    Salvatore DiMauro

15. **Peripheral Nerve Disorders 2**
    Arthur K. Asbury and
    P.K. Thomas

16. **Contemporary Behavioral
    Neurology**
    Michael R. Trimble and
    Jeffrey L. Cummings

17. **Headache**
    Peter J. Goadsby and
    Stephen D. Silberstein

18. **The Epilepsies 2**
    Roger J. Porter and
    David Chadwick

19. **The Dementias**
    John H. Growdon and
    Martin N. Rossor

20. **Hospitalist Neurology**
    Martin A. Samuels

21. **Neurologic Complications in
    Organ Transplant Recipients**
    Eelco F.M. Wijdicks

22. **Critical Care Neurology**
    David H. Miller and
    Eric C. Raps

23. **Neurology of Bladder, Bowel, and
    Sexual Dysfunction**
    Clare J. Fowler

24. **Muscle Diseases**
    Anthony H.V. Schapira and
    Robert C. Griggs

25. **Clinical Trials in Neurologic
    Practice**
    José Biller and
    Julien Bogousslavsky

26. **Mitochondrial Disorders in
    Neurology 2**
    A.H.V. Schapira and
    Salvatore DiMauro

27. **Multiple Sclerosis 2**
    W. Ian McDonald and
    John H. Noseworthy

28. **Motor Neuron Disorders**
    Pamela J. Shaw and
    Michael J. Strong

29. **Prevention and Treatment of
    Ischemic Stroke**
    Scott E. Kasner and
    Philip B. Gorelick

Prevention and Treatment of Ischemic Stroke

Edited by

Scott E. Kasner, M.D.
Associate Professor, Department of Neurology
Director, Comprehensive Stroke Center
University of Pennsylvania Medical Center
Philadelphia, Pennsylvania

and

Philip B. Gorelick, M.D., M.P.H., F.A.C.P.
John S. Garvin Professor and Head
Department of Neurology and Rehabilitation
University of Illinois College of Medicine at Chicago
Chicago, Illinois

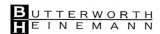

An Imprint of Elsevier

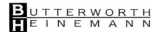

An Imprint of Elsevier, Inc.

The Curtis Center
Independence Square West
Philadelphia, Pennsylvania 19106

NOTICE

Medicine is an ever-changing field. Standard safety precautions must be followed, but as new research and clinical experience broaden our knowledge, changes in treatment and drug therapy may become necessary or appropriate. Readers are advised to check the most current product information provided by the manufacturer of each drug to be administered to verify the recommended dose, the method and duration of administration, and contraindications. It is the responsibility of the licensed prescriber, relying on experience and knowledge of the patient, to determine dosages and the best treatment for each individual patient. Neither the publisher nor the editor assumes any liability for any injury and/or damage to persons or property arising from this publication.

Library of Congress Cataloging-in-Publication Data

Prevention and treatment of ischemic stroke / [edited by] Scott Eric Kasner, Philip B. Gorelick. – 1st ed.
    p. ; cm. – (Blue books of practical neurology ; 29)
    Includes bibliographical references and index.
    ISBN 0-7506-7464-4
    1. Cerebrovascular disease. 2. Cerebral ischemia. I. Kasner, Scott Eric. II. Gorelick, Philip B. III. Series.
    [DNLM: 1. Cerebrovascular Accident–therapy. 2. Brain Infarction. 3. Cerebrovascular Accident–prevention & control. 4. Risk Factors. 5. Thrombolytic Therapy. WL 355 P9442 2004]
RC388.5.P657 2004
616.8'1–dc21

Acquisitions Editor: Susan F. Pioli
Developmental Editor: Laurie Anello
Project Manager: Mary Stermel

Printed in the United States of America

Last digit is the print number: 9   8   7   6   5   4   3   2   1

To my wife Margie, for everything.
– Scott E. Kasner

In dedication to my wonderful children, David and Alissa, and loving
wife, Bonnie, and their promise to make the world a better place.
– Philip B. Gorelick

Contents

Contributing Authors   ix
Series Preface   xiii
Preface   xv

1. Prevention and Treatment of Ischemic Stroke:
   A Practical Perspective   1
   Scott E. Kasner and Philip B. Gorelick

2. Primary Prevention of Stroke by Modification of Selected
   Risk Factors   5
   Michael A. Sloan

3. Etiologies and Mechanisms of Ischemia   55
   Enrique C. Leira and Harold P. Adams Jr.

4. Diagnostic Evaluation of Transient Ischemic Attack and
   Ischemic Stroke   67
   Andrei V. Alexandrov and John Y. Choi

5. Cardioembolic Stroke   79
   Richard K. T. Chan and Patrick M. Pullicino

6. Large-Vessel Atherosclerosis   99
   Sarah T. Pendlebury and Peter M. Rothwell

7. Small-Vessel Occlusive Disease   123
   Oscar Benavente

8. Unusual Causes of Stroke   139
   Serge A. Blecic and Julien Bogousslavsky

9. Antithrombotic Therapy for Secondary Prevention of
   Ischemic Stroke   175
   Pierre Fayad and Sanjay P. Singh

10. Risk Factor Modification for Secondary Prevention   197
    Sean Ruland

11. Rapid Clinical Evaluation   211
    Chelsea S. Kidwell and Jeffrey L. Saver

12. Rapid Diagnostic Evaluation   237
    David S. Liebeskind

13. Thrombolytic Therapies   267
    Fahmi M. Al-Senani and James C. Grotta

14. Antithrombotic Therapy for Acute Ischemic Stroke   283
    Brett L. Cucchiara and Scott E. Kasner

15. Emerging Therapies for Ischemic Stroke   303
    Y. Dennis Cheng, Lama Michel Al-Khoury, and Justin A. Zivin

16. Supportive Care of the Acute Stroke Patient   329
    Julio A. Chalela and Jason W. Todd

17. Medical Complications of Stroke   349
    Devin L. Brown, Teresa L. Smith, and Karen C. Johnston

18. Neurological Deterioration in Acute Stroke   363
    Devin L. Brown, Teresa L. Smith, and Karen C. Johnston

19. Rehabilitation After Stroke   377
    Alexander W. Dromerick

Index   393

Contributing Authors

Harold P. Adams Jr., M.D.
Professor, Department of Neurology, University of Iowa College of Medicine, Iowa City, Iowa

Lama Michel Al-Khoury, M.D.
Stroke Fellow, Department of Neurology/Neurosciences, University of California at San Diego, San Diego

Fahmi M. Al-Senani, M.D.
Associate Consultant, Department of Neurosciences, King Faisal Specialist Hospital and Research Center, Riyadh, Saudi Arabia

Andrei V. Alexandrov, M.D.
Assistant Professor and Director, Cerebrovascular Ultrasound, Stroke Treatment Team, Department of Neurology, University of Texas Medical School, Houston

Oscar Benavente, M.D., F.R.C.P.(C.)
Associate Professor, Department of Medicine/Neurology, University of Texas Health Science Center, San Antonio

Serge Blecic, M.D.
Associate Professor of Neurology, Department of Neurology, Free University of Brussels, Brussels, Belgium; Head of the Stroke Unit, Department of Neurology, Erasme Hospital, Free University of Brussels, Brussels, Belgium

Julien Bogousslavsky
Professor and Chairman, Department of Neurology, Centre Hospitalier, Universitaire Vaudois, Lausanne, Switzerland

Devin L. Brown, M.D.
Fellow, Stroke and Cardiovascular Disease, Department of Neurology, University of Virginia School of Medicine, Charlottesville, Virginia

Julio A. Chalela, M.D.
Staff Clinician–Director of Clinical Stroke Service, Section on Stroke Diagnostics and Therapeutics, National Institute of Neurological Disorders and Stroke (NINDS)/National Institutes of Health (NIH), Bethesda, Maryland

Richard K. T. Chan, M.B.B.S., F.R.C.P.(Edin.)
Assistant Professor of Neurology and Neurosurgery, Department of Neurology, State University of New York at Buffalo, Buffalo; Director, Stroke Program at Kaleida Health System, Department of Neurology, Buffalo General Hospital, Buffalo

Y. Dennis Cheng, M.D., Ph.D.
Stroke Fellow, Department of Neuroscience, University of California at San Diego, San Diego

John Y. Choi, M.D.
Assistant Professor, Stroke Treatment Team, Department of Neurology, Uniformed Services University of the Health Sciences, Bethesda, Maryland

Brett L. Cucchiara, M.D.
Clinical Instructor, Department of Neurology, University of Pennsylvania Medical Center, Philadelphia

Alexander W. Dromerick, M.D.
Associate Professor of Neurology, Department of Neurology, Washington University School of Medicine, St. Louis; Medical Director of Rehabilitation Services, Barnes-Jewish Hospital, St. Louis

Pierre Fayad, M.D.
Reynolds Centennial Professor and Chairman, Department of Neurological Sciences, University of Nebraska Medical Center, College of Medicine and Nebraska Health System, Omaha; Reynolds Centennial Professor and Chairman, Department of Neurological Sciences, Nebraska Health System, Omaha

Philip B. Gorelick, M.D., M.P.H.
Professor and Director, Center for Stroke Research, Department of Neurological Sciences, Rush Medical College and Rush Medical Center, Chicago

James C. Grotta M.D.
Professor, Department of Neurology, University of Texas Medical School, Houston

Karen C. Johnson, M.D., M.Sc.
Associate Professor of Neurology and Health Evaluation Sciences, Department of Neurology and Health Evaluation Sciences, University of Virginia School of Medicine, Charlottesville, Virginia

Scott E. Kasner, M.D.
Associate Professor, Department of Neurology, University of Pennsylvania, Philadelphia; Director, Comprehensive Stroke Center, University of Pennsylvania Medical Center, Philadelphia

Chelsea S. Kidwell, M.D.
Associate Professor, Department of Neurology, UCLA Medical Center, Los Angeles

David S. Liebeskind, M.D.
Assistant Professor, Department of Neurology, University of Pennsylvania School of Medicine, Philadelphia

Enrique C. Leira, M.D.
Assistant Professor and Co-Director of Souers Stroke Institute, Department of Neurology, Saint Louis University School of Medicine, St. Louis

Sarah T. Pendlebury, Ph.D., M.R.C.P.
Special Registrar, Department of Clinical Geratology, Radcliffe Infirmary, Oxford, United Kingdom

Patrick M. Pullicino, M.D.
Professor and Chairman, Department of Neurology and Neurosciences, New Jersey Medical School (NJMS), University of Medicine and Dentistry of New Jersey (UMDNJ), Newark, New Jersey

Peter M. Rothwell, M.D., Ph.D., F.R.C.P.
Reader in Clinical Neurology, Department of Clinical Neurology, University of Oxford, Oxford, United Kingdom; Consultant Neurologist, Department of Clinical Neurology, Radcliffe Infirmary, Oxford, United Kingdom

Sean Ruland, D.O.
Assistant Professor of Neurology and Neurological Surgery, Department of Neurological Sciences, Rush Medical College, Chicago; Assistant Attending, Department of Neurology, Rush-Presbyterian-St. Luke's Medical Center, Chicago

Jeffrey L. Saver, M.D.
Professor, Department of Neurology, David Geffen School of Medicine, University of California at Los Angeles, Los Angeles; Neurology Director, Stroke Center, UCLA Medical Center, Los Angeles

Sanjay P. Singh, M.D.
Assistant Professor, Department of Neurological Sciences, University of Nebraska Medical Center, Omaha; Director, Epilepsy Program, Department of Neurological Sciences, Nebraska Health System, Omaha

Michael A. Sloan, M.D.
Associate Professor, Department of Neurological Sciences and Neurosurgery, Rush-Presbyterian-St. Luke's Medical Center, Chicago; Director, In-Patient Stroke Service, Department of Neurological Sciences, Rush-Presbyterian-St. Luke's Medical Center, Chicago; Director, Cerebrovascular Ultrasonography Laboratory, Rush-Presbyterian-St. Luke's Medical Center, Chicago

Teresa L. Smith, M.D.
Clinical Instructor of Neurology, and Fellow of Neuro-Critical Care, Department of Neurology, University of Virginia School of Medicine, Charlottesville, Virginia

Jason W. Todd, M.D.
Clinical Fellow, Section on Stroke Diagnostics and Therapeutics, National Institute of Neurological Disorders and Stroke (NINDS), Bethesda, Maryland

Justin A. Zivin, M.D., Ph.D.
Professor, Department of Neurosciences, University of California at San Diego, La Jolla, California

Series Preface

The *Blue Books of Practical Neurology* denotes the series of monographs previously named the *BIMR Neurology* series, which was itself the successor of the *Modern Trends in Neurology* series. As before, the volumes are intended for use by physicians who grapple with the problems of neurological disorders on a daily basis, be they neurologists, neurologists in training, or those in related fields such as neurosurgery, internal medicine, psychiatry, and rehabilitation medicine.

Our purpose is to produce monographs on topics in clinical neurology in which progress through research has brought about new concepts of patient management. The subject of each book is selected by the Series Editors using two criteria: first, that there has been significant advance in knowledge in that area and, second, that such advances have been incorporated into new ways of managing patients with the disorders in question. This has been the guiding spirit behind each volume, and we expect it to continue. In effect, we emphasize research, both in the clinic and in the experimental laboratory, but principally to the extent that it changes our collective attitudes and practices in caring for those who are neurologically afflicted.

Arthur K. Asbury
Anthony H.V. Schapira
Series Editors

Preface

The third volume of *Blue Books of Practical Neurology* series was entitled *Cerebral Vascular Disease* and was published in 1982. It emphasized the natural history of stroke and its mechanisms. The next volume on this topic was number 12, *Stroke: Populations, Cohorts, and Clinical Trials,* published in 1993, which provided a detailed view of the potential targets and methods for effective treatment and prevention of stroke. The volume in your hands capitalizes on the fruits of these former labors, as we now have truly **practical** evidence and advice to provide to the multitude of clinicians who care for patients with stroke. Clinical research in stroke has grown exponentially over the past decade, but clinical practice has lagged substantially behind the available evidence. We have therefore asked our authors to provide specific and practical evidence-based approaches to stroke treatment and prevention. However, it is quite clear that there are many clinical questions that have not been answered, and many others that are beyond current research methodology. In these situations, we have asked the authors to "go out on a limb"—to offer their own recommendations when the evidence is lacking.

We thank all of the authors for their outstanding contributions; the Series Editors Arthur K. Asbury and Anthony H. V. Schapira for inviting us to join the ranks of the *Blue Books of Practical Neurology;* and the publishers Susan F. Pioli and Laurie Anello, in particular, for bringing this book to life.

1

Prevention and Treatment of Ischemic Stroke: A Practical Perspective

Scott E. Kasner and Philip B. Gorelick

DEFINITIONS

Stroke remains a broadly defined term, which includes ischemic stroke, intracerebral hemorrhage, subarachnoid hemorrhage, and cerebral venous thrombosis. This volume addresses only ischemic stroke. Ischemic stroke can be subclassified in many ways; one widely used system defines five major stroke subtypes according to the etiological mechanism: large-vessel athero-thromboembolism, cardioembolism, small-vessel occlusive disease, nonathero-sclerotic unusual causes of stroke, and cryptogenic (i.e., infarct of unknown cause) stroke.[1] The first three of these account for the vast majority (up to 90%) of all ischemic strokes and are therefore the major thrust of this volume.

EPIDEMIOLOGY

In the United States, it is estimated that there are approximately 600,000 to 750,000 strokes annually, of which 80 to 85 percent are ischemic.[2,3] Stroke ranks third among causes of death and first among causes of long-term disability. Nearly 25 percent of people who have a stroke will die within a year, and another 15 to 30 percent will be permanently disabled. Given the high incidence and mortality of stroke, it should be apparent that interventions with relatively small incremental benefit may affect a large number of people. Furthermore, the incidence of stroke increases with age, roughly doubling every 5 to 10 years beyond age 55,[2] and therefore stroke poses an increasing burden on the public health system as the population ages. Stroke risk is also higher in people of African and some of Hispanic origin. Although age, sex, race, and ethnicity are nonmodifiable, these factors should call attention to those people for whom

1

aggressive prevention measures and care are needed to minimize the risk and the complications of stroke.

PREVENTION OF ISCHEMIC STROKE

Stroke prevention may be targeted at two basic levels: the "mass approach" for the population at large and the "high-risk approach" for those in the population who are believed to be at greater risk.[4] Stroke-preventive strategies may be further conceptualized as being stratified into two major categories: generic or mechanism-specific. Generic prevention relates to the management of the modifiable vascular risk factors, such as hypertension, diabetes mellitus, lipid disorders, smoking, and so forth, all of which may cause injury to the large and small cerebral blood vessels and the coronary and peripheral arteries, regardless of the specific causes of stroke. Generic primary prevention is addressed in Chapter 2, whereas secondary prevention is addressed in Chapters 9 and 10. Mechanism-specific prevention addresses specific causes, such as carotid artery stenosis or atrial fibrillation, but does not address the systemic processes of atherosclerosis or other cardiovascular injury. Consequently, these mechanism-specific interventions require appropriate diagnosis of the proximate cause of stroke. The etiologies and mechanisms of stroke are defined further in Chapter 3, the diagnostic techniques are summarized in Chapter 4, and the mechanism-specific preventative strategies are discussed in Chapters 5 through 8.

ACUTE STROKE DIAGNOSIS AND TREATMENT

Treatment of acute stroke has been transformed by the advent of thrombolytic therapy. Newer therapies also appear on the horizon, but the overwhelming evidence supports the "time is brain" tenet and suggests that early intervention is needed for any therapy to improve outcome. Consequently, rapid diagnosis is needed, and the clinical and radiological tools for evaluation are evolving accordingly. The traditional approach has consisted of general physical and neurological examinations, a computed tomography (CT) of the brain, and a few basic blood tests, but these may be improved on. Chapters 11 and 12 describe these methods and newer approaches that provide a framework for expedited diagnosis and initiation of acute stroke therapies. In patients who are eligible, thrombolysis can improve outcome, but it is associated with a risk of hemorrhagic complications. This risk can be minimized with careful adherence to standard protocols. Chapter 13 describes the state-of-the-art approach to thrombolysis and the relevant considerations in clinical practice. For those who do not receive thrombolysis, antiplatelet agents and possibly anticoagulant medications remain the mainstay of early stroke therapy for most patients. The evidence for and against the use of these agents is summarized in Chapter 14. Emerging therapies, although not fully tested, provide promise for alternatives to existing therapy and the possibilities of multimodal or combination therapy. These novel putative treatments are described in Chapter 15.

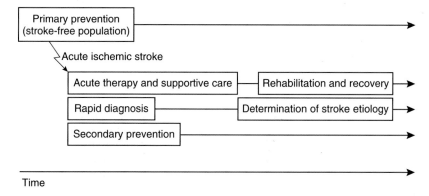

Figure 1.1 The continuum of stroke care. Primary prevention measures are implemented in the healthy stroke-free population to limit the risk of stroke (*upper bar*). If an acute stroke occurs, several issues must be implemented in parallel (*lower bars*): treatment (acute therapy and supportive care, followed by rehabilitation), diagnostic evaluation (initial rapid diagnosis followed by determination of etiology), and secondary prevention (which ultimately depends on both etiology and recovery).

In the days to weeks after stroke, patients are at risk of suffering from a host of medical and neurological complications, many of which are preventable and can worsen the outcome of the stroke. Many of these basic issues have been rigorously evaluated in recent years, and Chapters 16 to 18 offer guidelines about how to organize and implement supportive care of the stroke patient to prevent and treat these complications. Finally, patients with neurological deficits and disability may improve after their initial hospital-based treatment. Rehabilitation of the stroke patient and advances in this field are outlined in Chapter 19.

THE CONTINUUM OF STROKE CARE

Effective prevention and treatment of stroke require a comprehensive approach to each and every patient and span the full continuum of care (Figure 1.1). Clinical research has yielded a wealth of information to guide us in these efforts, and it is our hope that this text will help clinicians at all levels to transform evidence into clinical reality.

References

1. Adams HP, Bendixen BH, Kappelle LJ, et al. Classification of subtype of acute ischemic stroke. Definitions for use in a multicenter clinical trial. Stroke 1993;24:35–41.
2. Wolf PA, D'Agostino RB. Epidemiology of Stroke. In HJM Barnett, JP Mohr, BM Stein, FM Yatsu (eds), Stroke: Pathophysiology, Diagnosis, and Management (3rd ed). New York: Churchill Livingstone, 1998;3–28.
3. Broderick J, Brott T, Kothari R, et al. The Greater Cincinnati/Northern Kentucky Stroke Study: preliminary first-ever and total incidence rates of stroke among blacks. Stroke 1998;29:415–421.
4. Gorelick PB. Community Mass and High Risk Strategies. In PB Gorelick, MA Alter (eds), The Prevention of Stroke. New York: Parthenon, 2002;115–121.

cho

2
Primary Prevention of Stroke by Modification of Selected Risk Factors

Michael A. Sloan

Stroke is a major public health problem. It is the second leading cause of mortality worldwide; the leading cause of death in China and Japan; the third leading cause of death in most developed nations; and a major cause of hospital admission, morbidity, mortality, and long-term disability.[1] In the United States in 1999, there were an estimated 731,000 new and recurrent strokes,[2] with 167,366 deaths, 4.6 million stroke survivors, and 1.1 million functionally limited adults.[3] Major cardiovascular risk factors and associated health conditions have been identified.[3–7] The economic impact of stroke in the United States is enormous; in 1999, the estimated direct and indirect cost of stroke was $51 billion.[8] From an international perspective, stroke mortality in 1990 ranged from approximately 60 per 100,000 in the United States to 500 to 600 per 100,000 in the former republics of the Union of Soviet Socialist Republics.[9] Recent epidemiological data suggest that the decline in stroke-related mortality has leveled off.[10] These data are concerning in view of demographic trends predicting a substantial increase in the population of aged, stroke-prone individuals over the next few decades.

Recent reviews[11–22] have summarized the evidence regarding primary prevention of stroke by modification of established and potential stroke risk factors. The current prevalence of many of these risk factors is shown in Table 2.1.[3–7] As such, guidelines and advice regarding their proper use are now available.[11,13–15] This chapter provides an evidence-based update on the epidemiology, pathophysiology, and management of selected risk factors, such as hypertension, hyperlipidemia, smoking, alcohol use, diabetes mellitus, insulin resistance and metabolic syndrome, obesity, hyperhomocyst(e)inemia, inflammation/infection, and illicit drug use and abuse for primary stroke prevention. For each risk factor, data on strength of association, population attributable risk, treatment effect, and recommendations for stroke prevention are summarized in Tables 2.2 and 2.3.

Table 2.1 Prevalence of selected modifiable/potentially modifiable stroke risk factors by race/ethnicity and gender

Risk Factor	Non-Hispanic White Male (%)	Female (%)	Non-Hispanic Black Male (%)	Female (%)	Hispanic/Mexican American Male (%)	Female (%)	American Indian/Alaska Native Male (%)	Female (%)	Asian/Pacific Islander Male (%)	Female (%)	Age Group
Hypertension	25.2	20.5	36.7	36.6	24.2	22.4	—	—	—	—	≥20 years
	—	—	—	—	—	—	26.8	27.5	—	—	45–74 years
	—	—	—	—	—	—	—	—	9.7	8.4	Age-adjusted
Hyperlipidemia											
T-chol >200 mg/dL	52	49	45	46	53	48	—	—	—	—	20–74 years, age-adjusted
T-chol >240 mg/dL	18	20	15	18	18	17	—	—	—	—	20–74 years, age-adjusted
LDL chol >130 mg/dL	49.6	43.7	46.3	41.6	43.6	41.6	—	—	—	—	20–74 years, age-adjusted
HDL chol <40 mg/dL	40.5	14.5	24.3	13.0	40.1	18.4	—	—	—	—	≥20 years
Active smoking	25.5	23.1	28.7	20.8	24	12.3	40.9	40.8	24.3	7.1	≥18 years
Diabetes mellitus											
Diagnosed	5.4	4.7	7.6	9.5	8.1	11.4	—	—	—	—	≥20 years
	—	—	—	—	—	—	43.5	52.4	17	—	45–74 years
	—	—	—	—	—	—	—	—	17	—	71–93 years
Undiagnosed	3.0	2.1	2.8	4.7	5.8	3.9	—	—	—	—	≥20 years
	—	—	—	—	—	—	—	—	19	—	71–93 years
Dec gluc tol	9.4	4.8	8.0	6.8	12.1	6.7	—	—	—	—	≥20 years
	—	—	—	—	—	—	14.2	17.4	—	—	45–74 years
	—	—	—	—	—	—	—	—	32	—	71–93 years
Overweight/obesity											
BMI >25	61.5	46.8	58.4	68.3	69.3	69.3	25.9	31.3			20–74 years / 45–74 years
BMI >30	20.8	23.2	21.3	38.2	24.8	36.1	35.5	41.2			20–74 years / 45–74 years
Metabolic syndrome (≥3 components)	25.0	23.0	16.0	25.0	28.0	36.0					≥20 years, age-adjusted

Data adapted from references 3, 5, and 7.

BMI = body mass index; Dec gluc tol = decreased glucose tolerance; HDL chol = high-density lipoprotein cholesterol; LDL chol = low-density lipoprotein cholesterol; T-chol = total cholesterol.

DIASTOLIC AND ISOLATED SYSTOLIC HYPERTENSION

Hypertension, defined as systolic pressure 140 mm Hg or greater or diastolic pressure 90 mm Hg or greater or use of antihypertensive medication, is a disorder typically associated with increased mean arterial pressure and peripheral resistance. In 1999, it affected about 50 million Americans age 6 years and older or about one of four U.S. adults.[3] The prevalence of hypertension increases with age. In the United States, persons who are African American, with lower educational and income levels tend to have higher blood pressures.[3] For individuals age 40 to 70 years, each incremental increase of 20 mm Hg systolic blood pressure or 10 mm Hg diastolic blood pressure doubles the risk of cardiovascular disease across the entire blood pressure range from 115/75 to 185/115 mm Hg.[16] Patients with blood pressures of 120/80 to 139/89 mm Hg should be considered prehypertensive and require health promoting lifestyle modifications to prevent cardiovascular disease.[17] In patients with stage 1 hypertension (140/90 to 159/99 mm Hg) and additional cardiovascular risk factors, it is estimated that a sustained 12 mm Hg systolic blood pressure reduction would prevent 1 death for every 11 patients treated; if cardiovascular disease or end-organ damage is present, only 9 patients would require treatment to achieve this benefit.[18]

Hypertension is the preeminent risk factor for both ischemic and hemorrhagic stroke, with a population attributable risk of 35 to 50 percent, depending on age.[19,23] The Framingham Study observed that the age-adjusted relative risk of stroke among those with definite hypertension (blood pressure >160/95 mm Hg) was 3.1 for men and 2.9 for women.[24] A meta-analysis of nine prospective studies following 420,000 patients over 10 years showed that the risk of stroke increases in proportion to systolic and diastolic blood pressures, with the relationship being "direct, continuous, and independent of other risk factors." For every 7.5 mm Hg increase in diastolic blood pressure, there was a 46 percent increase in stroke risk.[25] A more recent meta-analysis of 450,000 patients showed that each 10 mm Hg increase in diastolic blood pressure multiplied the stroke risk by 1.84 (95% confidence interval [CI] 1.80 to 1.90), with some attenuation of the effect with increasing age (Figure 2.1).[26] In the Northern Manhattan Stroke Study (NOMASS), hypertension was a strong, independent risk factor for whites (odds ratio [OR] 1.8), African Americans (OR 2.0), and Hispanics (OR 2.1).[27] In the Baltimore-Washington Cooperative Young Stroke Study, the age-adjusted ORs (95% CI) of ischemic stroke for history of hypertension in patients age 15 to 44 years were white males 1.6 (0.7 to 3.2), white females 2.5 (1.1 to 5.9), African-American males 3.8 (1.8 to 7.9), and African-American females 4.2 (2.4 to 7.5).[28] A recent meta-analysis of 124,774 patients in 18 cohort studies from the People's Republic of China and Japan showed a stronger relationship between blood pressure and stroke (especially hemorrhagic) in east Asian populations. There was a lower risk of nonhemorrhagic stroke (OR 0.61, 95% CI = 0.57 to 0.66) and hemorrhagic stroke (OR 0.54, 95% CI = 0.50 to 0.58) for each 5-mm decrease in diastolic blood pressure.[29]

Isolated systolic hypertension (ISH) (>160 mm Hg systolic, <90 mm Hg diastolic) is an important risk factor for stroke in the elderly.[30–35] This disorder is mainly due to decreased elasticity of large arteries, as suggested by an increasing degree of blunting of the dicrotic notch in the pulse wave. The prevalence of ISH rises curvilinearly with age, averaging 8 percent in sexagenarians and

Table 2.2 Selected modifiable/potentially modifiable stroke risk factors: Prevalence, relative risk, attributable risk, and treatment effect

Risk Factor	Prevalence (%)	Relative Risk	Population Attributable Risk[a]	Positive Clinical Trial?	Treatment Effect/Risk Reduction
Hypertension	25–40	3–5	High	Yes	42–44%
50 years	20	4.0	High		
60 years	30	3.0	Medium		
70 years	40	2.0	Medium		
80 years	55	1.4	Medium		
90 years	60	1.0	Low		
Systolic hypertension		1.22		Yes	30–44%
60 years	8				
80 years	25				
Hyperlipidemia (total cholesterol >240 mg/dL, 6.21 mmol/L)	25–30	1.8 (240–279 mg/dL) 2.6 (>280 mg/dL)	Medium	Yes	30% with statins; patients with coronary artery disease
Cigarette smoking	20–40	1.5–1.8	Low	Yes	After cessation: 50% in 1 year; baseline after 2–5 years
Heavy alcohol consumption (>5 drinks per day)	2–5	1.6–2.2	Low	No	20% (men), 60% (young women), 1–2 drinks per day

Diabetes mellitus	5–11	1.8–6.0	Low	No	44% reduction in hypertensive diabetics with blood pressure control
Insulin resistance	22	1.5–2.1	Low	No	See text
20–29 years	6.7				
30–39 years	12.5				
40–49 years	22				
50–59 years	33				
60–69 years	43.5				
70–79 years	42				
Overweight/obesity		1.75–2.37	Medium	No	See text
BMI 25–29.9	37.1				
BMI ≥30	20.9				
BMI ≥40	2.3				
Hyperhomocysteinemia	21–47	1.3–2.3	Medium	No	See text
Drug abuse (cocaine)	3–14		Low	No	See text
Overall		1.8–7.0			
<24 hours		25–∞			

Data and table format are derived from references 3, 11–14, 19, and text.

BMI = body mass index.

[a] For population attributable risk, low = <15%, medium = 15–39%, high = 40+% (see references 11–13).

Table 2.3   Primary prevention of cardiovascular disease and stroke: Goals and interventions for (potentially) modifiable risk factors[a]

Risk Factor	Goal	Interventions
Hypertension Level of evidence—I; grade of recommendation—A	<140/90 mm Hg; <130/80 mm Hg if renal insufficiency, congestive heart failure are present; <130/80 mm Hg if diabetes is present	1. Promote healthy lifestyle modification 2. Weight reduction (ideal, desirable weight: BMI = 18.5–24.9) 3. Reduce sodium intake (<6 g/day) 4. Increase consumption of fruits, vegetables, grains, and nonfat/low-fat dairy products, unsaturated fatty acids (fish, vegetables, legumes, nuts) 5. Moderate alcohol intake 6. Appropriate level of physical activity (ideal: ≥30 min moderate intensity >3/wk) 7. Initiate drug therapy if lifestyle modification ineffective, presence of multiple risk factors
Hyperlipidemia Level of evidence—I, grade of recommendation—A (for patients with coronary artery disease)	Primary: ≤1 risk factor: goal LDL <160 mg/dL ≥2 risk factors and <20% 10-year CAD risk: goal LDL <130 mg/dL ≥2 risk factors, ≥20% 10-year CAD increase risk, diabetes: goal LDL <100 mg/dL Other targets: triglycerides >150 mg/dL, HDL cholesterol <40 mg/dL (men), <50 mg/dL (women)	1. If LDL is above goal range, initiate dietary/lifestyle changes: <7% calories from saturated fat, total cholesterol <200 mg/dL, dietary options (plant stanols/sterols <2 g/day, increased viscous (soluble) fiber 10–25 g/day), weight reduction, physical activity 2. If not successful after 12 weeks, start statin therapy 3. If not successful after 12 weeks despite dose adjustments, consider combination therapy (statin + resin, statin + niacin) 4. To reduce triglycerides, initiate lifestyle changes 5. If not successful, increase statin dose, add niacin or fibrate 6. To raise HDL, initiate/intensify lifestyle changes 7. If not successful, consider drugs to raise HDL—niacin, fibrates, statins
Smoking Level of evidence—III, grade of recommendation—C (however, observational epidemiological studies are compelling)	Complete cessation No environmental exposure to tobacco smoke	1. Firmly advise smoking cessation at every clinical encounter 2. Help the smoker develop a plan for smoking cessation 3. Offer counseling 4. Refer to special programs 5. Pharmacotherapy bupropion, nicotine-replacement products) 6. Advise avoidance of secondhand smoke

Risk factor	Goal	Recommendations
Alcohol consumption Level of evidence—IV, grade of recommendation—C (supported by case-control and cohort studies)	Moderate intake	1. Firmly advise that if one drinks, no more than 1 (women) and 2 (men) drinks/day at every clinical encounter 2. Offer counseling 3. Refer to Alcoholics Anonymous, faith-based rehabilitation program

Diabetes mellitus
Level of evidence—I, grade of recommendation—A (for control of hypertension in diabetics)
	Normal fasting plasma glucose (<110 mg/dL)
	Near normal HbA1c (<7%)
		1. Step 1: diet, weight loss, and exercise
		2. Step 2: usually oral hypoglycemic drugs—sulfonylureas, metformin, ancillary use of acarbose, thiazolidinedione
		3. Step 3: insulin
		4. Treat other cardiovascular risk factors aggressively
		  a. Blood pressure <130/80 mm Hg
		  b. LDL <100 mg/dL (2.6 mmol/L)
		  c. HDL >40 mg/dL (1.1 mmol/L) in men, >50 mg/dL (1.3 mmol/L) in women
		  d. Triglycerides <150 mg/dL (1.7 mmol/L)

Overweight and obesity Level of evidence—IV, grade of recommendation—C	Normal or near normal BMI	1. Reduce caloric intake (0.5–1.0 kcal below maintenance requirements (≤ 25 kg/m^2) 2. Behavioral modification 3. Exercise 4. Pharmacological agents
Illicit drug abuse Level of evidence—IV, grade of recommendation—C	Complete cessation	1. Firmly advise cessation of drug use at every clinical encounter 2. Offer counseling 3. Refer to treatment program

Adapted from references 11–19, 97, 170, 173.

BMI = body mass index; CAD = coronary artery disease; HbA1c = glycosylated hemoglobin; HDL = high-density lipoprotein; LDL = low-density lipoprotein.

[a]Interventions for alcohol consumption, obesity, and illicit drug use are not evidence-based in terms of primary stroke prevention but do reflect good clinical practice.

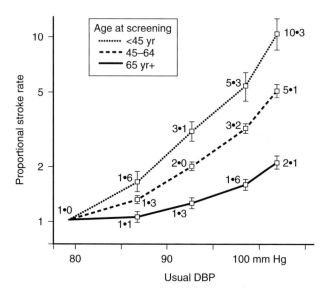

Figure 2.1 Proportional stroke risk, by age and usual diastolic blood pressure (DBP). Floating absolute risk, adjusted for study, sex, total cholesterol, history of coronary heart disease (CHD), and ethnicity.
(Reproduced with permission from Prospective Studies Collaboration. Cholesterol, diastolic blood pressure, and stroke: 13,000 strokes in 450,000 patients in 45 prospective cohorts. Lancet 1995;346:1647–1653.)

exceeding 25 percent in persons 80 years and older. In the Framingham Study,[31] individuals with ISH had a twofold to fourfold increased stroke risk compared with normotensives, after taking age and vascular rigidity into account. This relationship was somewhat stronger in women. In the Honolulu Heart Program,[32] the relative risk of stroke in Japanese-Americans resulting from ISH varied by age group; 4.8 in men age 45 to 54 years and 1.2 in men age 55 to 68 years. In a recent prospective ambulatory blood pressure monitoring cohort study of 519 elderly hypertensives from Tochigi, Japan,[30] a morning systolic blood pressure surge (>55 mm Hg vs. <55 mm Hg) was associated with a higher prevalence of multiple silent infarcts on baseline magnetic resonance imaging (MRI) (57% vs. 37%, $p = 0.004$) and incidence of stroke over 1 to 68 (mean 41) months follow-up (19% vs. 7.3%, $p = 0.004$). Stroke risk from the morning systolic blood pressure surge was increased after matching for age and 24-hour blood pressure (relative risk [RR] = 2.7, 95% CI = 1.1 to 6.8, $p = 0.04$), and was independent of 24-hour blood pressure, nocturnal blood pressure dipping status, and baseline prevalence of silent cerebral infarcts ($p = 0.008$). In the NHANES I long-term follow-up study,[33] stroke risk was increased in individuals with ISH (RR = 2.7, 95% CI = 2.0 to 3.4) and borderline ISH (systolic blood pressure = 140 to 159 mm Hg) (RR = 1.4, 95% CI = 1.1 to 1.8). In this population, the risk of stroke was independently associated with older age, diabetes mellitus, and systolic blood pressure 180 mm Hg or higher. In a recent meta-analysis of 15,693 patients in eight clinical trials, a 10 mm Hg higher initial systolic blood pressure was associated with a 22 percent increase in stroke.[36]

In the Systolic Hypertension in the Elderly Program (SHEP),[34] lacunar stroke was associated with a history of diabetes (RR = 3.03, 95% CI = 1.70 to 5.40) and smoking (RR = 3.04, 95% CI = 1.73 to 5.37), atherosclerotic stroke was associated with presence of carotid bruit (RR = 5.75, 95% CI = 2.50 to 13.24) and embolic stroke was associated with older age (RR = 1.65 per 5 years, 95% CI = 1.25 to 2.18).

The Joint National Committee on the Prevention, Detection, Evaluation, and Treatment of High Blood Pressure (JNC VI), citing data from the Third National Health and Nutrition Examination Survey (NHANES III), reported that of all individuals with hypertension, 31.6 percent are unaware of its presence, 27.4 percent are controlled on medication, 26.2 percent are uncontrolled on medication, and 14.8 percent are not taking antihypertensive medications.[35] In the United States, common reasons for lack of blood pressure control have included lack of access to health care and noncompliance with treatment. These observations may be explained in part by a disproportionate disease burden among racial and ethnic minorities. In NHANES III, most cases of uncontrolled hypertension were individuals with mild ISH who had health insurance. Independent predictors of lack of awareness of hypertension were age 65 years or older, male sex, non-Hispanic African-American race, and lack of physician visits within the preceding 12 months.[37] Of great concern are recent data showing that many U.S. physicians may not diagnose or treat systolic blood pressures between 140 to 160 mm Hg or diastolic blood pressures between 90 to 100mm Hg or are not meeting guideline targets for blood pressure management.[38–41]

Effective drug treatment of combined systolic and diastolic hypertension substantially reduces stroke risk. A meta-analysis of 14 unconfounded randomized treatment trials of antihypertensive drug therapy in 37,000 patients followed for a mean of 5 years showed highly significant reductions in fatal, nonfatal, and total strokes (each $2p < 0.0001$). A mean reduction in diastolic blood pressure of 5 to 6 mm Hg led to a 42 percent reduction in stroke incidence (Figure 2.2; $2p < 0.0001$).[42] A more recent meta-analysis of individual patient data from clinical trials using primarily thiazide diuretics and beta blockers by the INDANA Investigators showed similar reductions in fatal and total stroke risk in both men and women.[43] In east Asian populations, a mean reduction in diastolic blood pressure of 5 mm Hg is predicted to reduce age- and sex-adjusted stroke incidence by 44 percent.[29]

Four recent meta-analyses[44–47] and three recent clinical trials[48–50] have examined the effects of newer antihypertensive drugs on stroke prevention. Placebo-controlled trials have shown significant reductions in fatal or nonfatal stroke risk as follows: angiotensin-converting enzyme (ACE) inhibitors—30 percent, calcium channel antagonists—39 percent, and angiotensin-II type-1 receptor blocker—25 percent.[44,48] However, despite significant heterogeneity between trials comparing different antihypertensive agents and regimens, a meta-regression across 27 trials involving 136,124 patients showed that the observed ORs could be explained by the achieved differences in systolic pressure.[46] Three meta-analyses[44–46] suggest that there are no apparent significant differences among treatment regimens using different drug classes or intensities. These observations have recently been confirmed by the Antihypertensive and Lipid-Lowering Treatment to Prevent Heart Attack (ALLHAT) trial, in which there were no significant differences in overall stroke risk in 33,357 patients

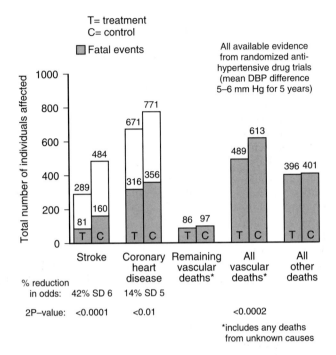

Figure 2.2   Crudely summated results of the unconfounded randomized trials of antihypertensive drug therapy. All were evenly randomized: total 37,000 individuals, mean diastolic blood pressure (DBP) at entry 99 mm Hg, mean DBP difference during follow-up 5 to 6 mm Hg, and mean time from entry to vascular event 2 to 3 years.
(Reproduced with permission from Collins R, Peto R, MacMahon S, et al. Blood pressure, stroke, and coronary heart disease: part 2: short-term reductions in blood pressure: overview of randomised drug trials in their epidemiologic context. Lancet 1990;335:827–835.)

randomized to receive either chlorthalidone (diuretic), amlodipine (calcium channel antagonist) or lisinopril (ACE inhibitor).[49] In a prespecified secondary analysis, stroke prevention in African-Americans was favored by use of chlorthalidone over lisinopril (OR = 1.40, 95% CI = 1.17 to 1.68).[49] However, systolic blood pressures were significantly higher in patients treated with lisinopril in ALLHAT, confirming the observation[51] that African-Americans have a lesser response to and may have required a higher dose of ACE inhibitor to achieve the same effect on stroke prevention. In the Losartan Intervention For Endpoint reduction in hypertension (LIFE) study comparing losartan (angiotensin-II receptor blocker) with atenolol (beta blocker),[48] losartan was associated with reduced fatal and nonfatal stroke risk (RR = 0.75, 95% CI = 0.63 to 0.89) and adverse events despite similar reductions in blood pressure. In the family practitioner-based Second Australian National Blood Pressure (ANBP2) study comparing enalapril (ACE inhibitor) with hydrochlorthiazide,[50] there were similar reductions in blood pressure and stroke risk, although there were more fatal strokes in the enalapril group. However, a recent network meta-analysis[47] of first-line antihypertensive agents in 42 clinical trials involving 192,478 hypertensive patients shows that low-dose diuretics are more effective than placebo (OR = 0.71, 95% CI = 0.63 to 0.81) and ACE inhibitors (0.86, 95% CI = 0.77 to 0.97) for stroke prevention.

Effective drug treatment of ISH substantially reduces stroke risk in the elderly by 30 percent (Figure 2.3; $p < 0.0001$).[36] The Systolic Hypertension in the Elderly Program (SHEP) trial,[52] comparing chlorthalidone with placebo, showed that active treatment reduced all strokes by 36 percent ($p < 0.001$). Treatment effect was observed within one year for hemorrhagic strokes, but not until the second year for ischemic (especially lacunar) strokes (Figure 2.4).[53] In the Systolic Hypertension in Europe (Syst-Eur) trial,[54] treatment with hydrochlorothiazide, with or without the addition of enalapril, and nitrendipine significantly reduced the risk of total stroke by 42 percent ($p = 0.003$) and nonfatal stroke by 44 percent ($p = 0.007$). In the Swedish Trial of Old Patients with Hypertension (STOP-Hypertension),[55] treatment with individuals age 70 to 84 years with thiazide and amiloride or beta blocker led to significant reduction stroke morbidity and mortality. In the Systolic Hypertension in China (Syst-China) trial,[56] comparing nitrendipine with or without captopril and/or hydro-chlorothiazide, there was a trend ($p = 0.07$) for reduced stroke in men. In the Swedish Trial of Old Patients with Hypertension-2 (STOP-2) trial,[57] similar stroke rates were found in patients taking conventional antihypertensive agents

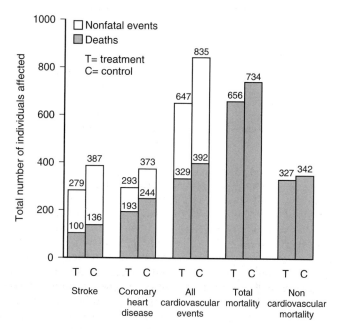

Figure 2.3 Summarized results in older patients with isolated systolic hypertension enrolled in eight trials of antihypertensive drug treatment. Analysis included 15,693 patients. Blood pressure at entry averaged 174 mm Hg systolic and 83 mm Hg diastolic. During follow-up (median 3.8 years), mean difference in blood pressure between treated and control patients was 10.4 mm Hg systolic and 4.1 mm Hg diastolic.

(Reproduced with permission from Staessen JA, Gasowski J, Wang JG, et al. Risks of untreated and treated isolated systolic hypertension in the elderly: meta-analysis of outcome trials. Lancet 2000;355:865–872.)

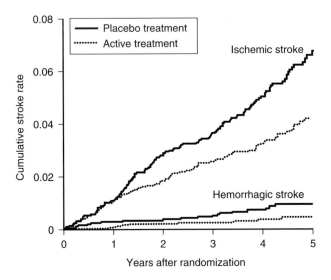

Figure 2.4   Kaplan-Meier event curves for ischemic and hemorrhagic strokes by treatment group. Seventeen strokes of unknown type are omitted. Three additional strokes were also omitted (one for a participant in the active treatment group and two participants in the placebo group). These three strokes occurred after the participants had completed 5 years in the trial.
(Reproduced with permission from Perry HM, Davis BR, Price TR, et al. Effect of treating isolated systolic hypertension on the risk of developing various types and subtypes of stroke: the Systolic Hypertension in the Elderly Program (SHEP). JAMA 2000;284:465–471.)

(22%), ACE inhibitors (20%), and calcium channel antagonists (20%). In patients age 80 years and older, antihypertensive treatment reduces stroke risk by 34 percent (95% CI = 8% to 52%).[58]

The initial treatment of hypertension has been reviewed.[17,35,59,60] If lifestyle interventions (lower body weight; exercise; reduced sodium intake; adequate quantities of fruits and vegetables; and adequate intake of potassium, calcium, and magnesium) are not successful, pharmacological therapy is considered. In general, the choice and dosage of initial antihypertensive therapy is based on a number of considerations, including age, race-ethnicity, coexisting medical conditions, anticipated side effects, and so on. Both diuretics and ACE inhibitors are effective in reducing adverse cardiovascular outcomes. The conflicting main results in ALLHAT and ANBP2 have given rise to controversy, but may in part be explained by differences in baseline characteristics (e.g., proportion of whites vs. African-Americans), baseline frequency of cardiovascular risk factors, and choice and dosage of agents.[60] In general, low-dose diuretics are recommended as first-line pharmacotherapy in uncomplicated hypertension for primary stroke prevention.[47] Younger whites have a better response to ACE inhibitors and beta blockers, whereas African-Americans respond better to diuretics or calcium channel antagonists. Patients with diabetes, renal disease, or both can benefit from an ACE inhibitor or angiotensin-II receptor blocker. Combination diuretic/ACE inhibitor therapy can be useful for a patient with congestive heart failure. Patients with angina or myocardial infarction may benefit from a long-acting dihydropyridine calcium channel antagonist or ACE inhibitor, respectively. For each medication, adequate and tolerable dosages should be used. There are no data regarding the ability of antihypertensive agents to reduce cerebrovascular risk associated with morning blood pressure surges.[61]

HYPERLIPIDEMIA

Increased total blood cholesterol level, defined as greater than 200 mg/dL, was present in an estimated 102,340,000 U.S. adults. Levels were greater than 240 mg/dL (high coronary risk) in an estimated 41,260,000 U.S. adults in 1999. Among Americans age 18 and older, the median percentage of those individuals who have been told by a professional that they have elevated blood cholesterol are whites 29.7 percent, African-Americans 26.0 percent, Hispanics 25.6 percent, Asian/Pacific Islanders 27.3 percent, and American Indians/Alaska Natives 26 to 28.6 percent.[3]

The relationships between elevated cholesterol and its treatment and stroke have become clearer. One meta-analysis of 450,000 patients from 45 prospective cohort studies showed that, after adjustment for age, gender, diastolic pressure, history of coronary artery disease, or ethnicity, there was no significant association between cholesterol and stroke, except in screened patients younger than age 45 years. In meta-analysis, there was no clear distinction between ischemic and hemorrhagic stroke, and most strokes were fatal.[26] However, several studies suggested an inverse association between serum cholesterol and occurrence of and higher mortality from hemorrhagic stroke in persons with total cholesterol levels less than 160 mg/dL. [62–64] In a meta-analysis of 124,774 east Asians, there were trends suggesting a decrease in ischemic stroke risk (OR = 0.77, 95% CI = 0.57 to 1.06) and an increase in hemorrhagic stroke risk (OR = 1.27, 95% CI = 0.84 to 1.91) for every 20 mg/dL decrease in cholesterol concentration[29]. The Honolulu Heart Study[65] found a continuous and progressive association between serum cholesterol level and increasing risk of ischemic stroke, with a relative risk of 1.4 comparing highest and lowest quartiles. The Multiple Risk Factor Intervention Trial (MRFIT)[66] screened 350,977 men and demonstrated a significant direct association between serum cholesterol level and mortality from nonhemorrhagic stroke ($p = 0.007$), as well as a threefold higher risk of death from intracranial hemorrhage in men with total serum cholesterol level less than 160 mg/dL. In the Women's Pooling Project of 24,343 women without prior cardiovascular disease,[67] there was a positive continuous relation between cholesterol level and nonhemorrhagic stroke death in women younger than 55 years old (RR = 1.23, 95% CI = 1.02 to 1.49). In addition, African-American women had an increased risk of stroke-related death (RR = 1.76, 95% CI = 1.10 to 2.81), particularly in the top versus lowest cholesterol quintile (RR = 2.58, 95% CI = 1.05 to 6.32). In the Atherosclerosis Risk in Communities (ARIC) study of 14,175 persons age 45 to 64 years,[68] there were weak and inconsistent associations between ischemic stroke and each lipid measurement (low-density lipoprotein [LDL] cholesterol, high-density lipoprotein [HDL] cholesterol, apolipoprotein B, apolipoprotein A-1, and triglycerides) in men, but there was a consistent decrease in ischemic stroke risk with higher HDL-cholesterol levels and increased risk with lower triglyceride levels in women. An inverse association between HDL cholesterol and risk of ischemic stroke was shown in the Oxfordshire Community Study, in which stroke risk was significantly reduced by approximately one third in individuals with higher HDL levels.[69] In the Northern Manhattan Stroke Study,[70,71] a protective dose-response effect was observed between HDL and ischemic stroke in the elderly and among whites, African-Americans, and Hispanics. Three studies[72–74] have shown that the degree and progression of carotid atherosclerosis are directly related to total- and LDL-cholesterol levels and inversely related to HDL-cholesterol levels. In a nested case-control study of three rural Japanese communities involving 9,174 individuals,[75] a one standard deviation (SD) increase in linoleic acid was associated with reduced risk of total stroke (OR = 0.72, 95% CI = 0.59 to 0.89), ischemic stroke (OR = 0.66, 95% CI = 0.49 to 0.88), and lacunar infarction (OR = 0.63, 95% CI = 0.46 to 0.88) but not hemorrhagic stroke (OR = 0.81, 95% CI = 0.59 to 1.12).

Before the introduction of HMG-CoA reductase, or statin, agents that reduce LDL cholesterol, two early meta-analyses of 11 randomized clinical trials involving more than 36,000 patients using other lipid-lowering strategies showed no benefit in terms of reducing stroke risk.[76,77] The vascular and other nonlipid actions of statins have been reviewed[78–81] and updated.[82–83] Oxidation of LDL cholesterol produces oxidized LDL, which impairs endothelial-dependent vasodilation, induces apoptosis of human endothelial cells, generates an inflammatory response, inhibits platelet-derived nitric oxide synthase to promote thrombus formation, promotes tissue factor expression, and contributes to macrophage foam cell formation. Statins exhibit a variety of antiatherosclerotic and antithrombotic effects to varying degrees by agent (Figure 2.5, Table 2.4). These include reducing macrophage activity, smooth muscle cell replication, lipid content, inflammation, metalloproteinases, and cell death or increasing collagen content within plaque leading to improved plaque stability; reduced tissue factor expression; reversal of endothelial cell dysfunction; reduced platelet aggregation; and reduction of levels or activity of prothrombotic substances (thrombin-antithrombin III complex, fibrinopeptide A, thrombomodulin, and plasminogen activator inhibitor-1; reduced activation of factors II, V, and XIII; enhanced inactivation of factor Va). In addition, statins appear to have neuroprotective properties.[81] In the mid-1990s, four trials[84–87] demonstrated that use of lovastatin and pravastatin can slow the progression or induce regression of carotid intima-media thickness or plaque on serial high-resolution B-mode carotid ultrasonography examinations. General treatment of lipid disorders has been reviewed.[88]

A number of trials in patients with or at risk for coronary artery disease, with elevated or normal cholesterol levels, have shown consistent benefits in reducing stroke risk.[89–97] The Scandinavian Simvastatin Survival Study (4S)[89] first showed in a post hoc analysis that simvastatin reduced total stroke risk by 30 percent. The West of Scotland Coronary Prevention Study (WOSCOPS),[90] a study of primary prevention, showed no clear overall benefit in stroke prevention from pravastatin, perhaps because of low event rates. More recent studies using pravastatin (CARE, LIPID)[91–96] have shown a 23 percent (95% CI = 6% to 37%) reduction in ischemic stroke and no difference in hemorrhagic stroke or unknown stroke type (Figure 2.6). In the LIPID trial,[95] there was a 20 percent stroke risk reduction over 8 years of follow-up. Two recent meta-analyses of

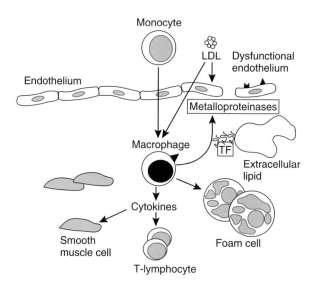

Figure 2.5 Vascular actions of statins. Uptake and endogenous synthesis of cholesterol by macrophages lead to foam cell formation. Release of metalloproteinases by macrophages leads to weakening of the plaque cap and thrombosis. Macrophages elaborate cytokines, which stimulate smooth muscle cell and lymphocyte proliferation, as well as elaboration of tissue factor (TF) expression. In plaque statins appear to attenuate macrophage activation, smooth muscle replication, and TF expression and render plaque more stable and less likely to undergo thrombotic disruption. Statins also ameliorate the endothelial dysfunction that accompanies hypercholesterolemia.
(Reproduced with permission from Delanty N, Vaughn CJ. Vascular effects of statins in stroke. Stroke 1997;28:2315–2320.)

16 trials using lovastatin, simvastatin or pravastatin with more than 29,000 randomized patients[98,99] have demonstrated a 29 to 31 percent (95% CI = 14% to 43%) reduction in stroke risk and 28 percent (95% CI = 16% to 37%) reduction in risk of cardiovascular death, without an increase in noncardiovascular death or cancer. Statistically significant benefits were seen in the secondary prevention trials (OR = 0.68, 95% CI = 0.55 to 0.85) but not in the primary prevention trials (OR = 0.80, 95% CI = 0.54 to 1.16). It is unclear whether the reduction in stroke risk in these studies is due to reduction in heart disease and subsequent cerebral embolism or some other mechanism.[98,99] In the Air Force/Texas Coronary Atherosclerosis Prevention Study (AFCAPS/TexCAPS) primary prevention trial in 6605 men and women,[100] there was a 25 percent reduction (95% CI = 19% to 38%, $p = 0.003$) in fatal and nonfatal cardiovascular events (stable angina, transient ischemic attack, ischemic stroke, peripheral arterial disease) in patients who received lovastatin. The study was underpowered to specifically address primary prevention of stroke. In a pre-specified secondary analysis of the MRC/BHF Heart Protection Study of 20,536 high-risk individuals with coronary disease, peripheral arterial disease, or diabetes,[101] patients receiving simvastatin had a 25 percent stroke risk reduction (95% CI = 15% to 34%, $p < 0.0001$) compared with patients receiving placebo. In the Myocardial

Table 2.4   Comparison of statins on potential mechanisms influencing plaque stabilization and thrombosis

Mechanisms	Statins					
	Atorvastatin	*Cerivastatin*	*Fluvastatin*	*Lovastatin*	*Pravastatin*	*Simvastatin*
Antiatherosclerotic						
Endothelial dilatation	—	—	—	←→	←→	↑, ↔ →
Macrophage cholesterol ester accumulation	—	—	—	—	→	—
LDL oxidation resistance	—	—	—	←→→	←	←, ↔ →
Tissue antioxidant capacity	— →	— →	— →	—	—	→ →, ↔
Smooth muscle cell proliferation	→	→	→	→	↕	←, ↔
Antithrombotic						
Tissue factor	—	—	→	—	↕	→ →
TEPI activity	—	—	—	— ↑, →, ↔	— →, ↔	→ →, ↔
Platelet aggregation and deposition	—	—	—	←, →, ↔	→, ↕	↕ ↕
Fibrinogen	←	—	—	←, →, ↔	→→→	↕ ↕
Blood viscosity	—	—	—	←, →		↕ ↕
Plasma viscosity	—	—	—	→, ↔		
Fibrinolysis						
PAI-1	←	—	←	←, ↑	→←	←←
Lp(a)	—	—	↕	←, →		

Adapted from Rosenson RS, Tangney CC. Antiatherothrombotic properties of statins: implications for cardiovascular event reduction. JAMA 1998;279:1643–1650.

LDL = low-density lipoprotein; Lp(a) = lipoprotein(a); PAI-1 = plasminogen activator inhibitor 1; TEPI = tissue factor pathway inhibitor; — = data not available; ↑ = increase; ↓ = decrease; ↔ = no effect.

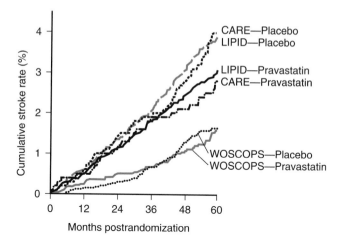

Figure 2.6 Occurrence of any stroke (fatal or nonfatal) by clinical trial and treatment assignment.
(Reproduced with permission from Byington RP, Davis BR, Plehn JF, et al. Reduction of stroke events with pravastatin: the Prospective Pravastatin Pooling (PPP) Project. Circulation 2001;103:387–392.)

Ischemia Reduction with Aggressive Cholesterol Lowering (MIRACL) study of 3086 patients,[102] use of atorvastatin was associated with a 50 percent reduction (95% CI = 26% to 99%) in stroke risk compared with placebo (12 events vs. 24 events, respectively). In the ALLHAT Lipid Lowering Trial (ALLHAT-LLT),[103] there was no difference in stroke risk between the pravastatin and usual care groups. This finding may be explained by the nonblinded trial design, which may have led to increased use of statins in the usual care group and increased nonpharmacological interventions to lower cholesterol levels in the pravastatin group, reduced adherence (e.g., lower degree of reduction in LDL cholesterol) and large degree of crossover.[104] In addition, the Veteran Affairs HDL Intervention Trial (VA-HIT)[105] recently showed that use of gemfibrozil resulted in a 31 percent (95% CI = 2% to 52%) reduction in stroke risk in patients with coronary artery disease, low HDL cholesterol, and LDL cholesterol less than 140 mg/dL.

Recently, there has been great interest in the efficacy and effectiveness of statin use among elderly, stroke-prone individuals. In the Pravastatin in elderly persons at risk of vascular disease (PROSPER) trial involving 5804 individuals age 70 to 82 years,[106] pravastatin use was associated with reduced hazard of the combined endpoint of coronary death, nonfatal myocardial infarction, and fatal or nonfatal stroke (hazard ratio [HR] = 0.85, 95% CI = 0.74 to 0.96, p = 0.014), but there was no reduced hazard of stroke (HR = 1.03, 95% CI = 0.81 to 1.31, p = 0.8). Lack of effect on stroke risk may be explained by lack of statistical power (41%) because of low stroke rates and short (average 3.2 years) duration of follow-up.[107] In the 34,501 individuals age 65 years and older enrolled in the New Jersey Medicaid and Pharmaceutical Assistance to the Aged and Disabled cohort programs,[108] persistence with statin use declines substantially over time, particularly in the first 6 months of treatment. In an administrative database from Ontario from 1994 to 1998,[109] 2-year adherence rates (e.g., statin prescription dispensed at least every 120 days after the index prescription for 2 years) among three cohorts age 66 years and older was low. Among the three cohorts, two year adherence rates were 40.1 percent for acute coronary syndromes ($n = 22,379$), 36.1 percent for chronic coronary artery disease ($n = 36,106$), and 25.4 percent for primary prevention ($n = 85,020$). Data from 138,001 patients in the National Registry of Myocardial Infarction-3[110] suggest that patients who are older than 65 years (OR = 0.82, 95% CI = 0.78 to 0.86), who have a history of hypertension (OR = 0.92, 95% CI = 0.89 to 0.95), and who are undergoing coronary artery bypass surgery (OR = 0.58, 95% CI = 0.55 to 0.60) are significantly less likely to be given lipid-lowering medications at the time of hospital discharge.

At this writing, data are not available on the use of statin drugs in asymptomatic patients for primary stroke prevention or specifically for secondary stroke prevention. In addition, data are insufficient to determine whether lipoprotein (a) [Lp(a)], an apolipoprotein homologous with plasminogen, is an independent risk factor for stroke.[11,13]

ACTIVE AND PASSIVE CIGARETTE SMOKING

Cigarette smoking is a major public health problem. For the years 1990 to 1994, an average of 430,700 Americans died from smoking-related illnesses; one of five cardiovascular deaths can be attributed to smoking. In 1998, the societal cost of smoking-related illness was estimated to be $130 billion. The population attributable risk of stroke associated with all forms of cigarette smoking is believed to be 36 percent (18% current smoking, 6% former smoking, and 12% environmental tobacco smoke exposure).[13]

Tobacco smoking, whether active or passive, has a number of adverse biological and vascular effects.[11–14,111–113] It causes reduced blood vessel distensibility and compliance, leading to increased arterial wall stiffness and elevated blood pressure. Smoking causes increased hematocrit levels, increased fibrinogen levels, increased platelet aggregability, increased blood viscosity, increased blood coagulability, decreased HDL-cholesterol levels, and endothelial dysfunction, the latter of which have been linked to atherosclerosis. Bacterial endotoxin has been identified as an active component of cigarette smoke,[114] and smokers have elevated plasma levels of endotoxin.[115] Cigarette smoking is an independent determinant of carotid intima-media thickness,[116–120] a significant predictor of severe extracranial internal carotid artery atherosclerosis[121–123] and stroke.[117,120] Passive smoking is associated with greater progression of intima-media thickness in patients with diabetes and hypertension[119] and increased likelihood of new carotid plaque formation in patients with chronic infections.[123]

Several prospective cohort[124–128] and case-control[129,130] studies have shown that cigarette smoking is an independent stroke risk factor. A meta-analysis of 32 studies demonstrated an overall RR of 1.5 (95% CI = 1.4 to 1.6).[131] There were important differences according to age (<55 years: RR = 2.94 [95% CI = 2.40 to 3.59]; 55 to 74 years: RR = 1.75 [95% CI = 1.56 to

1.97]; ≥75 years: RR = 1.11 [95% CI = 0.96 to 1.28]), gender (men: RR = 1.43 [95% CI = 1.35 to 1.52]; women: RR = 1.72 [95% CI = 1.59 to 1.86)]), and number of cigarettes smoked per day, with a relative risk of 1.82 (95% CI = 1.70 to 1.96) with ≥20 cigarettes per day. In addition, there were differences in risk between the various stroke subtypes: ischemic stroke RR = 1.92 (95% CI = 1.71 to 2.16), intracerebral hemorrhage RR = 0.74 (95% CI = 0.56 to 0.98), and subarachnoid hemorrhage RR = 2.93 (95% CI = 2.48 to 3.46). In the Physician's Health Study,[128] recent data suggest that male current smokers who consume ≥20 cigarettes per day have an increased risk of total hemorrhagic stroke (OR = 2.36, 95% CI = 1.38 to 4.02), intracerebral hemorrhage (OR = 2.06, 95% CI = 1.08 to 3.96), and subarachnoid hemorrhage (OR = 3.12, 95% CI = 1.26 to 8.18) when compared with never smokers. Data from several observational studies[124,127,132] have demonstrated a reduction in stroke risk after cessation of smoking. Stroke risk was substantially reduced within 2 years of smoking cessation,[124,132] whereas stroke risk may be at the level of nonsmokers 2 to 5 years after smoking cessation.[124] The benefit of stroke risk reduction may appear rapidly after smoking cessation.[124,132,133] Current smokers also have a relative risk of 1.88 (95% CI = 1.13 to 3.13) for silent cerebral infarction.[134]

Passive smoking is also of concern with respect to stroke risk. One study[135] found a relative risk of 1.82 (95% CI = 1.34 to 2.49) in nonsmokers and exsmokers exposed to environmental tobacco smoke. Another study[136] found a relative risk of 1.5 to 1.9 in individuals whose spouses smoke cigarettes compared with individuals who live on the same street.

Several approaches are somewhat effective in smoking cessation.[137,138] Physician intervention, typically via a brief (e.g., up to 3 minutes) period of counseling, is twice as effective as no intervention. Individual or group counseling using cognitive behavioral methods supplemented with written or visual materials, particularly if for greater than 4 weeks, is effective in assisting smokers with coping strategies during smoking cessation. The U.S. Food and Drug Administration has approved sustained-release bupropion (antidepressant with dopaminergic and noradrenergic activity) and four nicotine-replacement products (gum, transdermal patch, nasal spray, and vapor inhaler) for smoking cessation. The randomized, double-blind, placebo-controlled clinical trials involving patients motivated to quit smoking typically included counseling with drug treatment, leading to smoking cessation rates of 40 to 60 percent at the end of the treatment protocol and 25 to 30 percent at 1 year. In a randomized, placebo-controlled trial in African Americans,[138] sustained-release bupropion for 7 weeks was associated with improved abstinence from cigarettes (17%, 95% CI = 9.7 to 22.4), greater mean reduction in depression, and less weight gain than with placebo. Longer treatment is likely necessary in patients with psychiatric conditions (especially depression and schizophrenia), alcohol or substance abuse, strong nicotine dependence, low level of support, and lack of self-confidence.

ALCOHOL USE

Excess alcohol use and dependence is a significant public health problem. In 1995, there were an estimated 107,800 alcohol-related deaths, with an economic cost of $100 billion.[139] Both ischemic and hemorrhagic stroke have been associated with excess alcohol use.[140–142] Alcohol use has a variety of systemic effects that may cause stroke.[143] For example, cerebral ischemia may occur in the setting of cardiovascular effects (hypertension, "holiday heart" with cardiomyopathy, congestive heart failure, and atrial fibrillation); hematological effects (increased platelet reactivity to adenosine diphosphate (ADP); "rebound thrombocytosis" or "rebound platelet hyperaggregability" following alcohol withdrawal; shortened bleeding time; increased factor VIII-related antigen, ristocetin cofactor, and coagulant activity; and decreased fibrinolytic activity) and cerebral vasospasm-induced reduction in cerebral blood flow. Hemorrhagic stroke may occur in association with chronic, sustained, or acute hypertension; and in alcoholic cirrhotics with decreased circulating levels of clotting factors, excessive fibrinolysis, qualitatively abnormal fibrinogens, and laboratory evidence of disseminated intravascular coagulation. However, light to moderate alcohol consumption may increase HDL-cholesterol levels, reduce platelet aggregation, and reduce fibrinogen levels.[144,145]

A review article[140] and meta-analysis of 19 cohort studies and 16 case-control studies[142] have summarized the epidemiological associations between alcohol and stroke. Compared with abstainers, ingestion of more than 60 grams of alcohol (5 drinks) per day is associated with an increased overall risk of total stroke (RR = 1.64, 95% CI = 1.39 to 1.93), ischemic stroke (RR = 1.69, 95% CI = 1.34 to 2.15), and hemorrhagic stroke (RR = 2.18, 95% CI = 1.48 to 3.20); less than 12 grams of alcohol per day is associated with reduced risk of total stroke (RR = 0.83, 95% CI = 0.75 to 0.91) and ischemic stroke (RR = 0.80, 95% CI = 0.67 to 0.96); and 12 to 24 grams of alcohol per day is associated with reduced risk of ischemic stroke (RR = 0.72, 95% CI = 0.57 to 0.91). Results for more than 60 g/day are similar by gender (men: RR = 1.76, 95% CI = 1.57 to 1.98; women: RR = 4.29, 95% CI = 1.30 to 14.14) and for study design (cohort: RR = 1.63, 95% CI = 1.49 to 1.79; case-control: RR = 1.98, 95% CI = 1.35 to 2.92).[141]

For ischemic stroke, chronic heavy drinking and acute alcohol intoxication are associated with increased stroke risk in young adults.[146] In middle-age and older adults, this relationship may be present in men but is confounded by other risk factors, such as cigarette smoking.[147,148] A J-shaped nonlinear association has been observed for the relation between moderate alcohol consumption and ischemic stroke in whites but not Japanese (Figure 2.7).[140,142] In the Northern Manhattan Stroke Study,[149] moderate alcohol consumption was associated with reduced stroke risk in a largely African-American and Hispanic population. In the U.S. Physicians Health Study,[150] light to moderate alcohol consumption was associated with reduced risk of total stroke (RR = 0.79, 95% CI = 0.66 to 0.94) and ischemic stroke (RR = 0.77, 95% CI = 0.63 to 0.94). In the Stroke Prevention in Young Women Study,[151] up to 24 grams of alcohol per day in the past year was associated with reduced ischemic stroke risk (<12 g/day: OR = 0.57, 95% CI = 0.38 to 0.86; 12 to 24 g/day: OR = 0.38, 95% CI = 0.17 to 0.86) compared with never drinkers, particularly with less than 12 grams of wine per week. For hemorrhagic stroke, cohort studies[152–155] have shown that there is a direct, linear dose-response relationship between the amount of alcohol consumed and the risk of intracranial hemorrhage (see Figure 2.7). These findings have been shown for both intracerebral hemorrhage and subarachnoid hemorrhage in the large Kaiser Permanente health plan.[156]

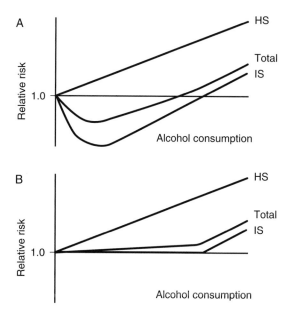

Figure 2.7 Proposed relation between moderate drinking and ischemic stroke (IS), hemorrhagic stroke (HS), and total stroke. Model A refers to whites, whereas Model B refers to Japanese; both models assume that IS accounts for 80 percent of total stroke.
(Reproduced with permission from Camargo CA. Moderate alcohol consumption and stroke: The epidemiological evidence. Stroke 1989;20:1611–1626.)

DIABETES MELLITUS AND INSULIN RESISTANCE

Diabetes mellitus is becoming an increasingly significant public health problem. The overall prevalence of diabetes increased from 4.9 percent in 1990 to 7.3 percent in 2000; 798,000 new cases are diagnosed each year. An estimated 5.6 million Americans have undiagnosed diabetes, and an estimated 13.8 million Americans have impaired fasting glucose.[3] Patients with diabetes have an increased prevalence of hypertension, obesity, and abnormal lipids. Diabetes may lead to stroke via premature large- and small-vessel atherosclerosis via glycosylation-induced vascular injury, adverse effects on cholesterol metabolism, and accelerated atherosclerotic plaque formation.[157]

Case-control and prospective studies have shown a relative risk of stroke in diabetics of 1.8 to nearly 6.0.[13] The Framingham study[158] found a significant and independent association between diabetes in older women. The Honolulu Heart Program[159] found a twofold higher stroke risk in diabetic Hawaiian Japanese men. Other studies have shown similar results.[27,148,160–162] In the Northern Manhattan Stroke Study,[27] diabetes was associated with an increased stroke risk (OR = 1.7, 95% CI = 1.3 to 2.2), with prevalence rates of diabetes as high as 22 percent in elderly African Americans and 20 percent in elderly Hispanics. The risk of first stroke in a patient with Type II diabetes can be predicted.[163]

Randomized controlled trials of intensive treatment of Type I (insulin)[164,165] and Type II (sulfonylurea and/or insulin)[166–168] diabetes leads to a statistically significant reduction in microvascular (neuropathy, nephropathy, retinopathy) but not macrovascular complications. In the Steno–2 Study,[169] a randomized, open, parallel comparison between targeted, intensified, multifactorial intervention with conventional treatment for modifiable cardiovascular risk factors among 160 patients showed reduced hazard of cardiovascular disease (cardiovascular mortality, nonfatal myocardial infarction or stroke, coronary- or peripheral-artery revascularization, or amputation as a result of ischemia) (HR = 0.47, 95% CI = 0.24 to 0.73) in patients receiving the multifactorial intervention. The study design did not permit an assessment of which specific intervention was most beneficial,[169,170] and there was limited power to detect an effect specifically for stroke prevention. However, the UK Prospective Diabetes Study Group[167] showed that blood pressure control (<150/85 mm Hg) significantly reduced the risk of stroke by 44 percent ($p = 0.01$). In the 3,577 diabetic patients in the MICRO-HOPE substudy of the Heart Outcomes Prevention Evaluation (HOPE) trial,[168] use of the ACE-inhibitor ramipril was associated with 25 percent (95% CI = 12% to 36%, $p = 0.0004$) reduction in the primary outcome of myocardial infarction, stroke and cardiovascular death and a 33 percent (95% CI = 10% to 50%) reduction in stroke. This benefit was present after adjustment for the minor blood pressure reduction by ramipril.

The management of diabetes mellitus has recently been reviewed.[170–173] Target levels of risk factors in diabetic patients have been published.[170,173] Recent data suggest that diabetes may be prevented. In a secondary analysis of the WOSCOPS trial,[174] use of pravastatin was associated with a reduced hazard of Type II diabetes (HR = 0.70, 95% CI = 0.50 to 0.99, $p = 0.042$) in men age 45 to 64 years. In a prespecified subgroup analysis of the LIFE trial,[48] use of losartan was associated with a reduced hazard of new-onset diabetes (HR = 0.75, 95% CI = 0.63 to 0.88, $p = 0.001$).

Insulin resistance is a physiological state of defective glucose transport into cells by decreased activation of transport proteins, particularly GLUT-4, despite the presence of normal insulin levels, leading to defective muscle glycogen synthesis.[175,176] It is present in almost all patients with Type II diabetes and approximately 50 percent of nondiabetic ischemic stroke patients.[177] Insulin resistance is associated with abnormal fibrinolysis, enhanced platelet aggregation, altered vascular endothelial function, systemic inflammation, cellular adhesion, and atherogenesis.[178–182] Definitions for the insulin resistance syndrome or multiple metabolic syndrome have been published (Table 2.5)[97,183–185] The World Health Organization (WHO) classification scheme appears to perform slightly better than the National Cholesterol Education Program (NCEP) classification scheme in predicting cardiovascular and all-cause mortality,[184] although their relative merits with respect to prediction of stroke are unclear at this time. In NHANES III Syndrome X, or multiple metabolic syndrome, consisting of insulin resistance (fasting glucose ≥110 mg/dL or 6.1 mmol/L), abdominal obesity (waist circumference >102 centimeters in men and >88 centimeters in women), hypertension (≥130/85 mm Hg), low HDL cholesterol (<40 mg/dL or 1.04 mmol/L in men and <50 mg/dL or <1.29 mmol/L in women), hypertriglyceridemia (>150 mg/dL or 1.69 mmol/L), and vascular disease, occurred in 22 percent of U.S. adults age 20 years and older.[7] In the Insulin Resistance in Atherosclerosis (IRAS) study of

Table 2.5   Modified NCEP and WHO definitions of the metabolic syndrome in men[a]

NCEP Definition	Modified WHO Definition

At least 3 of the following:
  Fasting plasma glucose ≥110 mg/dL
  Abdominal obesity
    Definition 1: Metabolic syndrome,
      NCEP definition with waist
      girth >102 cm
    Definition 2: Metabolic syndrome,
      NCEP definition with waist
      girth >94 cm
  Serum triglycerides ≥150 mg/dL
  Serum HDL cholesterol <40 mg/dL
  Blood pressure ≥130/85 mm Hg
    or medication
	Hyperinsulinemia (upper quartile of the
	    nondiabetic population) or fasting plasma
	    glucose ≥110 mg/dL
	AND
	At least 2 of the following:
	  Abdominal obesity
	    Definition 1: Metabolic syndrome, WHO
	      definition with waist-hip ratio >0.90 or
	      BMI ≥30
	    Definition 2: Metabolic syndrome, WHO
	      definition with waist girth ≥94 cm
	  Dyslipidemia (serum triglycerides≥150 mg/dL
	    or HDL cholesterol <35 mg/dL)
	  Hypertension (blood pressure ≥ 140/90 mm Hg
	    or medication)

Adapted from Lakka H-M, Laaksonen DE, Laaka TA, et al. The metabolic syndrome and total and cardiovascular disease mortality in middle-aged men. JAMA 2002;288:2709–2716.

BMI = body mass index (calculated as weight in kilograms divided by the square of height in meters); HDL = high-density lipoprotein; NCEP = National Cholesterol Education Program; WHO = World Health Organization.

[a]To convert plasma glucose from mg/dL to mmol/L, multiply by 0.0555; to convert serum triglycerides from mg/dL to mmol/L, multiply by 0.0113; and to convert serum HDL cholesterol from mg/dL to mmol/L, multiply by 0.0259.

1,397 healthy adults using an insulin-enhanced often sampled glucose tolerance test,[186] a significant ($p < 0.05$) positive correlation between insulin resistance and carotid intima-media thickness was found in both non-Hispanic whites and African Americans. In a cross-sectional study from Goteberg, Sweden,[187] similar findings were observed using the gold-standard hyperinsulinemic euglycemic clamp technique.

Two case-control studies[188,189] and three prospective observational studies[190–192] have carefully examined the association between insulin resistance and ischemic stroke. In one study[188] using the oral glucose tolerance test, ischemic stroke patients had higher insulin levels at fasting ($p = 0.05$), 2 hours ($p < 0.001$), and 3 hours ($p < 0.001$) than healthy age-matched controls. In another case-control study,[189] nonobese, nonhypertensive, and nondiabetic patients with athero-thrombotic infarction had significantly greater insulin resistance than controls. In a prospective 10-year follow-up study of 1521 Finnish men,[190] the adjusted relative risks for stroke in the three highest quartiles of fasting insulin, compared with the lowest quartile, were 1.6 (95% CI = 0.7 to 3.7), 0.9 (95% CI = 0.4 to 2.5), and 2.0 (95% CI = 0.9 to 4.4). In the Helsinki Policemen Study of 970 men age 35 to 64 years with 22 years of follow-up,[191] the age-adjusted relative risk for stroke was 2.12 (95% CI = 1.28 to 3.49) for patients in the highest quintile of insulin compared with the lowest four quintiles. After adjustment for cardiovascular risk factors, the relative risk was 1.54 (95% CI = 0.90 to 2.62). In the Atherosclerosis Risk in Communities (ARIC) Study of 12,728 healthy nondiabetic adults age 45 to 64 years with 6 to 9 years follow-up,[192] patients in the highest quartile of fasting plasma insulin levels had an adjusted relative risk of ischemic stroke of 2.11 (95% CI = 1.2 to 3.4) compared with patients in the lowest quartile. In the Saltzburg Atherosclerosis Prevention Program in Subjects at High Individual Risk (SAPHIR),[193] males with abdominal body fat distribution carrying the T allele of the C825T dimorphism in exon 10 of the *GNB3* gene coding for the beta-3 subunit of G proteins had lower insulin sensitivity, and the T allele was associated with a greater frequency of advanced carotid artery plaques in both men and women.

Thiazolidinedione agents activate a subclass of nuclear receptor, the peroxisome proliferator activator receptor (PPAR), and ameliorate many biochemical and hemostatic aspects of the insulin resistance syndrome.[194,195] Two studies[196,197] suggest that these agents effectively prevent progression of early carotid atherosclerosis in diabetic patients. It is not known if these agents are useful for primary or secondary stroke prevention.

OVERWEIGHT AND OBESITY

Overweight and obesity are the most common nutritional disorders in the U.S. adult population. In the 195,005 individuals age 18 years and older participating in the Behavioral Risk Factor Surveillance System in 2001,[5] overweight status (body mass index [BMI] = 25 to 29.9 kg/m^2) affected 37.1 percent (78.6 million) and obesity (>30 kg/m^2) affected 20.9 percent (44.3 million), with prevalence increasing with advancing age. Each year, an estimated 300,000 U.S. adults die of causes related to obesity.[3,198] There are well-established relations among increasing degrees of obesity, major cardiovascular risk factors, and poor health (Table 2.6).[5,199] Obese and insulin-resistant individuals have endothelial dysfunction and endothelial resistance to insulin's effect on enhancement of endothelium-dependent vasodilation.[200] The prevalence of overweight and obesity are increasing in U.S. children, adolescents, and adults.[4–6]

Several studies[201–204] have examined the relationship between the distribution and severity of obesity and stroke. In 774 Finnish men enrolled in the Kuopio Ischaemic Heart Disease Risk Factor Study,[201] increasing abdominal obesity was associated with accelerated carotid atherosclerosis by increased maximal intima-media thickness on B-mode ultrasound and plaque height (waist-to-hip ratio [WHR] $p = 0.007$ for linear trend and $p = 0.005$ for linear trend, respectively) and waist circumference ($p = 0.011$ for linear trend and $p = 0.003$ for linear trend, respectively). These associations were more prominent with higher LDL-cholesterol levels. In 28,643 individuals enrolled in the U.S. Health Professionals Follow-up Study,[202] the age-adjusted multivariate relative risk of stroke for extreme quintiles of WHR (<0.89 vs. ≥0.98) was 2.36 (95% CI = 1.21 to 4.64, $p < 0.001$). In 5062 women enrolled in the Progetto ATENA Study in Naples, Italy,[204] there was a graded and independent association between general and abdominal obesity, as measured by BMI and WHR, and increased common carotid intima-media thickness and area. In 116,759 women enrolled in the U.S. Nurse's Health Study,[203] the multivariate RR of ischemic stroke associated with increasing BMI was BMI = 27 to 28.9 kg/m^2: RR = 1.75 (95% CI = 1.17 to 2.59); BMI = 29 to 31.9 kg/m^2: RR = 1.90 (95% CI = 1.28 to 2.82); BMI ≥32 kg/m^2: RR = 2.37 (95% CI = 1.60 to 3.50) compared with BMI less

Table 2.6   Relation between body mass index and selected risk factors, behavioral risk factor surveillance system, 2001[a]

Variable	Body Mass Index				
	Total (N = 195,005)	Normal (n = 84,469)	Overweight (n = 70,231)	Obese, Class 2 (n = 35,767)	Obese, Class 3 (n = 4,538)
Diabetes					
Yes, % (SE)	7.9 (0.11)	4.1 (0.12)	7.3 (0.18)	14.9 (0.70)	25.6 (1.16)
Age adjusted		1.00	1.59 (1.47–1.72)	3.66 (3.38–3.96)	8.51 (7.41–9.78)
Fully adjusted		1.00	1.59 (1.46–1.73)	3.44 (3.17–3.74)	7.37 (6.39–8.50)
High blood pressure					
% (SE)	25.7 (0.17)	15.9 (0.21)	27.8 (0.29)	40.9 (0.45)	50.9 (1.32)
Age adjusted		1.00	1.88 (1.79–1.96)	3.72 (3.53–3.93)	7.03 (6.25–7.90)
Fully adjusted		1.00	1.82 (1.74–1.91)	3.50 (3.31–3.70)	6.38 (5.67–7.17)
High cholesterol					
% (SE)	31.0 (0.20)	23.5 (0.29)	34.1 (0.34)	39.4 (0.50)	36.2 (1.34)
Age adjusted		1.00	1.53 (1.46–1.60)	1.93 (1.83–2.04)	1.87 (1.65–2.11)
Fully adjusted		1.00	1.50 (1.43–1.57)	1.91 (1.80–2.01)	1.88 (1.67–2.13)
Asthma					
% (SE)	11.0 (0.12)	9.9 (0.18)	10.0 (0.20)	13.9 (0.31)	22.6 (1.12)
Age adjusted		1.00	1.05 (0.99–1.12)	1.55 (1.45–1.65)	2.77 (2.43–3.16)
Fully adjusted		1.00	1.14 (1.08–1.22)	1.62 (1.52–1.73)	2.72 (2.38–3.12)
Arthritis					
% (SE)	23.0 (0.16)	17.7 (0.21)	23.7 (0.28)	32.1 (0.41)	44.2 (1.31)
Age adjusted		1.00	1.24 (1.18–1.29)	1.92 (1.83–2.03)	4.55 (4.04–5.11)
Fully adjusted		1.00	1.38 (1.31–1.44)	2.03 (1.92–2.14)	4.41 (3.91–4.97)
General health					
% Fair or poor (SE)	15.2 (0.15)	11.8 (0.19)	14.1 (0.23)	22.5 (0.41)	37.6 (1.28)
Age adjusted		1.00	1.10 (1.05–1.17)	2.01 (1.89–2.14)	4.80 (4.27–5.40)
Fully adjusted		1.00	1.06 (1.00–1.12)	1.81 (1.70–1.93)	4.19 (3.68–4.76)

Adapted from Mokdad AH, Ford ES, Bowman BA, et al. Prevalence of obesity, diabetes, and obesity-related health risk factors, 2001. JAMA 2003;289:76–79.
[a]Full model is adjusted for age, education, smoking, sex, and race or ethnicity.

than 21 kg/m^2. In a multivariate analysis adjusted for BMI at age 18 years, weight gain from age 18 years to 1976 was associated with an increased risk of ischemic stroke (11 to 19.9 kilograms: RR = 1.69, 95% CI = 1.26 to 2.29; ≥20 kg: RR = 2.52, 95% CI = 1.80 to 3.52).

Multidisciplinary treatment of obesity has been reviewed.[205–209] Obese adults can lose 0.5 kg/week by decreasing their daily caloric intake by 500 to 1000 kcal below maintenance requirements. Behavioral strategies have been described.[205,207,208] Adding exercise to caloric restriction may not help much in the short term but is the component most likely to promote long-term maintenance of a reduced weight. Pharmacological treatment has been reviewed.[209] FDA-approved agents for short-term (12 weeks) include benzphetamine, phendimetrazine, phentermine, diethylpropion, sibutramine, and orlistat. These agents have the potential for adverse drug interactions with diverse central nervous system acting agents,[209] so they must be used with care. Although significant weight reduction has a number of systemic and cardiovascular benefits, there are no data showing that weight reduction independently reduces the risk of stroke.

HYPERHOMOCYST(E)INEMIA, VITAMINS, AND ANTIOXIDANTS

The term *homocyst(e)ine* is used to define the combined pool of homocysteine, homocystine, mixed disulfides involving homocysteine and homocysteine thiolactone found in the plasma of patients with hyperhomocyst(e)inemia.[210] Homocyst(e)ine is a sulfur-containing amino acid formed during the metabolism of methionine. Homocyst(e)ine is metabolized by one of two pathways, remethylation and transsulfuration, which require the vitamin B_{12}-dependent enzyme methionine synthase and vitamin B_6-dependent rate-limiting enzyme cystathionine β-synthase, respectively (Figure 2.8).[210] Defects of cystathionine β-synthase; the 677C→T substitution in the gene for methylene tetrahydrofolate reductase (MTHFR); deficiencies in folic acid, B_{12}, and B_6; age ≥70 years; renal insufficiency; ≥4 cups of coffee per day; methionine loading; and drugs such as methotrexate, 6-azauridine, nicotinic acid, and bile acid sequestrants are all associated with mild to moderate hyperhomocyst(e)inemia (15 to 100 μmol/L).[210–212] Homocyst(e)ine levels may be altered by alcohol, smoking, and physical inactivity.[213] Methionine loading may lead to increased homocysteine levels and to activated coagulation (increased levels of fibrinopeptide A and prothrombin fragment 1.2), modify the adhesive properties of the endothelium or circulating adhesion molecule levels, and impair hemodynamic and rheological responses to L-arginine, the natural precursor of nitric oxide.[214] In NHANES III,[215] reference ranges (95th percentile) for U.S. adults were associated with low vitamin levels and are as follows: men age older than 60 years 15.3 μmol/L; age 40 to 59 years: men 12.9 μmol/L, women 10.2 μmol/L; men age 20 to 39 years 11.4 μmol/L. Mild hyperhomocyst(e)inemia has been reported to occur in 5 to 7 percent of the general U.S. population.[216,217] Severe hyperhomocyst(e)inemia (>100 μmol/L) and homocystinuria are most often caused by mutations in cystathionine β-synthase. In one study of 1111 individuals from a farming community in southwest Japan,[218] mean total homocysteine

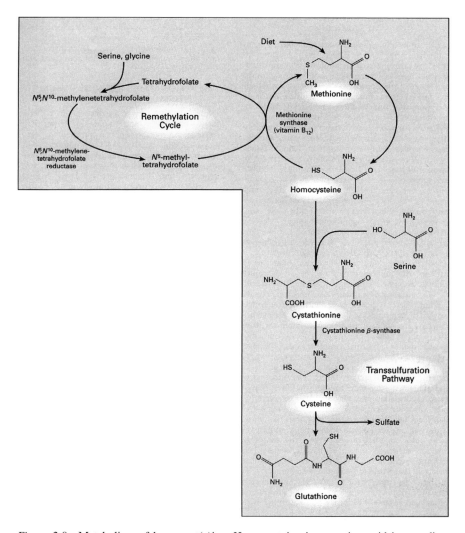

Figure 2.8 Metabolism of homocyst(e)ine. Homocysteine is an amino acid intermediate formed during the metabolism of methionine, an essential amino acid derived from dietary protein. It is metabolized by one of two pathways: remethylation and transsulfuration. In the remethylation cycle, homocysteine is salvaged by acquiring a methyl group in a reaction catalyzed by the vitamin B_{12}–dependent enzyme methionine synthase. The donor in this reaction is N5-methyltetrahydrofolate, and the enzyme N5, N10-methylenetetrahydrofolate reductase functions as a catalyst in the remethylation cycle. Under conditions in which excess methionine is present or cysteine synthesis is required, homocysteine enters the transsulfuration pathway. In the transsulfuration pathway, homocysteine condenses with serine to form cystathionine in a reaction catalyzed by the vitamin B_6–dependent rate-limiting enzyme cystathionine β-synthase. Cystathionine is subsequently hydrolyzed to form cysteine, which may in turn be incorporated into glutathione or further metabolized to sulfate and excreted in the urine.
(Reproduced with permission from Welch GN, Loscalzo J. Homocysteine and atherothrombosis. N Engl J Med 1998;338:1042–1050.)

level was 10.9 µmol/L, with 8 percent of men and 0.9 percent of women having levels ≥20 µmol/L.

Postulated mechanisms of the adverse vascular effects of homocyst(e)ine are shown in Figure 2.9.[210] The ARIC study[219] found an OR of 3.15 for intima-media thickness in the top versus bottom quintile of homocyst(e)ine concentrations (>10.5 µmol/L vs. <5.88 µmol/L). In the Framingham study,[220] the OR for carotid stenosis greater than 25 percent was 2.0 (95% CI = 1.4 to 2.9) for people with homocyst(e)ine levels greater than 14.4 µmol/L compared with those with homocyst(e)ine levels less than 9.1 µmol/L. In a Japanese study,[218] a multivariate regression analysis showed that total homocyst(e)ine levels were significantly related to carotid intima-media thickness. Two other studies[221,222] have suggested an association between increasing homocyst(e)ine levels and large-artery atherosclerotic stroke and, to a lesser extent, with small-vessel disease[221] or microangiopathic stroke.[222]

A meta-analysis of epidemiological studies and cardiovascular disease, including stroke,[223] suggested that moderate elevation of plasma or serum homocyst(e)ine is independently associated with an increased risk of cardiovascular disease, but expressed concern that data from prospective studies were not consistent. Since then, a number of observational and genetic epidemiological studies more clearly suggest that elevated homocyst(e)ine levels may be an independent risk factor for stroke.[224–236] In the Physician's Health Study,[224] there was a small but statistically nonsignificant association (OR = 1.2, 95% CI = 0.7 to 2.0) between elevated plasma homocysteine and risk of ischemic stroke. In NHANES III,[225] elevated homocysteine was associated with a risk of nonfatal stroke (OR = 2.3, 95% CI = 1.2 to 4.6). In the Stroke Prevention in Young Women Study,[226] elevated homocysteine was associated with ischemic stroke (OR = 1.6, 95% CI = 1.1 to 2.5) after adjustment for traditional vascular risk factors, vitamin use, and poverty status. In a case-control study of young (<50 years of age) ischemic stroke patients from Singapore,[227] cases had higher mean fasting homocyst(e)ine levels (13.7 vs. 10.8, $p < 0.001$), lower mean vitamin B_{12} levels (299.5 vs. 394.5, $p < 0.001$), and higher levels were associated with large-artery atherosclerotic strokes. In a logistic regression analysis model, for every 1 µmol/L increase in log homocyst(e)ine, the adjusted OR for ischemic stroke was 5.17 (95% CI = 1.96 to 13.63). In a nested case-control substudy of the 3090 individuals enrolled in the Bezafibrate Infarction Prevention secondary prevention study cohort in Israel,[228] an increase of one natural log unit in homocysteine concentration was associated with an increased risk of incident ischemic stroke (OR = 3.3, 95% CI = 1.2 to 10.2). In a recent meta-analysis of 13 studies of various designs involving 1113 stroke events,[229] a 25 percent lower than usual homocyst(e)ine level was associated with reduced ischemic stroke risk (OR = 0.81, 95% CI = 0.69 to 0.95).

One study of ischemic stroke patients[230] showed an association between MTHFR genotype and serum homocysteine concentration and an interaction with serum folate concentration. The MTHFR A677V allele has been associated with severe greater than 75 percent carotid stenosis (OR = 2.4, 95% CI = 1.1 to 5.3),[231] moderately elevated homocysteine after methionine loading with increased risk of ischemic stroke in young women (OR = 4.8, 95% CI = 1.4 to 6.7),[169] risk of cervical carotid artery dissection (17.88 ± 7.53 µmol/L vs. 6.00 µ0.99 µmol/L, $p < 0.001$),[233] and risk of silent stroke (>15.1 µmol/L: age-adjusted OR = 4.5, 95% CI = 1.5 to 13.5; gender adjusted OR = 4.7, 95%

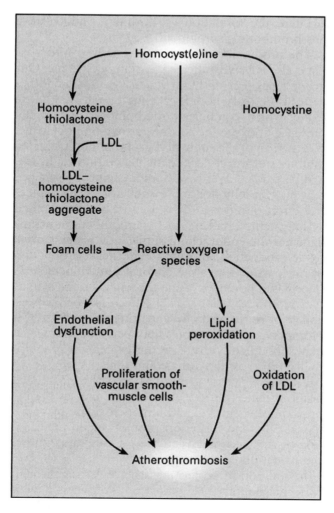

Figure 2.9 Postulated adverse vascular effects of homocyst(e)ine. The postulated effects involve oxidative damage to vascular endothelial cells and increased proliferation of vascular smooth-muscle cells after oxidative metabolism of homocysteine to homocystine and homocysteine thiolactone. Oxidative modification of low-density lipoprotein (LDL) promotes the formation of foam cells, which in turn yields another source of reactive oxygen species.
(Reproduced with permission from Welch GN, Loscalzo J. Homocysteine and atherothrombosis. N Engl J Med 1998;338:1042–1050.)

CI = 1.6 to 13.8; adjusted for hypertension and creatinine clearance OR = 6.0, 95% CI = 1.9 to 19.3; and adjusted for smoking and alcohol consumption OR = 4.5, 95% CI = 1.5 to 13.3).[234] However, a recent meta-analysis of homocyst(e)ine, MTHFR 677C→T polymorphism and risk of ischemic stroke from 19 studies involving 6750 individuals[235] showed that the TT genotype was weakly associated with ischemic stroke risk (OR = 1.23, 95% CI = 0.96 to 1.58, $p = 0.10$). A recent case-control study from Northern Ireland[236] has confirmed this observation.

Homocyst(e)ine levels can be reduced. Fortification of enriched grain products with folic acid can lead to a decrease in mean homocyst(e)ine levels and prevalence of elevated homocyst(e)ine levels in the population.[237] The use of B vitamin complex (B_{12}, B_6, folate) is positively associated with reduction of homocysteine levels[238] and carotid atherosclerotic plaque progression.[239] The use of vitamin E and vitamin C may also block the adverse effects of hyperhomocysteinemia on endothelial function.[214] Three ongoing trials, the Bergen Vitamin Study, Vitamins in Stroke Prevention (VISP), and Vitamins to Prevent Stroke Study (VITATOPS), will determine whether vitamin supplementation will lower homocyst(e)ine levels and reduce the risk of stroke.

Diets that are high in fruits and vegetables, sources of antioxidant nutrients vitamin C, vitamin E, and beta-carotene, have been suggested to be associated with a lower risk of cardiovascular disease.[240–243] The antioxidants may work by reducing the oxidation of LDL cholesterol to oxidized LDL, a compound that has been associated with accelerated endothelial damage, monocyte/macrophage recruitment, uptake of LDL cholesterol by foam cells, abnormal vascular tone, induction of growth factors, and autoantibodies to oxidized LDL, thus leading to reduced atheroma formation.[240–241] However, data are inconsistent on the ability of antioxidants to reduce the occurrence of cardiovascular disease and stroke.[244–249] The Heart Outcomes Prevention Evaluation (HOPE) Study[248] and the MRC/BHF Heart Protection Study[249] showed no difference in the occurrence of nonfatal or fatal stroke between patients who took vitamin C, vitamin E, or beta-carotene and those who did not. One study[250] suggested that ingestion of at least five daily portions of fruits and vegetables significantly increases levels of plasma antioxidants alpha-carotene, beta-carotene, lutein, beta-cryptoxanthin, and ascorbic acid and slightly reduces blood pressure levels. Consumption of fruits and vegetables, especially cruciferous and green leafy vegetables and citrus fruit and juice, may be protective against stroke. The Nurses' Health Study and Health Professionals' Follow-Up Study[251] found that the relative risk of stroke was 0.69 (95% CI = 0.52 to 0.92) for persons in the highest quintile of fruit and vegetable ingestion. An increment of one serving per day was associated with a six percent reduction in stroke risk. Whether these discrepant results reflect suboptimal dosage or potency of antioxidant preparations, improper form of vitamin E,[212,252] differences in study design, or other factors remains to be determined.

Recent data suggest that consumption of fish oils (long-chain n-3 polyunsaturated fatty acids [PUFAs]) or oily fish may reduce vascular and stroke risk.[253,254] In a randomized trial of 188 patients awaiting carotid endarterectomy,[253] patients who ingested fish (n-3) oils were more likely to have higher levels of n-3 PUFAs and thick fibrous caps and a lesser degree of plaque inflammation (i.e., improved plaque stability at surgery) than in patients receiving placebo or sunflower oil (n-6 oil). In the Health Professional Follow-Up Study of 43,671 men age 40 to 75 years,[254] ingestion of fish at least once a month was associated with reduced ischemic stroke risk (RR = 0.56, 95% CI = 0.38 to 0.83) but not reduced hemorrhagic stroke risk (RR = 1.36, 95% CI = 0.48 to 3.82).

INFLAMMATION/INFECTION

It has been estimated that only one half of cardiovascular disease risk is explained by traditional risk factors.[212] In addition, it has increasingly been recognized that atherosclerosis is, in the aggregate, an inflammatory disease.[255] The response-to-injury hypothesis of atherosclerosis has recently been modified to emphasize the importance of endothelial dysfunction and permeability related to elevated and modified LDL cholesterol, free radicals caused by cigarette smoking, hypertension, and diabetes; genetic alterations; elevated plasma homocyst(e)ine concentrations; inflammatory factors; infectious agents; and combinations. Endothelial dysfunction is associated with reduced formation of nitric oxide and vasoconstriction. Modification of LDL cholesterol by oxidation, glycation, aggregation, association with proteoglycans or incorporation into immune complexes is a major cause of injury to endothelium and underlying smooth muscle. Endothelial injury leads to increased adhesiveness to leukocytes and platelets at the injury site (upregulation of various adhesion molecules such as intercellular adhesion molecule-1 [ICAM-1], vascular-cell adhesion molecules [VCAMs], and selectins); procoagulant activity (tissue factor); and formation of vasoactive molecules, cytokines, and growth factors. Inflammatory mediators, such as tumor necrosis factor-alpha, interleukin-1, and macrophage colony-stimulating factor, increase binding of LDL to endothelium and smooth muscle cells. The renin-angiotensin system is involved in vascular remodeling, generation of oxidative stress, and inflammation in the atherosclerotic process by effects on adhesion molecules, growth factors, and chemoattractant molecules in the subendothelial compartment.[256,257] Angiotensin-II, the principal product of the renin-angiotensin system, is a potent vasoconstrictor and hypertensive agent, stimulates smooth muscle cell growth and contraction, increases inflammation, and oxidation of LDL cholesterol.

If the inflammatory response is not successful in removing the offending agent(s), the process can continue indefinitely and lead to smooth muscle cell migration and proliferation; remodeling of the vessel wall; release of hydrolytic enzymes, cytokines, chemokines (monocyte chemotactic protein 1, osteopontin), and growth factors; further vessel wall damage; and focal necrosis.[255] The atherosclerotic vessel wall contains soluble adhesion molecules that indicate an active inflammatory process. Carotid endarterectomy specimens contain a greater expression of ICAM-1 in symptomatic and higher grade stenotic plaques.[258] Activation of matrix-degrading metalloproteinases may be an important mechanism in plaque destabilization and symptom production.[259]

Inflammatory processes are often accompanied by an acute phase protein response, defined as an increase (positive) or decrease (negative) in plasma concentration by at least 25 percent, largely resulting from a change in hepatocyte production stimulated by interleukin-6.[260] Substantial changes in plasma concentrations of these acute phase reactants may occur in the setting of infection, trauma, surgery, burns, tissue infarction, immune- or crystal-mediated inflammatory conditions, and advanced cancer. However, the concentrations of these proteins do not increase to a similar degree (Figure 2.10). Acute-phase reactants are believed to have the potential to influence one or more stages of the inflammatory process. The acute-phase response is procoagulant, with interleukin-6 as the principal procoagulant cytokine and mediators including

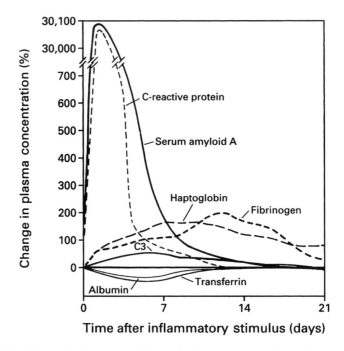

Figure 2.10   Characteristic patterns of change in plasma concentrations of some acute-phase proteins after a moderate inflammatory stimulus.
(Reproduced with permission from Gabay C, Kushner I. Acute-phase proteins and other systemic responses to inflammation. N Engl J Med 1999;340:448–454.)

fibrinogen, plasminogen-activator inhibitor-1, and possibly C-reactive protein (CRP).[261] CRP can bind phosphocholine and thus recognize foreign pathogens or phospholipid components of damaged cells, induce inflammatory cytokines and tissue factor expression on monocytes, and activate the complement system. However, in transgenic mice that produce large amounts of CRP, the net effect is anti-inflammatory resulting from prevention of neutrophil adhesion and production of superoxide radical and stimulation of mononuclear cell production of interleuken-1 receptor antagonist.[260] As such, the acute phase response may not always be beneficial to the organism.

The relationship between cardiovascular risk factors, cardiovascular disease, cerebrovascular disease, and inflammatory markers (such as CRP, fibrinogen, adhesion molecules, and others) has been actively studied.[262–293] Several studies revealed that CRP levels correlated with the presence of cardiovascular risk factors[262] and could add predictive power beyond LDL-cholesterol levels for future cardiovascular events (e.g., myocardial infarction) in men and women.[263–265] In a nested case-control study of the Physician's Health Study,[267] addition of CRP to standard lipid screening significantly improved the prediction of risk of peripheral arterial disease (intermittent claudication, peripheral arterial revascularization procedures). In the Rotterdam Study,[288] CRP levels (highest vs. lowest quartile) predicted progression of atherosclerosis at various arterial sites: carotid (OR = 1.9, 95% CI = 1.1 to 3.3); aortic (OR = 1.7, 95% CI = 1.0 to 3.0); iliac (OR = 2.0, 95% CI = 1.2 to 3.3); lower extremity (OR = 1.9, 95% CI = 1.0 to 3.7); and generalized (OR = 4.5, 95% CI = 2.3 to 8.5). In a transesophageal echocardiographic study of randomly selected stroke-free community subjects,[289] each unit increase in leukocyte count was associated with an increased risk of thick (>4 millimeter) aortic plaque (OR = 1.38, 95% CI = 1.05 to 1.79) after multivariate adjustment, irrespective of gender or age. Fibrinogen has been suggested as a risk factor for stroke,[268,269] because fibrinogen levels may be elevated in patients with transient ischemic attacks[270] or in patients at risk of stroke[271] and during stroke rehabilitation[272]; it also may be significantly higher in stroke survivors who have a second cardiovascular event within 2 years[272,277] or with progression of carotid stenosis.[273] Increasing levels of cholesterol are associated with elevated levels of inflammation-sensitive proteins (ISPs) (fibrinogen, haptoglobin, ceruloplasmin, orosomucoid).[285]

Inflammatory markers have been associated with an increased risk of stroke. In a Swedish study of 6071 healthy men age 28 to 61 years,[287] systolic and diastolic blood pressures were positively associated with elevated levels of ISPs. In men with high ISPs and systolic blood pressures greater than or equal to 140 mm Hg, the risk of stroke was increased (RR = 4.3, 95% CI = 2.3 to 7.8) compared with men who had systolic blood pressures less than 120 mm Hg and low ISPs. The stroke risk associated with high ISPs extended over the first 10 years of follow-up. In 1462 individuals with 12 to 14 year follow-up in the Framingham Study,[276] CRP levels (highest vs. lowest quartile) were associated with increased risk of ischemic stroke and transient ischemic attack in men (RR = 2.0, 95% CI = 1.10 to 3.79, $p = 0.027$) and women (RR = 2.7, 95% CI = 1.59 to 4.79, $p = 0.003$), with an independent effect in women remaining after multivariate adjustment. In a prospective observational study from Glasgow,[266] higher CRP concentration was an independent predictor of mortality (HR = 1.23 per additional natural log unit, 95% CI = 1.13 to 1.35, $p = 0.02$), particularly if CRP was greater than 10.1 mg/L. In 473 incident strokes in the Villa Pini Stroke Data Bank cohort,[275,277] elevated levels of inflammatory markers measured within 24 hours of stroke onset (highest vs. lowest tertile) were associated with increased hazard of cardiovascular events (D-dimer >1327 μg/L vs. <312 μg/L: $p = 0.0349$, log-rank; CRP >33 mg/L vs. <5 mg/L: $p < 0.0001$, log-rank; fibrinogen >6.17 g/L vs. <3.78 g/L: $p < 0.0001$, log-rank). CRP levels at admission (HR = 2.78, 95% CI = 1.45 to 5.33, $p = 0.0021$) and discharge (HR = 9.42, 95% CI = 4.27 to 19.05, $p < 0.0001$) were predictors of new vascular events or death at one year. Use of ticlopidine was associated with decreased risk in lower and middle tertiles. Increased levels of soluble intercellular adhesion molecules have been associated with prediction of carotid atherosclerosis[278,279] and acute stroke.[280,281] In 3090 individuals enrolled in the Bezafibrate Infarction Prevention (BIP) Study cohort,[282] elevated levels of soluble ICAM-1 (highest vs. other quartiles) was associated with an increased relative stroke risk after adjustment for risk factors and fibrinogen level (RR = 2.1, 95% CI = 1.1 to 4.2), with the highest risk for large, disabling cardioembolic strokes. In a case-control study of 110 patients with cerebral small-vessel disease (SVD) or ischemic leukoaraiosis and 50 community controls,[283] SVD patients had elevated levels of ICAM-1, thrombomodulin, and tissue factor pathway inhibitor whereas leukoaraiosis patients had lower levels of tissue factor pathway inhibitor and a higher tissue factor/tissue factor pathway inhibitor ratio.

Statin agents have been shown to reduce CRP levels.[261,291–293] In 472 randomly selected participants in the CARE study,[292] pravastatin use was associated with a 37.8 percent reduction in mean CRP levels ($p = 0.002$) over 5 years in an analysis stratified by age, body mass index, smoking status, blood pressure, and baseline lipid levels. In 1702 individuals enrolled in the Pravastatin Inflammation/CRP Evaluation (PRINCE) study,[291] pravastatin use was associated with a 16.9 percent reduction ($p < 0.001$) in CRP levels at 24 weeks independent of baseline or end-of-study lipid levels. In a retrospective analysis of 5742 individuals enrolled in the AFCAPS/TexCAPS trial,[293] lovastatin therapy reduced CRP levels by 14.8 percent ($p < 0.001$) in patients with low-to-intermediate levels of LDL cholesterol independently of its effect on the lipid profile, leading to reduced risk of coronary events. It is unknown if these effects are relevant to adhesion molecules, procoagulant substances, and primary or secondary stroke prevention.

Evidence supporting an association between infection and atherosclerosis has been reviewed.[212,294–297] Recently, five infectious agents (*Chlamydia pneumoniae, Helicobacter pylori,* cytomegalovirus, Epstein-Barr virus, and herpes simplex virus type 2) and endotoxin have been implicated in atherogenesis.[212,297–304] Diverse animal and experimental studies suggest that *C. pneumoniae* can infect macrophages, endothelial cells and vascular smooth muscle cells, induce formation of foam cells, and modify other lipid- and inflammatory-related processes.[212,297] In a recent study of 46 patients undergoing carotid endarterectomy for symptomatic internal carotid stenosis,[298] *C. pneumoniae*-specific DNA was found in 82.6 percent of atherosclerotic plaques and 86.9 percent of leukocytes, and was associated with increased CRP levels compared with *C. pneumonia*-negative plaques ($p < 0.05$). A recent analysis of 10 published studies[212] suggests that acute or chronic *C. pneumoniae* infection may increase stroke risk, although the mechanism is unclear. *H. pylori* seropositivity has been associated with degree of carotid stenosis and ischemic cerebrovascular disease.[212,300–302] In the Bruneck study,[300] seropositivity to the *H. pylori* cytotoxin-associated gene (*CagA*) product was associated with increased carotid intima-media thickness and atherosclerosis risk and was amplified by elevated CRP levels. Cytomegalovirus infection has been associated with increased carotid intima-media thickness.[303] The endotoxin receptor CD14 can enhance the endotoxin-neutralization capacity of plasma. In the Carotid Atherosclerosis Progression Study,[304] the *CC* genotype of the endotoxin receptor CD14-159 polymorphism was independently associated with increased common carotid artery intima-media thickness in smokers and exsmokers (OR = 2.02, 95% CI = 1.23 to 3.34, $p = 0.006$). In another study,[299] the number of infectious agents to which an individual has been exposed may be associated with progression of carotid intimal-medial thickness (4 to 5: OR = 1.8, 95% CI = 1.1 to 2.9; 6 to 8: OR = 3.8, 95% CI = 1.6 to 8.8; compared with 0 to 3).

Infections may trigger onset of or be associated with ischemic stroke.[295,296,305–310] One study[305] reported that febrile and nonfebrile infectious/inflammatory syndromes may precede onset of ischemic stroke, particularly within a 1-week time window. In a case-control study,[307] recent infection, primarily of bacterial origin, significantly increased the risk of cerebrovascular ischemia in patients age 51 to 70 years after adjustment for conventional stroke risk factors (OR = 4.6, 95% CI = 1.9 to 11.3). In another case-control study,[308] recent bacterial and viral infection (within 1 week) was independently associated with ischemic stroke risk (OR = 2.9, 95% CI = 1.31 to 6.4, p = 0.009), particularly in younger patients and independent of common inflammatory/coagulation abnormalities. However, another study[306] showed that patients with infection/inflammation within 1 week of ischemic stroke onset have lower mean levels of activated protein C (APC), elevated plasma C4b binding protein, and lower ratio of active tissue plasminogen activator to plasminogen activator inhibitor than other neurological in-patients and community controls. In the NHANES I and follow-up study of 9962 adults age 25 to 74 years,[309] patients with periodontitis had an increased risk of incident ischemic stroke (RR = 2.11, 95% CI = 1.30 to 2.42) and total stroke (RR = 1.66, 95% CI = 1.15 to 2.39) irrespective of gender and race. In 41,380 men enrolled in the Health Professionals' Follow-up Study,[310] increased stroke risk was observed in individuals with baseline periodontal disease history (HR = 1.33, 95% CI = 1.03 to 1.70) and lower baseline tooth count (<24 vs. ≥25 teeth: HR = 1.57, 95% CI = 1.24 to 1.98).

It is important to treat clinically evident inflammatory/infectious disorders. At this writing, there are no data to specifically support treatment of stroke-prone individuals with anti-inflammatory agents, statins, or antimicrobial drugs for primary stroke prevention.

ILLICIT DRUG USE/ABUSE

The problem of illicit drug abuse is an important public health problem in young adults that has reached national and international proportions.[311] The illicit drugs which have been most often observed in temporal association with stroke include cocaine (both alkaloidal "crack" and hydrochloride forms), heroin, amphetamines, and marijuana. The mechanisms of both ischemic and hemorrhagic stroke have recently been reviewed.[311] Mechanisms of ischemic stroke include arterial vasoconstriction (vasospasm, vasculopathy, and vasculitis), foreign body embolization, structural heart disease (arrhythmias, cardiomyopathy, myocardial infarction, and endocarditis), SVD, and prothrombotic tendencies (reduced fibrinolysis, increased platelet activation/aggregation, anticardiolipin antibodies, and in situ thrombosis). Mechanisms of hemorrhagic stroke include chronic/acute hypertension, unmasking preexisting lesions (aneurysms, arteriovenous malformations), lesion induction (microaneurysms, other), vasculopathy/vasculitis, endocarditis, immune perturbations, hemostatic defects (decreased clotting factors, thrombocytopenia/prolonged bleeding time), drug interactions (ethanol, heparin, and monoamine oxidase [MAO] inhibitors), reperfusion, or a combination of effects.

The relation between illicit drug use and stroke is becoming more clear. A number of case series[312–321] and single hospital[312,322–325] or population-based[326–328] case-control studies of the relation between illicit drug abuse and stroke are now available (Table 2.7). In one study[324] using a statistical method incorporating multiple imperfect sources of information regarding cocaine use (structured interview, toxicological screen, chart review), showed that the OR for the risk of any stroke with cocaine use in one single-hospital case-control study may vary from 1.59 to 2.35, depending on the sensitivity and specificity of the information source and whether the assumption of conditional independence of information sources was satisfied. In the population-based Stroke

Table 2.7   Association between illicit drug use and stroke

Author, Reference	Year(s) of Study	Age Group (y)	Any Stroke	IS	ICH	SAH
			n/N (%)	n/N (%)	n/N (%)	n/N (%)
A. Case Series						
Kaku[312]	1979–1988	15–44	73/214 (34.1)	—	—	—
Sloan[313]	1988–1989	15–49	7/51 (13.7)	—	—	4/26 (15.4)
Mitsias[314]	1989–1991	—	16/51 (29)	—	—	—
Adams[316]	1987–1993	15–45	—	7/329 (2.1)	—	—
Sloan/BWYSSG[317,318]	1988, 1991	15–45	—	—	18/67 (27)	11/38 (28.9)
Qureshi[319]	1990–1994	15–45	—	—	18/67 (27)	11/38 (28.9)
Sloan/BWYSSG[320]	1988, 1991	15–45	—	—	26/195 (13.3)	—
Simpson[321]	1980s	—	—	—	—	17/150 (11.3)
B. Case Control Studies			OR (95% CI)	OR (95% CI)	OR (95% CI)	OR (95% CI)
Kaku[312]	1979–1988	15–44	6.5 (3.1–13.6)	—	—	—
		<35	11.2 (3.2–42.5)	—	—	—
Stroke within 6 hours of drug use	—	—	49.4 (6.4–379)	—	—	—
Qureshi[322] ("crack" cocaine)	1994–1996	20–39	1.9 (0.7–5.10)	1.2 (0.4–3.8)	—	—
Sloan[323] (cocaine)	1992–1996	18–65	1.83 (0.95–3.8)	1.92 (0.59–6.3)	2.96 (1.35–6.5)	0.56 (0.18–1.76)
Sloan/BWYSSG[326]	1992–1996	—	—	—	—	—
Current cocaine	—	15–45	—	3.4 (1.4–8.3)	—	—
Cocaine within 24 hours of stroke	—	—	∞ (2.6–∞)	—	—	—
Pettiti/KP[327]	1991–1994	15–44	—	—	—	—
Cocaine—any	—	—	13.9 (2.8–69.4)	—	—	—
Cocaine—powder/paste	—	—	19.7 (2.3–166.3)	—	—	—
Cocaine—"crack"	—	—	11.2 (1.1–118.8)	—	—	—
HSP[328] (cocaine within 3 days)	—	15–49	—	—	—	24.97 (3.95–∞)
Pettiti/KP[327] (amphetamine)	1991–1994	15–44	3.8 (1.2–12.6)	—	—	—
Sloan[325] (current marijuana)	1992–1996	18–65	1.38 (0.73–2.61)	1.19 (0.51–2.80)	1.16 (0.46–2.93)	1.63 (0.70–3.82)

BWYSSG = Baltimore Washington Cooperative Young Stroke Study Group; HSP = Hemorrhagic Stroke Project; ICH = intracerebral hemorrhage; IS = ischemic stroke; KP = Kaiser Permanente project; *n* = number of drug-associated cases; *N* = total number of cases; OR = odds ratio; SAH = subarachnoid hemorrhage; 95% CI = 95% confidence interval.

Prevention in Young Women Study,[326] the age-adjusted risk of ischemic stroke with current cocaine use was OR = 3.4 (95% CI = 1.4 to 8.3, $p = 0.006$) and risk of cocaine use within 24 hours of ischemic stroke onset was OR = infinity (8 cases, 0 controls, 95% CI = 2.6 to infinity, $p = 0.001$). The risk of ischemic stroke from current cocaine use after adjustment for age and cerebrovascular risk factors was OR = 2.0 (95% CI = 0.7 to 5.8), with confounding resulting from current smoking and hypertension. The population-based Kaiser Permanente study[327] showed that after adjustment for cerebrovascular risk factors, use of cocaine or amphetamine in young women was associated with a significant increase in stroke risk (OR = 7.0, 95% CI = 2.8 to 17.9). In patients age 18 to 49 years from the 44 hospitals from several U.S. cities involved in the Hemorrhagic Stroke Project,[328] cocaine use within 3 days of onset of subarachnoid hemorrhage (3% cases, 0% controls) was associated with a marked increase in risk (OR = 24.97, 95% CI = 3.95 to infinity). The varying estimates of stroke risk attributable to cocaine use may in part be explained by the greater prevalence of drug use in inner city hospitals with resultant lower risk estimates than in population-based studies, ascertainment bias in population-based controls, and other factors mentioned previously. A recent study[325] found that current marijuana use did not increase the risk of all stroke or any stroke subtype.

SUMMARY AND RECOMMENDATIONS

In this chapter, current data pertaining to several major established and emerging stroke risk factors and their pathophysiology have been reviewed. According to the American Heart Association,[15] screening for vascular risk factors in adults should begin at age 20 and be updated at every clinical encounter. Blood pressure, body mass index, waist circumference, and pulse should be recorded at least every 2 years. Fasting glucose and lipoprotein concentrations should be obtained every 5 years, or every 2 years in the presence of other risk factors. For persons older than age 40, risk factor profiles for coronary heart disease should be assessed every 5 years, or more frequently if ≥2 risk factors are present. For persons age 55 and older, the clinician can use the Framingham Stroke Risk Score[329] to estimate the individual's 10-year probability of stroke. It is important to recognize that this scoring system was developed in a predominately white population. Until similar scoring systems from other race/ethnic groups are available, it may be used to provide a minimum estimate of the individual's level of stroke risk when dealing with an individual from a high-risk race-ethnic group. It is reasonable to pursue a more aggressive approach to risk factor control in individuals with multiple stroke risk factors or at high risk of stroke, because these individuals would be most likely to benefit from this strategy.

The prevalence, strength of association, public health importance (as suggested by population attributable risk), and the known treatment effect, that is, stroke risk reduction by appropriate interventions, for each risk factor are shown in Table 2.1. The goals and types of interventions, as well as level of evidence and grade of recommendation for each recommendation,[13] are shown in Table 2.2. Data presented herein suggest that antihypertensive and hypolipidemic therapies and smoking cessation strategies are either underused or less than optimally effective. Measures to increase adherence to prescribed therapies must be developed, improved, and more systematically implemented to realize the maximum benefits of efficacious preventative treatments for these risk factors. Effective treatments are needed to prevent stroke in patients with diabetes, insulin resistance, and hyperhomocyst(e)inemia. It is good clinical practice that individuals should be firmly advised to avoid the twin scourges of excess alcohol consumption and illicit drug abuse; affected persons should be supported with counseling and treatment programs. Finally, it is clear that complex interrelationships and interactions exist between risk factors, with overlapping pathophysiological derangements. In addition, some medications appear to have multiple actions that may be useful for stroke prevention beyond their known major pharmacological effects. Ongoing research will provide more data in this regard. Aggressive, multifaceted intervention to modify multiple coexisting risk factors may ultimately be the optimal approach for primary stroke prevention.

Acknowledgment

This work was supported in part by grant 1RO1 NS33430 (To PB Gorelick).

References

1. Bonita R. Stroke Prevention: A Worldwide Perspective. In JW Norris, V Hachinski (eds), Stroke Prevention. New York: Oxford University Press, 2001;259–274.
2. Broderick J, Brott T, Kothari R, et al. The Greater Cincinnati/Northern Kentucky Stroke Study: preliminary first-ever and total incidence rates of stroke among blacks. Stroke 1998;29:415–421.
3. American Heart Association. 2002 Heart and Stroke Statistical Update. Dallas, Texas: American Heart Association, 2001.
4. Flegal KM, Carroll MD, Ogden CL, et al. Prevalence and trends in obesity among US adults, 1999-2000. JAMA 2002;288:1723–1727.
5. Mokdad AH, Ford ES, Bowman BA, et al. Prevalence of obesity, diabetes, and obesity-related health risk factors, 2001. JAMA 2003;289:76–79.
6. Ogden CL, Flegal KM, Carroll MD, et al. Prevalence and trends in overweight among US children and adolescents, 1999-2000. JAMA 2002;288:1728–1732.
7. Ford ES, Giles WH, Dietz WH. Prevalence of the metabolic syndrome among US adults: findings from the Third National Health and Nutrition Examination Survey. JAMA 2002;287:356–359.
8. American Heart Association. Economic Cost of Cardiovascular Disease. Available at: http://www.americanheart.org/statistics/10econom.html. Accessed September 2000.
9. Sarti C, Rastenyte D, Cepaitis Z, et al. International trends in mortality from stroke, 1968 to 1994. Stroke 2000;31:1588–1601.
10. Gillum RF, Sempos CT. The end of the long-term decline in stroke mortality in the United States? Stroke 1997;28:1527–1529.
11. Gorelick PB, Sacco RL, Smith DB, et al. Prevention of a first stroke. A review of guidelines and a multidisciplinary consensus statement from the National Stroke Association. JAMA 1999;281:1112–1120.
12. Benson RT, Sacco RL. Stroke prevention: hypertension, diabetes, tobacco, and lipids. Neurol Clin 2000;19:309–319.
13. Goldstein LB, Adams R, Becker K, et al. Primary prevention of ischemic stroke. A statement for healthcare professionals from the Stroke Council of the American Heart Association. Stroke 2001;32:280–299.
14. Strauss SE, Majumdar SR, McAlister FA. New evidence for stroke prevention. Scientific review. JAMA 2002;288:1388–1395.

15. Pearson TA, Blair SN, Daniels SR, et al. AHA guidelines for primary prevention of cardiovascular disease and stroke: 2002 update. Consensus panel guide to comprehensive risk reduction for adult patients without coronary or other atherosclerotic vascular diseases. Circulation 2002;106:388–391.
16. Lewington S, Clarke R, Qizilbash N, et al. Age-specific relevance of usual blood pressure to vascular mortality. Lancet 2002;360:1903–1913.
17. Chobanian AV, Bakris GL, Black HR, et al. and the National High Blood Pressure Education Program Coordinating Committee. The seventh report of the National Committee on Prevention, Detection, Evaluation, and Treatment of High Blood Pressure. JAMA 2003;289:2560–2572.
18. Ogden LG, He J, Lydick E, et al. Long-term absolute benefit of lowering blood pressure in hypertensive patients according to the JNC VI risk stratification. Hypertension 2000;35:539–543.
19. Whisnant JP. Effectiveness versus efficacy of treatment of hypertension for stroke prevention. Neurology 1996;46:301–307.
20. Hankey GJ, Warlow CP. Treatment and secondary prevention of stroke: evidence, costs, and effects on individuals and populations. Lancet 1999;354:1457–1463.
21. Hart RG, Bailey RD. An assessment of guidelines for prevention of ischemic stroke. Neurology 2002;59:977–982.
22. Leys D, Deplanque D, Mounier-Vehier C, et al. Stroke prevention: management of modifiable vascular risk factors. J Neurol 2002;249:507–517.
23. MacMahon S, Rodgers A. The epidemiological association between blood pressure and stroke: implications for primary and secondary prevention. Hypertens Res 1994;17:S23–S32.
24. Wolf PA, Cobb JL, D'Agostino RB. Epidemiology of Stroke. In HJM Barnett, JP Mohr, BM Stein BM, et al. (eds), Stroke—Pathophysiology, Diagnosis, and Management. New York: Churchill Livingstone, 1992;3–27.
25. MacMahon S, Peto R, Cutler J, et al. Blood pressure, stroke, and coronary heart disease. Part 1: prolonged differences in blood pressure: prospective observational studies corrected for the regression dilution bias. Lancet 1990;335:765–774.
26. Prospective Studies Collaboration. Cholesterol, diastolic blood pressure, and stroke: 13,000 strokes in 450,000 patients in 45 prospective cohorts. Lancet 1995;346:1647–1653.
27. Sacco RL, Boden-Albala B, Abel G, et al. Race-ethnic disparities in the impact of stroke risk factors: the Northern Manhattan Stroke Study. Stroke 2001;32:1725–1731.
28. Rohr J, Kittner SJ, Feeser B, et al. Traditional risk factors and ischemic stroke in young adults: the Baltimore-Washington Cooperative Young Stroke Study. Arch Neurol 1996;53:603–607.
29. Eastern Stroke and Coronary Heart Disease Collaborative Research Group. Blood pressure, cholesterol, and stroke in eastern Asia. Lancet 1998;352:1801–1807.
30. Kario K, Pickering TG, Umeda Y, et al. Morning surge in blood pressure as a predictor of silent and clinical cerebrovascular disease in elderly hypertensives: a prospective study. Circulation 2003;107:1401–1407.
31. Kannel WB, Wolf PA, McGee DL, et al. Systolic blood pressure, arterial rigidity, and risk of stroke: the Framingham Study. JAMA 1981;245:1225–1229.
32. Petrovich H, Curb JD, Bloom-Marcus E. Isolated systolic hypertension and risk of stroke in Japanese-American men. Stroke 1995;26:25–29.
33. Qureshi AI, Suri MFK, Mohammad Y, et al. Isolated and borderline isolated systolic hypertension relative to long-term risk and type of stroke: a 20-year follow-up of the National Health and Nutrition Survey. Stroke 2002;33:2781–2788.
34. Davis BR, Vogt T, Frost PH, et al. Risk factors for stroke and type of stroke in persons with isolated systolic hypertension. Systolic Hypertension in the Elderly Program Cooperative Research Group. Stroke 1998;29:1333–1340.
35. Joint National Committee. The sixth report of the Joint National Committee on Prevention, Detection, Evaluation, and Treatment of High Blood Pressure. Arch Intern Med 1997;157:2413–2446.
36. Staessen JA, Gasowski J, Wang JG, et al. Risks of untreated and treated isolated systolic hypertension in the elderly: meta-analysis of outcome trials. Lancet 2000;355:865–872.
37. Hyman DJ, Pavlik VN. Characteristics of patients with uncontrolled hypertension in the United States. N Engl J Med 2001;345:479–486.
38. Hyman D, Pavlik VN. Self-reported hypertension treatment practices among primary care physicians: blood pressure thresholds, drug choices, and the role of guidelines and evidence-based medicine. Arch Intern Med 2000;160:2281–2286.
39. Berlowitz D, Ash A, Hickey R, et al. Inadequate management of blood pressure in a hypertensive population. N Engl J Med 1998;339:1957–1963.
40. Hyman D, Pavlik VN, Vallbona C. Physician role in the lack of awareness and control of hypertension. Clin Hypertens 2000;2:324–330.

41. Alexander M, Tekawa I, Hunkeler E, et al. Evaluating hypertension control in a managed care setting. Arch Intern Med 1999;159:2673–2677.
42. Collins R, Peto R, MacMahon S, et al. Blood pressure, stroke, and coronary heart disease: part 2: short-term reductions in blood pressure: overview of randomised drug trials in their epidemiologic context. Lancet 1990;335:827–835.
43. Gueyffer F, Boutitie F, Boissel J-P, et al. Effect of antihypertensive drug treatment on cardiovascular outcomes in women and men: a meta-analysis of individual patient data from randomized, controlled trials. Ann Intern Med 1997;126:761–767.
44. Blood Pressure Lowering Treatment Trialists' Collaboration. Effects of ACE inhibitors, calcium antagonists, and other blood-pressure-lowering drugs: results of prospectively designed overviews of randomized trials. Lancet 2000;355:1955–1964.
45. Pahor M, Psaty BM, Alderman MH, et al. Health outcomes associated with calcium antagonists compared with other first-line antihypertensive therapies: a meta-analysis of randomised controlled trials. Lancet 2000;355:1945–1954.
46. Staessen JA, Wang J-G, Thijs L. Cardiovascular protection and blood pressure reduction: a meta-analysis. Lancet 2001;358:1305–1315.
47. Psaty BM, Lumley T, Furberg CD, et al. Health outcomes associated with various antihypertensive therapies used as first-line agents: a network meta-analysis. JAMA 2003;289:2534–2544.
48. Dahlof B, Devereux RB, Kjeldsen SE, et al. Cardiovascular morbidity and mortality in the Losartan Intervention For Endpoint reduction in hypertension study (LIFE): a randomized trial against atenolol. Lancet 2002;359:1004–1010.
49. The ALLHAT Officers and Coordinators for the ALLHAT Collaborative Research Group. Major outcomes in high-risk hypertensive patients randomized to angiotensin-converting enzyme inhibitor or calcium channel blocker vs diuretic. The Antihypertensive and Lipid-Lowering Treatment to Prevent Heart Attack Trial (ALLHAT). JAMA 2002;288:2981–2997.
50. Wing LM, Reid CM, Ryan P, et al. A comparison of outcomes with angiotensin-converting-enzyme inhibitors and diuretics for hypertension in the elderly. N Engl J Med 2003;348:583–592.
51. Exner DV, Dries DL, Domanski MJ, et al. Lesser response to angiotensin-converting-enzyme inhibitor therapy in black as compared with white patients with left ventricular dysfunction. N Engl J Med 2001;344:1351–1357.
52. SHEP Cooperative Research Group. Prevention of stroke by antihypertensive drug treatment in older persons with isolated systolic hypertension: final results of the Systolic Hypertension in the Elderly Program (SHEP). JAMA 1991;265:3255–3264.
53. Perry HM, Davis BR, Price TR, et al. Effect of treating isolated systolic hypertension on the risk of developing various types and subtypes of stroke: the Systolic Hypertension in the Elderly Program (SHEP). JAMA 2000;284:465–471.
54. Staessen JA, Fagard R, Thijs L, et al. Randomised double-blind comparison of placebo and active treatment for older patients with isolated systolic hypertension. The Systolic Hypertension in Europe (Syst-Eur) Trial Investigators. Lancet 1997;350:757–764.
55. Dahlof B, Lindholm L, Hansson L, et al. Morbidity and mortality in the Swedish Trial in Old Patients with Hypertension (STOP-Hypertension). Lancet 1991;338:1281–1285.
56. Wang J-G, Staessen JA, Gong L, et al. Chinese trial on isolated systolic hypertension in the elderly. Systolic Hypertension in China (Syst-China) Collaborative Group. Arch Intern Med 2000;160:211–220.
57. Hansson L, Lindholm LH, Ekbom T, et al. Randomised trial of old and new antihypertensive drugs in elderly patients; the Swedish Trial in Old Patients with Hypertension-2 study. Lancet 2000;354:1744–1745.
58. Gueyffier F, Bulpitt C, Boissel JP, et al. Antihypertensive drugs in very old people. A subgroup meta-analysis of randomised controlled trials. INDANA Group. Lancet 1999;353:793–796.
59. August P. Initial treatment of hypertension. N Engl J Med 2003;348:610–617.
60. Frohlich ED. Treating hypertension—what are we to believe? N Engl J Med 2003;348:639–641.
61. Kaplan NM. Morning surge in blood pressure. Circulation 2003;107:1347.
62. Ueshima H, Iida M, Shimamoto T, et al. Multivariate analysis of risk factors for stroke: eight-year follow-up study of farming villages in Akita, Japan. Prev Med 1980;9:722–740.
63. Kagan A, Popper JS, Rhoades GG. Factors related to stroke incidence in Hawaii Japanese men: the Honolulu Heart Study. Stroke 1980;11:14–21.
64. Lindenstrom E, Boysen G, Nyboe J. Influence of total cholesterol, high density lipoprotein cholesterol, and triglycerides on risk of cerebrovascular disease: the Copenhagen City Heart Study. BMJ 1994;309:11–15.
65. Benfante R, Yano K, Hwang LJ, et al. Elevated serum cholesterol is a risk factor for both coronary heart disease and thromboembolic stroke in Hawaiian Japanese men: implications of shared risk. Stroke 1994;25:814–820.

66. Iso H, Jacobs DR, Wentworth D, et al. Serum cholesterol levels and six-year mortality from stroke in 350,977 men screened for the multiple risk factor intervention trial. N Engl J Med 1989;320:904–910.
67. Horenstein RB, Smith DE, Mosca L. Cholesterol predicts stroke mortality in the Women's Pooling Project. Stroke 2002;33:1863–1868.
68. Shahar E, Chambless LE, Rosamond WD, et al. Plasma lipid profile and incident ischemic stroke: the Atherosclerosis Risk in Communities (ARIC) Study. Stroke 2003;34:623–631.
69. Qizilbash N, Jones L, Warlow C, et al. Fibrinogen and lipid concentrations as risk factors for transient ischaemic attacks and minor stroke. BMJ 1991;303:605–609.
70. Kargman DE, Tuck C, Berglund LF, et al. High density lipoprotein: A potentially modifiable stroke risk factor: the Northern Manhattan Stroke Study. Neuroepidemiology 1996;15:20S.
71. Kargman DE, Tuck C, Berglund LF, et al. Elevated high density lipoprotein levels are more important in atherosclerotic ischemic stroke subtypes: the Northern Manhattan Stroke Study. Ann Neurol 1998;44:442–443.
72. O'Leary DH, Anderson KM, Wolf PA, et al. Cholesterol and carotid atherosclerosis in older persons: the Framingham Study. Ann Epidemiol 1992;2:147–153.
73. Salonen R, Seppanen K, Rauramaa R, et al. Prevalence of carotid atherosclerosis and serum cholesterol levels in eastern Finland. Atherosclerosis 1988;8:788–792.
74. Fine-Edelstein JS, Wolf PA, O'Leary DH, et al. Precursors of extracranial carotid atherosclerosis in the Framingham Study. Neurology 1994;44:1046–1050.
75. Iso H, Sato S, Umemura U, et al. Linoleic acid, other fatty acids, and risk of stroke. Stroke 2002;33:2086–2093.
76. Atkins D, Psaty B, Koepsell T, et al. Cholesterol reduction and risk factors for stroke in men: a meta-analysis of randomized, controlled trials. Ann Intern Med 1993;119:136–145.
77. Hebert PR, Gaziano JM, Hennekins CH. An overview of trials of cholesterol lowering and risk of stroke. Arch Intern Med 1995;155:50–55.
78. Delanty N, Vaughn CJ. Vascular effects of statins in stroke. Stroke 1997;28:2315–2320.
79. Rosenson RS, Tangney CC. Antiatherothrombotic properties of statins: implications for cardiovascular event reduction. JAMA 1998;279:1643–1650.
80. Rosenson RS, Lowe GDO. Effects of lipids and lipoproteins on thrombosis and rheology. Atherosclerosis 1998;140:271–280.
81. Vaughan CJ, Delanty N. Neuroprotective properties of statins in cerebral ischemia and stroke. Stroke 1999;30:1969–1973.
82. Crisby M, Nordin-Fredriksson G, Shah PK, et al. Pravastatin treatment increases collagen content and decreases lipid content, inflammation, metalloproteinases, and cell death in human carotid plaques: implications for plaque stabilization. Circulation 2001;103:926–933.
83. Undas A, Brummel KE, Musial J, et al. Simvastatin depresses blood clotting by inhibiting activation of prothrombin, factor V, and factor XIII and enhancing factor Va inactivation. Circulation 2001;103:2248–2253.
84. Furberg CD, Adams HP, Applegate WB, et al. Effect of lovastatin on early carotid atherosclerosis and cardiovascular events. Asymptomatic Carotid Artery Progression Study (ACAPS) Research Group. Circulation 1994;90:1679–1687.
85. Hodis HN, Mack WJ, LaBree L, et al. Reduction in carotid arterial wall thickness using lovastatin and dietary therapy: a randomized, controlled clinical trial. Ann Intern Med 1996;124:548–556.
86. Crouse JR, Byington RP, Bond MG, et al. Pravastatin, Lipids, and Atherosclerosis in the Carotid Arteries (PLAC-II). Am J Cardiol 1995;75:455–459.
87. Salonen R, Nyyssonen K, Porkkala E, et al. Kuopio Atherosclerosis Prevention Study (KAPS). A population-based primary prevention trial of the effect of LDL lowering on atherosclerotic progression in carotid and femoral arteries. Circulation 1995;92:1758–1764.
88. Knopp RH. Drug treatment of lipid disorders. N Engl J Med 1999;341:498–511.
89. Scandinavian Simvastatin Survival Study Group. Randomised trial of cholesterol lowering in 4444 patients with coronary heart disease: the Scandinavian Simvastatin Survival Study (4S). Lancet 1994;344:1383–1389.
90. Shepard J, Cobbe SM, Ford I, et al. Prevention of coronary heart disease with pravastatin in men with hypercholesterolemia. West of Scotland Coronary Prevention Study Group. N Engl J Med 1995;333:1301–1307.
91. Sacks FM, Pfeffer MA, Moye LA, et al. The effect of pravastatin on coronary events after myocardial infarction in patients with average cholesterol levels. Cholesterol and Recurrent Events Trial Investigators. N Engl J Med 1996;335:1001–1009.
92. Plehn JF, Davis BR, Sacks FM, et al. Reduction of stroke incidence after myocardial infarction with pravastatin: the Cholesterol and Recurrent Events (CARE) Study. The CARE Investigators. Circulation 1999;99:216–223.

93. The Long-Term Intervention with Pravastatin in Ischaemic Disease (LIPID) Study Group. Prevention of cardiovascular events and death with pravastatin in patients with coronary heart disease and a broad range of initial cholesterol levels. N Engl J Med 1998;339:1349–1357.

94. White HD, Simes RJ, Anderson NE, et al. Pravastatin therapy and the risk of stroke. N Engl J Med 2000;343:317–326.

95. The LIPID Study Group. Long-term effectiveness and safety of pravastatin in 9014 patients with coronary heart disease and average cholesterol concentrations: the LIPID trial follow-up. Lancet 2002;359:1379–1387.

96. Byington RP, Davis BR, Plehn JF, et al. Reduction of stroke events with pravastatin: the Prospective Pravastatin Pooling (PPP) Project. Circulation 2001;103:387–392.

97. Expert Panel on Detection, Evaluation, and Treatment of High Blood Cholesterol in Adults. Executive summary of the Third Report of the National Cholesterol Education Program (NCEP) Expert Panel on Detection, Evaluation, and Treatment of High Blood Cholesterol in Adults (Adult Treatment Panel III). JAMA 2001;285:2486–2497.

98. Blauw GJ, Lagaay AM, Smelt AHM, et al. Stroke, statins, and cholesterol: a meta-analysis of randomized, placebo-controlled, double-blind trials with HMG-CoA reductase inhibitors. Stroke 1997;28:946–950.

99. Hebert PR, Gaziano JM, Chan KS, et al. Cholesterol lowering with statin drugs, risk of stroke, and total mortality: an overview of randomized trials. JAMA 1997;278:313–321.

100. Downs JR, Clearfield M, Weis S, et al. Primary prevention of acute coronary events with lovastatin in men and women with average cholesterol levels: results of AFCAPS/TexCAPS. Air Force/Texas Coronary Atherosclerosis Prevention Study. JAMA 1998;279:1615–1622.

101. Heart Protection Study Collaborative Group. MRC/BHF Heart Protection Study of cholesterol lowering with simvastatin in 20 536 high-risk individuals: a randomized placebo-controlled trial. Lancet 2002;360:7–22.

102. Schwartz GG, Olsson AG, Ezekowitz MD, et al. Effects of atorvastatin on early recurrent ischemic events in acute coronary syndromes: the MIRACL Study: a randomized controlled trial. JAMA 2001;285:1711–1718.

103. The ALLHAT Officers and Coordinators for the ALLHAT Collaborative Research Group. Major outcomes in moderately hypercholesterolemic, hypertensive patients randomized to pravastatin vs usual care: the Antihypertensive and Lipid-Lowering Treatment to Prevent Heart Attack Trial (ALLHAT-LLT). JAMA 2002;288:2998–3007.

104. Pasternak RC. The ALLHAT Lipid Lowering Trial—less is less. JAMA 2002;288:3042–3044.

105. Bloomfield Rubins H, Davenport J, Babikian V, et al. Reduction in stroke with gemfibrozil in men with coronary heart disease and low HDL cholesterol: the Veterans Affairs HDL Intervention Trial (VA-HIT). Circulation 2001;103:2828–2833.

106. Shepard J, Blauw GJ, Murphy MB, et al. Pravastatin in elderly individuals at risk of vascular disease (PROSPER): a randomised controlled trial. Lancet 2002;360:1623–1630.

107. Collins R, Armitage J. High-risk elderly patients PROSPER from cholesterol-lowering therapy. Lancet 2002;360:1618–1619.

108. Benner JS, Glynn RJ, Mogun H, et al. Long-term persistence in use of statin therapy in elderly patients. JAMA 2002;288:455–461.

109. Jackevicius CA, Mamdani M, Tu JV. Adherence with statin therapy in elderly patients with and without acute coronary syndromes. JAMA 2002;288:462–467.

110. Fonarow GC, French WJ, Parsons LS, et al. Use of lipid-lowering medications at discharge in patients with acute myocardial infarction: data from the National Registry of Myocardial Infarction 3. Circulation 2001;103:38–44.

111. Wolf PA. Cigarettes, alcohol and stroke. N Engl J Med 1986;315:1087–1089.

112. Howard G, Wagenknecht LE. Environmental tobacco smoke and measures of subclinical vascular disease. Environ Health Perspect 1999;107(suppl 6):837–840.

113. Glantz SA, Parmley WW. Even a little secondhand smoke is dangerous. JAMA 2001;286:462–463.

114. Hasday JD, Bascom R, Costa JJ, et al. Bacterial endotoxin is an active component of cigarette smoke. Chest 1999;115:829–835.

115. Wiedermann CJ, Kiechl S, Dunzendorfer S, et al. Association of endotoxemia with carotid atherosclerosis and cardiovascular disease: prospective results from the Bruneck Study. J Am Coll Cardiol 1999;34:1975–1981.

116. Heiss G, Sharrett AR, Barnes R, et al. Carotid atherosclerosis measured by B-mode ultrasound in populations: associations with cardiovascular risk factors in the ARIC study. Am J Epidemiol 1991;134:250–256.

117. O'Leary DH, Polak JF, Kronmal RA, et al. Distribution and correlates of sonographically detected carotid artery disease in the Cardiovascular Health Study. The CHS Collaborative Research Group. Stroke 1992;23:1752–1760.

118. Howard G, Burke GL, Szklo M, et al. Active and passive smoking are associated with increased carotid wall thickness. Arch Intern Med 1994;154;1277–1282.

119. Howard G, Wagenknecht LE, Burke GL, et al. Cigarette smoking and the progression of atherosclerosis: the Atherosclerosis Risk in Communities (ARIC) Study. JAMA 1998;279:119–124.

120. O'Leary DH, Polak JF, Kronmal RA, et al. Carotid-artery intima and media thickness as a risk factor for myocardial infarction and stroke in older adults: the Cardiovascular Health Study. N Engl J Med 1999;340:14–22.

121. Sacco RL, Roberts JK, Boden-Albala B, et al. Race-ethnicity and determinants of carotid atherosclerosis in a multiethnic population. The Northern Manhattan Stroke Study. Stroke 1997;28:929–935.

122. Mast H, Thompson JL, Lin IF, et al. Cigarette smoking as a determinant of high-grade carotid artery stenosis in Hispanic, black and white patients with stroke or transient ischemic attack. Stroke 1998;29:908–912.

123. Kiechl S, Werner P, Egger G, et al. Active and passive smoking, chronic infections, and the risk of carotid atherosclerosis: prospective results from the Bruneck Study. Stroke 2002;33:2170–2176.

124. Wolf PA, D'Agostino RB, Kannel WB, et al. Cigarette smoking as a risk factor for stroke: the Framingham study. JAMA 1988;259:1025–1029.

125. Abbott RD, Yin Y, Reed DM, et al. Risk of stroke in male cigarette smokers. N Engl J Med 1986; 315:717–720.

126. Colditz GA, Bonita R, Stampfer MJ, et al. Cigarette smoking and risk of stroke in middle-aged women. N Engl J Med 1988;318:937–941.

127. Robbins AS, Manson JE, Lee I-M, et al. Cigarette smoking and stroke in a cohort of U.S. male physicians. Ann Intern Med 1994;120:458–462.

128. Kurth T, Kase CS, Berger K, et al. Smoking and the risk of hemorrhagic stroke in men. Stroke 2003;34:1151–1155.

129. Bonita R, Scragg R, Stewart A, et al. Cigarette smoking and the risk of premature stroke in men and women. BMJ 1986;293:6–8.

130. Gorelick PB, Rodin MB, Langenberg P, et al. Weekly alcohol consumption, cigarette smoking, and the risk of ischemic stroke: results of a case-control study at three urban medical centers in Chicago, Illinois. Neurology 1989;39:339–343.

131. Shinton R, Beevers G. Meta-analysis of relation between cigarette smoking and stroke. BMJ 1989;298:789–794.

132. Kawachi I, Colditz GA, Stampfer MJ, et al. Smoking cessation and decreased risk of stroke in women. JAMA 1993;269:232–236.

133. Wannamethee SG, Shaper AG, Whincup PH, et al. Smoking cessation and the risk of stroke in middle-aged men. JAMA 1995;274:155–160.

134. Howard G, Wagenknecht LE, Cai J, et al. Cigarette smoking and other risk factors for silent cerebral infarction in the general population. Stroke 1998;29:913–917.

135. Bonita R, Duncan J, Truelsen T, et al. Passive smoking increases the risk of stroke. Tobacco Control 1999;7:156–160.

136. You RX, Thrift AG, McNeil JJ, et al. Ischemic stroke risk and passive exposure to spouses' cigarette smoking. Melbourne Stroke Risk Factor Study (MERFS) Group. Am J Public Health 1999;89:572–575.

137. Rigotti NA. Treatment of tobacco use and dependence. N Engl J Med 2002;346:506–512.

138. Ahluwalia JS, Harris KJ, Catley D, et al. Sustained-release bupropion for smoking cessation in African-Americans: a randomized controlled trial. JAMA 2002;288:468–474.

139. Archer L, Grant BF, Dawson DA. What if Americans drank less? The potential effect on the prevalence of alcohol abuse and dependence. Am J Public Health 1995;85:61–66.

140. Camargo CA. Moderate alcohol consumption and stroke: the epidemiological evidence. Stroke 1989;20:1611–1626.

141. Gorelick PB. The status of alcohol as a risk factor for stroke. Stroke 1989;20:1607–1610.

142. Reynolds K, Lewis LB, Nolen JDL, et al. Alcohol consumption and risk of stroke: a meta-analysis. JAMA 2003;289:579–588.

143. Gorelick PB. Alcohol and stroke. Stroke 1987;18:268–271.

144. Thornton J, Symes C, Heaton K. Moderate alcohol intake reduces bile cholesterol saturation and raises HDL cholesterol. Lancet 1983;2:819–822.

145. Pellegrini N, Pareti FI, Stabile F, et al. Effects of moderate consumption of red wine on platelet aggregation and haemostatic variables in healthy volunteers. Eur J Clin Nutr 1996;50:209–213.

146. Hillbom M, Kaste M. Does ethanol intoxication promote brain infarction in young adults? Lancet 1978;2:1181–1183.

147. Gorelick PB, Rodin MB, Langenberg P, et al. Is acute alcohol ingestion a risk factor for ischemic stroke? Results of a controlled study in middle-aged and elderly stroke patients at three urban medical centers. Stroke 1987;18:359–364.

148. Boysen G, Nyboe J, Appleyard M, et al. Stroke incidence and risk factors for stroke in Copenhagen, Denmark. Stroke 1988;19:1345–1353.
149. Sacco RL, Elkind ME, Boden-Albala B. The protective effect of moderate alcohol consumption on ischemic stroke. JAMA 1999;281:53–60.
150. Berger K, Ajani UA, Kase CS, et al. Light to moderate alcohol consumption and the risk of stroke among U.S. male physicians. N Engl J Med 1999;341:1557–1564.
151. Malarcher AM, Giles WH, Croft JB, et al. Alcohol intake, type of beverage, and the risk of cerebral infarction in young women. Stroke 2001;32:77–83.
152. Donahue RP, Abbott RD, Reed DM, et al. Alcohol and hemorrhagic stroke: the Honolulu Heart Program. JAMA 1986;255:2311–2314.
153. Klatsky AL, Armstrong MA, Friedman GD. Alcohol use and subsequent cerebrovascular disease hospitalizations. Stroke 1989;20:741–746.
154. Caicoya M, Rodriguez T, Corrales C, et al. Alcohol and stroke: a community case-control study in Asturias, Spain. J Clin Epidemiol 1999;52:677–684.
155. Thrift A, Donnan G, McNeil J. Heavy drinking, but not moderate or intermediate drinking, increases the risk of intracerebral hemorrhage. Epidemiology 1999;10:307–312.
156. Klatsky AL, Armstrong MA, Friedman GD, et al. Alcohol drinking and risk of hemorrhagic stroke. Neuroepidemiology 2002;21:115–122.
157. Masharani U, Karem JH. Diabetes Mellitus and Hypoglycemia. In LH Tierney, SJ McPhee, MA Papadakis (eds), Current Medical Diagnosis and Treatment. New York, McGraw Hill 2002;1203–1250.
158. Kannel WB, McGee DL. Diabetes and cardiovascular disease: the Framingham study. JAMA 1979;241:2035–2038.
159. Burchfiel CM, Curb JD, Rodriguez BL, et al. Glucose intolerance and 22-year stroke incidence: the Honolulu Heart Program. Stroke 1994;25:951–957.
160. Abbott RD, Donahue RP, MacMahon SW, et al. Diabetes and the risk of stroke: the Honolulu Heart Program. JAMA 1987;257:949–952.
161. Barrett-Connor E, Khaw K. Diabetes mellitus: an independent risk factor for stroke. Am J Epidemiol 1988;128:116–124.
162. Noto D, Barbagallo CM, Cavera G, et al. Leucocyte count, diabetes mellitus, and age are strong predictors of stroke in a rural population in southern Italy: an 8-year follow-up. Atherosclerosis 2001;17:225–231.
163. Kothari V, Stevens RJ, Adler AI, et al. UKPDS 60: risk of stroke in type 2 diabetes estimated by the UK Prospective Diabetes Study Group Risk Engine. Stroke 2002;33:1776–1781.
164. The Diabetes Control and Complications Trial Research Group. The effect of intensive treatment of diabetes on the development and progression of long-term complications in insulin-dependent diabetes mellitus. N Engl J Med 1993;329:977–986.
165. The Diabetes Control and Complications Trial (DCCT) Research Group. Effect of intensive diabetes management on macrovascular events in the Diabetes Control and Complications Trial. Am J Cardiol 1995;75:894–903.
166. UK Prospective Diabetes Study (UKPDS) Group. Intensive blood-glucose control with sulphonylureas or insulin compared with conventional treatment and risk of complications in patients with type 2 diabetes (UKPDS 33). Lancet 1998;352:837–853.
167. UK Prospective Diabetes Study Group. Tight blood pressure control and risk of macrovascular and microvascular complications in type 2 diabetes: UKPDS 38. BMJ 1998;317:703–713.
168. Heart Outcomes Prevention Evaluation Study Investigators. Effects of ramipril on cardiovascular and microvascular outcomes in people with diabetes: results of the HOPE study and MICRO-HOPE substudy. Lancet 2000;355:253–259.
169. Gaede P, Vedel P, Larsen N, et al. Multifactorial intervention and cardiovascular disease in patients with type 2 diabetes. N Engl J Med 2003;348:383–393.
170. Solomon CG. Reducing cardiovascular risk in type 2 diabetes. N Engl J Med 2003;348:457–459.
171. Inzucchi SE. Oral hypoglycemic therapy for type 2 diabetes: scientific review. JAMA 2002;287:360–372.
172. Holmboe ES. Oral antihyperglycemic therapy for type 2 diabetes: clinical applications. JAMA 2002;287:373–376.
173. American Diabetes Association. Standards of medical care for patients with diabetes. Diabetes Care 2003;26(suppl 1):S33–S50.
174. Freeman DJ, Norrie J, Sattar N, et al. Pravastatin and the development of diabetes mellitus: evidence for a protective treatment effect in the West of Scotland Coronary Prevention Study. Circulation 2001;103:357–362.
175. Krentz AJ. Insulin resistance. BMJ 1996;313:1385–1389.

176. Shulman GI. Cellular mechanisms of insulin resistance. J Clin Invest 2000;106:171–176.
177. Reaven GM. Insulin resistance in noninsulin-dependent diabetes: does it exist and can it be measured? Am J Med 1983;86:3–17.
178. van Loon BJP. The cardiovascular risk factor plasminogen activator inhibitor type I is related to insulin resistance. Metabolism 1993;42:945–949.
179. Imperatore G, Riccardi G, Iovine C, et al. Plasma fibrinogen: a new factor of the metabolic syndrome. Diabetes Care 1998;21:649–654.
180. Trovati M, Anfossi G. Insulin, insulin resistance, and platelet function: similarities with insulin effects on cultured vascular smooth muscle cells. Diabetologia 1998;41:609–622.
181. Hak AE, Pols HAP, Stehouwer CDA, et al. Markers of inflammation and cellular adhesion molecules in relation to insulin resistance in nondiabetic elderly: the Rotterdam Study. J Clin Endocrinol Metab 2001;86:4398–4405.
182. Stout RW. Insulin and atheroma: 20-yr perspective. Diabetes Care 1990;13:631–654.
183. Balkau B, Charles MA. Comment on the provisional report from the WHO consultation: European Group for the Study of Insulin Resistance (EGIR). Diabet Med 1999;16:442–443.
184. Lakka H-M, Laaksonen DE, Laaka TA, et al. The metabolic syndrome and total and cardiovascular disease mortality in middle-aged men. JAMA 2002;288:2709–2716.
185. Liese AD, Mayer-Davis EJ, Haffner SM. Development of the multiple metabolic syndrome: an epidemiologic perspective. Epidemiol Rev 1998;20:157–172.
186. Howard G, O'Leary DH, Zaccaro D, et al. Insulin sensitivity and atherosclerosis. Circulation 1996;93:1809–1817.
187. Agewall S, Fagergerg B, Attvall S, et al. Carotid artery wall intima-media thickness is associated with insulin-mediated glucose disposal in men at high and low coronary risk. Stroke 1995;26: 956–960.
188. Gertler MM, Leetma HE, Koutrouby RJ, et al. The assessment of insulin, glucose and lipids in ischemic thrombotic cerebrovascular disease. Stroke 1975;6:77–84.
189. Shinozaki K, Naritomi H, Shimizu T, et al. Role of insulin resistance associated with compensatory hyperinsulinemia in ischemic stroke. Stroke 1996;27:37–43.
190. Lakka H-M, Lakka TA, Toumilehto J, et al. Hyperinsulinemia and the risk of cardiovascular death and acute coronary and cerebrovascular events in men: the Kuopio Ischaemic Heart Disease Risk Factor Study. Arch Intern Med 2000;160:1160–1168.
191. Pyorala M, Miettinen H, Laasko M, et al. Hyperinsulinemia and the risk of stroke in healthy middle-aged men: the 22 year follow-up results of the Helsinki Policemen Study. Stroke 1998;29:1860–1868.
192. Folsom AR, Rasmussen ML, Chambless LE, et al. Prospective associations of fasting insulin, body fat distribution, and diabetes with risk of ischemic stroke. Diabetes Care 1999;22:1077–1083.
193. Wascher TC, Paulweber B, Malaimare L, et al. Associations of a human G protein beta-3 subunit dimorphism with insulin resistance and carotid atherosclerosis. Stroke 2003;34:605–609.
194. Jha RJ. Thiazolidinediones—the new insulin enhancers. Clin Exp Hypertension 1999;21:157–166.
195. Parulkar AA, Pendergrass ML, Granda-Ayala R, et al. Nonhypoglycemic effects of thiazolidinediones. Ann Intern Med 2001;134:61–71.
196. Minamikawa J, Tanaka S, Yamauchi M, et al. Potent inhibitory effect of troglitazone on carotid arterial wall thickness in type 2 diabetes. J Clin Endocrinol Metab 1998;83:1818–1820.
197. Koshiyama H, Shimono D, Kuwamura N, et al. Inhibitory effect of pioglitazone on carotid arterial wall thickness in type 2 diabetes. J Clin Endocrinol Metab 2001;86:3452–3456.
198. Allison DB, Fontaine KR, Manson JE, et al. Annual deaths attributable to obesity in the United States. JAMA 1999;282:1530–1538.
199. National Task Force on the Prevention and Treatment of Obesity. Overweight, obesity, and health risk. Arch Int Med 2000;160:898–904.
200. Steinberg HO, Chaker H, Leaming R, et al. Obesity/insulin resistance is associated with endothelial dysfunction: implications for the syndrome of insulin resistance. J Clin Invest 1996;97:2601–2610.
201. Lakka TA, Lakka H-M, Salonen R, et al. Abdominal obesity is associated with accelerated progression of carotid atherosclerosis in men. Atherosclerosis 2001;154:497–504.
202. Walker SP, Rimm EB, Ascherio A, et al. Body size and fat distribution as predictors of stroke among U.S. men. Am J Epidemiol 1996;144:1143–1150.
203. Rexrode KM, Hennekens CH, Willett WC, et al. A prospective study of body mass index, weight change, and risk of stroke in women. JAMA 1997;277:1539–1545.
204. De Michele M, Panico S, Iannuzzi A, et al. Association of obesity and central fat distribution with carotid artery wall thickening in middle-aged women. Stroke 2002;33:2923–2928.
205. NIH Technology Assessment Conference Panel. Methods for voluntary weight loss and control. Ann Intern Med 1993;119:764–770.

206. Expert Panel on the Identification, Evaluation, and Treatment of Overweight and Obesity in Adults. Executive summary of the clinical guidelines on the identification, evaluation, and treatment of overweight and obesity in adults. Arch Intern Med 1998;158:1855–1867.
207. McGuire MT, Wing RR, Klem ML, et al. Behavioral strategies of individuals who have maintained long-term weight losses. Obes Res 1999;7:334–341.
208. Wadden TA, Foster GD. Behavioral treatment of obesity. Med Clin North Am 2000;84:441–461.
209. Yanovski SZ, Yanovski JA. Obesity. N Engl J Med 2002;346:591–602.
210. Welch GN, Loscalzo J. Homocysteine and atherothrombosis. N Engl J Med 1998;338:1042–1050.
211. Diaz-Arrastia R. Homocysteine and neurologic disease. Arch Neurol 2000;57:1422–1428.
212. Gorelick PB. Stroke prevention therapy beyond antithrombotics: unifying mechanisms in ischemic stroke pathogenesis and implications for therapy. Stroke 2002;33:862–875.
213. Sacco RL, Roberts JK, Jacobs BS. Homocysteine as a risk factor for ischemic stroke: an epidemiologic story in evolution. Neuroepidemiology 1998;17:167–173.
214. Napo F, De Rosa N, Marfella R, et al. Impairment of endothelial functions by acute hyperhomocysteinemia and reversal by antioxidant vitamins. JAMA 1999;281:2113–2118.
215. Selhub J, Jacques PF, Rosenberg IH, et al. Serum total homocysteine concentrations in the Third National Health and Nutrition Examination Survey (1991-1994): population reference ranges and contribution of vitamin status to high serum concentrations. Ann Intern Med 1999;131:331–339.
216. Ueland PM, Refsum H. Plasma homocysteine, a risk factor for vascular disease: plasma levels in health, disease, and drug therapy. J Lab Clin Med 1989;114:473–501.
217. McCully KS. Homocysteine and vascular disease. Nat Med 1996;2:386–389.
218. Adachi H, Hirai Y, Fujiura Y, et al. Plasma homocysteine levels and atherosclerosis in Japan: epidemiological study by use of carotid ultrasonography. Stroke 2002;33:2177–2181.
219. Malinow MR, Nieto FJ, Szklo M, et al. Carotid intima-medial wall thickening and plasma homocyst(e)ine in asymptomatic adults. Circulation 1993;87:1107–1113.
220. Selhub J, Jacques PF, Bostom AG, et al. Association between plasma homocysteine concentrations and extracranial carotid-artery stenosis. N Engl J Med 1995;332:286–291.
221. Eikelboom JW, Hankey GJ, Anand SS, et al. Association between high homocysteine and ischemic stroke due to large- and small-artery disease but not other etiologic subtypes of ischemic stroke. Stroke 2000;31:1069–1075.
222. Fassbender K, Mielke O, Bertsch T, et al. Homocysteine in cerebral macroangiopathy and microangiopathy. Lancet 1999;353:1586–1587.
223. Eikelboom JW, Lonn E, Genest J Jr, et al. Homocyst(e)ine and cardiovascular disease: a critical review of the epidemiologic evidence. Ann Intern Med 1999;131:363–375.
224. Verhoef P, Hennekens CH, Malinow R, et al. A prospective study of plasma homocysteine and risk of ischemic stroke. Stroke 1994;25:1924–1930.
225. Giles WH, Croft J, Greenlund KJ, et al. Total homocysteine concentration and risk of nonfatal stroke: results from the Third National Health and Nutrition Examination Survey. Stroke 1998;29:2473–2477.
226. Kittner SJ, Giles WH, Macko RF, et al. Homocyst(e)ine and risk of cerebral infarction in a biracial population: the Stroke Prevention in Young Women Study. Stroke 1999;30:1554–1560.
227. Tan NC-K, Venketasubramanian N, Saw S-M, et al. Hyperhomocyst(e)inemia and risk of ischemic stroke among young Asian males. Stroke 2002;33:1956–1962.
228. Tanne D, Haim M, Goldbourt U, et al. Prospective study of serum homocysteine and risk of ischemic stroke among patients with preexisting coronary heart disease. Stroke 2003;34: 632–636.
229. The Homocysteine Studies Collaborators. Homocysteine and the risk of ischemic heart disease and stroke: a meta-analysis. JAMA 2002;288(16):2015–2022.
230. Markus HS, Ali N, Swaminathan R, et al. A common polymorphism in the methylenetetrahydrofolate reductase gene, homocysteine, and ischemic cerebrovascular disease. Stroke 1997;28: 1739–1743.
231. Bova I, Chapman J, Sylantiev C, et al. The A677V methylenetetrahydrofolate reductase gene polymorphism and carotid atherosclerosis. Stroke 1999;30:2180–2182.
232. Kristensen B, Malm J, Nilsson TK, et al. Hyperhomocysteinemia and hypofibrinolysis in young adults with ischemic stroke. Stroke 1999;30:974–980.
233. Gallai V, Caso V, Paciaroni M, et al. Mild hyperhomocyst(e)inemia: a possible risk factor for cervical artery dissection. Stroke 2001;32:714–718.
234. Matsui T, Arai H, Yuzuriha T, et al. Elevated plasma homocysteine levels and risk of silent brain infarction in elderly people. Stroke 2001;32:1116–1119.
235. Kelly PJ, Rosand J, Kistler JP, et al. Homocysteine, MTHFR 677C→T polymorphism, and risk of ischemic stroke: results of a meta-analysis. Neurology 2002;59:529–536.

236. McIlroy SP, Dynan KB, Lawson JT, et al. Moderately elevated plasma homocysteine, methylenetetrahydrofolate reductase genotype, and risk for stroke, vascular dementia, and Alzheimer disease in Northern Ireland. Stroke 2002;33:2351–2356.

237. Jacques PF, Selhub J, Bostom AG, et al. The effect of folic acid fortification on plasma folate and total homocysteine concentrations. N Engl J Med 1999;340:1449–1454.

238. Woodside JV, Yarnell JW, McMaster D, et al. Effect of B-group vitamins and antioxidant vitamins on hyperhomocysteinemia: a double-blind, randomized, factorial-design, controlled trial. Am J Clin Nutr 1998;67:858–866.

239. Hackam DG, Peterson JC, Spence JD. What level of plasma homocysteine should be treated? Effects of vitamin therapy on progression of carotid atherosclerosis in patients with homocysteine levels above and below 14 umol/L. Am J Hypertens 2000;13:105–110.

240. Manson JE, Gaziano JM, Jonas MA, et al. Antioxidants and cardiovascular disease: a review. J Am Coll Nutr 1993;12:426–432.

241. Hennekens CH, Gaziano JM, Manson JE, et al. Antioxidant vitamin-cardiovascular disease hypothesis is still promising, but still unproven: the need for randomized trials. Am J Clin Nutr 1995;62(suppl):1377S–1380S.

242. Delanty N, Dichter MA. Oxidative injury in the nervous system. Acta Neurol Scand 1998;98: 145–153.

243. Todd S, Woodward M, Tunstall-Pedoe H, et al. Dietary antioxidant vitamins and fiber in the etiology of cardiovascular disease and all-causes mortality: results from the Scottish Heart Health Study. Am J Epidemiol 1999;150:1073–1080.

244. Stephens NG, Parsons A, Schofield PM, et al. Randomized controlled trial of vitamin E in patients with coronary disease: Cambridge Heart Antioxidant Study (CHAOS). Lancet 1996;347:781–786.

245. Rapola JM, Virtano J, Ripatti S, et al. Randomised trial alpha-tocopherol and beta-carotene supplements on incidence of major coronary events in men with previous myocardial infarction. Lancet 1997;349:1715–1720.

246. GISSI-Prevenzione Investigators. Dietary supplementation with n-3 polyunsaturated fatty acids and vitamin E after myocardial infarction: results of the GISSI-Prevenzione trial. Lancet 1999;354:447–457.

247. Ascherio A, Rimm EB, Hernan MA, et al. Relation of consumption of vitamin E, vitamin C, and carotenoids to risk for stroke among men in the United States. Ann Intern Med 1999;130:963–970.

248. The Heart Outcomes Prevention Evaluation Study Investigators. Vitamin E supplementation and cardiovascular events in high-risk patients. N Engl J Med 2000;342:154–160.

249. Heart Protection Study Collaborative Group. MRC/BHF Heart Protection Study of antioxidant vitamin supplementation in 20 536 high-risk individuals: a randomised placebo-controlled trial. Lancet 2002;360:23–33.

250. John JH, Ziebland S, Yudkin P, et al. Effects of fruit and vegetable consumption on plasma antioxidant concentrations and blood pressure: a randomised controlled trial. Lancet 2002;359: 1969–1974.

251. Joshipura KJ, Ascherio A, Manson JE, et al. Fruit and vegetable intake in relation to risk of ischemic stroke. JAMA 1999;282:1233–1239.

252. Warnholtz A, Munzel T. Why do antioxidants fail to provide clinical benefit? Curr Control Trials Cardiovasc Med 2000;1:38–40.

253. Thies F, Garry JMC, Yaqoob P, et al. Association of n-3 polyunsaturated fatty acids with stability of atherosclerotic plaques: a randomised controlled trial. Lancet 2003;361:477–485.

254. He K, Rimm EB, Merchant A, et al. Fish consumption and the risk of stroke in men. JAMA 2002;288:3130–3136.

255. Ross R. Atherosclerosis—an inflammatory disease. N Engl J Med 1999;340:115–126.

256. Rossi GP, Rossi A, Sacchetto A, et al. Hypertensive cerebrovascular disease and the renin-angiotensin system. Stroke 1995;26:1700–1706.

257. Farmer JA, Torre-Amione G. The renin angiotensin system as a risk factor for coronary artery disease. Curr Atheroscler Rep 2001;3:117–124.

258. DeGraba TJ, Siren AL, Penix L, et al. Increased endothelial expression of intercellular adhesion molecule-1 in symptomatic versus asymptomatic human carotid atherosclerotic plaque. Stroke 1998;29:1405–1410.

259. Johnson JL, Jackson CL, Angelini GD, et al. Activation of matrix-degrading metalloproteinases by mast cell proteinases in atherosclerotic plaques. Arterioscler Thromb Vasc Biol 1998;18: 1707–1715.

260. Gabay C, Kushner I. Acute-phase proteins and other systemic responses to inflammation. N Engl J Med 1999;340:448–454.

261. Munford RS. Statins and the acute-phase response. N Engl J Med 2001;344:2016–2018.

262. Rohde LEP, Hennekens CH, Ridker PM. Survey of C-reactive protein and cardiovascular risk factors in apparently healthy men. Am J Cardiol 1999;84:1018–1022.
263. Ridker PM, Cushman M, Stampfer MJ, et al. Inflammation, aspirin, and the risk of cardiovascular disease in apparently healthy men. N Engl J Med 1997;336:973–979.
264. Ridker PM, Hennekens CH, Buring JE, et al. C-reactive protein and other markers of inflammation in the prediction of cardiovascular disease in women. N Engl J Med 2000;342:836–842.
265. Ridker PM, Rifai N, Rose L, et al. Comparison of C-reactive protein and low-density lipoprotein cholesterol levels in the prediction of first cardiovascular events. N Engl J Med 2002;347: 1557–1565.
266. Muir KW, Weir CJ, Alwan W, et al. C-reactive protein and outcome after ischemic stroke. Stroke 1999;30:981–985.
267. Ridker PM, Stampfer MJ, Rifai N. Novel risk factors for systemic atherosclerosis: a comparison of C-reactive protein, fibrinogen, homocysteine, lipoprotein (a), and standard cholesterol screening as predictors of peripheral arterial disease. JAMA 2001;285:2481–2485.
268. Wilhelmsen L, Svardsudd K, Korsan-Bengtsen K, et al. Fibrinogen as a risk factor for stroke and myocardial infarction. N Engl J Med 1984;311:501–505.
269. Ernst E, Resch KL. Fibrinogen as a cardiovascular risk factor. Ann Intern Med 1993;118:956–963.
270. Coull BM, Beamer N, de Garmo P, et al. Chronic hyperviscosity in subjects with acute stroke, transient ischemic attack, and risk factors for stroke. Stroke 1991;22:162–168.
271. Tanne D, Benderly M, Goldbourt U, et al. A prospective study of plasma fibrinogen levels and the risk of stroke among participants in the Bezafibrate Infarction Prevention (BIP) Study. Am J Med 2001;111:457–463.
272. Resch KL, Ernst E, Matrai A, et al. Fibrinogen and viscosity as risk factors for subsequent cardio-vascular events in stroke survivors. Ann Intern Med 1992;117:371–375.
273. Grotta JC, Yatsu FM, Pettigrew K, et al. Prediction of carotid stenosis progression by lipid and hematologic measurements. Neurology 1989;39:1325–1331.
274. Di Napoli M, Papa F, Bocola V. Prognostic influence of increased C-reactive protein and fibrinogen levels in ischemic stroke. Stroke 2001;32:133–138.
275. Di Napoli M, Papa F, Bocola V. C-reactive protein in ischemic stroke: an independent prognostic factor. Stroke 2001;32:917–924.
276. Rost NS, Wolf PA, Kase CS, et al. Plasma concentration of C-reactive protein and risk of ischemic stroke and transient ischemic attack: the Framingham Study. Stroke 2001;32: 2575–2579.
277. Di Napoli M, Papa F for the Villa Pini Stroke Data Bank Investigators. Inflammation, hemostatic markers, and antithrombotic agents in relation to long-term risk of new cardiovascular events in first-ever ischemic stroke patients. Stroke 2002;33:1763–1771.
278. Hwang SJ, Ballantyne CM, Sharrett AR, et al. Circulating adhesion molecules VCAM-1, ICAM-1, and E-selectin in carotid atherosclerosis and incident coronary heart disease cases: the Atherosclerosis Risk in Communities (ARIC) study. Circulation 1997;96:4219–4225.
279. Rohde LE, Lee RT, Rivero J, et al. Circulating cell adhesion molecules are correlated with ultrasound-based assessment of carotid atherosclerosis. Arterioscler Thromb Vasc Biol 1998;18: 1765–1770.
280. Blann A, Kumar P, Krupinski J, et al. Soluble intercellular adhesion molecule-1, E-selectin, vascu-lar cell adhesion molecule-1 and von Willebrand factor in stroke. Blood Coagul Fibrinolysis 1999;10:277–284.
281. Shyu KG, Chang H, Lin CC. Serum levels of intercellular adhesion molecule-1 and E-selectin in patients with ischaemic stroke. J Neurol 1997;244:90–93.
282. Tanne D, Haim M, Boyko V, et al. Soluble intercellular adhesion molecule-1 and risk of future ischemic stroke: a nested case-control study from the Bezafibrate Infarction Prevention (BIP) Study Cohort. Stroke 2002;33:2182–2186.
283. Hassan A, Hunt BJ, O'Sullivan M, et al. Markers of endothelial dysfunction in lacunar stroke and ischaemic leukoaraiosis. Brain 2003;126:424–432.
284. Blann AD, Ridker PM, Lip GYH. Inflammation, cell adhesion molecules, and stroke: tools in pathophysiology and epidemiology? Stroke 2002;33:2141–2143.
285. Engstrom G, Lind P, Hedblad B, et al. Effects of cholesterol and inflammation-sensitive plasma proteins on incidence of myocardial infarction and stroke in men. Circulation 2002;105: 2632–2637.
286. Muir KW. Inflammation, blood pressure, and stroke: an opportunity to target primary prevention? Stroke 2002;33:2732–2733.
287. Engstrom G, Lind P, Hedblad B, et al. Long-term effects of inflammation-sensitive plasma proteins and systolic blood pressure on incidence of stroke. Stroke 2002;33:2744–2749.

288. van der Meer IM, de Maat MPM, Hak AE, et al. C-reactive protein predicts progression of athero-sclerosis measured at various sites in the arterial tree: the Rotterdam Study. Stroke 2002;33: 2750–2755.
289. Elkind MSV, Sciacca R, Boden-Albala B, et al. Leukocyte count is associated with aortic arch plaque thickness. Stroke 2002;33:2587–2592.
290. Magyar MT, Szikszai Z, Balla J, et al. Early-onset carotid atherosclerosis is associated with increased intima-media thickness and elevated serum levels of inflammatory markers. Stroke 2003;34:58–63.
291. Albert MA, Danielson E, Rifai N, et al. Effect of statin therapy on C-reactive protein levels: the Pravastatin Inflammatory/CRP Evaluation (PRINCE): a randomized trial and cohort study. JAMA 2001;286:64–70.
292. Ridker PM, Rifai N, Pfeffer MA, et al. Long-term effects of pravastatin on plasma concentration of C-reactive protein. The Cholesterol and Recurrent Events (CARE) Investigators. Circulation 1999;100:230–235.
293. Ridker PM, Rifai N, Clearfield M, et al. Measurement of C-reactive protein for the targeting of statin therapy in the primary prevention of acute coronary events. N Engl J Med 2001;344: 1959–1965.
294. Nieto FJ. Infections and atherosclerosis: new clues from an old hypothesis? Am J Epidemiol 1998;148:937–948.
295. Bornstein NM, Bova IY, Korczyn AD. Infections as triggering factors for ischemic stroke. Neurology 1997;49(suppl 4):S45–S46.
296. Grau AJ. Infection, inflammation, and cerebrovascular ischemia. Neurology 1997;49(suppl 4): S47–S51.
297. Kalayoglu MV, Libby P, Byrne GI. Chlamydia pneumoniae as an emerging risk factor in cardiovascular disease. JAMA 2002;288:2724–2731.
298. Prager M, Turel Z, Speidel WS, et al. Chlamydia pneumoniae in carotid artery atherosclerosis: a comparison of its presence in atherosclerotic plaque, healthy vessels, and circulating leukocytes from the same individuals. Stroke 2002;33:2756–2761.
299. Espinola-Klein C, Rupprecht H-J, Blankenberg S, et al. Impact of infectious burden on progression of carotid atherosclerosis. Stroke 2002;33:2581–2586.
300. Mayr M, Kiechl S, Mendall MA, et al. Increased risk of atherosclerosis is confined to CagA-positive Helicobacter pylori strains: prospective results from the Bruneck Study. Stroke 2003;34:610–615.
301. Ameriso SF, Fridman EA, Leiguarda RC, et al. Detection of Helicobacter pylori in human athero-sclerotic plaques. Stroke 2001;32:385–391.
302. Markus HS, Mendall MA. Helicobacter pylori infection: a risk factor for ischemic cerebrovascular disease and carotid atheroma. J Neurol Neurosurg Psychiatry 1998;64:104–107.
303. Nieto FJ, Adam E, Sorlie P, et al. Cohort study of cytomegalovirus infection as a risk factor for carotid intimal-medial thickening, a measure of subclinical atherosclerosis. Circulation 1996;94: 922–927.
304. Risley P, Jerrard-Dunne P, Sitzer M, et al. Promoter polymorphism in the endotoxin receptor (CD14) is associated with increased carotid atherosclerosis only in smokers: the Carotid Athero-sclerosis Progression Study. Stroke 2003;34:600–604.
305. Macko RF, Ameriso SF, Barndt R, et al. Precipitants of brain infarction: roles of preceding infection/inflammation and recent psychological stress. Stroke 1996;27:1999–2004.
306. Macko RF, Ameriso SF, Gruber A, et al. Impairments of the protein C system and fibrinolysis in infection-associated stroke. Stroke 1996;27:2005–2011.
307. Grau AJ, Buggle F, Heindl S, et al. Recent infection as a risk factor for cerebrovascular ischemia. Stroke 1995;26:373–379.
308. Grau AJ, Buggle F, Becher H, et al. Recent bacterial and viral infection is a risk factor for cerebrovascular ischemia: clinical and biochemical studies. Neurology 1998;50:196–203.
309. Wu T, Trevisan M, Genco RJ, et al. Periodontal disease and risk of cerebrovascular disease: the First National Health and Nutrition Examination Survey and Its Follow-up Study. Arch Intern Med 2000;160:2749–2755.
310. Joshipura KJ, Hung H-C, Rimm EB, et al. Periodontal disease, tooth loss, and incidence of ischemic stroke. Stroke 2003;34:47–52.
311. Sloan MA, Kittner SK, Price TR. Illicit Drug Use/Abuse and Stroke. In MD Ginsburg, J Bogousslavsky (eds), Cerebrovascular Disease: Pathophysiology, Diagnosis, and Management. Malden, Massachusettes:Blackwell Science, 1998;1589–1609.
312. Kaku DA, Lowenstein DH. Emergence of recreational drug abuse as a major risk factor for stroke in young adults. Ann Intern Med 1990;113:821–827.

313. Sloan MA, Kittner SJ, Rigamonti D, et al. Occurrence of stroke associated with use/abuse of drugs. Neurology 1991;41:1358–1364.
314. Mitsias P, Lee N, Ramadan NM, et al. Ischemic cerebrovascular disease in the young. Stroke 1992;23:143.
315. Peterson PL, Roszler M, Jacobs I, et al. Neurovascular complications of cocaine abuse. J Neuropsychiatry Clin Neurosci 1991;3:143–149.
316. Adams HP, Kapelle LJ, Biller J, et al. Ischemic stroke in young adults. Arch Neurol 1995;52:491–495.
317. Kittner SJ, Stern BJ, Wozniak MA, et al. Cerebral infarction in young adults: the Baltimore-Washington Cooperative Young Stroke Registry. Neurology 1998;50:890–894.
318. Sloan MA, Kittner SJ, Feeser BR, et al. Illicit drug-associated ischemic stroke in the Baltimore-Washington Young Stroke Study. Neurology 1998;50:1688–1693.
319. Qureshi AI, Safdar K, Patel M, et al. Stroke in young black patients: risk factors, subtypes, and prognosis. Stroke 1995;26:1995–1998.
320. Sloan MA, Kittner SJ, Feeser B, et al. Mechanisms of drug-associated intracerebral hemorrhage in the Baltimore-Washington Cooperative Young Stroke Study. Circulation 1996;94(suppl 1):I–390.
321. Simpson RK, Contant CF, Fischer DK, et al. Epidemiological characteristics of subarachnoid hemorrhage in an urban population. J Clin Epidemiol 1991;44:641–648.
322. Qureshi AI, Akbar MS, Czander E, et al. Crack cocaine use and stroke in young patients. Neurology 1997;48:341–345.
323. Sloan MA, Duh S-H, Magder LS, et al. Association between cocaine use and stroke: results of a case-control study. Neurology 1998;50(suppl):A247.
324. Magder LS, Sloan MA, Duh S-H, et al. Utilization of multiple imperfect assessments of the dependent variable in a logistic regression analysis. Statist Med 2000;19:99–111.
325. Sloan MA, Duh S-H, Magder LS, et al. Marijuana and the risk of stroke. Stroke 1999;30:255.
326. Sloan MA, Kittner SJ, Magder L, et al. Is cocaine a risk factor for ischemic stroke in young women? The Stroke Prevention in Young Women Study. Neuroepidemiology 1997;16:13–14.
327. Pettiti DB, Sidney S, Quesenberry C, et al. Stroke and cocaine or amphetamine use. Epidemiology 1998;9:596–600.
328. The Hemorrhagic Stroke Project Investigators. Major risk factors for aneurysmal SAH in the young are modifiable. Stroke 2003;34:243.
329. Wolf PA, D'Agostino RB, Belanger AJ, et al. Probability of stroke: a risk profile from the Framingham Study. Stroke 1991;22:312–318.

3
Etiologies and Mechanisms of Ischemia

Enrique C. Leira and Harold P. Adams Jr.

The causes of ischemic stroke are numerous.[1] The heterogeneous nature of stroke is reflected by the diversity of affected patients. Although the common final result is cerebral ischemia, this can result from a variety of different pathogenic mechanisms. The pathogenic mechanisms that can lead to cerebral ischemia are outlined in Table 3.1. When categorizing ischemic stroke, one can differentiate events that result from atherosclerotic or nonatherosclerotic arterial lesions, cardiac embolization, prothrombotic hematological disorders, or systemic hypoperfusion.

ARTERIAL STROKES

Arterial lesions can cause stroke through two basic mechanisms: hypoperfusion and artery-to-artery embolism. Hypoperfusion typically results from a stenotic area that compromises the distal blood flow. This area of lumen reduction can result from a lesion of the arterial wall (e.g. atherosclerotic plaque), dissection, compression of the vessel or arterial vasospasm. In addition, arterial lesions can also cause stroke through migration of either thrombus or fragments of an intrinsic arterial lesion (e.g., atherosclerotic plaque), a mechanism leading to artery-to-artery embolism. Both pathogenic mechanisms can coexist and clinical features can suggest either mechanism. Clinical and imaging findings of a branch cortical infarction usually point to artery-to-artery embolization. In general, embolic infarctions usually have a more abrupt onset than those caused by hypoperfusion. On the other hand, clinical and imaging evidence of a stroke in a watershed pattern usually suggests hypoperfusion as the likely stroke mechanism. However, it is very difficult to determine clinically whether a particular stroke was caused by hypoperfusion, artery-to-artery embolization, or both. In fact, borderline perfusion with impaired collateral flow may allow symptoms to occur with embolization, when the patient might have remained asymptomatic if normal flow had been present.

Table 3.1 Overview of mechanisms of ischemic stroke

Arterial disorders
  Large artery atherosclerosis
  Small vessel disease
  Nonatherosclerotic
    Noninflammatory
    Inflammatory (infectious and noninfectious)
Cardioembolism
  High-risk lesions
  Medium-risk lesions
Hematological disorders
  Hypercoagulable states
    Acquired (e.g., paraneoplastic)
    Primary (e.g., lupus anticoagulant)
  Hyperviscosity syndromes (e.g., polycythemia)
  Severe anemia
Systemic hypoperfusion (low-flow infarctions)

Table 3.2 summarizes the most common arteriopathies causing stroke. By far the most common is atherosclerosis. Atherosclerosis can affect large caliber arteries, either extracranially or intracranially. Atherosclerosis can also affect the small penetrating terminal branches of the cerebral arteries.

Strokes attributed to the large-artery atherosclerotic lesions (LAA) are also known as atherothromboembolic and account for approximately 25 percent of the strokes. The location of the arterial lesion might be influenced by ethnicity. Whites tend to have more extracranial disease, whereas persons of African or Asian descent may have more atherosclerotic lesions of the intracranial vessels.[2] Atherothromboembolic strokes have distinct clinical features. The medical history usually elicits the risk factors for atherosclerosis, such as hypertension, hyperlipidemia, diabetes, or smoking. These types of strokes may be preceded by transient cerebral or retinal ischemic events in the same

Table 3.2 Arterial disorders causing stroke

Atherosclerosis
  Large arteries (atherothrombotic)
  Small vessel (lipohyalinosis)
Nonatherosclerotic, noninflammatory
  Arterial dissection
  Fibromuscular dysplasia
  Moya-Moya
  Other (e.g., Ehlers-Danlos, Marfan syndrome, postradiation, CADASIL, homocystinuria, NF type I)
Nonatherosclerotic, inflammatory
  Infectious (e.g., syphilis, HIV, Lyme, herpes zoster, HSV, tuberculosis, cysticercosis)
  Noninfectious (e.g., isolated CNS, Takayasu, GCA, cocaine)

CADASIL = cerebral autosomal dominant arteriopathy with subcortical infarcts and leukoencephalopathy; CNS = central nervous system; GCA = giant cell arteritis; HIV = human immunodeficiency virus; HSV = herpes simplex virus; NF = neurofibromatosis.

vascular distribution. Those transient attacks are the result of either hypoperfusion or embolism from the more proximal arterial lesion. These strokes might be precipitated by conditions that result in a reduction in blood flow, such as when there is a reduction of the systemic blood pressure. The diagnosis of LAA is made by correlating compatible clinical findings with diagnostic ancillary tests. Other causes, such as a cardioembolic source, need to be excluded. Among those diagnostic ancillary tests that can demonstrate this type of arteriopathy are carotid ultrasound, magnetic resonance angiography, and conventional angiography. Transcranial Doppler might be also used to indirectly detect a stenotic lesion of a major intracranial artery. The results of these diagnostic tests are not specific for atherosclerosis but corroborate that an obstructive lesion exists.

Lacunes ("small lakes") may be caused by disease of small penetrating terminal arteries. Lacunar lesions account for approximately 25 percent of strokes. Hypertension and diabetes are well-recognized risk factors for this form of arteriopathy. The underlying pathological mechanism can be either microatheromas, microembolism, or lipohyalinosis (concentric hyaline microarterial wall thickening) in small arteries of 40 to 200 μ diameter.[3] These branches, which lack collateral circulation,[4] perfuse such subcortical structures as the internal capsule, thalamus, basal ganglia, and pons. Lacunes typically are 3 to 7 mm in diameter and often present as distinct clinical syndromes. The most common is pure motor hemiparesis. These syndromes reflect the unique lesion localization and usually consist of focal neurological symptoms that spare consciousness and cortical functions.[4]

Lacunar or small vessel strokes are typically diagnosed by correlating a suggestive clinical syndrome with ancillary studies, especially brain imaging. The development of diffusion-weighted magnetic resonance imaging allows the visualization of acute lacunar infarction, which is often missed by conventional computerized tomography. The diagnosis is supported when ancillary tests exclude an alternative cause for the infarction[5] such as a large-artery lesion or cardiac source of embolism.

Other less common forms of arteriopathies can cause stroke including noninflammatory vasculopathies (e.g., dissections), infectious vasculitis (e.g., syphilis), and noninfectious vasculitis (e.g., giant cell arteritis). Dissections result from extravasations of blood into the arterial wall. The resultant hematoma can compromise the lumen or produce an aneurysmal dilatation. Dissections can cause stroke by either a hemodynamic mechanism or artery-artery embolism from thrombotic fragments.[6] Dissection can occur in the extracranial portions of the internal carotid, typically above the level of the carotid bifurcation; in the vertebral arteries; and in the intracranial circulation. Dissections can occur after trauma[7] that may be trivial. They can also be spontaneous,[8] particularly in persons with underlying connective tissue abnormalities.[9] Dissection is an important cause of stroke in young adults. It should be considered when a stroke occurs in a patient who does not have overt risk factors for an ischemic event. Besides typical stroke symptoms, dissections may be characterized by ipsilateral neck or head pain. Carotid and vertebral artery dissections may also cause an ipsilateral Horner syndrome. A history of trauma to the head or neck may be elicited.

Other noninflammatory vasculopathies causing stroke are Moya-Moya, fibromuscular dysplasia, connective tissue abnormalities (e.g., Ehlers-Danlos or

Marfan syndrome), cerebral autosomal dominant arteriopathy with subcortical infarcts and leukoencephalopathy (CADASIL),[10] homocystinuria, or neurofibromatosis type I.

The inflammatory vasculitides are another group of uncommon arteriopathies that may cause stroke.[11] Different types of vasculitis preferentially affect different caliber vessels, including large arteries (e.g., Takayasu disease), medium-size vessels (e.g., giant cell arteritis), or small muscular arteries (e.g., isolated angiitis of the nervous system). Central nervous system (CNS) vasculitis can occur either as an isolated disease (e.g., isolated angiitis of the nervous system) or as a manifestation of a multisystemic vasculitis.[12] Circulating immune complexes accumulate in the arterial wall and trigger an inflammatory cellular response. The cellular infiltration, proliferation, and necrosis can lead to a stenosis or occlusion of the artery. It may also precipitate thrombus that can embolize distally. The inflammatory response affecting the arterial wall may promote secondary dissection. Inflammatory vasculitis may also occur in association with infection. Among those infectious causes are syphilis, HIV, Lyme, herpes zoster, herpes simplex, tuberculosis, and cysticercosis.

Patients with stroke caused by vasculitis often present with headaches resulting from meningeal artery involvement. Because vasculitis is often a multifocal process, an encephalopathy may occur in conjunction with recent multiple subacute strokes. The presence of constitutional symptoms, an elevated sedimentation rate, or C-reactive protein favor this diagnosis. However, these abnormalities may not be present in patients with isolated CNS angiitis. The cerebrospinal fluid may show an inflammatory reaction (leucocytosis and elevated protein) in patients with intracranial vasculitis. The diagnosis is further supported by neuroimaging studies showing multiple acute and subacute ischemic lesions, as well as diffuse angiographic abnormalities. The diagnosis can be confirmed by meningeal biopsy. The diagnostic yield from conventional arteriography and meningeal biopsy might be limited.[13]

CARDIOEMBOLIC STROKES

Cardiac emboli occlude cerebral vessels either transiently or permanently. A common fate of embolus is to recanalize or to fragment and migrate to distal branches.[14] This explains why embolic stroke deficits may improve or fluctuate. Stroke may result from several cardiac problems[15] including disturbances in the cardiac rhythm, valvular disease, cardiac wall motion abnormalities, cardiac tumors, endocarditis, and right-to-left shunt facilitating paradoxical embolization. Cardiac abnormalities causing stroke have been classified as "high-risk" and "medium-risk" depending on the perceived risk for embolism[16] (Tables 3.3 and 3.4). Although there is general agreement about the embolic potential of high-risk lesions, the propensity for embolization with medium-risk lesions is more controversial.[17–19]

The most common source of cardiac embolism is atrial fibrillation, which accounts for approximately one half of the cardioembolic strokes.[15] Atrial fibrillation is associated with stagnation of blood in the left atrium, which in turns predisposes to thrombus formation, especially in the left atrial appendage.[20] In general, the risk of stroke is highest if atrial fibrillation

Table 3.3   High-risk cardiac sources of embolization

Mechanical prosthetic valve
Rheumatic mitral stenosis
Atrial fibrillation
Left atrial/atrial appendage thrombus
Sick sinus syndrome
Recent myocardial infarction (<4 wk)
Left ventricular thrombus
Dilated cardiomyopathy
Akinetic left ventricular segment
Atrial myxoma
Infective endocarditis

Reprinted with permission from Adams HP Jr, Bendixen BH, Kappelle LJ, et al. Classification of subtype of acute ischemic stroke. Definitions for use in a multicenter clinical trial. TOAST. Trial of Org 10172 in Acute Stroke Treatment. Stroke 1993;24:35–41.

accompanies a structural cardiac lesion (e.g., rheumatic mitral stenosis). Thrombus can also form after a myocardial infarction,[21] particularly within 4 weeks of the event and with infarctions located in the anterior wall of the heart.[20] Similarly, dilated cardiomyopathy has an estimated embolization risk of 2 to 4 percent per year, which may be higher in those with a left ventricular thrombus or coexistent atrial fibrillation.[20] Cardiac tumors, such as myxomas or papillary fibroelastoma, can result in stroke by either tumor fragmentation or superimposed thrombus formation.[20] Infective endocarditis is another high-risk lesion for stroke. Vegetations measuring more than 10 mm and those that are mobile pose the highest risk for embolism.[22] Other high-risk cardiac lesions include rheumatic mitral stenosis and mechanical valves, especially mitral

Table 3.4   Medium-risk cardiac sources of embolism

Mitral valve prolapse
Mitral annulus calcification
Mitral stenosis without atrial fibrillation
Left atrial turbulence (smoke)
Atrial septal aneurysm
Patent foramen ovale
Atrial flutter
Lone atrial fibrillation
Bioprosthetic cardiac valve
Nonbacterial thrombotic endocarditis
Congestive heart failure (EF > 28%)
Hypokinetic left ventricular segment
Myocardial infarction (>4 wk, <6 mo)

Reprinted with permission from Adams HP Jr, Bendixen BH, Kappelle LJ, et al. Classification of subtype of acute ischemic stroke. Definitions for use in a multicenter clinical trial. TOAST. Trial of Org 10172 in Acute Stroke Treatment. Stroke 1993;24:35–41.

EF = ejection fraction.

prostheses. Right-to-left cardiac shunts can cause strokes by allowing thrombus in the venous circulation to directly enter the arterial system bypassing the lung, particularly if a Valsalva maneuver transiently increases the pressure gradient between the right and left cardiac chambers.

HEMATOLOGICAL STROKES

Hematological disorders are a relatively uncommon cause of stroke in the general population, although they are more relevant in younger patients.[23] Several different prothrombotic hematological abnormalities that lead to arterial or venous thrombosis and can result in stroke are outlined in Table 3.5. For example, increased cellularity (e.g., leukemia) can lead to hyperviscosity syndromes. Disorders of the red blood cells (e.g., sickle cell disease) can lead to ischemic stroke by interfering with neuronal oxygenation. Deficiencies in the factors that inhibit thrombosis (e.g., protein C deficiency) or that promote fibrinolysis (e.g., plasminogen activator deficiency) can lead to thrombotic cerebral events. A hematological disorder should be suspected in patients with a personal or familiy history of recurrent arterial or venous thrombosis. It should also be suspected in stroke patients of young age or with an unclear cause for the stroke.

SYSTEMIC HYPOPERFUSION (LOW-FLOW INFARCTIONS)

Ischemic stroke can also result from systemic hypoperfusion, which can be the consequence of pump failure (e.g., cardiac arrest or cardiac arrhythmia), hypovolemia (e.g., severe dehydration), or vasodilatation (e.g., sepsis). Individual asymmetries in the collateral arterial supply or underlying focal cerebral stenosis have to be invoked to explain focal cerebral infarctions from systemic hypoperfusion.[24]

Table 3.5   Hematological abnormalities causing stroke

Cellular
   Platelet disorders (e.g., thrombocytosis)
   Red blood cell disorders (e.g., polycythemia vera)
   White blood cell disorders (e.g., leukemia)
Hyperviscosity
   Plasma cell disorders (e.g., myeloma)
   Hemoglobin disorders (e.g., sickle cell)
   Waldenstrom macroglobulinemia
   Cryoglobulinemia
Procoagulant states
   Inherited (e.g., antithrombin III deficiency, plasminogen deficiency, antiphospholipid antibody syndrome)
   Acquired (e.g., alcohol intoxication, snake bite, cancer, birth control medication, postpartum)

IMPORTANCE OF DETERMINING SUBTYPE IN ISCHEMIC STROKE

Table 3.6 summarizes the reasons for establishing the most likely cause of ischemic stroke. The most important reason is because the diagnosis influences management decisions to prevent recurrent strokes. The recommended secondary prevention strategy varies with the subtype of stroke. For example, a large-artery atherosclerotic stroke in the extracranial internal carotid might be best treated with endarterectomy and antiplatelet drugs, whereas a cardioembolic infarction is best treated with anticoagulants. Therefore, the accuracy of the stroke subtype determination will have an impact on choosing the appropriate measures for secondary prevention. Because the care of stroke patients usually involves different teams of physicians in sequential order (e.g., acute stroke team, rehabilitation team, outpatient primary care physician, etc.) it is important not only to accurately determine the subtype but also to convey that information adequately to colleagues. Merely reporting the results of the ancillary tests does not substitute for a clear subtype diagnosis. Those test results can be conflicting and adequate clinical integration is always needed. When a patient is described in a medical record as having had a "left middle cerebral infarction," that statement suggests uncertainty about the etiological diagnosis and workup. On the other hand, the same patient described as having had an "atherothrombotic left middle cerebral artery infarction" conveys the impression that such a patient has been carefully studied and that appropriate secondary prevention strategies can be pursued.

In the future, diagnosis of stroke subtype may be important to select patients for acute therapies. At present the only acute therapy approved in ischemic stroke is intravenous recombinant tissue plasminogen activator (rt-PA) for selected stroke patients within 3 hours of ischemic stroke onset. The results of the two large studies that were used to seek approval of such treatment suggest that rt-PA benefits all stroke subtypes, despite prior physiopathological concerns that such therapy may not improve lacunar infarctions.[25] Although presently the determination of stroke subtype may not influence acute therapy, this may change in the near future. In a Trial of ORG 10172 in Acute Stroke Treatment (TOAST) secondary analysis, patients with stroke secondary to LAA appeared to benefit from treatment with intravenous danaparoid.[26] Another study demonstrated a benefit of intra-arterial pro-urokinase with angiographically documented occlusion of the middle cerebral artery. If such treatment becomes accepted, imaging of the arterial tree may be mandatory to make a subtype diagnosis before considering such therapy.

Subtype diagnosis is also useful for determining the short-term prognosis, because there are differences in regard to the stroke subtype.[27] For example, large-artery atherothrombotic infarctions may have the highest risk for early

Table 3.6   Reasons for determining the subtype of ischemic stroke

---

Establish appropriate secondary prevention measures
Determine eligibility for acute therapies
Estimate risk of early recurrence
Facilitate research

---

recurrence,[28] whereas cardioembolic infarctions have the highest mortality rate.[29] On the other hand, lacunar infarctions have a more benign prognosis.[30]

Finally, ischemic stroke subtype determination is of vital importance for future stroke research. Clinical trialists are aware that ischemic stroke is a heterogeneous disease and that future therapies may only benefit certain stroke subtypes. An adequate determination of stroke subtype should, therefore, favor progress in the field of therapy for acute stroke.

STANDARDIZATION OF STROKE SUBTYPE DETERMINATION

Physicians often disagree on the subtype diagnosis of ischemic stroke.[31] This is an obvious impediment to the advancement of research in stroke because disagreements can lead to misclassification of patients and subsequent errors in the interpretation of results. For this reason several standard classifications of stroke subtypes have been developed.[16,32,33] One of the most accepted is the classification designed for TOAST.[16] Although this classification scheme was initially designed for research, the TOAST classification has gained acceptance in clinical practice. It is reliable with good interphysician agreement.[31] The TOAST classification identifies 11 categories of ischemic stroke (Table 3.7). These categories include the combination of the three major stroke subtypes (atherothrombotic, cardioembolic, and lacunar). Epidemiological studies have shown that at least 70 percent of the strokes in the general population fall in one of these three categories.[34] The classification includes in the group "other," the

Table 3.7   Stroke subtypes in the TOAST classification

Atherothrombotic
  Probable (clinical data and studies consistent with LAA, others excluded)
  Possible (clinical data and studies consistent with LAA, but others not excluded)
Cardioembolic
  Probable (clinical data and studies consistent with cardioembolism, others excluded)
  Possible (clinical data and studies consistent with cardioembolism, but others not
    excluded; or medium-risk cardiac lesion but no other cause found)
Lacunar
  Probable (clinical data and studies consistent with lacunar, others excluded)
  Possible (clinical data and studies consistent with lacunar, but others not excluded)
Other determined etiology
  Probable (clinical data and studies consistent with subtype, others excluded)
  Possible (clinical data and studies consistent with subtype, but others not excluded)
Undetermined etiology
  Complete evaluation
  Incomplete evaluation
Multiple possible etiologies

Reprinted with permission from Adams HP Jr, Bendixen BH, Kappelle LJ, et al. Classification of subtype of acute ischemic stroke. Definitions for use in a multicenter clinical trial. TOAST. Trial of Org 10172 in Acute Stroke Treatment. Stroke 1993;24:35–41.
LAA = large artery atherosclerotic lesions; TOAST = Trial of Org 10172 in Acute Stroke Treatment.

remaining different diagnostic alternatives. All four options can b with the modifiers "possible" and "probable," depending on whethe evaluation for an alternative diagnosis was carried out. The TOAS' tion also includes the category "undetermined" with the modifiers "complete" or "incomplete" for those cases in which a definite diagnosis is not possible. Finally the category "multiple possible etiologies" was created for those cases in which the physician is unable to determine which mechanism caused the stroke. Other classifications of subtypes used, such as the Oxfordshire Community Stroke Project that distinguishes four major types (total and partial anterior circulation infarction, lacunar infarction, and posterior circulation infarction), also have good interobserver reliability.[33]

DETERMINING SUBTYPE OF ISCHEMIC STROKE

The determination of a stroke subtype is based on a combination of the clinical history, physical findings, neuroimaging studies, and results of ancillary testing. The clinical presentation and the patient's general health including risk factors usually suggest an initial working diagnosis of the subtype.[35,36] Unfortunately this initial impression is often wrong, even among physicians with expertise in stroke.[37,38] A more accurate stroke subtype diagnosis is determined after reviewing the imaging studies and ancillary studies. The tests more commonly used to determine stroke subtype are listed in Table 3.8. A judicious approach to test ordering is recommended rather than a shotgun approach. Figure 3.1 illustrates a diagnostic algorithm based on the TOAST classification to reach the four major subtype diagnoses. This algorithm does not include the category "undetermined" in which the subtype cannot be diagnosed despite a complete

Table 3.8   Tests used to determine stroke subtype

Brain imaging
  Magnetic resonance imaging brain
  Computerized tomography scan brain
Vascular imaging
  Carotid ultrasound
  Magnetic resonance angiography
  Computerized tomographic angiography
  Conventional Angiography
  Transcranial Doppler
Cardiac studies
  ECG
  Holter monitoring
  Transthoracic echocardiography
  Transesophageal echocardiography
Hematological studies (PT, PTT, lupus anticoagulant)
Serological studies (RPR)
Meningeal and temporal artery biopsy

ECG = electrocardiogram; PT = prothrombin time; PTT = partial thromboplastin time; RPR = rapid plasma reagin.

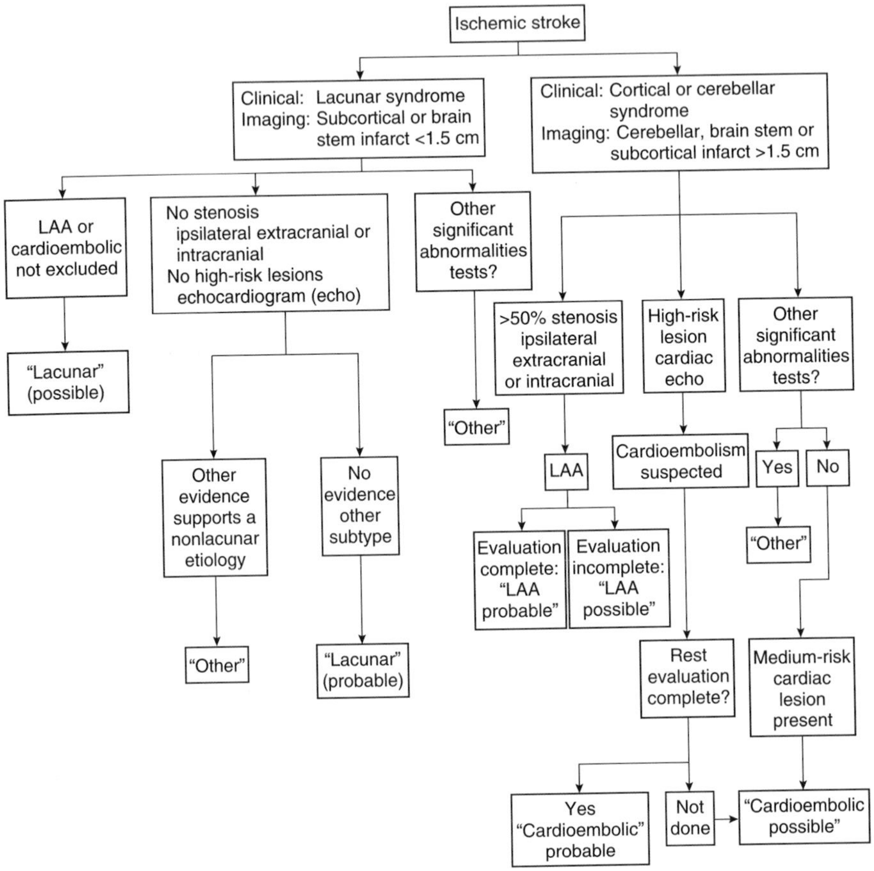

Figure 3.1   Algorithm to diagnose ischemic stroke subtype based on the Trial of ORG 10172 in Acute Stroke Treatment (TOAST) classification.
(Reprinted with permission from Adams HP Jr, Bendixen BH, Kappelle LJ, et al. Classification of subtype of acute ischemic stroke. Definitions for use in a multicenter clinical trial. TOAST. Trial of Org 10172 in Acute Stroke Treatment. Stroke 1993;24:35–41.)

or incomplete evaluation. It also does not include the category "multiple possible etiologies" in which the diagnosis cannot be made due to the coexistence of several mechanisms.

PITFALLS IN THE DIAGNOSIS OF STROKE SUBTYPE

The diagnosis of the stroke subtype is made by association of clinical findings with ancillary studies and, therefore, is always based on circumstantial evidence. This limitation is inherent to the subtype determination strategy and is evidenced by the frequent disagreement among physicians about subtype determinations.[31] It can be explained by the wide practice variations in the tests ordered for a workup, as well as in disagreement of what constitutes a medium- or high-risk cardiac lesion. This problem has improved but has not been eliminated by the standardized stroke subtype determination systems.

FUTURE TRENDS IN STROKE SUBTYPE DIAGNOSIS

We anticipate that stroke subtypes will have more influence on acute therapeutic decisions. Although the current TOAST subtype strategy could be used in the acute setting, this is logistically difficult due to the lack of availability of carotid ultrasound and echocardiography in that setting. Magnetic resonance imaging and magnetic resonance angiography performed acutely increase the accuracy of the initial stroke subtype clinical diagnosis.[39] It is likely that these techniques will play an important role in stroke subtype determination in the near future.

References

1. Mohr JP. Classification and mechanisms of cerebrovascular disease. Ann Epidemiol 1993;3:454–457.
2. Sacco RL, Kargman DE, Gu Q, Zamanillo MC. Race-ethnicity and determinants of intracranial atherosclerotic cerebral infarction. The Northern Manhattan Stroke Study. Stroke 1995;26:14–20.
3. Lammie GA. Pathology of small vessel stroke. Br Med Bull 2000;56:296–306.
4. Kappelle LJ, van Gijn J. Lacunar infarcts. Clin Neurol Neurosurg 1986;88:3–17.
5. Gan R, Sacco RL, Kargman DE, et al. Testing the validity of the lacunar hypothesis: the Northern Manhattan Stroke Study experience. Neurology 1997;48:1204–1211.
6. Bogousslavsky J, Despland PA, Regli F. Spontaneous carotid dissection with acute stroke. Arch Neurol 1987;44:137–140.
7. Emmerich J, Fiessinger JN. Stroke from traumatic arterial dissection. Lancet 1999;354:160.
8. Mokri B, Schievink WI, Olsen KD, Piepgras DG. Spontaneous dissection of the cervical internal carotid artery. Presentation with lower cranial nerve palsies. Arch Otolaryngol Head Neck Surg 1992;118:431–435.
9. Schievink WI, Mokri B. Familial aorto-cervicocephalic arterial dissections and congenitally bicuspid aortic valve. Stroke 1995;26:1935–1940.
10. Joutel A, Tournier-Lasserve E. [Molecular basis and physiopathogenic mechanisms of CADASIL: a model of small vessel diseases of the brain]. J Soc Biol 2002;196:109–115.
11. Ferro JM. Vasculitis of the central nervous system. J Neurol 1998;245:766–776.
12. Hinchey JA, Sila CA. Cerebrovascular complications of rheumatic disease. Rheum Dis Clin North Am 1997;23:293–316.
13. Kendall B. Cerebral angiography in vasculitis affecting the nervous system. Eur Neurol 1984;23:400–406.
14. Helgason CM. Cardioembolic stroke: topography and pathogenesis. Cerebrovasc Brain Metab Rev 1992;4:28–58.
15. Cardiogenic brain embolism. Cerebral Embolism Task Force. Arch Neurol 1986;43:71–84.
16. Adams HP Jr, Bendixen BH, Kappelle LJ, et al. Classification of subtype of acute ischemic stroke. Definitions for use in a multicenter clinical trial. TOAST. Trial of Org 10172 in Acute Stroke Treatment. Stroke 1993;24:35–41.
17. Di Pasquale G, Labanti G, Urbinati S, et al. The role of echocardiography in the evaluation of patients with ischemic stroke. Acta Neurol Belg 1996;96:322–328.
18. Manning WJ. Role of transesophageal echocardiography in the management of thromboembolic stroke. Am J Cardiol 1997;80(4C):19D–28D.
19. Beattie JR, Cohen DJ, Manning WJ, Douglas PS. Role of routine transthoracic echocardiography in evaluation and management of stroke. J Intern Med 1998;243:281–291.
20. Di Tullio MR, Homma S. Mechanisms of cardioembolic stroke. Curr Cardiol Rep 2002; 4(2):141–148.

21. Martin R, Bogousslavsky J. Mechanism of late stroke after myocardial infarct: the Lausanne Stroke Registry. J Neurol Neurosurg Psychiatry 1993;56:760–764.
22. Di Salvo G, Habib G, Pergola V, et al. Echocardiography predicts embolic events in infective endocarditis. J Am Coll Cardiol 2001;37:1069–1076.
23. Hart RG, Kanter MC. Hematologic disorders and ischemic stroke. A selective review. Stroke 1990;21:1111–1121.
24. Weiller C, Ringelstein EB, Reiche W, Buell U. Clinical and hemodynamic aspects of low-flow infarcts. Stroke 1991;22:1117–1123.
25. Tissue plasminogen activator for acute ischemic stroke. The National Institute of Neurological Disorders and Stroke rt-PA Stroke Study Group. N Engl J Med 1995;333:1581–1587.
26. Adams HP Jr, Bendixen BH, Leira E, et al. Antithrombotic treatment of ischemic stroke among patients with occlusion or severe stenosis of the internal carotid artery: a report of the Trial of Org 10172 in Acute Stroke Treatment (TOAST). Neurology 1999;53:122–125.
27. Grau AJ, Weimar C, Buggle F, et al. Risk factors, outcome, and treatment in subtypes of ischemic stroke: the German stroke data bank. Stroke 2001;32:2559–2566.
28. Moroney JT, Bagiella E, Paik MC, et al. Risk factors for early recurrence after ischemic stroke: the role of stroke syndrome and subtype. Stroke 1998;29:2118–2124.
29. Petty GW, Brown RD Jr, Whisnant JP, et al. Ischemic stroke subtypes: a population-based study of functional outcome, survival, and recurrence. Stroke 2000;31:1062–1068.
30. Landi G, Cella E, Boccardi E, Musicco M. Lacunar versus non-lacunar infarcts: pathogenetic and prognostic differences. J Neurol Neurosurg Psychiatry 1992;55:441–445.
31. Gordon DL, Bendixen BH, Adams HP Jr, et al. Interphysician agreement in the diagnosis of subtypes of acute ischemic stroke: implications for clinical trials. The TOAST Investigators. Neurology 1993;43:1021–1027.
32. Bamford J, Sandercock P, Dennis M, et al. Classification and natural history of clinically identifiable subtypes of cerebral infarction. Lancet 1991;337:1521–1526.
33. Lindley RI, Warlow CP, Wardlaw JM, et al. Interobserver reliability of a clinical classification of acute cerebral infarction. Stroke 1993;24:1801–1804.
34. Kolominsky-Rabas PL, Weber M, Gefeller O, et al. Epidemiology of ischemic stroke subtypes according to TOAST criteria: incidence, recurrence, and long-term survival in ischemic stroke subtypes: a population-based study. Stroke 2001;32:2735–2740.
35. Timsit SG, Sacco RL, Mohr JP, et al. Early clinical differentiation of cerebral infarction from severe atherosclerotic stenosis and cardioembolism. Stroke 1992;23:486–491.
36. Arboix A, Oliveres M, Massons J, et al. Early differentiation of cardioembolic from atherothrombotic cerebral infarction: a multivariate analysis. Eur J Neurol 1999;6:677–683.
37. Madden KP, Karanjia PN, Adams HP Jr, Clarke WR. Accuracy of initial stroke subtype diagnosis in the TOAST study. Trial of ORG 10172 in Acute Stroke Treatment. Neurology 1995;45:1975–1979.
38. Pullicino PM. Pathogenesis of lacunar infarcts and small deep infarcts. Adv Neurol 1993;62:125–140.
39. Lee LJ, Kidwell CS, Alger J, et al. Impact on stroke subtype diagnosis of early diffusion-weighted magnetic resonance imaging and magnetic resonance angiography. Stroke 2000;31:1081–1089.

4

Diagnostic Evaluation of Transient Ischemic Attack and Ischemic Stroke

Andrei V. Alexandrov and John Y. Choi

Transient ischemic attack (TIA) is a medical emergency because there are well-documented measures to prevent stroke when they are implemented in a timely manner. The complete resolution of focal cerebral ischemic symptoms within 24 hours has been used to separate strokes from TIAs. However, most TIAs resolve within minutes, and advanced neuroimaging studies demonstrate that longer lasting symptoms are likely to be strokes. Therefore clinical history aided by diagnostic tests remain important for diagnosis. Knowledge of the central nervous system anatomy is essential to determine whether the symptom is referable to the anterior circulation, potentially a marker for carotid disease, or the posterior circulation (vertebrobasilar system).

TIAs have a more serious prognostic implication then previously appreciated. After a TIA occurs, about 10 percent of these patients will have a stroke in the next 3 months, and almost one half of these strokes will develop within the first 2 days of the initial symptoms.[1] Because TIAs are a highly predictive risk factor for permanent neurological deficit and disability, patients with TIA must be evaluated in a timely and comprehensive manner when the diagnosis is suspected. In the United States, health care providers and systems may not always practice these measures.[2–5]

In addition, appropriate clinical decisions during a possible TIA in the setting of effective ischemic stroke therapy with intravenous (IV) recombinant tissue plasminogen activator (rt-PA) are necessary. In a patient with ischemic neurological deficits within a 3-hour onset, appropriate action is to expedite workup for thrombolytic therapy. No readily available test currently exists that will immediately confirm infarction versus TIA in the acute period. The most likely diagnostic test candidate will be magnetic resonance imaging (MRI) technology. One must recognize that outcomes are better the earlier that thrombolytic therapy is instituted.[6] The maxim is, "Strive for early action in conjunction with early identification of stroke victims." More severe ischemic stroke deficits are aggressively treated to avoid future disability. Milder ischemic stroke deficits may have measurable and persistent impact on quality of life[7] and also warrant consideration for thrombolytic treatment, because the National Institutes of Neurological Disorders and Stroke (NINDS) rt-PA Stroke Trial did not exclude patients with mild stroke. Symptoms persisting for more than 1 hour are suggestive of stroke. Only 2.6 percent of patients in the placebo group of the NINDS rt-PA Stroke study recovered completely within 24 hours.[8] On the other hand, stroke symptoms lasting for more than 3 hours may not necessarily point to a completed stroke because at least 15 percent of these patients experience progression or fluctuation of the neurological deficit.[9] In some situations, this may represent a hemodynamically significant major artery stenosis, blood flow fluctuation at the small vessel level, or thrombus propagation or lysis.

Although a sense of less urgency occurs with patients presenting beyond the first 3 hours of stroke symptom onset, the threat of a stroke or progression of symptoms within hours after hospital admission necessitates that key elements of the diagnostic workup such as neuroimaging to rule out hemorrhage be completed as soon as possible. The remainder of the diagnostic evaluation can be completed within the next 24 to 48 hours. This chapter discusses a general diagnostic algorithm for TIA and ischemic stroke patients and provides illustrations of how this process can be tailored in select cases to provide timely information for therapeutic decision making.

DIAGNOSTIC ALGORITHM

The major consideration is whether a TIA or stroke has occurred. The preventive measures are similar although attention to addressing rehabilitation needs and treatment of poststroke depression may need to be consolidated for the stroke patients. Mild subdural hematomas or intracerebral hemorrhages may also mimic TIA. In rare cases, a sentinel bleed may present with focal neurological deficits, necessitating the need for neuroimaging or lumbar puncture to rule out subarachnoid hemorrhage. The lumbar puncture may demonstrate xanthochromia or bloody cerebrospinal fluid. Sentinel bleeds should be considered in the setting of an abrupt severe headache with or without neurological symptoms. Metabolic derangements such as hypoglycemia or infections particularly in the setting of a patient who has prior neurological deficits from, for example, previous strokes may appear to have TIAs. Seizure activity with or without a Todd postictal paralysis and complicated migraine headaches are part of the differential diagnosis. Psychogenic disease may have similar presentations. Therefore the algorithm consists of the following questions:

Question 1. Is the focal neurological deficit of a vascular (i.e., ischemic or hemorrhagic) or nonvascular origin?
Question 2. Is this event a TIA or stroke?
Question 3. If cerebral ischemia is suspected, what is the mechanism of this event?

Question 1. Is the Focal Neurological Deficit of a Vascula, (i.e., Ischemic or Hemorrhagic) or Nonvascular Origin?

To answer this question, a careful history must be taken from the ¡ tives, and any other key informants. A neurological examination is ..d, and brain imaging is obtained on admission. Recognition of con..1on TIA symptoms (Table 4.1) does not require in-depth neurological expertise.[10] The role of the paramedics, triage workers, and emergency department personnel is to quickly recognize the condition and provide urgent access to a neurologist. Because of frequent rotations among paramedics and other personnel involved in the initial patient assessment, stroke teams should provide continuing education to maintain the knowledge and skills necessary to quickly identify patients with stroke symptoms. The emphasis should be made on common symptoms at presentation (Table 4.1) because this information will help to identify most patients with stroke symptoms.

After clinical assessment confirms TIA or persistent stroke symptoms, a noncontrast brain computed tomography (CT) scan is usually the procedure of choice because of short scanning times, wide availability at most emergency centers, and rapid visualization of conditions that contraindicate administration of thrombolytic therapy. Such conditions include intracerebral, subdural, or subarachnoid hemorrhages; brain tumors; and some large infarctions. Occasionally, subacute or chronic subdural hematomas may be difficult to diagnose because they appear isodense. Sentinel bleeds may not readily appear on brain CTs, and subarachnoid blood may dissipate over several days. Brain CTs may not show brain tissue damage in patients with TIAs, and posterior fossa

Table 4.1 Frequency of most common transient ischemic attack symptoms at presentation[a]

Symptom	%
Unilateral weakness (hemiparesis), heaviness, or clumsiness	50
Unilateral sensory symptoms	35
Slurred speech (dysarthria)	23
Transient monocular blindness (TMB, or amaurosis fugax)	18
Difficulty speaking (aphasia)	18
Unsteadiness (ataxia)	12
Dizziness (vertigo)	5
Visual field defect (hemianopsia)	5
Double vision (diplopia)	5
Bilateral limb weakness	4
Difficulty swallowing (dysphagia)	1
Crossed motor and sensory loss	1

Reprinted with permission from Flaker GC, McGowan DJ, Boechler M, et al. Underutilization of antithrombotic therapy in elderly rural patients with atrial fibrillation. Am Heart J 1999;137:307–312.

TIA = transient ischemic attack; TMB = transient monocular blindness.

[a]Note that patients can have more than one symptom present, that is, left middle cerebral artery ischemia can produce hemiparesis, aphasia, and hemianopsia. Patients with more severe symptoms at onset tend to arrive at the emergency department earlier whereas patients with mild isolated symptoms, that is, TMB may be delayed.

visualization with CT is often suboptimal. CTs detect early ischemic processes after several hours because cytotoxic tissue edema has to evolve to become visible on CT (Figure 4.1). There is a correlation between duration of TIA and appearance of a low-density clinically relevant area on CT. However, only 10 percent of patients with TIAs lasting less than 60 minutes have evidence of infarction on CT.[11] Frank hypoattenuation or hypodensity of brain tissues is a sign of cerebral infarction and irreversible tissue injury.

On the other hand, MRI is more sensitive in visualizing the location and extent of acute cerebral ischemia with diffusion-weighted images. The posterior fossa is much better visualized with this technology compared with CT. Subdural hematomas are visualized reasonably well even in subacute and chronic phases unlike brain CT. MRI diffusion uses the apparent diffusion coefficient (ADC) to generate a map showing brain areas of restricted water molecule movement consistent with ischemia and to create a diffusion-weighted image that clearly shows the ischemic areas (Figure 4.2). This technology has demonstrated persistent focal brain lesions despite symptom resolution in almost half of patients with a clinical diagnosis of TIA.[12] However, diffusion is not 100 percent sensitive for ischemia and may miss lacunar infarctions as well as larger infarctions particularly in the posterior fossa in the acute period. After the critical ischemic insult, pseudonormalization may occur after 1 week with reduction of the diffusion signal abnormality, although ADC maps may be useful for dating the age of cerebral lesions. Diffusion changes may be reversible in ischemia with rapid restoration of circulation. Diffusion signal abnormality may be caused by other conditions: brain abscess, subdural empyema, septic emboli, ventriculitis, encephalitis (e.g., herpes), active demyelinating plaque, and brain contusion. ADC maps may be helpful to distinguish these injuries versus ischemic insult. MRI perfusion studies are required to appreciate cerebral blood flow dynamics. Mismatch of diffusion and perfusion, that is, a large perfusion defect with no or little diffusion abnormality, has been suggested to provide information of the brain at risk for developing cerebral infarction.

MRI studies do have some disadvantages. CT scans have been proven clearly to be very sensitive to hemorrhage compared with MRI. Most centers still do not have MRI available at all times of day for unscheduled studies. Cardiac

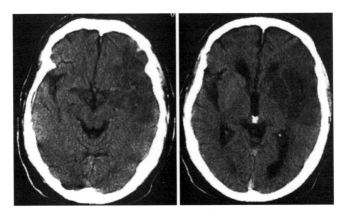

Figure 4.1   Irreversibly damaged tissue on a noncontrast brain computed tomography (CT) scan in a patient with ischemic stroke.

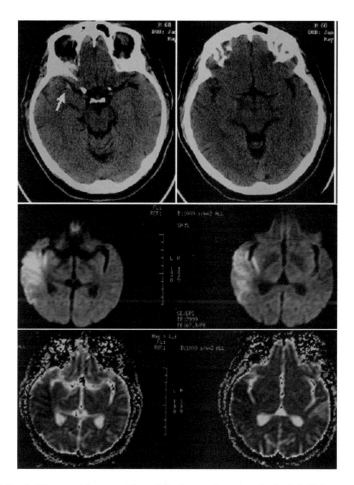

Figure 4.2 A 52-year-old man with rapidly improving neurological deficit over the first 2 hours after symptom onset and the National Institutes of Health Stroke Scale (NIHSS) score of 4 points at 12 hours after symptom onset. Computed tomography (CT) demonstrates hyperdense middle cerebral artery (MCA) without parenchymal ischemic changes (*upper row*). Positive diffusion weighted images demonstrate stroke localization in the right MCA (*middle*), and apparent diffusion coefficient (ADC) map (*bottom row*).

pacemakers and cranial metallic objects such as ferromagnetic aneurysm clips and shrapnel are contraindications for MRI. Scan quality can easily be degraded when a patient cannot remain still in the scanner. Compared with CT, acquiring MRI scans in the intubated patient is logistically more difficult. For additional information about neuroimaging of acute stroke, see Chapter 12.

Question 2. Is This Event a TIA or Stroke?

The definition of TIA, as a resolution of focal neurological deficits within 24 hours, is incongruent with a proactive approach to acute stroke management.

It is inappropriate to wait for symptoms to resolve spontaneously to avoid treatment or diagnostic testing. This rationale is flawed because patients may have neurological worsening while waiting and no diagnostic tests to clarify the cause of the event. Evidence-based medicine should be practiced. Presently, most TIAs are known to last less than 60 minutes.[13,14] Therefore it is practical to consider patients showing persistent and anatomically appropriate abnormalities on T2 MRI despite symptom resolution as having a stroke. If the patient has resolving neurological deficits and the brain MRI does not show diffusion abnormalities, this is more suggestive of transient ischemia. Brain CT may show findings suggestive of irreversible cellular damage at 6 hours but more often a few days after the insult.

Question 3. If Cerebral Ischemia Is Suspected, What Is the Mechanism of This Event?

To answer this question, a variety of tests must be performed (Table 4.2). This investigation starts in the emergency center with determination of vital signs and monitoring of blood pressure, heart rate, tissue oxygenation, a 12-lead electrocardiogram (ECG), and blood workup. The essential investigations include complete blood count with differential and platelet count, erythrocyte sedimentation rate, prothrombin time (PT), partial thromboplastin time (PPT), plasma glucose level, blood urea nitrogen, serum creatinine, lipid analysis, luetic serology, and urinalysis.[15] Telemetry or a Holter monitor may be considered to rule out serious arrhythmias. Atrial fibrillation may be discovered for the first time as well as metabolic causes such as hypoglycemia that could be the cause of the neurological deficit. A chest x-ray film should be obtained on admission to rule out a widened mediastinum suggestive of an aortic aneurysm or cancerous disease. Brain CT and MRI should also be obtained.

The other elements of the diagnostic workup are vascular ultrasound (carotid, transcranial) and echocardiography. Carotid ultrasound is a noninvasive, safe, readily available, and well-established procedure to evaluate for extracranial stenosis.[16,17] A representative case is shown in Figure 4.3. The quality of the test is user-dependent. It may fail to visualize the vessel if the carotid bifurcation is located above the mandible or excessive neck adipose tissue is present. The subclavian artery may sometimes be insonated to obtain flow information. Antegrade or retrograde flow in the vertebral arteries may also be determined. Although dissections can be noted on carotid ultrasound, MRI or magnetic resonance angiography (MRA) or conventional cerebral angiography are considered more sensitive and definitive tests. MRI is effective in showing the transmural hematoma characteristic for dissections ("crescent moon" sign), and conventional angiography can show the vessel flap or distinctive flow patterns associated with dissection.

Transcranial Doppler (TCD) can provide real-time information for intracranial blood flow in a noninvasive, readily available manner. Signal evidence of tight stenosis (Figure 4.4) or occlusion is highly suggestive of continuing ischemia and collateral flow patterns can be obtained.[18] TCD is a sensitive technology for showing right-to-left shunting with IV agitated saline injection. High-intensity signals (HITS) are noted and may be as indicative as transesophageal echocardiography (TEE) for diagnosing a patent foramen ovale and

Table 4.2   Immediate and subsequent diagnostic studies for patients with transient ischemic attack or stroke

---

Immediate clinical assessment
  Vital signs
  General physical examination
  Neurological examination
Immediate diagnostic studies (in emergency department)
  Complete blood count with differential
  Platelet count
  Prothrombin time
  Partial thromboplastin time
  Serum chemistries
  12-lead ECG
Chest x-ray
  Noncontrast head CT scan
Subsequent diagnostic studies, if clinically indicated (after admission to an
  observation or stroke unit)
  Blood cultures
  Drug screen
  Carotid/vertebral duplex ultrasound
  Transcranial Doppler
  Transesophageal echocardiography
  Holter monitor
  Magnetic resonance (MR) imaging/MR angiogram
  Cerebral digital subtraction angiography
  Electroencephalography
  Lumbar puncture
  Special hematologic studies (protein S, protein C, antithrombin III, anticardiolipin,
    sickle cell screen)
  Erythrocyte sedimentation rate
  Fluorescent treponemal antibody absorption test

CT = computed tomography; ECG = electrocardiogram; TIA = transient ischemic attack.

may be better than TEE for evaluating pulmonary shunting.[19] Anterior and posterior circulation vessels can be studied. TCD limitations include poor insonation windows in about 15 percent and quality of studies being user-dependent.[18,19] Only the major cerebral blood vessels can be insonated by TCD.

Transthoracic echocardiography is readily available, is noninvasive, and visualizes the heart's left ventricle for possible thrombus formation or decreased wall motion as well as the aortic valve for function or calcification. Obese persons may have suboptimal studies. However, in stroke patients TEE has definite advantages.[20] TEE visualizes the mitral valve, left atrium, and right-to-left shunts. This study is the gold standard for patent foramen ovale evaluation and can evaluate for possible sources of emboli such as atrial septal aneurysm, left atrial flow stasis (atrial "smoke"), aortic arch atherosclerotic disease, and mitral valve strands. Disadvantages include longer delays to obtain this study, need for sedation, and patient discomfort because a probe must be inserted. This test may not technically be possible to carry out in persons with esophageal stricture disease. Rarely esophageal perforation or aspiration may occur.

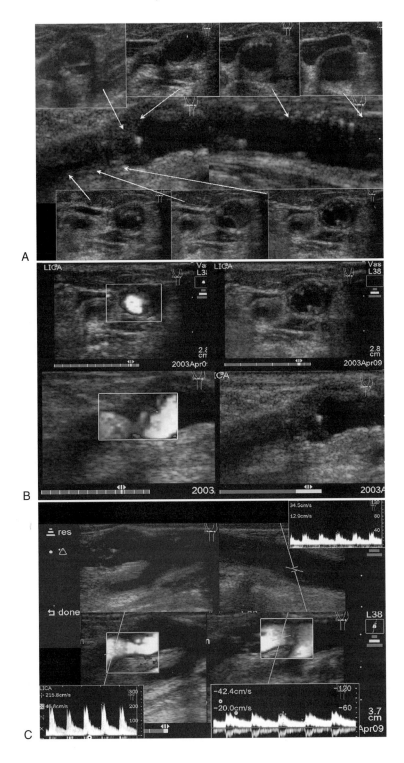

Color Plate 1

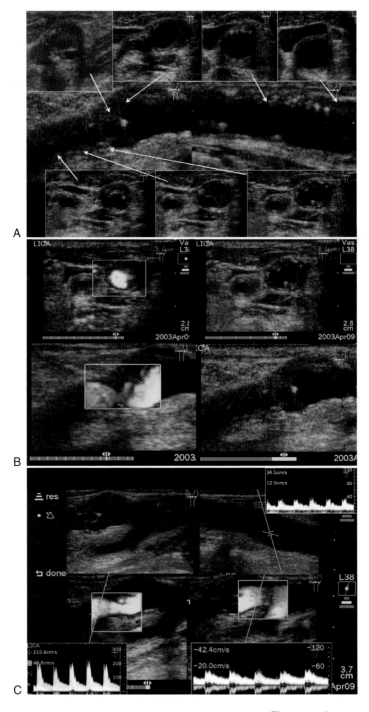

Figure caption on next page

Figure 4.3 Carotid duplex findings in a 75-year-old woman with carotid bruit. Upper panel A shows brightness-mode (B-mode) longitudinal images of the carotid bifurcation with evidence of heterogenous plaque with irregular surface. Middle panel B shows B-mode and power-mode images of the transverse and longitudinal planes of the plaque and residual lumen. Lower panel C shows angle-corrected Doppler velocity spectra in the common carotid artery (CCA), proximal internal carotid artery (ICA), and at the site of maximal narrowing. Interpretation: atherosclerotic left ICA diameter stenosis of 60 to 70 percent (peak systolic velocity 216 centimeters per second, ICA/CCA peak systolic velocity ratio 6.1 without elevation of the diastolic velocity at the site of the stenosis).

Color Plate 2

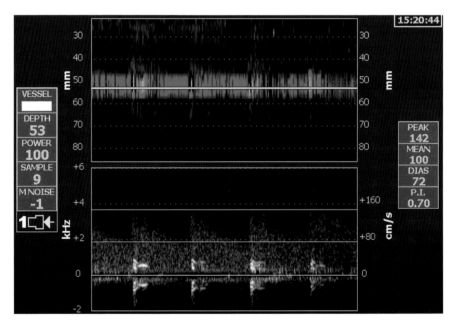

Figure 4.4 Transcranial Doppler findings in a 26-year-old man with hemodynamically significant right M1 middle cerebral artery (MCA) stenosis and fluctuating neurological deficit. (From left to right) Upper images show power-motion Doppler (PMD) findings of disturbed flow in the M1 segment and identification of the right M2 MCA flow signal. Lower images show spectral Doppler velocity measurements at presumed 0-degree angle of insonation. The right M1 MCA segment has focal significant velocity increase of 100 cm per second (ratio 2:1 with contralateral MCA, image not shown), and thrombolysis in brain ischemia (TIBI) flow grade 4 with harmonic bruit. The right M2 MCA segment has absence of systolic upstroke, a blunted TIBI flow grade 2 signal with mean flow velocity of approximately 20 centimeters per second.

Figure 4.3 Carotid duplex findings in a 75-year-old woman with carotid bruit. Upper panel A shows brightness-mode (B-mode) longitudinal images of the carotid bifurcation with evidence of heterogenous plaque with irregular surface. Middle panel B shows B-mode and power-mode images of the transverse and longitudinal planes of the plaque and residual lumen. Lower panel C shows angle-corrected Doppler velocity spectra in the common carotid artery (CCA), proximal internal carotid artery (ICA), and at the site of maximal narrowing. Interpretation: atherosclerotic left ICA diameter stenosis of 60 to 70 percent (peak systolic velocity 216 centimeters per second, ICA/CCA peak systolic velocity ratio 6.1 without elevation of the diastolic velocity at the site of the stenosis). *(See Color Insert.)*

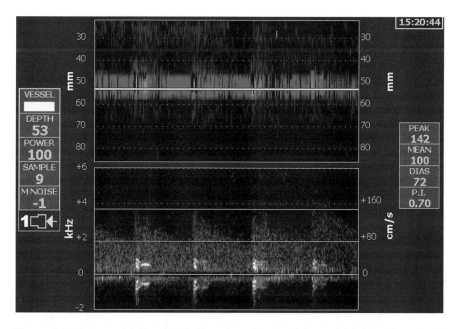

Figure 4.4 Transcranial Doppler findings in a 26-year-old man with hemodynamically significant right M1 middle cerebral artery (MCA) stenosis and fluctuating neurological deficit. (From left to right) Upper images show power-motion Doppler (PMD) findings of disturbed flow in the M1 segment and identification of the right M2 MCA flow signal. Lower images show spectral Doppler velocity measurements at presumed 0-degree angle of insonation. The right M1 MCA segment has focal significant velocity increase of 100 cm per second (ratio 2:1 with contralateral MCA, image not shown), and thrombolysis in brain ischemia (TIBI) flow grade 4 with harmonic bruit. The right M2 MCA segment has absence of systolic upstroke, a blunted TIBI flow grade 2 signal with mean flow velocity of approximately 20 centimeters per second. *(See Color Insert.)*

In the evaluation of cerebral ischemic disease, assessment of the cerebral blood vessels can be made by MRA, TCD, CT angiography (CTA), and conventional angiography.[21,22] MRA and TCD technology have been previously discussed. The MRI technique, gadolinium bolus angiography, allows visualization of the origins of the great vessels at the aortic arch, where stenosis may occur, and provides flow information. CTA is an alternative for patients who may have a contraindication to MRI or as a preferred screening test for acute stroke. CTA effectively visualizes the major arteries noninvasively and can demonstrate stenosis or occlusion in a timely manner.[21] However, the contrast load is high, which excludes patients with significant renal impairment or dye allergies, and the study requires technical support for reconstruction of images. The gold standard for cerebral blood vessel visualization remains invasive digital subtraction cerebral angiography (DSA). Cerebral angiography shows the distal vasculature in better detail than the other imaging methods, and it is the procedure of choice leading to additional interventions such as intra-arterial thrombolysis and clot manipulation by catheter. DSA is the preferred modality to diagnose vessel disorders such as fibromuscular dysplasia, aneurysms, and moyamoya disease.[23] However, angiography is invasive with the risk of stroke, bleeding (femoral artery or retroperitoneal), and infection. This study is expensive and time-consuming to execute.

In short, CT and MRI are performed to determine lesion location in the brain parenchyma and vascular distribution of the lesion. Angiographic modalities and ultrasound screening are used to determine the presence and location of extracranial or intracranial arterial occlusion or stenosis, and cardiac imaging techniques are used to reveal cardiac or aortic arch pathology. These various tests are performed in combination to determine pathogenic mechanisms of cerebral ischemia. Stroke pathogenic mechanisms can be classified using the Trial of Org 10172 in Acute Stroke Treatment (TOAST) criteria.[24] Briefly, stroke pathogenic mechanisms are divided into the following groups:

1. Large-vessel atherosclerotic occlusive disease if angiography or carotid ultrasound show a greater than 50 percent stenosis or occlusion of an extracranial or intracranial artery.
2. Embolic stroke if a potential cardiac source of brain embolism is found.
3. Lacunar stroke if a typical subcortical syndrome, that is, pure motor paresis, is present with a normal CT or characteristic lesions on CT or MRI attributable to small-vessel disease.
4. Other causative mechanisms, that is, arterial dissection, coagulopathy, and so forth.
5. Undetermined mechanism, if no obvious cause of the stroke symptoms is found after standard diagnostic workup. This type is also called "cryptogenic."

(See also Chapter 3).

CONCLUSION

There are several diagnostic approaches in evaluating TIAs. First, rapid recognition and evaluation of a symptomatic patient is required. TIAs are serious events and are predictive of stroke. Knowledge of the advantages and disadvantages of diagnostic tests is essential to provide optimal and outcome-driven treatment. Sophisticated MRI studies have provided some means to differentiate TIAs from stroke, but the availability of advanced MRI technology must be improved for routine use among patients being admitted to hospitals or daily observation units. Continued investment in neuroimaging and vascular screening and diagnostic tests will improve patient access to timely diagnostic workup and early administration of appropriate stroke prevention therapies.

References

1. Johnston SC, Gress DR, Browner WS, Sidney S. Short-term prognosis after emergency department diagnosis of TIA. JAMA 2000;284:2901–2906.
2. Goldstein LB, Samsa GP, Bonito AJ, et al. New transient ischemic attack and stroke. Outpatient management by primary care physicians. Arch Intern Med 2000;160:2941–2946.
3. Morgenstern LB, Steffen-Batey L, Smith MA, et al. Barriers to acute stroke therapy and stroke prevention in Mexican Americans. Stroke 2001;321:360–364.
4. Flaker GC MD, McGowan DJ, Boechler M, et al. Underutilization of antithrombotic therapy in elderly rural patients with atrial fibrillation. Am Heart J 1999;137:307–312.
5. Stafford RS, Singer DE. Recent national patterns of warfarin use in atrial fibrillation. Circulation 1998;97:1231–1233.
6. Marler JR, Tilley BC, Lu M, et al. Early stroke treatment associated with better outcome: the NINDS rt-PA Stroke Study. Neurology 2000;55:1649–1655.
7. Acharya AB, Edwards DF, Hahn MG, et al. What is the outcome in patients not given tPA because of a low NIHSS Score? Abstract Presentation, American Stroke Association Meeting, Phoenix, Arizona, 2003.
8. The National Institutes of Neurological Disorders and Stroke rt-PA Stroke Study Group. Tissue plasminogen activator for acute ischemic stroke. N Engl J Med. 1995;333:1581–1587.
9. Grotta JC. The Significance of Clinical Deterioration in Acute Carotid Distribution Cerebral Infarction. In M Reivich, HI Hurtig (eds), Cerebrovascular Diseases. New York: Raven Press. 1983;109–120.
10. Warlow CP, Dennis MS, van Gijn J, et al. Stroke: A Practical Guide (2nd ed). Oxford: Blackwell Science, 2001:35.
11. Koudstaal PJ, van Gijn J, Frenken CW, et al. TIA, RIND, minor stroke: a continuum, or different subgroups? J Neurol Neurosurg Psychiatry 1992;55:95–97.
12. Kidwell CS, Alger JR, Di Salle F, et al. Diffusion MRI in patients with transient ischemic attacks. Stroke 1999;30:1174–1180.
13. Hankey GJ, Warlow CP. Transient Ischemic Attacks of the Brain and Eye. London: WB Saunders, 1994.
14. Johnston SC. Clinical practice. Transient ischemic attack. N Engl J Med 2002;347:1687–1692.
15. Biller J, Love BB. Ischemic Cerebrovascular Disease. In WG Bradley, RB Daroff, GM Fenichel, CD Marsden (eds), Neurology in Clinical Practice. Boston: Butterworth-Heinemann, 2000;1125–1166.
16. Blakely DD, Oddone EZ, Hasselbad V, et al. Noninvasive carotid artery testing. A meta-analytic review. Ann Intern Med 1995;122:360–367.
17. Kent KC, Kuntz KM, Patel MR, et al. Perioperative imaging strategies for carotid endarterectomy. An analysis of morbidity and cost-effectiveness in symptomatic patients. JAMA 1995;274:888–893.
18. Alexandrov AV, Demchuk A, Wein T, Grotta JC. The yield of transcranial Doppler in acute cerebral ischemia. Stroke 1999;30:1605–1609.
19. Babikian VL, Feldmann E, Wechsler LR, et al. Transcranial Doppler ultrasonography: year 2000 update. J Neuroimaging 2000;10:101–115.
20. McNamara RL, Lima JA, Whelton PK, Powe NR. Echocardiographic identification of cardiovascular sources of emboli to guide clinical management of stroke: a cost-effectiveness analysis. Ann Intern Med. 1997;127:775–787.
21. Wildermuth S, Knauth M, Brandt T, et al. Role of CT angiography in patient selection for thrombolytic therapy in acute hemispheric stroke. Stroke 1998;29:935–938.

22. Kenton AR, Martin PJ, Abbott RJ, Moody AR. Comparison of transcranial color-coded sonography and magnetic resonance angiography in acute stroke. Stroke 1997;28:1601–1606.
23. Lownie S. Conventional Angiography. In HJM Barnett, JP Mohr, BM Stein, FM Yatsu (eds), Stroke: Pathophysiology, Diagnosis, and Management (3rd ed). New York: Churchill-Livingstone, 1998; 257–283.
24. Adams HP, Bendixen BH, Kappelle LJ, et al. Classification of subtype of acute ischemic stroke. Definitions for use in a multicenter clinical trial. TOAST. Trial of Org 10172 in Acute Stroke Treatment. Stroke 1993;24:35–41.

5
Cardioembolic Stroke

Richard K.T. Chan and Patrick M. Pullicino

Community- and hospital-based studies consistently show that 20 to 25 percent of ischemic strokes are cardiogenic in origin. This represents more than 100,000 new cardiogenic ischemic strokes in the United States each year. The incidence of cardiogenic stroke can be minimized by appropriate intervention by primary care physicians, cardiologists, and neurologists. In this chapter, we review the mechanisms and preventive treatment of cardiogenic stroke in selected cardiac conditions.

MECHANISM OF CARDIOGENIC STROKE

Cardiac conditions that increase, or are associated with an increase in, the risk of ischemic stroke are tabulated in Table 5.1. Regardless of the underlying cause, the mechanisms leading to the development of ischemic stroke involve either embolism or hypoperfusion.

The brain receives 20 percent of the cardiac output, and it is the organ that most commonly bears the brunt of systemic embolism. Cardioembolic stroke occurs when an embolus arising from, or via, the cardiac chambers occludes a cerebral arterial vessel. Endocardial injuries, whether resulting from inflammation or ischemia, expose blood to thrombogenic materials at the endocardial surface. The resulting activation of platelets and the coagulation cascade leads to deposition of fibrin and formation of thrombus. The thrombus may become fragmented and give rise to free-floating emboli. Although intracardiac thrombus is an obvious source of emboli, it is not commonly found in patients with cardioembolic stroke. In most patients, an obvious intracardiac thrombus cannot be demonstrated, but embolism is inferred either because of a cardiac condition often associated with embolism (see Table 5.1) or because of a typical neuro-imaging appearance of embolic infarction. Anatomical and physiological changes (e.g., conditions that promote stagnation of blood flow, infection, presence of

Table 5.1   Cardiac diseases associated with stroke

	High Stroke Risk	Some Increase in Stroke Risk	No Increase in Stroke Risk
Common conditions	Atrial fibrillation	Acute myocardial infarction Congestive heart failure/low left ventricular ejection fraction Patent foramen ovale	Mitral valve prolapse Mitral annulus calcification Calcified aortic stenosis
Uncommon conditions	Mitral stenosis Prosthetic cardiac valve Left atrial/ventricular thrombus Infective endocarditis Nonbacterial thrombotic endocarditis Atrial myxoma	Atrial septal aneurysm Nonmyxomatous intracardiac tumor	Hypertrophic cardiomyopathy

foreign or thrombogenic material) promote thrombosis with formation of microthrombi that embolize distally.

Paradoxical embolism is another mechanism of cardioembolic stroke. For this to occur, three conditions must be present: a thrombus in the venous system, a potential connection between the right- and left-sided cardiac chambers, and a right-to-left flow across the connection. The heart, an innocent bystander in this case, serves as a conduit for the emboli from the venous to the arterial compartment of the circulatory system.

Hemodynamic disturbance leading to systemic hypoperfusion is another potential mechanism of cardiogenic stroke. Because of the inherent autoregulatory mechanisms of the cerebral vasculature, hypoperfusion is seldom the primary cause of a cerebral infarct. Cerebral hypoperfusion may be more severe distal to a coexisting arterial stenosis, particularly if the systemic hemodynamic change was severe and acute. In these cases, infarctions are found in the cerebral vascular watershed regions.

Understanding the underlying mechanism of cardiogenic stroke is important in planning a stroke prevention management strategy. In the following sections, we discuss the more common or important cardiac conditions and management options that reduce the risk of stroke.

ATRIAL FIBRILLATION

Atrial fibrillation (AF) is one of the most commonly encountered chronic medical conditions. In a recent study, the prevalence rose from 0.1 percent among individuals younger than 55 years to 9.0 percent in persons age 80 years or older.[1] The incidence rate of chronic AF is 0.5 to 2.0 per 1000 person-years and increases markedly with age.[2,3] Without appropriate management, patients with AF have an annual stroke risk in excess of 4 percent.[4–8] The annual risk increases to 12 percent if there is a history of ischemic cerebral event.[9] From a public health viewpoint, AF is probably the most important risk factor for cardiogenic stroke.

Most cases of AF are either idiopathic (but age-related) or secondary to ischemic heart disease. AF associated with rheumatic heart disease is distinctly uncommon today. Regardless of the underlying cause, AF may be persistent (chronic) or paroxysmal. There is still some uncertainty as to whether paroxysmal AF carries the same risk of systemic embolization as the persistent variety. For practical purposes, paroxysmal AF that occurs frequently or is long lasting is managed the same way as chronic AF.

AF is a recognized cause of cardioembolism. Blood in the fibrillating left atrium is not propelled in a normal manner to the left ventricle. The relative stagnation leads to activation of platelets and the coagulation cascade and results in the formation of free-floating thrombi. In some patients, stagnant blood in the vestigial atrial appendage leads to formation of a thrombus visible by echocardiographic examination. Once disseminated, the emboli occlude arteries in the cerebral or systemic vasculature.

The most important intervention to reduce the risk of stroke in patients with AF is the administration of warfarin. Other management options include a strategy to control the rhythm or the ventricular response rate. For rhythm control, sinus rhythm is restored using either electrical or pharmacological cardioversion. Successful cardioversion is possible in a limited proportion of patients; the success rate is higher in patients in whom AF is of fairly recent onset. For rate control, restoration of sinus rhythm is not attempted. Instead, medications (e.g., β-adrenergic antagonists, calcium channel blockers, digitalis, etc.) are administered to slow the ventricular response rate. Recent studies[10–13] did not show any obvious advantage of rhythm control over rate control, if the patients are adequately anticoagulated. These studies were not sufficiently powered to address the question of superiority, with respect to stroke risk reduction, of one approach versus the other.

Despite the body of evidence supporting its beneficial effect, anticoagulation is underused in patients with chronic AF. Warfarin is the anticoagulant most commonly employed for stroke prevention among patients with AF. Ximelagatran, a direct thrombin inhibitor, has the advantage of predictable antithrombotic effect without the need for frequent blood tests or dose adjustments; however, the safety and efficacy of ximelagatran in AF have not yet been established.[14] Studies suggest that adequate anticoagulation results in a 50 percent risk reduction in first-ever or recurrent stroke compared with aspirin, and a 67 percent risk reduction versus placebo. The reduction is significant despite a 2 to 4 percent annual risk of major hemorrhage. The benefit and risk of anticoagulant therapy are highly dependent on the intensity of anticoagulation. An international normalized ratio (INR) of more than 3.0 is associated with an unacceptably high risk of major hemorrhage and should be avoided. The desirable INR range has conventionally been set at 2.0 to 3.0, with a target INR of 2.5. Recent studies suggest that an INR between 1.6 to 2.6 has 90 percent of the maximal possible stroke-prevention effect and may be sufficient for individuals at high risk of hemorrhage, particularly elderly patients.[15] None of the studies to date gave clear indications of the optimal duration of anticoagulation. The studies do show that the risks and benefits of anticoagulation appear consistent during the study period. The available data suggest that anticoagulation should be given as long as possible, possibly life long, until a contraindication or a serious bleeding complication occurs.[16]

Patients who have AF and recent cerebral infarctions should be started on anticoagulation therapy as soon as it is safe to do so. In the International Stroke Trial, the long-term outcome was not improved by early anticoagulation, even among patients with AF. Other anticoagulant trials in the setting of acute ischemic stroke also suggest that anticoagulation should probably be delayed for 2 weeks because of the increased risk of intracerebral hemorrhage. This is particularly true if the infarct is large.

There are patients with AF who are not candidates for long-term anticoagulation. Warfarin use is contraindicated in patients with hemorrhagic tendency, frequent falls, or history of intracranial hemorrhages. In these individuals, antiplatelet therapy should be instituted. The 20 percent stroke risk reduction from antiplatelet therapy (aspirin) is significantly less than that obtained from warfarin but still substantial when compared with placebo. Antiplatelet therapy is also considered reasonable and adequate in some patients with AF. The AF trials consistently demonstrated that the risk of stroke was closely related to coexisting vascular risk factors. Several risk stratification schemes have been suggested, among which the CHAD2 index[17] appears to be the most accurate predictor of stroke. The CHAD2 score is obtained by assigning one point each for the presence of congestive heart failure, hypertension, age 75 years or older, and diabetes mellitus and by assigning two points for history of stroke or transient ischemic attack. The risk of stroke increased from 1.9 percent per year at 0 points to 18.2 percent per year at 6 points. Patients with AF but without any of the previously listed risk factors (i.e., CHAD2 score of 0) have a low risk of stroke, and aspirin may be sufficient for the purpose of primary stroke prevention. However, aspirin appears to reduce nondisabling, noncardioembolic stroke more than cardioembolic stroke in AF (see Chapter 9).

AF associated with hyperthyroidism is probably distinct, in terms of stroke risk, from idiopathic or ischemic heart disease–related AF. There are no data to suggest that the risk of systemic and cerebral embolism are increased in hyperthyroid patients with AF. Anticoagulation is usually not indicated, and aspirin is a reasonable choice of antithrombotic agent if needed. It is more important to normalize thyroid function to restore the normal sinus cardiac rhythm in these patients.

CORONARY ARTERY DISEASE

The risk factors for ischemic stroke are similar to those for coronary artery disease. Not surprisingly, patients with coronary artery disease are at risk of ischemic stroke, and vice versa. Optimal evaluation of patients with symptomatic coronary disease or cerebrovascular disease should include careful evaluation of the other vascular bed.

Current knowledge of the short- and long-term cerebrovascular outcome of patients with symptomatic coronary artery disease is derived from studies of patients with recent myocardial infarction. Earlier studies suggest that the risk of stroke approaches 3 percent in the first month following acute myocardial infarction. The risk of stroke is 6 percent among patients with anterior wall myocardial infarction, compared with 1 percent among patients with inferior wall infarction. Advances in the management of acute myocardial infarction have reduced the risk of ischemic stroke to approximately 1 percent in the first month.[18–20] Ischemic strokes that occur in the first 24 hours of myocardial infarction are mostly due to cerebral hypoperfusion from systemic hypotension. Cardioembolism becomes the predominant cause of ischemic stroke after the hyperacute phase, because of the development of intracardiac thrombus (from endothelial injury or ventricular aneurysm), AF, and/or dyskinesia of the ventricular wall (Figure 5.1). A small proportion of ischemic strokes in the early postmyocardial infarction period is related to medical procedures including coronary arteriography.

It is doubtful that ischemic stroke resulting from refractory systemic hypotension in the early postmyocardial infarction period can be prevented. Patients affected tend to have large or anterior wall myocardial infarction, with a high mortality rate. Embolic strokes that occur in the setting of acute myocardial infarction may be associated with the presence of left ventricular thrombus. The risk of cerebral embolism is higher in patients with left ventricular thrombus compared to those without a thrombus. The risk of cerebral and systemic embolism, if a left ventricular thrombus is visualized, is greastest in the initial weeks following acute myocardial infarction and falls sharply in the ensuing months. Parenteral anticoagulants could reduce the risk of embolic stroke; in one study, intravenous heparin reduced the risk of stroke from 2.9 percent to

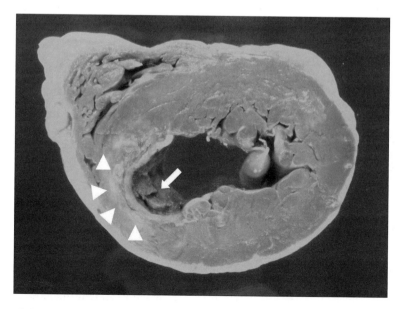

Figure 5.1 Left ventricular thrombus *(arrow)*. The underlying myocardium is thinned and shows changes of fibrosis resulting from remote infarction *(arrowhead)*.
Photograph courtesy of Peter Ostrow, SUNY Buffalo.

1.2 percent. Unfortunately, the modest reduction in stroke risk was overshadowed by the increased risk of major hemorrhage. Current data suggest that the routine use of anticoagulation following acute myocardial infarction for the purpose of stroke prevention is not recommended.

The introduction of thrombolytic therapy for acute myocardial infarction is accompanied by an increased risk of hemorrhagic stroke. The risk is less than 1 percent, but its occurrence is associated with an extremely high mortality rate.[21,22] Factors that increased the risk of hemorrhagic stroke included elevated blood pressure (systolic and/or diastolic), older age, and previous stroke.

After the acute phase of acute myocardial infarction, patients continue to experience a 0.5 to 1 percent annual risk of ischemic stroke. The cause and mechanism of stroke parallel those in the general population, where coexisting large-vessel atheromatous disease is the most common cause of ischemic stroke. Once cases of AF are excluded, there is no suggestion that there is a predominance of cardiogenic stroke following myocardial infarction. Patients who had a previous acute coronary event are usually prescribed antithrombotics to prevent recurrent myocardial infarction. Warfarin is seldom indicated for the purpose of stroke prevention once patients with AF (see previous section) and left atrial and left ventricular thrombus are excluded. When left atrial or left ventricular thrombi are detected in patients with previous myocardial infarction, anticoagulation is often administered to reduce the risk of systemic and cerebral embolization. Resolution of thrombi can be demonstrated in most, but not all, patients following anticoagulation. The optimal duration of anticoagulation in cases of intracardiac thrombus is not known.

The use of HMG Co-A reductase inhibitors (statins) is associated with a modest stroke risk reduction among patients with recent symptomatic coronary artery disease.[23-25] The beneficial effects may be independent of the cholesterol-lowering properties and may be related to the plaque-stabilizing and anti-inflammatory properties of these agents.[26,27]

Revascularization procedures for management of coronary artery disease may be complicated by stroke. Percutaneous transluminal coronary angioplasty (PTCA) without or with stenting performed electively or emergently (following acute myocardial infarction) is associated with up to 0.4 percent risk of ischemic stroke within the 30 days following the procedure.[28-33] Fatal stroke is distinctly uncommon, occurring at a rate of 0.41 per 1000 PTCAs performed.[34] Strokes following PTCA are often due to fragmented atherosclerotic plaque flicked off by the catheter or guide wires, or thrombus at the tip of the catheter. Intensive antiplatelet therapy did not appear to reduce the risk of strokes during PTCA.[35] The risk of stroke following coronary artery bypass graft (CABG) is much higher. Most of the strokes are due to emboli formed within the bypass conduit (platelet aggregates, thrombus, and air bubbles) or from atheromatous plaque during aortic manipulation. Some cases of strokes are due to cerebral hypoperfusion from systemic hypotension during the surgery. Advances in perfusion and operative techniques have lowered the stroke risk, which currently ranges from 0.5 to 5 percent in the 30 days following the procedure. Fatal stroke occurs in approximately 1 percent of patients who undergo CABG. Despite initial promise, off-pump CABG has not been shown to reduce fatal[36] or nonfatal[37] stroke risk.

Review of the literature suggests that approximately 9 percent of patients undergoing CABG have concomitant carotid artery disease.[38] The risk of perioperative stroke is higher in these patients (<2% in patients with no significant carotid disease; 3% in patients with unilateral 50% to 99% carotid stenosis; 5% in patients with bilateral 50% to 99% carotid artery stenosis; and 7% to 11% in patients with carotid artery occlusion.) Although carotid artery stenosis increases the risk of stroke resulting from hypoperfusion, it is not an important cause of perioperative stroke. Almost half of the CABG-related strokes occurred in patients without significant carotid artery disease, and 60 percent of cerebral infarction could not be attributed to carotid artery disease alone. The apparent relationship between carotid artery disease and perioperative stroke risk is likely due to the fact that carotid artery disease is often associated with the presence of aortic atheromatous plaque that may be fractured during intraoperative manipulation.

CONGESTIVE HEART FAILURE AND LOW CARDIAC OUTPUT STATE

Congestive heart failure is the second-most-common cause of cardiogenic stroke. Compared to age-match controls, the risk of stroke is four time higher among patients with congestive heart failure.[39] For every case of congestive heart failure identified, there are about four patients with impaired cardiac function but without overt signs of failure.[40] Measurement of left ventricular ejection fraction is a good way to identify individuals with impaired cardiac function, even in the absence of symptoms. Although the mortality rate is higher among individuals with congestive heart failure compared with asymptomatic individuals with low ejection fraction, the risk of stroke appears to be similar in the two groups. In patients without a prior stroke, the annual incidence approaches 2 percent. Patients with a prior stroke, however, have high recurrent stroke risks of 20 percent and 45 percent at 1 year and 5 years, respectively.[41,42]

Most cases of impaired left ventricular function and congestive heart failure are results of ischemic heart disease. The risk of stroke among patients with ischemic cardiomyopathy is not different than patients with cardiomyopathy from other causes (i.e., idiopathic or resulting from previous viral myocarditis, drugs, toxins including alcohol, infections, etc.). Most strokes in these patients are likely due to emboli formed in the poorly functioning left ventricle. It is possible that a small number of patients have watershed infarction resulting from systemic hypotension, particularly when there is concomitant stenosis of the cerebral arteries.

One would assume that improvement in left ventricular function would be followed by a reduction in stroke risk. Surprisingly, although multiple agents (including angiotensin-converting enzyme inhibitors, β-adrenergic antagonists, diuretics, inotropes, and vasodilators) have been shown to improve hemodynamic parameters or long-term survival, there is no documented effect on the incidence of stroke. The use of antithrombotic agents for stroke prevention, although logical, remains unproved.

There is a tendency for clinicians to prescribe oral anticoagulant for stroke prevention in patients with impaired left ventricular function of congestive heart failure, particularly for patients who have already suffered a stroke. The practice is based, to a large extent, on the experience gained from the AF trials. The risk of stroke, however, is lower in the case of impaired left ventricular function compared with AF. Because oral anticoagulation is also associated with a significant risk of major hemorrhage, the benefit (if any) gained from stroke prevention may be negated by the hemorrhagic complications. Antiplatelet agents, particularly aspirin, are commonly prescribed in patients with impaired left ventricular function and/or congestive heart failure resulting from ischemic heart disease. Aspirin has been shown to reduce the risk of recurrent stroke by about 15 to 20 percent in general, but it is unclear if the same magnitude of risk reduction could be seen in patients with low cardiac output state. There is also some concern that aspirin may attenuate the survival benefits conferred by angiotensin-converting enzyme inhibitors, although this is still controversial.[43,44]

Although major clinical trials are underway to determine the best antithrombotic agent for prevention of stroke and death in patients with low cardiac output, the following treatment algorithm may be appropriate. Patients with low left ventricular ejection fraction and/or symptoms of congestive heart failure should receive a comprehensive cardiac evaluation. If coronary reperfusion is needed and feasible, it should be attempted. Agents that improve cardiac function should be prescribed, including diuretics, nitrates, vasodilators, β-adrenergic antagonists, and angiotensin-converting enzyme inhibitors. If a potential emboligenic left atrial or left ventricular thrombus is demonstrated on echocardiography, long-term anticoagulation should be instituted unless contraindicated. In the remaining patients, long-term anticoagulation should only be instituted if the absolute stroke risk reduction to be achieved is large enough to make warfarin therapy worthwhile for the patient. Patients appear to be unwilling to take warfarin for risk reductions smaller than 4 percent.[45] Even at this level 25 patients have to be treated for 1 year to prevent one stroke. Assuming a 50 percent relative risk reduction with warfarin, treatment is not warranted with a stroke rate of less than 8 percent per year, and this has not been satisfactorily demonstrated in any subgroup of patients with low ejection fraction. For this reason, long-term anticoagulation for the purpose of stroke prevention is not indicated. However, there is tantalizing evidence to suggest that anticoagulation may reduce mortality in patients with left ventricular ejection fraction of 35 percent or lower. Clear indications for warfarin therapy will only emerge when large clinical trials define heart failure and low ejection fraction patients at high risk for stroke. The Warfarin Versus Aspirin in Reduced Cardiac Ejection Fraction (WARCEF) Study is an ongoing clinical trial that compares the effects of warfarin and aspirin in reducing stroke and mortality. Patients are still being recruited for the study, and the results are not expected before 2006.

CARDIOMYOPATHY

Cardiomyopathy is the third most common group of cardiac diseases encountered in clinical practice. Most cases are due to ischemic damage to the myocardium. Other causes include genetic diseases (muscle dystrophies, hypertrophic cardiomyopathy), infection (Chagas' disease, postviral myocarditis), drugs or chemicals (catecholamines, doxorubicin, ethanol), or autoimmunity (rheumatoid arthritis, hypereosinophilic syndromes). Some cases remain idiopathic. By itself, cardiomyopathy does not increase the risk of stroke. However, they are often associated with AF, low left ventricular ejection fraction, and congestive failure, which explains the slight predominance of cardiomyopathy among stroke patients. Readers are referred to the preceding sections for additional details.

PATENT FORAMEN OVALE

Contrast echocardiography demonstrates physiological shunting via a patent foramen ovale in more than 50 percent of young patients with otherwise unexplained stroke (Figure 5.2), compared with 10 to 18 percent in the normal population.[46–48] The intracardiac shunt contributes to development of focal cerebral ischemia by allowing embolic material in the right (venous) side of the heart to become disseminated in the left (arterial) side of the heart. Most of the emboli are believed to arise from thrombi forming in the venous bed, although concomitant venous thrombosis is seldom demonstrated in patients. Other embolic materials may account for cases of cerebral infarction related to scuba diving (air) and severe trauma (fat). A right-to-left shunt is required for the emboli to enter the systemic circulation. Such shunting can occur in Valsalva-provoking activities, which lead to a transient elevation in right atrial pressure.

There are many options for managing patients with patent foramen ovale and history of paradoxical embolization, including antiplatelet therapy, long-term oral anticoagulation, surgical closure, and percutaneous catheter closure. Anticoagulation and surgical closure were widely used in the 1980s and early 1990s, because of the uncertainty in the natural history. A review of five retrospective studies suggested that warfarin and surgical closure provided better protection against future episodes of embolization compared with aspirin.[49] Recently published prospective studies, however, suggest that the risk of recurrent stroke is low (0.6% to 1.8% per year).[50–52] Oral anticoagulation was not found to reduce the risk of recurrent stroke or death in one study. In view of the risk of major hemorrhage, the routine use of warfarin is not warranted. Based on current knowledge, it is reasonable to prescribe antiplatelet agents along with other nonpharmacological methods to reduce the risk of venous thrombosis to patients with patent foramen ovale to prevent recurrent paradoxical

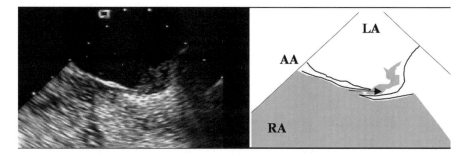

Figure 5.2   Patent foramen ovale (PFO). Contrast enhanced trans-esophageal echocardiogram showing bubbles (*shaded area*) flowing from the right atrium (RA) to the left atrium (LA) via the PFO (*arrow*).

embolic events. Short-term anticoagulation may be needed when the risk of deep venous thrombosis seems particularly high (e.g., postsurgical immobilization).

Attempts to identify risk factors for recurrent paradoxical embolization have yielded inconsistent and often conflicting results. Potential risk factors that were identified included large (>4 mm in diameter) patent foramen ovale, concomitant atrial septal aneurysm (ASA), and previous embolic events. In the absence of definitive data, we recommend that long-term anticoagulation, surgical closure, or percutaneous catheter closure be reserved for individuals with recurrent embolization (while receiving antiplatelet therapy) who have at least one of the potential risk factors listed previously. The role of long-term anticoagulation, surgical closure, or percutaneous catheter closure of patent foramen ovale is still unclear and requires further study.

ATRIAL SEPTAL ANEURYSM

ASAs are areas of localized bulging in the region of the fossa ovalis. Although some ASAs remain as a fixed atrial septal bulge into the right atrium, most protrude alternately into the left and right atria as the pressure gradient shifts. Despite multiple reports that linked ASA with systemic embolization, there is no clear evidence that ASA by itself is a significant risk factor for cerebral embolism. Most ASAs are associated with a patent foramen ovale, which may explain the prevalence of this anomaly in young patients with unexplained strokes. The interaction between ASA and patent foramen ovale is unclear—one recent study suggested that ASA increases the risk of recurrent stroke,[50] but another study showed no additional risk when both conditions were present.[52]

VALVULAR HEART DISEASE

In the preantibiotic era, rheumatic valvular disease was an important source of cerebral emboli. The risk of stroke is particularly high in patients with rheumatic mitral stenosis. Many of the affected patients have concomitant AF, and long-term anticoagulation has been recommended to reduce the risk of first-ever and recurrent embolism.[53] Patients with mitral stenosis but no AF are also at risk of systemic and cerebral embolism, probably because of the development of a prothrombotic state in the dilated atrium. Whether long-term anticoagulation is indicated in patients with mitral stenosis without AF is less clear. Surgical or percutaneous valvuloplasty can correct the hemodynamic abnormality caused by the narrow valve, but it is unclear if the procedure alone reduces the risk of stroke or other systemic embolic events.

Other diseases involving the native mitral and/or aortic valve have been suggested as potential sources of cardiac emboli at one time or other. Definitive proof is lacking. In the 1970s and 1980s, mitral valve prolapse was suggested as an important risk factor for cerebral embolism among young, otherwise healthy individuals. Several studies published in recent years, however, suggest that individuals with mitral valve prolapse are not at excessive risk of developing first-ever or recurrent ischemic cerebral events.[54–56] Mitral annulus calcification is commonly seen in patients with stroke, but the apparent increased risk of stroke could be explained by concomitant generalized atherosclerosis[57] or AF.[58] The same is true for calcified aortic stenosis.[59] Bicuspid aortic valve is probably not associated with an increased risk of stroke.

Prosthetic cardiac valves, unlike native cardiac valves, are associated with an increased risk of systemic and cerebral embolism. They may be broadly classified as either mechanical valves or bioprosthetic (tissue) valves. Examples of the former include the St. Jude medical bileaflet mechanical valve and tilting disk valves (Medtronic-Hall valves, Bjork-Shiley spherical disk valve, Bjork-Shiley Convexo Concave valve). Bioprosthetic valves are either harvested from porcine heart or crafted using pericardium from cadavers.

The risk of stroke is particularly high with mechanical valves that cause marked flow turbulence within the cardiac chambers. Embolism occurs when thrombus begins to form at the site of attachment of the prosthesis and grows in a centripetal fashion. The risk of valve thrombosis is high with infection (see the section on infective endocarditis) or when the patient is not adequately anticoagulated. The incidence of thromboembolism and stroke ranges from 1.4 percent per year to 4.7 percent per year, depending on the type of valve (mechanical vs. bioprosthetic), the number of valves, the location of the prosthetic valve (mitral vs. aortic), concomitant cardiac abnormality, and the intensity of anticoagulation. There is no clear evidence that one type of mechanical valve is superior to other valve types with respect to lower risk of thromboembolism, if the patients are adequately anticoagulated. Mechanical valves in the mitral position are associated with an increased risk of thromboembolism compared with comparable valve in the aortic position. Even with long-term anticoagulation, the risk of embolization cannot be eliminated; mechanical prosthetic mitral valves have a 3 percent annual risk of embolization, whereas mechanical prosthetic aortic valves have an annual risk of about 2 percent. The excess risk of thromboembolism (about 1% per year) of mechanical valve in the mitral position is probably related to disruption of atrioventricular conduction, associated AF, and impaired left ventricular function. Clinical studies confirmed that the risk of thromboembolism increased with increasing number of prosthetic valves in the heart. Long-term outcome following mechanical valve placement is poor without antithrombotic therapy.[60] Aspirin has not been shown to improve the outcome significantly, whereas long-term anticoagulation using warfarin is associated with improved survival and lower risk of thromboembolism. The optimal intensity of anticoagulation is not entirely clear, because many studies were performed before INR was developed and universally accepted. Based on available literature, the American College of Chest Physicians recommends that: (1) in patients with mechanical valve in the aortic position, anticoagulant be administered to achieve a target INR of 2.5 (range 2.0 to 3.0), if the left atrium is of normal size and the patient is in sinus rhythm; (2) in patients with mechanical valve in the mitral position, patients with mechanical valve in the aortic position associated with AF, or patients who have mechanical valves and additional risk factors, *either* administer anticoagulant to achieve a target INR of 3.0 (range 2.5 to 3.5) or adopt combination therapy with aspirin 80 to 100 mg daily and anticoagulant with target INR of 2.5 (range 2.0 to 3.0); (3) for patients with mechanical valves who suffer systemic embolism despite adequate therapy with anticoagulant, aspirin 80 to 100 mg per day combined with anticoagulants to achieve a target INR of 3.0 (range 2.5–3.5) should be administered.

The risk of systemic embolization is low with tissue replacement valves. The risk of embolic events appear to be highest in the first 3 months following surgery (without the use of oral anticoagulant, the risk is 6% for bioprosthetic valve in the mitral position and 2% for valves in the aortic positions). For this reason, anticoagulation, with a target INR of 2.5 (range 2.0 to 3.0) is suggested in the first 3 months. If the patient remains in sinus rhythm antiplatelet therapy (e.g., aspirin 80 mg per day) is usually sufficient to reduce the incidence of embolic events (average between 2% to 4% per year) in these patients.[61,62]

INFECTIVE ENDOCARDITIS

Osler first emphasized the relationship between infective endocarditis and central nervous system complications in 1885. Improvement in imaging techniques and new medical and surgical intervention has led to earlier recognition and a better prognosis in the last century. However, stroke remains a major cause of morbidity and mortality in affected patients.

In the earlier part of the 20th century, infective endocarditis was seen predominantly among individuals with rheumatic valvular heart disease. In the last few decades, patients with infective endocarditis tend to have prosthetic cardiac valves, are immunosuppressed, or are intravenous drug users. The pattern of responsible organisms has also shifted from predominantly low-virulent streptococci to more virulent strains of streptococci or staphylococci. Unusual organisms such as rickettsia and fungus are also being reported.

About 20 percent of patients experience stroke as a complication of infective endocarditis,[63–66] most (60% to 70%) occur by the time of presentation and recur at a rate of 0.5 percent per day thereafter. More than 90 percent of strokes associated with infective endocarditis are embolic cerebral infarctions. Most of these take the form of multiple discrete small subcortical infarcts on neuroimaging studies, although large wedge-shaped cortical infarcts can also be seen. A small proportion of strokes is hemorrhagic, and they are more likely in cases of acute bacterial endocarditis from *Staphylococcus aureus* infection among intravenous drug users.

Attempts have been made to define subgroups of patients with infective endocarditis who are at high risk of stroke. There is no apparent difference in the risk of recurrent stroke in native versus prosthetic valve, once the infection has taken hold. Cerebral embolism is more common within mitral valve involvement compared with aortic valve involvement. Large vegetation size is another predictor, although its predictive value is less consistent.

All patients with infective endocarditis require intensive antibiotic therapy regardless of whether a stroke has occurred. Anticoagulation (with heparin or a heparin-like product) is not recommended because of the high propensity for hemorrhagic transformation in tissues (including brain) with embolic infarction. The use of low-dose aspirin (<100 mg per day) may be reasonable to prevent growth of vegetation.[67] The timing of valve replacement, if needed, remains unsettled. A recent study[68] suggest that urgent valve replacement could be performed safely within 72 hours of cerebral embolism. However, if hemorrhagic transformation of cerebral infarction had occurred, it is best to postpone the valve replacement procedure to a later time.

A rare but potentially fatal complication of infective endocarditis is the development of mycotic aneurysms in the intracranial vessels.[69] A septic embolus becomes lodged at the point of arterial bifurcation, with subsequent inflammation of the arterial wall that leads to aneurysmal dilatation. Typically, the aneurysms are located distally. Most of the affected patients have a solitary mycotic aneurysm, although multiple aneurysms can be found in up to 29 percent of patients.[70] Typical clinical presentation include subarachnoid hemorrhage and intracerebral hemorrhage resulting from rupture of the affected segment of the artery. In patients who survive the initial cerebral insult, administration of appropriate antibiotics resulted in complete resolution of aneurysm in 33 percent, partial resolution with decreased diameter in 17 percent, and stabilization of aneurysm size in 33 percent of cases.[70] Surgical repair or endovascular intervention of mycotic aneurysm may be attempted for enlarging aneurysms, although their roles remains unsettled.

NONINFECTIVE THROMBOTIC ENDOCARDITIS

Noninfective endocarditis is also called marantic, verrucous, terminal, or paraneoplastic endocarditis. As its name implies, thrombus is formed on the endothelial surface (usually valvular) unrelated to any infective processes (Figure 5.3). Common predisposing conditions include systemic cancer (carcinoma of lung, pancreas, colon), autoimmune diseases (systemic lupus erythematosus), or immunosuppressive state (e.g., acquired immunodeficiency syndrome). Many cases are probably results of a hypercoagulable state, appearing as a continuum with Trousseau syndrome and diffuse intravascular coagulation in some patients. Its presence is clinically under-recognized. In

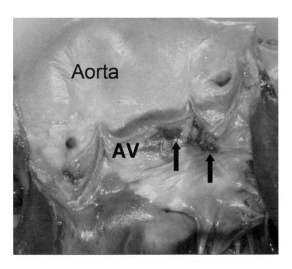

Figure 5.3 Noninfective endocarditis. Friable vegetations *(arrowheads)* are seen on the ventricular side of the aortic valves (AV).
Photographs courtesy of Peter Ostrow, SUNY Buffalo.

consecutive autopsy series, noninfective thrombotic endocarditis is present in 0.5 to 1.0 percent of cases, and it accounts for 27 percent of ischemic stroke in patients with cancer. Valvular excrescences are usually small, measuring less than 3 mm in diameter. At times, they grow to larger size and fragment easily. Advances in echocardiographic examination technique have resulted in more frequent and earlier diagnosis. Nearly one third of affected patients have clinical embolic events. Embolism to the brain is most common, and often takes the form of multiple small subcortical infarctions. Clinical manifestations range from focal neurological deficits to a diffuse encephalopathic state.

The best treatment for noninfective thrombotic endocarditis remains elusive. Because of the high propensity for embolization and fear of subsequent hemorrhagic transformation, long-term anticoagulation is generally avoided. Short-term use of heparin appears safe, but there is no clear indication that it prevents subsequent embolic events.[71,72] Treatment with an antiplatelet agent is probably reasonable for patients at high risk of hemorrhagic complications.

INTRACARDIAC NEOPLASM

Neoplasm that is found within, or protruding into, the cardiac chambers is a rare but important cause of stroke. Left atrial myxoma is probably the most common cardiac tumor associated with cerebral embolism. Most patients have symptoms of cardiac failure, and less than one third have symptoms of systemic or cerebral embolization.[73] Myxomas that are associated with embolization tend to be small but with a friable surface. Anticoagulation is not advisable in cases of cerebral embolism because of the high risk of hemorrhagic transformation. Surgical resection is always indicated.[74] Resection of the tumor leads to cessation of cerebral embolization.[75,76] Serial echocardiography is advisable because there is a small (5%) risk of recurrence after successful tumor resection.

ECHOCARDIOGRAPHIC FEATURES ASSOCIATED WITH STROKE RISK

Two echocardiographic features—spontaneous echocontrast and mitral valvular strands—seemed to be associated with an increased risk of stroke, although their significance has not been systemically studied. Spontaneous echocontrast refers to a smoke-like appearance in the cardiac chambers without external provocation (Figure 5.4). It is usually seen in the left atrium, in association with AF or left appendage thrombus. Similar findings can also be seen in the left ventricles, often associated with a low output state or an aneurysmal ventricular dilation. The pathological basis of this phenomenon is unclear, although it seems to reflect either stasis or a prothrombotic state. Initial speculation that it represents a collection of microthrombi is probably untrue because the anomaly may persist despite adequate anticoagulation. Spontaneous echocontrast is seldom seen in isolation, and it is unclear if it independently increases the risk of embolization.

Mitral valvular strands are a recently described entity.[77,78] The echocardiographic appearance (Figure 5.5) is that of a thin, mobile filament that moves

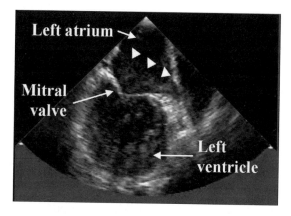

Figure 5.4 Spontaneous echocontrast in the left atrium is well demonstrated in this echocardiogram.

with each valvular movement. Its pathological basis remains unclear. The anomaly was encountered in a sizable proportion of young adults with unexplained stroke in several small studies. Further study is needed to clarify its role in stroke and method of treatment.

CONCLUSION

Although certain cardiac anomalies are risk factors for stroke (Table 5.1), not all stroke in patients with these anomalies are cardiogenic. Large-artery (aorta,

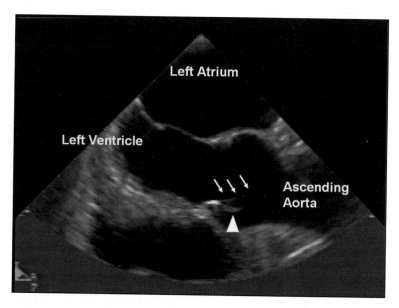

Figure 5.5 Mitral valvular strands *(arrows)* are seen in the left ventricles (LV).

carotid, vertebrobasilar, and middle cerebral) and small-artery (lacunar) infarctions must also be considered in the differential diagnosis. When a cardiac cause of stroke is identified, it seems intuitive that correction of the anomaly would reduce the risk of stroke. Unfortunately, corrective measures may be associated with a high risk of unacceptable side effects, and they may increase the risk of ischemic or hemorrhagic stroke. In the case of long-term anticoagulation with warfarin, the treatment itself may be so burdensome that the patient's quality of life is severely affected. Common sense dictates that the management plan should take into consideration the risk and cost (financial or otherwise) of intervention, balanced by the perceived benefits derived from that treatment. Risk stratification schemes[17,79] have been developed for patients with AF that define patients in whom the stroke risk is sufficiently high to warrant more aggressive clinical intervention. These are still being improved, but all future treatment of cardioembolic stroke with warfarin will likely be based on these risk stratification schemes.

Stroke may be the initial presentation of a cardiac condition. Economic progress among developing countries and the aging of the world's population will likely lead to an increase in the incidence and prevalence of cardiac diseases, particularly those related to age and affluent lifestyle. Neurologists and primary care physicians need to be prepared to handle the expected increase in stroke over the next few decades.

The challenges for clinicians and researchers in the next decade include better definition of stroke risk associated with various cardiac abnormalities and development or improvement of treatment to reduce the risk of strokes associated with these abnormalities. Advancement in electrophysiological methods and imaging technology will no doubt identify new phenomena that may be associated with increased risk of cardioembolism. It is tempting to attribute the risk of stroke to a new finding, but caution should be exercised. In the early days of echocardiography, prolapsed mitral valve was thought to be an important risk factor for systemic embolization, an assumption proven to be untrue in recent years. Another example is that of patent foramen ovale, best demonstrated by transesophageal echocardiogram, in which it was realized the risk of stroke was probably exaggerated when the phenomenon was first described. The role of valvular strands and atrial smoke with respect to the risk of systemic embolization and stroke still must be defined. Similar standards for validation will also apply to new phenomena that might be uncovered in the future.

The strategy to prevent cardioembolic strokes has to be refined. It is common knowledge that anticoagulation is beneficial in many patients with AF. Unfortunately, the lessons learned from clinical trials have not translated into widespread use in general practice. From a public health view, it is more important for patients with chronic AF (who are at high risk of stroke) to be anticoagulated than to discover potentially expensive treatments that will minimize the damage caused by embolic strokes. Although warfarin is considered to be standard treatment for patients with AF, better medications that are easier to administer and monitor must be developed. Newer medications such as ximelagatran hold great promise as the next-generation oral anticoagulant, but their roles will have to be studied.

There is a tendency to prescribe an anticoagulant to patients with cardioembolic strokes. However, AF is the only condition associated with cardioembolism in which the risk of stroke was reduced by such intervention. Compared with antiplatelet agents, warfarin (particularly at high INR range) is a stronger antithrombotic drug. Stronger antithrombotic effect, however, does not always translate into better stroke prevention. This was well demonstrated in the landmark Warfarin versus Aspirin in Recurrent Stroke Study (WARSS). The benefit of anticoagulant in cases of low cardiac output state or patent foramen ovale remains unproved. Clearly, clinical trials are needed to provide additional management guidance for these conditions. Unfortunately, it is unlikely that clinical trials will be conducted to determine the best stroke prevention strategy for every cardiac condition encountered in clinical settings. Ultimately, appropriate treatment will have to be based on the characteristics of the individual patients, the clinicians' understanding of the underlying cardiac disease, and a logical appraisal of the risk and benefit associated with the proposed treatment.

References

1. Go AS, Hylek EM, Phillips KA, et al. Prevalence of diagnosed atrial fibrillation in adults: national implications for rhythm management and stroke prevention: the Anticoagulation and Risk Factors in Atrial Fibrillation (ATRIA) Study. JAMA 2001;285:2370–2375.
2. Stewart S, Hart CL, Hole DJ, et al. Population prevalence, incidence, and predictors of atrial fibrillation in the Renfrew/Paisley study. Heart 2001;86:516–521.
3. Ruigomez A, Johansson S, Wallander MA, et al. Incidence of chronic atrial fibrillation in general practice and its treatment pattern. J Clin Epidemiol 2002;55:358–363.
4. Petersen P, Boysen G, Fodtfredsen J, et al. Placebo-controlled, randomized trial of warfarin and aspirin for prevention of thromboembolic complications in chronic atrial fibrillation. The Copenhagen AFASAK Study. Lancet 1989;1:175–179.
5. The Stroke Prevention in Atrial Fibrillation Investigators. Stroke Prevention in Atrial Fibrillation. Final results. Circulation 1991;84:527–539.
6. The Boston Area Anticoagulation Trial for Atrial Fibrillation Investigators. The effect of low-dose warfarin on the risk of stroke in patients with nonrheumatic atrial fibrillation. N Engl J Med 1990;323:1505–1511.
7. Connolly SJ, Laupacis A, Gent M, et al. Canadian Atrial Fibrillation Anticoagulation (CAFA) Study. J Am Coll Cardiol 1991;18:349–355.
8. Ezekowitz MD, Bridgers SL, James KE, et al. Warfarin in the prevention of stroke associated with nonrheumatic atrial fibrillation. N Engl J Med 1992;327:1406–1412.
9. European Atrial Fibrillation Trial Study Group. Secondary prevention in non-rheumatic atrial fibrillation after transient ischaemic attack or minor stroke. Lancet 1993;342:1255–1262.
10. Carlsson J, Miketic S, Windeler J, et al. Randomized trial of rate-control versus rhythm-control in persistent atrial fibrillation: the Strategies of Treatment of Atrial Fibrillation (STAF) study. Am J Coll Cardiol 2003;41:1690–1696.
11. Van Gelder IC, Hagens VE, Bosker HA, et al. A comparison of rate control and rhythm control in patients with recurrent persistent atrial fibrillation. N Engl J Med 2002;347:1834–1840.
12. Wyse DG, Waldo AL, DiMarco JP, et al. A comparison of rate control and rhythm control in patients with atrial fibrillation. N Engl J Med 2002;347:1825–1833.
13. Hohnloser SH, Kuck KH, Lilienthal J. Rhythm or rate control in atrial fibrillation—Pharmacological Intervention in Atrial Fibrillation (PIAF): a randomised trial. Lancet 2000;356:1789–1794.
14. Petersen P, Grind M, Adler J, et al. Ximelagatran versus warfarin for stroke prevention in patients with nonvalvular atrial fibrillation. SPORTIF II: a dose-guiding, tolerability, and safety study. J Am Coll Cardiol 2003;41:1445–1451.
15. Yasaka M, Minematsu K, Yamaguchi T. Optimal intensity of international normalized ratio in warfarin therapy for secondary prevention of stroke in patients with non-valvular atrial fibrillation. Intern Med 2001;40:1183–1188.
16. Caro JJ, Groome PA, Flegel KM. Atrial fibrillation and anticoagulation: from randomized trials to practice. Lancet 1993;341:1381–1384.
17. Gage BF, Waterman AD, Shannon W, et al. Validation of clinical classification schemes for predicting stroke: results from the National Registry of Atrial Fibrillation. JAMA 2001;285:2864–2870.

18. Van de Werf F, Cannon CP, Luyten A, et al. Safety assessment of single-bolus administration of TNK tissue-plasminogen activator in acute myocardial infarction: the ASSENT-1 trial. Am Heart J 1999;137:786–791.

19. Aversano T, Aversano LT, Passamani E, et al. Forman SA. Atlantic Cardiovascular Patient Outcomes Research Team (C-PORT). Thrombolytic therapy vs primary percutaneous coronary intervention for myocardial infarction in patients presenting to hospitals without on-site cardiac surgery: a randomized controlled trial. JAMA 2002;287:1943–1951.

20. Waters DD, Schwartz GG, Olsson AG, et al. Effects of atorvastatin on stroke in patients with unstable angina or non-Q-wave myocardial infarction: a Myocardial Ischemia Reduction with Aggressive Cholesterol Lowering (MIRACL) substudy. Circulation 2002;106:1690–1695.

21. Gurwitz JH, Gore JM, Goldberg RJ, et al. Risk for intracranial hemorrhage after tissue plasminogen activator treatment for acute myocardial infarction. Participants in the National Registry of Myocardial Infarction 2. Ann Intern Med 1998;129:597–604.

22. Mahaffey KW, Granger CB, Sloan MA, et al. Neurosurgical evacuation of intracranial hemorrhage after thrombolytic therapy for acute myocardial infarction: experience from the GUSTO-I trial. Global Utilization of Streptokinase and tissue-plasminogen activator (tPA) for Occluded Coronary Arteries. Am Heart J 1999;138:493–499.

23. Plehn JF, Davis BR, Sacks FM, et al. Reduction of stroke incidence after myocardial infarction with pravastatin: the Cholesterol and Recurrent Events (CARE) study. Circulation 1999; 99:216–223.

24. The LIPID Study Group. Long-term effectiveness and safety of pravastatin in 9014 patients with coronary heart disease and average cholesterol concentrations: the LIPID trial follow-up. Lancet 2002;359:1379–1387.

25. Waters DD, Schwartz GG, Olsson AG, et al. Effects of atorvastatin on stroke in patients with unstable angina or non-Q-wave myocardial infarction: a Myocardial Ischemia Reduction with Aggressive Cholesterol Lowering (MIRACL) substudy. Circulation 2002;106:1690–1695.

26. Bea F, Blessing E, Bennett B, et al. Simvastatin promotes atherosclerotic plaque stability in ApoE-deficient mice independently of lipid lowering. Arterioscler Thromb Vasc Biol 2002; 22:1832–1837.

27. Sukhova GK, Williams JK, Libby P. Statins reduce inflammation in atheroma of nonhuman primates independent of effects on serum cholesterol. Arterioscler Thromb Vasc Biol 2002;22:1452–1458.

28. The EPIC Investigators. Use of a monoclonal antibody directed against the platelet glycoprotein IIb/IIIa receptor in high-risk coronary angioplasty. N Engl J Med 1994;330:956–961.

29. The CAPTURE Investigators. Randomised placebo-controlled trial of abciximab before and during coronary intervention in refractory unstable angina: the CAPTURE study. Lancet 1997;349: 1429–1435.

30. The EPILOG Investigators. Platelet glycoprotein IIb/IIIa receptor blockade and low-dose heparin during percutaneous coronary revascularization. N Engl J Med 1997;336:1689–1696.

31. The EPISTENT Investigators. Randomised placebo-controlled and balloon-angioplasty-controlled trial to assess safety of coronary stenting with use of platelet glycoprotein-IIb/IIIa blockade. Lancet 1998;352:87–92.

32. The IMPACT-II Investigators. Randomised placebo-controlled trial of effect of eptifibatide on complications of percutaneous coronary intervention: IMPACT-II. Lancet 1997;349:1422–1428.

33. The RESTORE Investigators. Effects of platelet glycoprotein IIb/IIIa blockade with tirofiban on adverse cardiac events in patients with unstable angina or acute myocardial infarction undergoing coronary angioplasty. Circulation 1997;96:1445–1453.

34. Malenka DJ, O'Rourke D, Miller MA, et al. Cause of in-hospital death in 12,232 consecutive patients undergoing percutaneous transluminal coronary angioplasty. Am Heart J 1999;137: 632–638.

35. Akkerhuis KM, Deckers JW, Lincoff AM, et al. Risk of stroke associated with abciximab among patients undergoing percutaneous coronary intervention. JAMA 2001;286:78–82.

36. van Dijk D, Nierich AP, Jansen EW, et al. Early outcome after off-pump versus on-pump coronary bypass surgery: results from a randomized study. Circulation 2001;104:1761–1766.

37. Cheng W, Denton TA, Fontana GP, et al. Off-pump coronary surgery: effect on early mortality and stroke. J Thorac Cardiovasc Surg 2002;124:313–320.

38. Naylor AR, Mehta Z, Rothwell PM, et al. Carotid artery disease and stroke during coronary artery bypass: a critical review of the literature. Eur J Vasc Endovasc Surg 2002;23:283–294.

39. Kannel WB, Wolf PA, Verter J. Manifestations of coronary disease predisposing to stroke. The Framingham study. JAMA 1983;250:2942–2946.

40. Packer M, Cohn JN, Abraham WT, et al. Consensus recommendations for the management of chronic heart failure. Am J Cardiol 1999;83:1A–38A.

41. Sacco RL, Shi T, Zamanillo MC, et al. Predictors of mortality and recurrence after hospitalized cerebral infarction in an urban community: the Northern Manhattan stroke study. Neurology 1994;44:626–634.
42. Petty GW, Brown RD Jr, Whisnant JP, et al. Survival and recurrence after first cerebral infarction—a population-based study in Rochester, Minnesota, 1975 through 1989. Neurology 1998;50:208–216.
43. Cleland JGF, Bulpitt C, Falk RH, et al. Is aspirin safe for patients with heart failure? Br Heart J 1995;74:215–219.
44. SOLVD investigators. Effect of Enalapril on survival in patients with reduced left ventricular ejection fractions and congestive heart failure. N Engl J Med 1991;325:293–302.
45. Howitt A, Armstrong D. Implementing evidence based medicine in general practice: audit and qualitative study of antithrombotic treatment for atrial fibrillation. BMJ 1999;318:1324–1327.
46. Hagen PT, Scholz DG, Edwards WD. Incidence and size of patent foramen ovale during the first 10 decades of life: an autopsy study of 965 normal hearts. Mayo Clin Proc 1984;59:17–20.
47. Webster MWI, Smith HJ, Sharpe DN, et al. Patent foramen ovale in young stroke patients. Lancet 1988;2:11–12.
48. Lynch JJ, Schuchard GH, Gross CM, et al. Prevalence of right-to-left arterial shunting in a healthy population: Detection by Valsalva maneuver contrast echocardiography. Am J Cardiol 1984;53:1478–1480.
49. Orgera MA, O'Malley PG, Taylor AJ. Secondary prevention of cerebral ischemia in patent foramen ovale: systematic review and meta-analysis. South Med J 2001;94:699–703.
50. Mas JL, Arquizan C, Lamy C, et al. Patent Foramen Ovale and Atrial Septal Aneurysm Study Group. Recurrent cerebrovascular events associated with patent foramen ovale, atrial septal aneurysm, or both. N Engl J Med 2001;345:1740–1746.
51. Nedeltchev K, Arnold M, Wahl A, et al. Outcome of patients with cryptogenic stroke and patent foramen ovale. J Neurol Neurosurg Psychiatry 2002;72:347–350.
52. Homma S, Sacco RL, Di Tullio MR, et al. Effect of medical treatment in stroke patients with patent foramen ovale: patent foramen ovale in Cryptogenic Stroke Study. Circulation 2002;105:2625–2631.
53. Levine JH, Pauker S, Saltzman EW. Antithrombotic therapy in valvular heart disease. Chest 1989;95(suppl):98–106.
54. Orencia AJ, Petty GW, Khandheria B, et al. Risk of stroke with mitral valve prolapse in population-based cohort study. Stroke 1995;26:7–13.
55. Orencia AJ, Petty GW, Khandheria BK, et al. Mitral valve prolapse and the risk of stroke after initial cerebral ischemia. Neurology 1995;45:1083–1086.
56. Gilon D, Buonanno FS, Joffe MM, et al. Lack of evidence of an association between mitral-valve prolapse and stroke in young patients. N Engl J Med 1999;341:48–50.
57. Lin CS, Schwartz IS, Chapman I. Calcification of the mitral annulus fibrosus with systemic embolization. Arch Pathol Lab Med 1987;111:411–414.
58. Jespersen CM, Egeglad H. Mitral annulus calcification and embolism. Acta Med Scand 1987;222:37–41.
59. Boon A, Lodder J, Cheriex E, et al. Risk of stroke in a cohort of 815 patients with calcification of the aortic valve with or without stenosis. Stroke 1996;27:847–851.
60. Baudet EM, Oca CC, Roques XF, et al. A 5½ year experience with the St. Jude Medical cardiac valve prosthesis: early and late results of 737 valve replacements in 671 patients. J Thorac Cardiovasc Surg 1985;90:137–144.
61. Bloomfield P, Kitchin AH, Wheatley DJ, et al. A prospective evaluation of the Bjork-Shiley, Hancock, and Carpentier-Edwards heart valve prosthesis. Circulation 1986;11:42–47.
62. Chesebro JH, Adams PC, Fuster V. Antithrombotic therapy in patients with valvular heart disease and prosthetic heart valves. J Am Coll Cardiol 1986;8:41B–56B.
63. Pruitt AA, Rubin RH, Karchmer AW, et al. Neurologic complications of bacterial endocarditis. Medicine 1978;57:329–343.
64. Salgado AV, Furlan AJ, Keys TF, et al. Neurologic complications of endocarditis: a 12-year experience. Neurology 1989;39:173–178.
65. Hart RG, Foster JW, Luther MF, et al. Stroke in infective endocarditis. Stroke 1990;21:695–700.
66. Cabell CH, Pond KK, Peterson GE, et al. The risk of stroke and death in patients with aortic and mitral valve endocarditis. Am Heart J 2001;142:75–80.
67. Taha TH, Durrant SS, Mazeika PK, et al. Aspirin to prevent growth of vegetations and cerebral emboli in infective endocarditis. J Intern Med 1992;231:543–546.
68. Piper C, Wiemer M, Schulte HD, et al. Stroke is not a contraindication for urgent valve replacement in acute infective endocarditis. J Heart Valve Dis 2001;10:703–711.

69. Kanter MC, Hart RG. Mycotic aneurysms are rare in infective endocarditis. Ann Neurol 1990;28:590–591.
70. Corr P, Wright M, Handler LC. Endocarditis-related cerebral aneurysms: radiologic changes with treatment. AJNR Am J Neuroradiol 1995;16:745–748.
71. Lopez JA, Ross RS, Fishbein MC, et al. Nonbacterial thrombotic endocarditis: a review. Am Heart J 1987;113:773–784.
72. Rogers LR, Cho ES, Kempin S, et al. Cerebral infarction from non-bacterial thrombotic endocarditis. Clinical and pathological study including the effects of anticoagulation. Am J Med 1987;83: 746–756.
73. Pinede L, Duhaut P, Loire R. Clinical presentation of left atrial cardiac myxoma. A series of 112 consecutive cases. Medicine (Baltimore) 2001;80:159–72.
74. Maroon JC, Campbell RL. Atrial myxoma: a treatable cause of stroke. J Neurol Neurosurg Psychiatry 1969;32:129–133.
75. Sandok BA, von Estorff I, Giuliani ER. Subsequent neurological events in patients with atrial myxoma. J Neurol Neurosurg Psychiatry 1969;32:129–133.
76. Kawamura T, Muratani H, Inamura T, et al. Serial MRI of cerebral infarcts before and after removal of an atrial myxoma. Neuroradiology 1999;41:573–575.
77. Roberts JK, Omarali I, Di Tullio MR, et al. Valvular strands and cerebral ischemia. Effect of demographics and strand characteristics. Stroke 1997;28:2185–2188.
78. Nighoghossian N, Derex L, Perinetti M, et al. Course of valvular strands in patients with stroke: cooperative study with transesophageal echocardiography. Am Heart J 1998;136:1065–1069.
79. Pearce LA, Hart RG, Halperin JL. Assessment of three schemes for stratifying stroke risk in patients with nonvalvular atrial fibrillation. Am J Med 2000;109:45–51.

6
Large-Vessel Atherosclerosis
Sarah T. Pendlebury and Peter M. Rothwell

PATHOLOGICAL FEATURES OF ATHEROSCLEROSIS

Atherosclerosis is a multifocal disease affecting large and medium-size arteries particularly where there is branching, tortuosity, or confluence of vessels (Figure 6.1). Turbulence caused by changes in blood flow direction is thought to contribute to endothelial damage and ultimately plaque formation. Atheroma begins in childhood as fatty streaks. Over many years arterial smooth muscle cells proliferate, the intima is invaded by macrophages, fibrosis occurs, and cholesterol is deposited to form fibrolipid plaques.[1] Individuals with atheroma in one artery tend to have widespread vascular disease making them at high risk of angina, myocardial infarction, and claudication,[2,3] particularly white males who often have accompanying hypercholesterolemia.[4] There appear to be important racial differences in the distribution of atheroma, and race is an independent predictor of lesion location.[5] White males tend to develop atheroma in the extracranial cerebral vessels, the aorta, and coronary arteries, whereas intracranial large-vessel disease appears to be relatively more common in African-American, Hispanic, and Asian populations[6–10] and tends to affect younger patients[6,11,12] and those with type I diabetes mellitus.[4,6] Some sources report that women have more intracranial disease compared with men,[4] but this is disputed by others.[7]

Pathological, angiographic, and ultrasonic studies show that the most common extracranial sites for atheroma are the aortic arch, the proximal subclavian arteries, the carotid bifurcation (Figure 6.2), and the vertebral artery origins (Figure 6.3).[13–19] Plaques in the subclavian arteries often extend into the origin of the vertebral arteries and similar plaques may occasionally occur at the origin of the innominate arteries. Often, the second portion of the vertebral artery as it passes through the transverse foramen is also affected

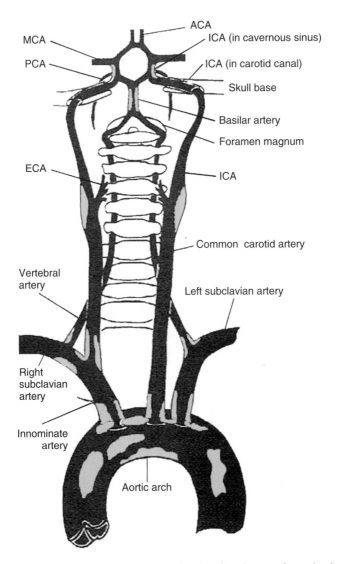

Figure 6.1   Schematic diagram showing the major sites for atheroma formation in the major extracranial and intracranial vessels.

but the atheroma, which tends to form a ladder-like arrangement opposite cervical discs and osteophytes, does not normally restrict the lumen size significantly.[20]

Intracranial arteries are morphologically different than extracranial arteries because they have no external elastic membrane, fewer elastic fibers in the media and adventitia, and a thinner intimal layer. The major sites for atheroma formation have been shown in pathological and angiographic studies.[11,12,21–23]

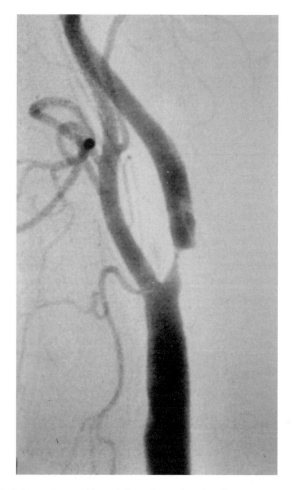

Figure 6.2 Digitally subtracted arterial angiography showing a severe stenosis of the internal carotid artery.

The carotid siphon, the proximal middle cerebral artery (MCA), and the anterior cerebral artery around the anterior communicating artery origin are the most common sites for intracranial atheroma formation in the anterior circulation. In the posterior circulation, the intracranial vertebral arteries are often affected just after they penetrate the dura and distally near the basilar artery origin. Plaques are also found in the proximal basilar artery (Figure 6.4) and also prior to the origin of the posterior cerebral arteries. The midbasilar segment may be affected around the origins of the cerebellar arteries. Occlusion of a branch artery at its origin by disease in the parent vessel seems to occur more commonly in the posterior circulation (e.g., basilar branch occlusion) than in the anterior circulation where occlusion of the small perforating arteries is usually caused by intrinsic small vessel disease.

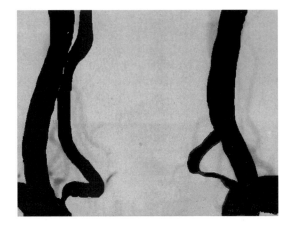

Figure 6.3   Digitally subtracted arterial angiography of the origins of both common carotid and vertebral arteries showing bilateral vertebral artery stenosis.

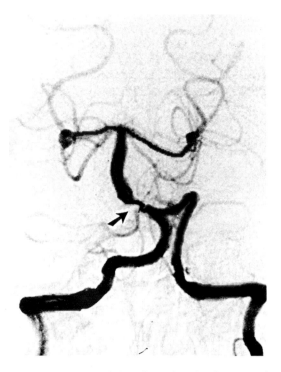

Figure 6.4   Digitally subtracted arterial angiography showing stenosis of the proximal basilar artery.

Atheromatous medium-size arteries at the base of the brain, particularly the vertebral and basilar arteries, may become affected by dolichoectasia. The arteries are widened, tortuous, and elongated and may be visualized on magnetic resonance imaging (MRI) or, if the walls are calcified, on computed tomography (CT). Dolichoectasia is usually found in elderly patients with hypertension and diabetes and may cause stroke through embolization of thrombus or by occlusion of small branch arteries.

LARGE-VESSEL ATHEROSCLEROSIS: STROKE MECHANISMS AND RISK OF STROKE

There are four principal mechanisms by which atherosclerotic lesions may cause ischemic stroke. First, thrombi may form on lesions and cause local occlusion. This will tend to occur at sites where plaques are common: at the origin of the internal carotid artery (ICA), for example, leading to carotid occlusion. Second, embolization of plaque debris or thrombus may block a more distal vessel. Emboli follow the prevailing direction of flow in a vessel; thus most emboli from the internal carotid arteries will travel to the retina or the anterior two thirds of the ipsilateral cerebral hemisphere. However, in patients with vascular disease, abnormal flow patterns may arise because of vessel occlusion and collateral flow. For example, infarction may occur ipsilateral to a chronically occluded ICA as emboli from the contralateral internal carotid pass via the anterior communicating artery. Emboli are usually the cause of obstruction of the anterior circulation intracranial vessels[24,25] at least in white males in whom intracranial disease is relatively rare. Third, small vessel origins may be occluded by growth of plaque in the parent vessel. This is seen particularly in the basilar artery and the subclavian artery around the vertebral origin. Finally, severe reduction in the diameter of the vessel lumen caused by plaque growth may lead to hypoperfusion of distal brain regions particularly in the border zones where blood supply is poorest. This may lead to watershed infarction of these regions particularly following severe hypotension or hypoxia.

Approximately 50 percent of ischemic strokes in whites are caused by atherothromboembolism.[26,27] Most of such strokes in whites (approximately 90%) are caused by atheroma in the extracranial vessels whereas intracranial disease appears to be equally important in African Americans and Hispanics.[6,7] Atheromatous disease in the ascending aorta and the aortic arch is increasingly recognized as a source of cerebral emboli and an independent risk factor for ischemic stroke in vivo.[18,28,29] In the anterior circulation, the risk of stroke is strongly related to the severity of ipsilateral carotid stenosis[30] and to whether the stenosis is symptomatic (15%, 5%, 2% for each successive year after the index event)[31,32] or asymptomatic (2% per year).[33] The annual stroke risk on medical treatment from stenosis involving the carotid siphon or the MCA was reported to be 7 to 10 percent in the EC/IC Bypass Study.[34,35] The natural history of extracranial vertebral artery stenosis has not been extensively studied, but anecdotal reports suggest that such lesions tend to be asymptomatic or to cause transient symptoms presumably because of the availability of collateral supply.[36] This view is supported by one study[37] of patients with 50 percent or greater unilateral vertebral artery stenosis that reported no definite verte-brobasilar transient ischemic attacks (TIAs) or vertebrobasilar territory infarcts in patients without coexistent basilar disease in a mean follow-up time of 4.6 years (medical treatment details were unclear). In those patients who do have stroke related to extracranial vertebral artery disease, the mechanism is usually intra-arterial embolism.[38] Intracranial posterior circulation disease appears to be associated with a higher risk of stroke than extracranial posterior circulation disease. In the study by Moufarrij et al[39] of 93 patients with symp-tomatic basilar and/or distal vertebral artery stenosis, 27 percent had verte-brobasilar territory ischemia over a mean of 6.1 years of follow-up on medical treatment. Bilateral vertebral artery and basilar artery stenosis seem to carry a worse prognosis than disease in the posterior cerebral artery, posterior inferior cerebellar artery, or a single intracerebral vertebral artery.[40]

It is important to note that the likelihood of stroke in patients with cerebral atheromatous disease varies with time: The risk of stroke is highest in the few days after a TIA or stroke and is likely to occur in the same arterial terri-tory.[31,41–43] This sudden increase in stroke risk is thought to be related to plaque activation. Atheromatous plaques are typically slow growing or quiescent for long periods but may suddenly develop ruptures, fissures, or hemorrhages.[44,45] These activated plaques trigger platelet aggregation and thrombus formation.[46] There is recent evidence to suggest that ulcerated carotid plaques are more likely than smooth plaques to be associated with vascular events in other territories such as the coronary arteries,[47] suggesting that plaque activation is a systemic phenomenon. Histological examples of smooth and ulcerated plaques are shown in Figure 6.5. The trigger for activation is not known but infective or inflammatory mechanisms have been put forward.

PREVENTION OF CEREBRAL ISCHEMIA ASSOCIATED WITH LARGE-VESSEL ATHEROSCLEROSIS

Overview

Strategies for prevention of stroke secondary to large artery atherosclerosis can be divided into lifestyle and medical treatments aimed at reducing atheroma and thrombus formation and surgical or endovascular techniques to remove lesions or augment flow. Primary prevention, prevention of first ever stroke or TIA, is designed to reduce the rate of development of atherosclerotic disease or to aug-ment flow in areas felt to be at high risk of ischemia. Prevention of subsequent stroke, secondary prevention, is targeted to the individual patient following appropriate investigation to determine the likely cause of the TIA or first stroke. Some secondary preventive measures are applicable to most stroke patients and include lifestyle changes (e.g., cessation of smoking, weight reduction, modifi-cation of excess alcohol intake, etc.). Specific secondary preventive treatments are particularly important in the case of strokes associated with large-vessel atherosclerosis (see later) because plaque activation results in TIAs or minor strokes occurring in the few days before a completed stroke. Consequently, assessment of patients with TIA must be rapid and comprehensive to enable treatment to be started as soon as possible.

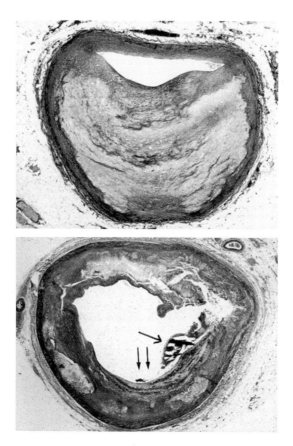

Figure 6.5   Examples of atherosclerotic plaques: the top picture shows a stable plaque with a thick fibrous cap and the bottom picture shows an unstable plaque with rupture of a thin fibrous cap and adherent thrombus *(arrows)*.

Medical Treatments

Primary Prevention

Primary prevention of atheroma is dealt with in more detail in Chapter 2. Briefly, it involves avoidance and/or treatment of the modifiable risk factors that are known to predispose to atheromatous disease such as hypertension, smoking, diabetes, and hypercholesterolemia.[48] Despite extensive research into atheroma it remains unclear why the risk factors for atheromatous stroke are quantitatively different than those for coronary disease. For example, hypertension is one of the major risk factors for stroke, whereas smoking and high cholesterol are more strongly implicated in heart disease. In addition, the mean age of stroke sufferers is higher than that of patients with coronary disease, and there are racial differences with African-American and Asian people tending to be more susceptible to stroke than coronary disease.[49] The tendency to treat stroke as a single entity rather than a group of pathologically distinct disorders may have resulted in the risk factors not being as well defined as those for coronary vascular disease.

Secondary Prevention

Antithrombotic therapy, directed toward reducing platelet aggregation and thrombus formation, is used widely and there is convincing evidence from randomized trials and meta-analyses that antiplatelet agents reduce the risk of recurrent stroke and vascular death[50,51] (see Chapter 9 on antithrombotic therapies and Chapter 10 on secondary prevention). Very few trials distinguish between subtypes of stroke and the results tend to be applied to all stroke patients, but because stroke patients have a high risk of vascular death this seems reasonable. [42] Most trial data concern aspirin but newer antiplatelet agents such as ticlopidine, clopidigrel,[52] or extended-release dipyridamole[53,54] (see Chapter 9) have also been shown to be effective. However, there is uncertainty as to whether they provide sufficient extra benefit over aspirin as first-line treatment to justify the additional cost. Currently, there is interest in the use of combination antiplatelet therapy particularly for patients perceived to be at high risk of recurrent ischemic events. There are a number of ongoing trials including the European/Australian Stroke Prevention in Reversible Ischaemia Trial (ESPRIT: aspirin and dipyridamole versus aspirin) and Management of ATherothrombosis with Clopidogrel in High-risk patients with recent TIA or ischemic stroke (MATCH: clopidogrel and aspirin versus clopidogrel).

As stated earlier, most trials did not distinguish between different vascular territories or mechanisms of stroke or only included patients with anterior circulation disease. There are few trial data specifically relating to antiplatelet agents in posterior circulation disease. The Canadian Cooperative Study[55] showed that aspirin reduced recurrent episodes of cerebral ischemia and death in patients with vertebrobasilar ischaemic episodes. The European Stroke Prevention Study (ESPS)[54] study of aspirin and immediate-release dipyridamole versus placebo appeared to show that patients with posterior circulation TIA benefited more than those with carotid disease (66% reduction versus 40% reduction in stroke) but the numbers were small.

Anticoagulation has been considered for secondary prevention of stroke for patients in sinus rhythm, and until recently patients with posterior circulation ischemic symptoms thought to be caused by severe vertebrobasilar disease were routinely anticoagulated largely as a result of several early studies. In 1946, Kubik and Adams[56] published a clinicopathological paper on a series of 18 patients with fatal basilar artery occlusion. Subsequently several retrospective case series of patients who were anticoagulated for apparent severe symptomatic vertebrobasilar disease appeared to show reduced symptoms and mortality.[57,58] However, these studies were flawed by modern standards in that diagnosis was made on the basis of clinical findings, angiograms were not performed, and there was no control group comparison being made with historical controls. A recent trial of aspirin versus warfarin for patients in sinus rhythm (WARSS)[59] in which patients were not selected as to stroke cause (but those with cardioembolic sources or >50 percent carotid stenosis were excluded), showed no additional benefit for warfarin at a mean international normalized ratio (INR) of 1.8 (target INR 1.4 to 2.8). Treatment with warfarin to a target

INR of 3 to 4.5 has been shown to be associated with significant harm caused by an increase in major bleeding complications especially intracerebral hemorrhage.[60] There is an ongoing trial, the ESPRIT trial (http://home.wxs.nl/~esprit/) that is allocating patients to aspirin, aspirin and extended-release dipyridamole, or warfarin (INR 2 to 3). In light of current evidence, antiplatelet agents should probably remain as first-line treatment antithrombotic therapy for extracranial posterior circulation disease.

There is uncertainty as to whether anticoagulation is preferable to antiplatelet treatment for the secondary prevention of ischemia related to intracranial atherosclerosis. A retrospective analysis of warfarin versus aspirin in 68 patients with a variety of symptomatic intracranial arterial stenoses appeared to show that warfarin was significantly better than aspirin in reducing the rate of stroke.[40] The NIH/NINDS is currently funding a randomized double-blind clinical trial of warfarin versus aspirin (WASID)[61] to determine whether warfarin (INR 2 to 3) or aspirin 1300 mg per day is more effective for preventing stroke or vascular death in patients with 50 to 99 percent stenosis of a major intracranial artery. Another study, the Aspirin versus Anticoagulants in Symptomatic Intracranial Stenosis of the Middle Cerebral Artery Trial (AVASIS) is comparing aspirin with coumarin (INR 2 to 3) in patients with symptomatic stenosis of the MCA.

As stated previously, the best antithrombotic therapy for intracranial disease is uncertain, but there is evidence that such therapy may not be as effective in intracranial disease as compared with extracranial disease in that patients are more likely to have ongoing ischemic episodes. Patients in the extracranial to intracranial (EC-IC) bypass study with symptomatic MCA stenosis who were randomized to medical treatment had annual ipsilateral stroke rates of 7.8 percent and total stroke rates of 9.5 percent.[35] In a more recent study,[62] 56 percent of patients with a significant intracranial stenosis in either the anterior or the posterior circulation who were receiving antithrombotic therapy had a recurrent ischemic event over a 3-year period. This has led to attempts to determine the characteristics of patients who fail antithrombotic therapy,[62] because it could be argued that such patients might benefit from surgical or endovascular intervention. Older age and the use of therapies other than warfarin appeared to be associated with treatment failure. However, the study analysis could be criticized because its design favored warfarin over antiplatelet therapies. For instance, patients who had ischemic events with subtherapeutic INR or intracranial hemorrhage associated with warfarin were not counted as treatment failures. Therefore the best medical therapy for symptomatic intracranial atherosclerosis remains unclear but should be clarified by the WASID study. This study also aims to identify those patients in whom the rate of subsequent stroke in the territory of the ischemic artery is sufficiently high to justify a subsequent trial of intracranial angioplasty or stenting versus best medical therapy.

There is evidence from trials to suggest that both blood pressure and cholesterol lowering are effective for secondary prevention of stroke. As in the antiplatelet trials, specific ischemic stroke subtypes were not examined but there is no reason to suppose that patients with large-artery atherosclerosis did not benefit. Data from the United Kingdom Transient Ischemic Attack (UKTIA) aspirin trial and the Antithrombotic Trialists' Collaboration had suggested that there is a strong linear relationship between usual blood pressure and risk of stroke in patients with previous minor stroke or TIA.[63] More recently, the Perindopril pROtection aGainst REcurrent Stroke Study (PROGRESS) trial of perindopril and indapamide[64] (see Chapter 10 on secondary prevention) showed that blood pressure reduction after stroke reduces the risk of subsequent stroke. However, many physicians are cautious about applying the PROGRESS results to patients with bilateral severe carotid stenosis or severe basilar or bilateral vertebral artery disease. Such patients may be at risk of watershed infarction if their existing poor cerebral blood flow is further compromised by reduction in systemic blood pressure.

There had been some evidence to suggest a positive association between cholesterol and ischemic stroke and a negative association between cholesterol and hemorrhagic stroke. In addition, studies of carotid atheroma showed that cholesterol-lowering drugs could slow or arrest atheroma progression.[63,65] Recently, the Heart Protection Study[66] (see Chapter 10 on secondary prevention) has shown that treatment with a statin to lower lipid levels reduced the risk of recurrent stroke in patients with previous stroke and coronary or peripheral vascular disease. This was the case even for patients with normal cholesterol levels.

Surgical Treatment

Surgical treatments for secondary prevention of stroke in patients with large-artery atherosclerosis can be divided into endarterectomy, in which plaque is removed from a vessel, and bypass or anastomotic procedures designed to augment flow. The evidence for surgery is considerably more extensive in anterior circulation disease than in posterior circulation disease.

Anterior Circulation: Symptomatic Carotid Disease

Significant atherosclerotic narrowing at, or around, the origin of the ipsilateral ICA is found in about 20 to 30 percent of patients with a TIA or an ischemic stroke. That the carotid plaque is responsible for many of these strokes has been demonstrated by the observation that endarterectomy of severe atherothrombotic stenosis markedly reduces the risk of subsequent ipsilateral carotid territory ischemic stroke.[31,32] More than 150,000 carotid endarterectomies are now performed each year in the United States, and rates continue to rise in Europe.[67,68]

There have been five randomized clinical trials (RCTs) of endarterectomy for symptomatic carotid stenosis.[69–73] The first two were small, included patients with noncarotid symptoms, and probably no longer reflect current surgical practice.[69,70] The larger Veteran's Administration (VA) trial (VA #309), reported a nonsignificant trend in favor of surgery[71] but was stopped early when the two largest trials, the European Carotid Surgery Trial (ECST) and the North American Symptomatic Carotid Endarterectomy Trial (NASCET), reported their preliminary results.[31,32] The analyses of these trials were stratified by the degree of stenosis of the symptomatic carotid artery, a powerful predictor of stroke risk on medical treatment. However, different methods of measurement of the degree of stenosis on prerandomization angiograms were used, the NASCET method underestimating stenosis compared with the ECST method. Stenoses reported to be 50 to 69 percent and 70 to 99 percent by the NASCET method are 65 to 81 percent and 82 to 99 percent respectively by the ECST method.[74]

In 1991, the ECST showed that surgery reduced the risk of stroke in patients with 70 to 99 percent stenosis.[31] The NASCET trial reported similar results in patients with 70 to 99 percent (ECST 82 to 99% stenosis).[32] The ECST also reported that surgery was harmful in patients with mild stenosis (0 to 29%) in whom the risk of stroke on medical treatment was too low to offset the operative risks.[31] In 1998, the ECST showed that there was no benefit from surgery in patients with 30 to 49 percent stenosis or 50 to 69 percent stenosis.[72] When the results of the ECST were stratified by decile of stenosis, endarterectomy was only significantly beneficial in patients with 80 to 99 percent stenosis: absolute reduction in risk of major stroke or death at 3 years was 11.6 percent ($p < 0.001$). This was consistent with the 10.1 percent ($p < 0.01$) reduction in major stroke or death at 2 years reported in NASCET in patients with 70 to 99 percent stenosis.[73] However, in contrast to the ECST, the NASCET reported a 6.9 percent ($p = 0.03$) absolute reduction in risk of disabling stroke or death in patients with 50 to 69 percent stenosis, although no benefit was seen in patients with 40 to 59 percent stenosis.[73] A subsequent reanalysis of the individual patient data from the ECST, with remeasurement of the degree of stenosis on the original angiograms and redefinition of outcome events in the same way as NASCET, yielded estimates of the effect of surgery that were highly consistent with NASCET.[75]

Thus both the ECST and NASCET have now demonstrated benefit in patients with [NASCET]50 to 69 percent stenosis as well as in patients with [NASCET]70 to 99 percent stenosis. One remaining uncertainty, also related to measurement of the degree of carotid stenosis, has been whether surgery is beneficial in patients with "near-occlusions" as identified in NASCET[76] or in patients with "abnormal post-stenotic narrowing" of the ICA as identified in the ECST.[77] These overlapping categories identify a subgroup of patients in whom it is not possible to measure the degree of stenosis using the NASCET method, either because the poststenotic ICA is narrowed or collapsed (Figure 6.6) or because poststenotic blood flow is markedly reduced. Both the ECST and NASCET have shown that, although these patients have very severe stenosis, they have a paradoxically low risk of stroke on medical treatment.[76,77] However, neither trial had sufficient power to determine the effect of endarterectomy in this subgroup.

There have been a number of systematic reviews of the overall results of the RCTs of endarterectomy for symptomatic stenosis.[78,79] However, in this case, they have been of limited value because of the methodological differences between the trials described previously. To properly compare and combine the results of the individual trials, definitions of outcome events must be matched and the same method of measurement of stenosis must be used. This has recently been done with data from the ECST, the NASCET, and the VA #309 trial (Carotid Endarterectomy Trialists' Collaboration).[80] These trials included all patients randomized in the last 20 years and more than 95 percent of patients ever randomized.

In 6092 randomized patients, with 35,000 patient-years of follow-up, surgery increased the 5-year risk of *any stroke or operative death* in patients with less than 30 percent stenosis ($n = 1746$, absolute risk reduction [ARR] = -2.6%, $p = 0.03$), had no significant effect in patients with 30 to 49 percent stenosis ($n = 1429$, ARR = 2.6%, $p = 0.7$), was of some benefit in patients with 50 to

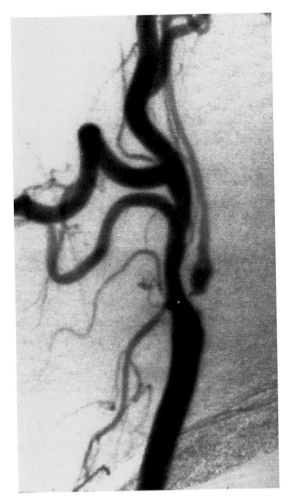

Figure 6.6 Digitally subtracted arterial angiography showing a near-occlusion of the internal carotid artery distal to a severe carotid stenosis.

69 percent stenosis ($n = 1549$, ARR = 7.8%, $p = 0.002$), and was highly beneficial in patients with more than 70 percent stenosis without near-occlusion ($n = 1095$, ARR = 15.3%, $p < 0.0001$) (stenosis measured by the NASCET method). However, there was no clear benefit ($n = 262$, ARR = −0.1%, $p = 0.6$) in patients with the most severe disease (near-occlusions).[81] The effect of surgery on each of the three main trial outcomes in the five stenosis groups is shown in Figure 6.7. Qualitatively similar results were seen for disabling stroke, but surgery had no consistent effect on survival. Operative mortality was 1.1 percent (95% confidence interval [CI] = 0.9 to 1.4) and the operative risk of stroke and death was 7.0 percent (95% CI = 6.2 to 8.0).

In the final reports of the ECST and NASCET, some subgroup analyses were attempted[72,73] but neither trial was powered to allow subgroup analysis. The Carotid Endarterectomy Trialists' Collaborative meta-analysis went on to

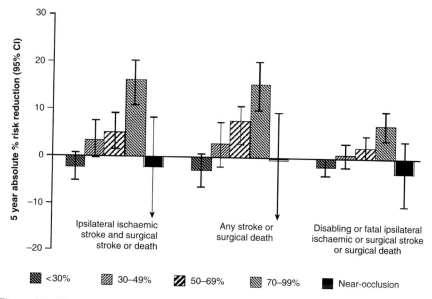

Figure 6.7 The effect of carotid endarterectomy on three outcomes in five carotid stenosis groups in a pooled analysis of all available randomized trials of carotid endarterectomy versus medical treatment for recently symptomatic carotid stenosis.
(Data derived from Rothwell PM, Gutnikov SA, Eliasziw M, et al. Pooled analysis of individual patient data from randomized controlled trials of endarterectomy for symptomatic carotid stenosis. Lancet 2003;361:107–116.)

determine the effect of surgery in a number of predefined clinically important subgroups and found statistically significant subgroup-treatment effect interactions in five of these subgroups. Benefit from surgery was greater in men than women, increased with age, decreased with time since presenting event, was greater in patients presenting with stroke than TIA, and was greater in patients with irregular or ulcerated carotid plaques than smooth plaques.[81] These data show that the patients who are most likely to benefit from endarterectomy for symptomatic carotid stenosis cannot be identified by the degree of stenosis alone. Several other clinical and angiographic characteristics influence the efficacy of surgery.

Anterior Circulation: Asymptomatic Carotid Disease

There have been seven RCTs of endarterectomy for asymptomatic carotid stenosis,[33] one of which is ongoing.[82] The initial studies were small and did not produce statistically significant results.[33] The VA study (VA #167) demonstrated a significant reduction in the risk of the combined outcome of stroke and TIA in the endarterectomy group in patients with NASCET 50 to 99 percent stenosis but did not have the power to demonstrate a reduction in the risk of stroke alone.[83] In 1995, the Asymptomatic Carotid Artery Study (ACAS)[84] demonstrated a clearly significant reduction in the risk of ipsilateral ischemic stroke in patients with NASCET 60 to 99 percent asymptomatic stenosis (assessed by angiography in the surgery group and Doppler ultrasound in the medical group), a reduction in the 5-year actuarial risk of ipsilateral ischemic stroke or operative death from 11 percent to 5.1 percent ($p < 0.001$). In other words, 17 operations are required to prevent one stroke or operative death over the next 5 years. The Asymptomatic Carotid Surgery Trial (ACST) is a large European RCT that is still recruiting and has now randomized in excess of 3000 patients.[82]

Thus there is evidence of benefit from endarterectomy in patients with asymptomatic stenosis, but the low short-term risk of stroke on medical treatment means that the reduction in the absolute risk of stroke with surgery is small. Although there are data to suggest that the long-term risk of ischemic stroke distal to an asymptomatic stenosis may be higher than previously considered,[85] the low short-term risk means that it is particularly important to determine the factors that identify high-risk individuals. However, because the operative risk of stroke and death resulting from endarterectomy for asymptomatic stenosis is lower than that for symptomatic stenosis,[86] the level of stroke risk without surgery that is required for the operation to be worthwhile may be slightly lower.

Anterior Circulation: Intracranial Disease

Lesions of the carotid artery distal to the bifurcation (intracranial carotid artery) and the MCA are surgically inaccessible, although they may be reached with angioplasty (see later). Until relatively recently, a bypass procedure was often performed in which a branch of the external carotid artery (usually the superficial temporal artery) was anastomosed via a skull burr hole to a cortical branch of the MCA. It was felt that this would improve blood flow in the MCA territory and thus reduce the risk of subsequent stroke. The procedure was evaluated in one randomized controlled trial, the EC-IC Bypass Study[34] that failed to show any benefit. However, it has been argued that the procedure might be of help in patients with maximal oxygen extraction or impaired cerebrovascular reactivity indicating poor existing collateral flow.[87–89] There is a randomized trial in this specific subgroup currently in progress.[90]

Posterior Circulation Disease

As noted earlier, surgery for carotid disease has been shown from two large randomized trials to be an effective treatment for secondary prevention of anterior circulation stroke in certain patients. Similar randomized controlled trials have not been performed in posterior circulation disease,[91] but despite this many surgical procedures continue to be undertaken. In general, surgery in the posterior circulation is technically more demanding than in the anterior circulation because of the smaller caliber of the posterior circulation arteries and the difficulty in obtaining surgical access. In addition, the fact that there is a single basilar artery supplying blood to the posterior circulation increases the risk of surgical treatment.

The most common surgical treatment for proximal vertebral artery disease is transposition of the vertebral artery into the ipsilateral common carotid artery and may be accompanied by carotid endarterectomy if carotid stenosis is also present. The vertebral artery may also be reimplanted into the subclavian or a vein or graft bypass inserted from the subclavian to the vertebral artery.[92–94] External carotid artery branches may also be anastomosed to the distal extracranial vertebral artery. Patency rates after these procedures are reported to be high[94] and morbidity and mortality to be low, but figures are likely to be biased because independent observer assessment is lacking. Further, and most importantly, the absence of control groups makes the risk benefit of such procedures unclear.

In contrast to carotid disease, vertebral artery endarterectomy is performed much less frequently than bypass procedures. Elective vertebral artery endarterectomy was first performed in 1958 by Crawford and DeBakey,[95] although it does not appear to have been widely adopted presumably because of its technical difficulty. Despite this large series of patients have been reported including that from Thevenet[96] of 212 vertebral endarterectomies in which 81 percent of postoperative angiograms showed normal vertebral arteries, 14 percent had irregularities or stenoses, and 5 percent had occlusions. It was reported that 77 percent of the patients became asymptomatic, and in 9 percent symptoms were much improved. However, it should be emphasized that the results are difficult to evaluate because there was no control group. In addition, the natural history of proximal vertebral artery disease is poorly understood. It is likely that complication rates from vertebral endarterectomy exceed those of carotid surgery because of the smaller vessel caliber meaning that there would need to be a concomitant larger benefit to make the procedure worthwhile in patients.

For intracranial disease, a number of different procedures are performed according to the exact location of the lesions. Anastomosis of the occipital artery to the posterior inferior cerebellar artery (PICA) is probably the most common. More distal occlusions often involve the use of superficial temporal artery anastomoses to the posterior cerebral artery (PCA) or superior cerebellar artery. None of these operations has been subject to a randomized trial but the lack of benefit from a similar bypass procedure in the anterior circulation[34] has meant that they are becoming less popular. Endarterectomy of the intracranial vertebral artery is feasible where the lesion is focal and proximal but requires microsurgical techniques and too few operations have been performed to allow assessment.

In the clinical syndrome of subclavian steal, stenosis or occlusion of the subclavian artery proximal to the vertebral artery origin leads to reverse flow in the vertebral artery to supply the distal subclavian artery and consequent ischemia in the vertebral territory. Symptoms consistent with posterior circulation TIA may be produced by exercising the ipsilateral arm, and examination shows unequal blood pressures in the arms and a possible subclavian bruit.[97,98] In such patients, surgical treatment of the subclavian stenosis is beneficial.

Endovascular Treatment

Extracranial Disease

Transluminal angioplasty was first reported in the limbs in 1964 by Dotter and Judkins[99] and subsequently used in the renal and coronary arteries but has been

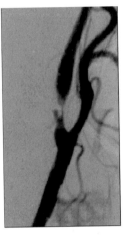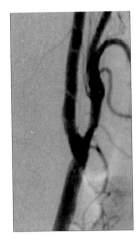

Figure 6.8   Digitally subtracted arterial angiography of the carotid bifurcation before *(left)* and after *(right)* carotid angioplasty.

introduced cautiously in the cerebral circulation because of fears of plaque rupture and embolism causing stroke. However, carotid angioplasty (Figure 6.8) and stenting are currently under investigation as a potential alternative to endarterectomy. Taken together, the three randomized controlled trials of angioplasty ± stenting versus endarterectomy that have been performed so far suggest that angioplasty ± stenting is associated with a higher procedural risk than endarterectomy and a higher rate of restenosis during follow-up.[100–102] However, improvements in cerebral protection devices may reduce the procedural risks,[103] and several randomized trials of angioplasty and stenting with cerebral protection versus endarterectomy are currently ongoing. The use of angioplasty is likely to increase in the future, but whether the increase will be confined to cases in which endarterectomy is technically difficult or whether it is more general will depend on the results of these trials.

Angioplasty of the proximal vertebral artery is technically fairly straightforward but is not widely performed. It is not currently undergoing the same rigorous assessment as carotid angioplasty but there are a few case series.[104–107] Higashida et al[107] reported endovascular treatment of 42 vertebrobasilar occlusive lesions of which 34 were in the proximal vertebral artery. There were two strokes and one vessel rupture and four cases of transient ischemia or vessel spasm. Because of the lack of randomized evidence there is ongoing uncertainty over the risks and benefits of endovascular treatment of proximal vertebral artery disease, and vertebral angioplasty tends to be reserved for patients who continue to have symptoms despite antithrombotic therapy or in whom occlusion is likely to lead to severe stroke (e.g., where a dominant vertebral artery is involved or where there are no patent posterior communicating arteries).

Intracranial Disease

Endovascular treatment for intracranial anterior circulation atherosclerosis has not been subject to clinical trials. The method is technically more difficult than in large-caliber extracranial vessels, but there are reports that it may be of benefit to patients in whom medical therapy has failed.[108] Marks et al[109] reported their experience with 23 patients with symptomatic intracranial stenoses of whom 20 had TIAs resistant to anticoagulation treatment. Percutaneous transluminal angioplasty (PTA) resulted in reduced stenosis in 21 patients, one stenosis could not be crossed, and there was one death related to MCA rupture. The stroke rate post PTA was 3.2 percent in the territory of the treated vessel and 4.8 percent for all strokes over a mean follow up period of 35.4 months. A further series was recently reported by Connors and Wojak.[110] In their last 50 cases, good clinical outcomes were reportedly achieved in 49 patients with 1 death caused by vessel perforation. Dissection occurred in 7 patients requiring thrombolysis.

Angioplasty has been used in the intracranial posterior circulation since at least 1980 when angioplasty of the basilar artery was reported by Sundt et al.[111] They used a surgical cut down to expose the distal extracranial vertebral artery into which the balloon catheter was inserted. However, subsequent reports showed significant mortality[112] and called for a moratorium on the use of the technique. At present there are no trial data and the indications for such procedures are unclear. Endovascular procedures on the small vessels of the posterior circulation, particularly involving the single basilar artery, may well remain high risk given the disastrous consequences of plaque embolism, blockage of perforating vessels, or prolonged vessel spasm.

FUTURE DEVELOPMENTS

Regarding medical treatments, it is possible that neuroprotective agents may be effective when administered immediately after a TIA or minor stroke. Animal experiments have shown that neuroprotective agents reduce infarct size when given as a pretreatment or immediately after stroke induction, but clinical trials in humans showed such agents to be ineffective when administered some hours after stroke onset. There are numerous reasons why animal data may not be extrapolated to humans but in this instance it may be the difference in timing of treatment that is crucial (see Chapter 15 on emerging therapies).[113] Treatment with neuroprotective agents following a TIA or minor stroke might increase neuronal resistance to ischemia and thus reduce the severity of a subsequent stroke.

There are ongoing studies designed to try and identify patients at particularly high risk of stroke from atherosclerotic disease. Several investigations that were unavailable at the time when the carotid surgery trials were designed are now beginning to be used in clinical practice and might be of value in identifying individual patients with symptomatic carotid stenosis who have a high risk of stroke on medical treatment. These include the detection of cerebral microemboli[114–117] and assessment of cerebral perfusion reserve.[89,118–120]

It is possible to detect platelet microemboli in the MCA distal to a carotid stenosis using transcranial Doppler ultrasound (TCD). TCD detection of microemboli has been shown to be reproducible in patients with carotid stenosis,[114,115] to correlate with risk factors for stroke,[116,117] and to be reduced considerably by endarterectomy.[115] These findings suggest that emboli detection might be useful in identifying patients at particularly high early risk of stroke. One small study has produced encouraging results,[121] but large prospective cohort studies are required. However, it is important to determine whether microemboli rates are independently predictive of stroke risk after adjustment for established risk factors. For example, microemboli rates are highest immediately after the last symptomatic ischemic event and then fall with time[116] and are highest in patients with ulcerated carotid plaques on angiography.[117] Both of these characteristics are known to be associated with an increased stroke risk and are included in the ECST risk model. It is important to determine what additional predictive power the inclusion of data on microemboli would provide and also how the rate of microemboli is related to subsequent operative risk.

Thromboembolism is the main mechanism by which carotid plaque causes cerebral ischemia. However, the risk of ischemic stroke, as opposed to TIA or clinically silent microemboli, depends to a significant extent on the degree to which blood flow to the ipsilateral cerebral hemisphere is reduced by the carotid stenosis. The absence of blood flow toward the symptomatic cerebral hemisphere in collateral vessels on angiography[122] and reduced cerebral perfusion reserve, as indicated by the inability to increase cerebral perfusion in response to raised levels of carbon dioxide,[89,114,118,119] are both associated with a high risk of stroke on medical treatment in patients with recently symptomatic severe carotid stenosis or occlusion. It is possible that measurement of cerebral perfusion might be useful in identifying patients with carotid stenosis who are at high risk of stroke.[119]

CONCLUSION

Prevention of cerebral ischemia associated with large-vessel atherosclerosis consists of primary measures to reduce the development of atheroma and secondary preventive measures to avoid a second or subsequent ischemic event. Secondary prevention is of particular importance to the stroke physician because of the high risk of stroke in the first few days after a first stroke or TIA. This high stroke risk is thought to be caused by an atheromatous plaque becoming ulcerated or ruptured and acting as a trigger for thrombus formation. Thus patients presenting with TIA or minor stroke require emergency assessment and treatment targeted to their specific clinical needs. Medical treatments are directed toward reducing the likelihood of thrombus formation and antiplatelet therapy has been proven in randomized trials to be effective at reducing stroke and vascular death. The place of anticoagulation in secondary prevention for patients in sinus rhythm is less clear cut. The WARSS trial of warfarin versus aspirin for patients in sinus rhythm suggested no additional benefit for warfarin. However, there is still significant uncertainty over the question of whether anticoagulation is preferable to aspirin in the case of intracranial vessel disease. This question is being addressed by the ongoing WASID trial. Furthermore, the arrival of newer antiplatelet agents means that questions remain regarding which antiplatelet agent to use and whether combination therapy may provide better antithrombotic results. Finally, blood pressure lowering and lipid lowering have shown to be beneficial in secondary prevention of stroke.

Surgical treatment in the form of endarterectomy for symptomatic large-vessel atherosclerosis of the anterior circulation has been proven to be effective in two large randomized trials. It is becoming clear, however, that surgery must be performed very soon after the index event to be beneficial. Presumably, this is because of the high stroke risk associated with plaque activation, this activated plaque being removed at surgery. The use of a bypass procedure, EC-IC bypass, in the anterior circulation has been shown to be ineffective in a randomized trial, but it is possible that there may be benefit to some patients because this trial did not distinguish between disease subtypes (i.e., intracranial ICA occlusion, MCA stenosis or occlusion, etc.). There are no randomized trial data for other surgical procedures, but despite this many such procedures continue to be performed. Trials are required to test these approaches against best medical therapy in patients at high risk of ongoing ischemic events.

Endovascular methods are beginning to be more widely used in the treatment of symptomatic large-vessel atherosclerosis, but more data from randomized controlled trials are required. As yet there are no trial data on use of this technique in other vessels, but angioplasty has been performed in the extracranial vertebral arteries and in the intracranial vessels. Case reports suggest that basilar artery procedures in particular may be a high risk. At present, these treatments should probably be reserved for patients with ongoing ischemic events despite best medical therapy and should be performed only by experienced specialists.

Editors' Note: The WASID study was terminated in August 2003. Results are expected to be published in 2004.

References

1. Ross R. Atherosclerosis—an inflammatory disease. N Engl J Med 1999;340:115–126.
2. Mitchell JRA, Schwartz CJ. Relationship between arterial disease in different sites: a study of the aorta and coronary, carotid and iliac arteries. BMJ 1962;1:1293–1301.
3. Hertzer NR, Young JR, Beven EG, et al. Coronary angiography in 506 patients with extracranial cerebrovascular disease. Arch Intern Med 1985;145:849–852.
4. Caplan LR, Gorelick PB, Hier DB. Race, sex and occlusive cerebrovascular disease: a review. Stroke 1986;17:648–655.
5. Inzitari D, Hachinski VC, Taylor DW, Barnett HJ. Racial differences in the anterior circulation in cerebrovascular disease. How much can be explained by risk factors? Arch Neurol 1990; 47:1080–1084.
6. Sacco RL, Kargman DE, Gu Q, Zamanillo MC. Race-ethnicity and determinants of intracranial atherosclerotic cerebral infarction. The Northern Manhattan Stroke Study. Stroke 1995; 26:14–20.
7. Wityk RJ, Lehman D, Klag M, et al. Race and sex differences in the distribution of cerebral atherosclerosis. Stroke 1996;27:1974–1980.
8. Leung SY, Ng TH, Yuen ST, et al. Pattern of cerebral atherosclerosis in Hong Kong Chinese. Severity in intracranial and extracranial vessels. Stroke 1993;24:779–786.
9. Feldmann E, Daneault N, Kwan E, et al. Chinese-white differences in the distribution of occlusive cerebrovascular disease. Neurology 1990;40:1541–1545.
10. Gorelick PB. Distribution of atherosclerotic cerebrovascular lesions. Effects of age, race, and sex. Stroke 1993;24:I16–I19.
11. Gorelick PB, Caplan LR, Hier DB, et al. Racial differences in the distribution of anterior circulation occlusive disease. Neurology 1984;34:54–59.
12. Gorelick PB, Caplan LR, Hier DB, et al. Racial differences in the distribution of posterior circulation occlusive disease. Stroke 1985;16:785–790.

13. Fisher CM. Occlusion of the carotid arteries. Archives of neurology and psychiatry 1954; 72:187–204.
14. Fisher CM. Occlusion of the internal carotid artery. Arch Neurol Psychiatry 1951;65:346–377.
15. Hutchinson EC, Yates PO. Caratico-vertebral stenosis. Lancet 1957;1:2–8.
16. Schwartz CJ, Mitchell JRA. Atheroma of the carotid and vertebral arterial systems. BMJ 1961; 2:1057–1063.
17. Hass WK, Fields WS, North RR. Joint study of extracranial arterial occlusion. II. Arteriography: techniques, sites, and complications. JAMA 1968;203:961–968.
18. Heinzlef O, Cohen A, Amarenco P. An update on aortic causes of ischemic stroke. Curr Opin Neurol 1997;10:64–72.
19. Hennerici M, Aulich A, Sandmann W, Freund HJ. Incidence of asymptomatic extracranial arterial disease. Stroke 1981;12:750–758.
20. Moosy J. Morphology, sites and epidemiology of cerebral atherosclerosis in research publications. Assoc Res Nerv Ment Dis 2002;51:1–22.
21. Cornhill JF, Akins D, Hutson M, Chandler AB. Localization of atherosclerotic lesions in the human basilar artery. Atherosclerosis 1980;35:77–86.
22. Castaigne P, Lhermitte F, Gautier JC. Arterial occlusions in the vertebrobasilar system. A study of 44 patients with post mortem data. Brain 1973;96:133–154.
23. Meyer JS, Sheehan S, Bauer RB. An arteriographic study of cerebrovascular disease in man. I. Stenosis and occlusion of the vertebro-basilar arterial system. Arch Neurol 1960; 2:27–45.
24. Lhermitte F, Gautier JC, Derouesne C. Nature of occlusions of the middle cerebral artery. Neurology 1970;20:82–88.
25. Ogata J, Masuda J, Yutani C, Yamaguchi T. Mechanisms of cerebral artery thrombosis: a histopathological analysis on eight necropsy cases. J Neurol Neurosurg Psychiatry 1994;57:17–21.
26. Sandercock PA, Warlow CP, Jones LN, Starkey IR. Predisposing factors for cerebral infarction: the Oxfordshire community stroke project. BMJ 1989;298:75–80.
27. Bamford J, Sandercock P, Dennis M, et al. Classification and natural history of clinically identifiable subtypes of cerebral infarction. Lancet 1991;337:1521–1526.
28. Amarenco P, Cohen A, Tzourio C, et al. Atherosclerotic disease of the aortic arch and the risk of ischemic stroke. N Engl J Med 1994;331:1474–1479.
29. Jones EF, Kalman JM, Calafiore P, et al. Proximal aortic atheroma. An independent risk factor for cerebral ischemia. Stroke 1995;26:218–224.
30. Rothwell PM, Gibson R, Warlow CP. Interrelation between plaque surface morphology and degree of stenosis on carotid angiograms and the risk of ischemic stroke in patients with symptomatic carotid stenosis. On behalf of the European Carotid Surgery Trialists' Collaborative Group. Stroke 2000;31:615–621.
31. MRC European Carotid Surgery Trial: interim results for symptomatic patients with severe (70-99%) or with mild (0-29%) carotid stenosis. European Carotid Surgery Trialists' Collaborative Group. Lancet 1991;337:1235–1243.
32. Beneficial effect of carotid endarterectomy in symptomatic patients with high-grade carotid stenosis. North American Symptomatic Carotid Endarterectomy Trial Collaborators. N Engl J Med 1991; 325:445–453.
33. Benavente O, Moher D, Pham B. Carotid endarterectomy for asymptomatic carotid stenosis: a meta-analysis. BMJ 1998;317:1477–1480.
34. Failure of extracranial-intracranial arterial bypass to reduce the risk of ischemic stroke. Results of an international randomized trial. The EC/IC Bypass Study Group. N Engl J Med 1985; 313:1191–1200.
35. Bogousslavsky J, Barnett HJ, Fox AJ, et al. Atherosclerotic disease of the middle cerebral artery. Stroke 1986;17:1112–1120.
36. Caplan LR. Proximal Extracranial Occlusive Disease: Subclavian, Innominate, and Proximal Vertebral Arteries. In Posterior Circulation Disease. Cambridge, Mass: Blackwell Science, 1996; 198–230.
37. Moufarrij NA, Little JR, Furlan AJ, et al. Vertebral artery stenosis: long-term follow-up. Stroke 1984;15:260–263.
38. Caplan LR, Amarenco P, Rosengart A, et al. Embolism from vertebral artery origin occlusive disease. Neurology 1992;42:1505–1512.
39. Moufarrij NA, Little JR, Furlan AJ, et al. Basilar and distal vertebral artery stenosis: long-term follow-up. Stroke 1986;17:938–942.
40. Chimowitz MI, Kokkinos J, Strong J, et al. The Warfarin-Aspirin Symptomatic Intracranial Disease Study. Neurology 1995;45:1488–1493.

41. Whisnant JP, Wiebers DO. Clinical Epidemiology of Transient Cerebral Ischaemic Attacks (TIA) in the Anterior and Posterior Cerebral Circulation. In TM Sundt Jr (ed), Occlusive Cerebrovascular Disease: Diagnosis and Surgical Management. Philadelphia: Saunders, 1987;60–65.
42. Dennis M, Bamford J, Sandercock P, Warlow C. Prognosis of transient ischemic attacks in the Oxfordshire Community Stroke Project. Stroke 1990;21:848–853.
43. Hankey GJ, Slattery JM, Warlow CP. The prognosis of hospital-referred transient ischaemic attacks. J Neurol Neurosurg Psychiatry 1991;54:793–802.
44. Torvik A, Svindland A, Lindboe CF. Pathogenesis of carotid thrombosis. Stroke 1989;20:1477–1483.
45. Ogata J, Masuda J, Yutani C, Yamaguchi T. Rupture of atheromatous plaque as a cause of thrombotic occlusion of stenotic internal carotid artery. Stroke 1990;21:1740–1745.
46. Ware JA, Heistad DD. Seminars in medicine of the Beth Israel Hospital, Boston. Platelet-endothelium interactions. N Engl J Med 1993;328:628–635.
47. Rothwell PM, Villagra R, Gibson R, et al. Evidence of a chronic systemic cause of instability of atherosclerotic plaques. Lancet 2000;355:19–24.
48. Goldstein LB, Adams R, Becker K, et al. Primary prevention of ischemic stroke: a statement for healthcare professionals from the Stroke Council of the American Heart Association. Stroke 2001;32:280–299.
49. Reed DM. The paradox of high risk of stroke in populations with low risk of coronary heart disease. Am J Epidemiol 1990;131:579–588.
50. Collaborative overview of randomised trials of antiplatelet therapy—I: prevention of death, myocardial infarction, and stroke by prolonged antiplatelet therapy in various categories of patients. Antiplatelet Trialists' Collaboration. BMJ 1994;308:81–106.
51. Antithrombotic Trialists' Collaboration. Collaborative meta-analysis of randomized trials of antiplatelet therapy for prevention of death, myocardial infarction and stroke in high risk patients. BMJ 2002;342:71–86.
52. A randomised, blinded, trial of clopidogrel versus aspirin in patients at risk of ischaemic events (CAPRIE). CAPRIE Steering Committee. Lancet 1996;348:1329–1339.
53. European Stroke Prevention Study. ESPS Group. Stroke 1990;21:1122–1130.
54. Sivenius J, Riekkinen PJ, Smets P, et al. The European Stroke Prevention Study (ESPS): results by arterial distribution. Ann Neurol 1991;29:596–600.
55. Barnett HJ. The Canadian Cooperative Study of Platelet Suppressive Drugs in Transient Cerebral Ischemia. In T Price and E Nelson (eds), Cerebrovascular Disease. Proceedings of the Eleventh Princeton Conference. New York: Raven Press, 1979;221.
56. Kubik CS, Adams RD. Occlusion of the basilar artery: a clinical and pathological study. Brain 1946;69:73–121.
57. Millikan CH, Siekert R, Shick R. Studies in cerebrovascular disease III. The use of anticoagulant drugs in the treatment of insufficiency or thrombosis within the basilar arterial system. Staff Meet Mayo Clin 2002;30:116–126.
58. Whisnant JP. Discussion in Cerebral Vascular Diseases. In CH Millikan, R Siekert, JP Whisnant JP (eds), Third Princeton Conference on Cerebrovascular Diseases. Orlando: Grune & Stratton, 1961; 56–157.
59. Redman AR, Allen LC. Warfarin versus aspirin in the secondary prevention of stroke: the WARSS Study. Curr Atheroscl Rep 2002;4:319–325.
60. Algra A, Francke CL, Koehler PJJ. A randomized trial of anticoagulants versus aspirin after cerebral ischaemia of presumed arterial origin. Ann Neurol 1997;42:857–865.
61. The following is a list of major ongoing studies about stroke. Information about other multicenter studies that might be included in this list should be submitted to the Stroke Editorial Office by the Principal Investigator. The list will appear in the February, June, and October issues of Stroke. Stroke 1999;30:2256–2261.
62. Thijs VN, Albers GW. Symptomatic intracranial atherosclerosis: outcome of patients who fail antithrombotic therapy. Neurology 2000;55:490–497.
63. Rodgers A, MacMahon S, Gamble G, et al. Blood pressure and risk of stroke in patients with cerebrovascular disease. The United Kingdom Transient Ischaemic Attack Collaborative Group. BMJ 1996;313:147.
64. Randomised trial of a perindopril-based blood-pressure-lowering regimen among 6,105 individuals with previous stroke or transient ischaemic attack. Lancet 2001;358:1033–1041.
65. Mercuri M, Bond MG, Sirtori CR, et al. Pravastatin reduces carotid intima-media thickness progression in an asymptomatic hypercholesterolemic Mediterranean population: the Carotid Atherosclerosis Italian Ultrasound Study. Am J Med 1996;101:627–634.
66. MRC/BHF Heart Protection Study of cholesterol lowering with simvastatin in 20,536 high-risk individuals: a randomised placebo-controlled trial. Lancet 2002;360:7–22.

67. Hsia DC, Moscoe LM, Krushat WM. Epidemiology of carotid endarterectomy among Medicare beneficiaries: 1985-1996 update. Stroke 1998;29:346–350.
68. Tu JV, Hannan EL, Anderson GM, et al. The fall and rise of carotid endarterectomy in the United States and Canada. N Engl J Med 1998;339:1441–1447.
69. Fields WS, Maslenikov V, Meyer JS, et al. Joint study of extracranial arterial occlusion. V. Progress report of prognosis following surgery or nonsurgical treatment for transient cerebral ischemic attacks and cervical carotid artery lesions. JAMA 1970;211:1993–2003.
70. Shaw DA, Venables GS, Cartlidge NE, et al. Carotid endarterectomy in patients with transient cerebral ischaemia. J Neurol Sci 1984;64:45–53.
71. Mayberg MR, Wilson SE, Yatsu F, et al. Carotid endarterectomy and prevention of cerebral ischemia in symptomatic carotid stenosis. Veterans Affairs Cooperative Studies Program 309 Trialist Group. JAMA 1991;266:3289–3294.
72. Randomised trial of endarterectomy for recently symptomatic carotid stenosis: final results of the MRC European Carotid Surgery Trial (ECST). Lancet 1998;351:1379–1387.
73. Barnett HJ, Taylor DW, Eliasziw M, et al. Benefit of carotid endarterectomy in patients with symptomatic moderate or severe stenosis. North American Symptomatic Carotid Endarterectomy Trial Collaborators. N Engl J Med 1998;339:1415–1425.
74. Rothwell PM, Gibson RJ, Slattery J, Warlow CP. Prognostic value and reproducibility of measurements of carotid stenosis. A comparison of three methods on 1001 angiograms. European Carotid Surgery Trialists' Collaborative Group. Stroke 1994;25:2440–2444.
75. Rothwell PM, Gutnikov S, Warlow CP, for the European Carotid Surgery Trialists' Collaboration. Re-analysis of the final results of the European Carotid Surgery Trial. Stroke 2003;34:514–523.
76. Morgenstern LB, Fox AJ, Sharpe BL, et al. The risks and benefits of carotid endarterectomy in patients with near occlusion of the carotid artery. North American Symptomatic Carotid Endarterectomy Trial (NASCET) Group. Neurology 1997;48:911–915.
77. Rothwell PM, Warlow CP. Low risk of ischemic stroke in patients with reduced internal carotid artery lumen diameter distal to severe symptomatic carotid stenosis: cerebral protection due to low poststenotic flow? On behalf of the European Carotid Surgery Trialists' Collaborative Group. Stroke 2000;31:622–630.
78. Goldstein LB, Hasselblad V, Matchar DB, McCrory DC. Comparison and meta-analysis of randomized trials of endarterectomy for symptomatic carotid artery stenosis. Neurology 1995;45:1965–1970.
79. Cina CS, Clase CM, Haynes RB. Carotid endarterectomy for symptomatic carotid stenosis (Cochrane review). The Cochrane Library Issue 3, 1999. Oxford: Update Software.
80. Rothwell PM, Gutnikov SA, Eliasziw M, et al. Pooled analysis of individual patient data from randomized controlled trials of endarterectomy for symptomatic carotid stenosis. Lancet 2003;361:107–116.
81. Rothwell PM, Mayberg MR, Warlow CP, Barnett HJ, for the Carotid Endarterectomy Trialists' Collaboration. Meta-analysis of individual patient data from randomised controlled trials of carotid endarterectomy for symptomatic stenosis: (3) the efficacy of surgery in important predefined subgroups. Cerebrovasc Dis 2000;10(suppl 2):1–109.
82. Halliday AW, Thomas D, Mansfield A. The Asymptomatic Carotid Surgery Trial (ACST). Rationale and design. Steering Committee. Eur J Vasc Surg 1994;8:703–710.
83. Hobson RW, Weiss DG, Fields WS, et al. Efficacy of carotid endarterectomy for asymptomatic carotid stenosis. The Veterans Affairs Cooperative Study Group. N Engl J Med 1993;328:221–227.
84. Endarterectomy for asymptomatic carotid artery stenosis. Executive Committee for the Asymptomatic Carotid Atherosclerosis Study. JAMA 1995;273:1421–1428.
85. Rothwell PM, Gutnikov S. The Asymptomatic Carotid Stenosis Study (ACSS): differences in time course of risk of ischaemic stroke distal to symptomatic and asymptomatic stenoses. Cerebrovasc Dis 1999;9(suppl 1):66.
86. Rothwell PM, Slattery J, Warlow CP. A systematic comparison of the risks of stroke and death due to carotid endarterectomy for symptomatic and asymptomatic stenosis. Stroke 1996;27:266–269.
87. Warlow CP. Extracranial to intracranial bypass and the prevention of stroke. J Neurol 1986;233:129–130.
88. Powers WJ, Grubb RL Jr, Raichle ME. Clinical results of extracranial-intracranial bypass surgery in patients with hemodynamic cerebrovascular disease. J Neurosurg 1989;70:61–67.
89. Grubb RL Jr, Derdeyn CP, Fritsch SM, et al. Importance of hemodynamic factors in the prognosis of symptomatic carotid occlusion. JAMA 1998;280:1055–1060.
90. Adams HP Jr, Powers WJ, Grubb RL Jr, et al. Preview of a new trial of extracranial-to-intracranial arterial anastomosis: the carotid occlusion surgery study. Neurosurg Clin N Am 2001;12:613.

91. Crawley F, Brown MM. Percutaneous transluminal angioplasty and stenting for vertebral artery stenosis (Cochrane review). The Cochrane Library Issue 4, 2000. Oxford: Update Software.
92. Berguer R, Kiefer E. Surgery of the Arteries to the Head. New York: Springer-Verlag, 1992.
93. Feldman AJ. Surgical Approach to Disease of the First Portion of the Vertebral Artery. In R Berguer, R Bauer (eds), Vertebrobasilar Arterial Occlusive Disease. New York: Raven, 1984;231–239.
94. Lee RE. Reconstruction of the Proximal Vertebral Artery. In R Berguer, LR Caplan (eds), Vertebrobasilar Arterial Disease. St. Louis: Quality Medical Publishers, 1992;211–224.
95. Walt A. The Story of Vertebrobasilar Surgery. In R Berguer R, R Bauer R (eds), Vertebrobasilar Arterial Occlusive Disease. New York: Raven, 1984;225–230.
96. Thevenet A. Endarterectomy of the Vertebral Artery. In R Berguer, LR Caplan (eds), Vertebrobasilar Arterial Disease. St. Louis: Quality Medical Publishers, 1992;224–235.
97. Bornstein NM, Norris JW. Subclavian steal: a harmless haemodynamic phenomenon? Lancet 1986;2:303–305.
98. Hennerici M, Klemm C, Rautenberg W. The subclavian steal phenomenon: a common vascular disorder with rare neurologic deficits. Neurology 1988;38:669–673.
99. Dotter CT, Judkins MP. Transluminal treatment of arteriosclerotic obstruction. Description of a new technique and a preliminary report of its application. Circulation 1964;30:654–670.
100. Endovascular versus surgical treatment in patients with carotid stenosis in the Carotid and Vertebral Artery Transluminal Angioplasty Study (CAVATAS): a randomised trial. Lancet 2001;357: 1729–1737.
101. Naylor AR, London NJ, Bell PR. Carotid and Vertebral Artery Transluminal Angioplasty Study. Lancet 1997;349:1324–1325.
102. Alberts MJ for the Publications Committee of the WALLSTENT. Results of a multicentre prospective randomised trial of carotid artery stenting vs. carotid endarterectomy. Stroke 2001;32:325.
103. Reimers B, Corvaja N, Moshiri S, et al. Cerebral protection with filter devices during carotid artery stenting. Circulation 2001;104:12–15.
104. Motarjeme A, Keifer JW, Zuska AJ. Percutaneous transluminal angioplasty of the brachiocephalic arteries. AJR Am J Roentgenol 1982;138:457–462.
105. Zeumer H. Vascular recanalizing techniques in interventional neuroradiology. J Neurol 1985; 231:287–294.
106. Schutz H, Yeung HP, Chiu MC, et al. Dilatation of vertebral-artery stenosis. N Engl J Med 1981;304:732.
107. Higashida RT, Tsai FY, Halbach VV, et al. Transluminal angioplasty for atherosclerotic disease of the vertebral and basilar arteries. J Neurosurg 1993;78:192–198.
108. Clark WM, Barnwell SL, Nesbit G, et al. Safety and efficacy of percutaneous transluminal angioplasty for intracranial atherosclerotic stenosis. Stroke 1995;26:1200–1204.
109. Marks MP, Marcellus M, Norbash AM, et al. Outcome of angioplasty for atherosclerotic intracranial stenosis. Stroke 1999;30:1065–1069.
110. Connors JJ III, Wojak JC. Percutaneous transluminal angioplasty for intracranial atherosclerotic lesions: evolution of technique and short-term results. J Neurosurg 1999;91:415–423.
111. Sundt TM Jr, Smith HC, Campbell JK, et al. Transluminal angioplasty for basilar artery stenosis. Mayo Clin Proc 1980;55:673–680.
112. Piepgras DG, Sundt TM Jr, Forbes GS, Smith HC. Balloon Catheter Transluminal Angioplasty for Vertebrobasilar Ischemia. In R Berguer, R Bauer (eds). Vertebrobasilar Arterial Occlusive Disease. New York: Raven, 1984;215–224.
113. Dorman PJ, Sandercock PA. Considerations in the design of clinical trials of neuroprotective therapy in acute stroke. Stroke 1996;27:1507–1515.
114. Markus H, Loh A, Brown MM. Computerized detection of cerebral emboli and discrimination from artifact using Doppler ultrasound. Stroke 1993;24:1667–1672.
115. Siebler M, Sitzer M, Rose G, et al. Silent cerebral embolism caused by neurologically symptomatic high-grade carotid stenosis. Event rates before and after carotid endarterectomy. Brain 1993; 116(Pt 5):1005–1015.
116. Forteza AM, Babikian VL, Hyde C, et al. Effect of time and cerebrovascular symptoms of the prevalence of microembolic signals in patients with cervical carotid stenosis. Stroke 1996;27:687–690.
117. Sitzer M, Muller W, Siebler M, et al. Plaque ulceration and lumen thrombus are the main sources of cerebral microemboli in high-grade internal carotid artery stenosis. Stroke 1995; 26:1231–1233.
118. Vernieri F, Pasqualetti P, Passarelli F, et al. Outcome of carotid artery occlusion is predicted by cerebrovascular reactivity. Stroke 1999;30:593–598.

119. Blaser T, Hofmann K, Buerger T, et al. Risk of stroke, transient ischemic attack, and vessel occlusion before endarterectomy in patients with symptomatic severe carotid stenosis. Stroke 2002; 33:1057–1062.
120. Markus H, Cullinane M. Severely impaired cerebrovascular reactivity predicts stroke and TIA risk in patients with carotid artery stenosis and occlusion. Brain 2001;124:457–467.
121. Molloy J, Markus HS. Asymptomatic embolization predicts stroke and TIA risk in patients with carotid artery stenosis. Stroke 1999;30:1440–1443.
122. Henderson RD, Eliasziw M, Fox AJ, et al. Angiographically defined collateral circulation and risk of stroke in patients with severe carotid artery stenosis. North American Symptomatic Carotid Endarterectomy Trial (NASCET) Group. Stroke 2000;31:128–132.

7

Small-Vessel Occlusive Disease (Lacunar Stroke)

Oscar Benavente

In 1901, Pierre Marie introduced the term *lacunar stroke* to describe a patient with a capsular infarct. Miller Fisher established the term *lacunar syndrome* in the early 1960s and correlated these distinct clinical syndromes with small infarcts in deep areas of the brain. Five lacunar syndromes were described, and the infarcts were supposed to result from occlusion of one of the perforating arteries.[1-4]

Lacunar strokes or small subcortical strokes are an important subtype of ischemic stroke, accounting for more than 25 percent of brain infarcts[5-13] (Table 7.1). They are particularly frequent in Hispanic Americans and African Americans.[14] Lacunes tend to occur at a younger age than other types of ischemic strokes[15] and are the most common cause of vascular dementia.[16,17]

Lacunes are commonly located in the basal ganglia, internal capsule, thalamus, or brain stem. Conventionally, their size ranges from 3 to 15 mm in diameter, and most are caused by occlusion of a single, small, deep penetrating artery.[3,18,19] Despite the fact that lacunar strokes are relatively small in size, they can cause severe neurological deficits because of their strategic location.

Any cause of brain ischemia (e.g., cardiogenic embolism or carotid stenosis) can occasionally cause a lacunar infarct.[20-23] However, most lacunar strokes result from diseases of the small cerebral penetrating arteries (size between 200 to 800 µm in diameter). Two pathological types of small-artery disease are responsible for most lacunes: (1) lipohyalinosis, characterized by segmental disorganization of the vessel wall with replacement by fibrin and collagen deposits (this condition is most likely secondary to the effect of chronic hypertension) and (2) microatheroma in which a small atheromatous plaque occludes the origin of the affected penetrating vessel, which tends to result in larger lesions. The latter is believed to be responsible for larger subcortical infarcts, whereas lipohyalinosis tends to affect smaller arteries leading to smaller subcortical infarcts.[19,24] Patchy or diffuse abnormalities in the deep cerebral white matter, which appear as hypodensities on computed tomography (CT) or

Table 7.1   Frequency of patients with lacunar stroke in case series

Study	No. of Patients with Ischemic Stroke	Lacunar Stroke (%)
Rothrock et al[11]	500	27
Mohr et al[12]	579	23
Yip et al[10]	676	29
Bamford et al[9]	515	21
Chamorro et al[5]	1273	26
Boon et al[8]	755	27
Kolominsky-Rabas et al[6]	583	26
Wolfe et al[7]	862	33
Bogousslavsky et al[13]	778	19
Vivo et al[111]	231	29
de Jong et al[88]	998	34
Aggregate	**7750**	**27**

high-intensity signals on T2-weighted magnetic resonance imaging (MRI) sequences are common findings in patients with lacunes.[25,26] Multiple lacunar strokes correlate with the extent of white matter abnormality on MRI[27–30] (Figure 7.1). It is likely that both conditions, white matter abnormalities and lacunar infarcts, reflect a shared pathophysiology (i.e., small cerebral artery disease).

LACUNAR SYNDROMES

The diagnosis of lacunar stroke is based on the description of the clinical syndrome, which is corroborated by the findings on brain imaging studies (CT or MRI). A lacunar stroke syndrome is identified based on the constellation of symptoms and/or signs resulting from lesions in areas of the brain supplied by the small penetrating arteries, without symptoms and/or signs of cortical dysfunction such as aphasia, visual field defect, apraxia, neglect, and so forth, after other structural lesions have been excluded (Table 7.2).

Classic lacunar syndromes are commonly accompanied by a small, deep infarction, and each syndrome typically is associated with specific locations.[31,32] Several clinical syndromes have been associated to lacunar stroke, but only five are well characterized: pure motor hemiparesis (PMH), sensorimotor stroke (SMS), pure sensory stroke (PSS), dysarthria clumsy hand syndrome, and ataxic hemiparesis.[2–4,18,19,33,34] Lacunar syndromes have an overall positive predictive value of 87 percent for detecting radiological lacunar infarct. The PSS has the highest positive predictive value and PMH the lowest (100% and 79%, respectively).[21]

Pure Motor Hemiparesis

PMH, also known as pure motor stroke, is the most common form of lacunar syndrome, accounting for more than half of the cases.[21,35,36] In the original

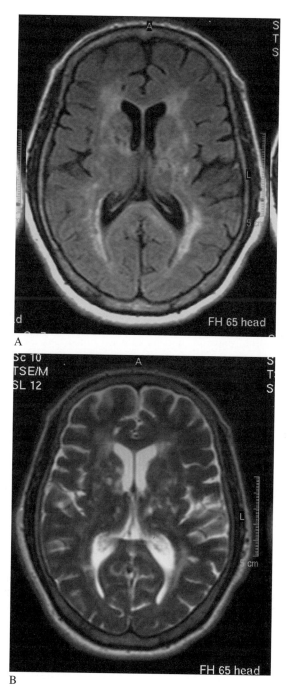

Figure 7.1 (A, B) Fluid-attenuated inversion-recovery (FLAIR) and T2-weighted magnetic resonance imaging (MRI) sequences: multiple lacunar infarcts and severe white matter abnormalities.

Table 7.2   Lacunar syndromes with possible lesion sites

Lacunar Syndrome	Lesion Site
Pure motor hemiparesis (PMH)	Internal capsule
	Pons
	Midbrain
	Corona radiata
Pure sensory stroke (PSS)	Thalamus
	Internal capsule
Sensory motor stroke	Thalamocapsular
Ataxic hemiparesis	Internal capsule
	Thalamus
	Pons
Dysarthria-clumsy hand	Pons
	Genu internal capsule

description of this syndrome, Fisher included "paralysis complete or incomplete of the face, arm and leg on one side without sensory signs, visual field defects, dysphasia or apractognosia."[4] Sensory symptoms may be present but not sensory signs.[4] Autopsy-based studies of patients with PMH showed focal lesions involving the internal capsule, corona radiata, pons, and medullary pyramid. However, the most common location for the infarct is in the posterior limb of internal capsule.[37–39] Most of the PMH are due to a lacunar infarct; however, with newer and more sensitive neuroimaging techniques it may be possible to detect other pathological processes responsible for this syndrome. The classical presentation of the complete PMH syndrome is paresis or paralysis equally affecting face, arm, and leg unilaterally and sparing sensation, vision, language, and behavior. The complete syndrome is rarely present, and in most cases only parts are involved such as face and arm. In the presence of monoparesis, the diagnosis of small subcortical stroke should be questioned, because it is almost never caused by a lacunar infarct.[40]

Lacunes involving the internal capsule tend to produce symptoms equally affecting the face, arm, and leg. When infarcts involve more posterior aspects of the capsule, the leg has a greater deficit than the arm and face. Lesions in the basis pons resulting in PMH produce almost identical syndromes to those from internal capsule infarcts.

Even in patients with complete PMH, other symptoms are commonly present, especially sensory disturbances, which are present in up to 40 percent of the cases. Nevertheless, the sensory examination remains normal.[41]

Pure Sensory Stroke

PSS accounts for less than 10 percent of all lacunar syndromes; however, it has the highest predictive value in the diagnosis of a lacunar infarct.[5,21] It is possible to find cases with persistent symptoms in the absence of objective signs.[2] The lesions causing PSS are the smallest of the symptomatic, small, subcortical strokes.[5,42] Most of the patients have an infarct in the thalamus, and the remainder have an infarct in the anterior limb of the internal capsule. Involvement of all sensory modalities is usually associated with large lacunes in the lateral thalamus; partial sensory impairment implies smaller lacunes at any level of the sensory pathway.[43]

In complete hemisensory syndromes, the sensory deficit typically extends over the entire hemibody, involving the face and proximal and distal limbs with a remarkable midline split. This type of hemisensory syndrome usually results from thalamic involvement. In cases of incomplete syndromes, the sensory disturbance may affect the face, arm, leg, cheeks, lips, unilateral intraoral and perioral sites, and fingers, the so-called cheiro-oral syndrome. The incomplete syndromes are usually the result of small infarcts.

Sensorimotor Stroke

SMS was not one of the original lacunar syndromes described by Fisher. This presentation is relatively uncommon; however, in another series of lacunar stroke patients it was reported as the second most common syndrome after PMH.[5] The most common locations of lacunar strokes responsible for this syndrome are in the posterior limb of the internal capsule, followed by the corona radiata, genu, and anterior limb of the internal capsule. The specificity of SMS to predict a lacunar stroke is not as high as other classic lacunar syndromes. In several series, it was found that only 20 percent of patients presenting with SMS had a lacunar stroke confirmed by CT or MRI.[44,45]

Ataxic Hemiparesis

Ataxic hemiparesis was originally described as ipsilateral ataxia with crural paresis.[46,47] The responsible lesion most commonly found is in the pons; however, the anterior limb of the internal capsule or corona radiata have also been implicated.[48]

The usual presentation includes mild to moderate leg weakness with very mild involvement of the upper extremities or face, accompanied by ipsilateral ataxia of the arm and leg. Usually, the degree of ataxia is more impressive than the motor deficit. Frequently, the symptoms develop over hours or days.[49] Based on the presenting symptoms and signs, it is almost impossible to differentiate between pontine and hemispheric lacunes.

Dysarthria Clumsy-Hand Syndrome

In patients with dysarthria clumsy-hand syndrome, dysarthria and ataxia of the upper limb are the prominent features. However, other symptoms and signs may be also present, such as facial weakness, dysphagia, and rarely a mild degree of limb weakness. The most common locations for this syndrome are the anterior limb of the internal capsule and the basis pontis.[1] Usually the functional recovery of these patients is good.

Hemichorea-Hemiballismus

Lacunar infarcts responsible for hemichorea-hemiballismus syndrome involve the head of the caudate nucleus, the subthalamic nucleus, or thalamus.[50] The symptoms are usually abrupt in onset, and occasionally hemiparesis occurs weeks or months before the involuntary movements.

RISK FACTORS

Risk factors for lacunar stroke such as advancing age, hypertension, and diabetes are similar to those for atherothrombotic stroke. Perhaps the exception is hyperlipidemia, which does not to appear to be a risk factor for small subcortical strokes.[51]

Although lacunar infarcts have a unique pathophysiological mechanism,[2,34,52] the vascular risk factors are not exclusive to small-vessel disease, because they are similar to those present in atherothrombotic strokes. Therefore it is still not clear what determines whether small or large vessels will be affected in the presence of comparable risk factors.

Hypertension

Hypertension is a powerful independent risk factor for stroke but particularly for lacunar stroke. There is a direct correlation between blood pressure level and stroke risk.[53] The prevalence of hypertension is higher in lacunar stroke patients than in other stroke subtypes, and it is estimated that about 70 percent of patients with lacunar stroke have a history of hypertension.[54-57] The risk of lacunar infarct is increased between fivefold to ninefold by hypertension.[58-60] In addition, hypertension appears to play a key role in the development and severity of cerebral small-artery disease. Autopsy-based studies show an association between a history of hypertension and the presence of lacunar infarcts, with diastolic hypertension (rather than systolic hypertension) as a stronger predictor for the development of multiple infarcts.[61,62]

Diabetes Mellitus

Diabetes mellitus (DM) is also a major risk factor for stroke in general. Case-controlled studies show DM as an independent risk factor for lacunes, with a prevalence ranging from 2 to 55 percent.[30,58-60] The overall prevalence of DM is not different in lacunar strokes when compared with other stroke subtypes. Therefore it is unlikely that DM is an exclusive risk factor for small-vessel disease.

Heart Disease

The data about ischemic heart disease (IHD) and lacunar stroke are conflicting. Several case-controlled studies showed that IHD was not a risk factor for lacunar infarct, whereas others found that IHD increased the risk of stroke by threefold.[59,60] Overall, between 8 to 40 percent of lacunar stroke patients have a history of coronary artery disease. Boiten et al[63] found IHD significantly less often in lacunar stroke patients when compared with nonlacunar stroke patients. Thus despite the paucity of data in this area, it seems that cardiac emboli are an unlikely cause of lacunar infarct.

INVESTIGATIONS FOR LACUNAR STROKES

Neuroimaging Studies

On CT scan or T1-weighted imaging (MRI), a lacunar infarct appears as an area of hypodensity; on T2-weighted sequence, a lacunar infarct appears as an area of hyperintensity. The area of infarct is well demarcated in the region supplied by penetrating arteries (basal ganglia, internal capsule, corona radiata, or brain stem). Lacunar infarct is usually defined as measuring less than 1.5 cm in diameter.

The sensitivity of CT scan to detect a lesion in patients with a classical lacunar syndrome ranges from 10 to 50 percent.[64] On the contrary, MRI can demonstrate a lacunar infarct in up to 95 percent of patients presenting with a lacunar syndrome.[65] Diffusion-weighted imaging (DWI) is extremely sensitive in detecting early small subcortical infarcts, with a sensitivity of about 95 percent and specificity of 94 percent in detecting lacunar infarcts within the first 48 hours of symptom onset[31,66,67] (Figure 7.2). MRI with DWI is the preferred neuroimaging technique to visualize lacunar strokes, particularly during the acute stage and for those located in brain stem and cerebellum.

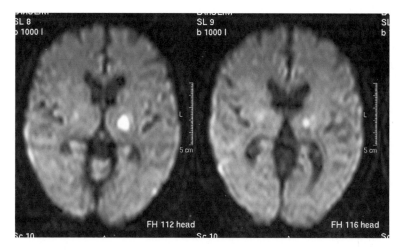

Figure 7.2 Patient presented with pure motor hemiparesis (PMH). Magnetic resonance imaging (MRI) with diffusion-weighted imaging (DWI) was performed 12 hours after symptom onset. Acute area of infarction in left internal capsule.

Carotid Imaging Studies

Searching for ipsilateral carotid stenosis in hemispheric stroke is justified only if the results will influence therapeutic management or give information about prognosis. The notion that lacunar infarcts could be caused by embolization from the internal carotid artery is still controversial but plausible.[68–70] Several case studies of lacunar stroke patients, in which carotid stenosis measurement and definition was not uniform, found that 5 to 19 percent of patients had significant ipsilateral carotid stenosis (>70%).[63,71–75] Carotid stenosis was not equally distributed among lacunar stroke patients; patients with multiple lacunes tended to have a lower frequency of carotid stenosis than those with a single lacune,[71] and those with strokes in the centrum semiovale had a higher frequency of ipsilateral stenosis when compared with lacunes located in the basal ganglia.[20]

Cardioembolic Source

Some patients with documented lacunar stroke have associated cardio-embolic disease. In these cases, it is unclear whether these findings are purely coincidental or represent the cause of the infarct.[55,58,76] Recent studies found that approximately 5 percent of patients with documented lacunar stroke have a cardiac source of embolism, particularly atrial fibrillation.[21,77–79]

At least one fourth of patients with radiological confirmed lacunar stroke are likely to have infarcts resulting from non–small-vessel disease (i.e., cardio-embolic or large-artery atherosclerosis).[21] Therefore given the uncertainty about the stroke mechanism, patients with lacunar strokes should be routinely investigated for other stroke causes that will influence their management poststroke, such extracranial large-artery atherosclerotic disease and potential cardio-embolic sources.

PROGNOSIS OF PATIENTS WITH LACUNAR STROKE

The prognosis of patients with lacunar stroke should be considered under four categories: mortality related to stroke, stroke recurrence, cognitive decline, and progression of asymptomatic disease.

Mortality Associated to Lacunar Strokes

The early mortality associated with lacunes is almost nil; studies that looked at this issue found a 30-day case-fatality rate ranging from 0 to 2 percent.[9,15,57,80] This can be explained by the small size of the infarct and the relatively mild stroke disability present in lacunar stroke patients. The long-term risk of death following a lacunar stroke averages 3 percent per year.[15,80] Overall, survival has been found to be more favorable in patients with lacunar infarcts than with other stroke subtypes.

Stroke Recurrence

Small subcortical strokes often cause relatively mild neurological disability;[15,81] however, multiple or recurrent lacunes can give rise to more severe clinical manifestations including lacunar state *(état lacunaire)* and vascular dementia. Prospective studies showed that the rate of recurrent stroke among patients with lacunar stroke ranged from 4 to 11 percent[9,15,57,82–86] (Table 7.3). Most recurrent strokes (about 60%) in lacunar stroke patients are also lacunes.[30] The event rate was not uniform across all studies, and most likely it was influenced by the severity of small-vessel disease or additional risk factors. For instance, preliminary reports from the Secondary Prevention of Small Subcortical Stroke (SPS3) pilot study showed that patients with symptomatic recent lacunes, assigned to antiplatelet therapy plus strict control of hypertension, had an early recurrent stroke rate higher than previously reported, particularly among Hispanic Americans, 15 percent per year (95% confidence interval [CI] 8 to 29) versus 6 percent per year (95% CI 1 to 22) in non-Hispanic Americans.[30,87] The presence of white matter abnormalities also predicts a high recurrent rate of stroke in this stroke subtype.[29,30,83]

Thus among lacunar stroke patients there are subgroups at different risks for stroke recurrence.[27,88] Risk-stratification schemes should be developed to characterize lacunar stroke patients at high versus low risk for recurrent stroke, and, based on these risks, the appropriate therapy balancing risk and benefit could be selected.

Small Subcortical Strokes and Risk of Vascular Dementia

Cognitive impairment following stroke has been recognized as an important outcome in stroke survivors. Patients with lacunar stroke are at risk of developing vascular dementia. Lacunar infarct is the most common stroke subtype that

Table 7.3   Recurrent ischemic stroke in patients with lacunar stroke

Study	No. of Patients	Recurrent Stroke (% per year)
Bamford et al[9]	102	11
Sacco et al[57]	78	10
Clavier et al[82]	172	4
Samuelsson et al[94]	81	7
Miyao et al[83]	190	9
Boiten and Lodder[15]	103	5
Salgado et al[85]	145	7
Petty et al[84]	72	7
WARSS[a,86]	1237	8
SPS3 pilot study[b,30]	80	10
Aggregate	**2260**	**8**

WARSS, Warfarin-Aspirin Recurrent Stroke Study.
[a]Outcome: stroke or death in patients assigned to aspirin or warfarin.
[b]Patients randomized to aspirin, clopidogrel, or both.

predisposes to vascular dementia;[16,17,89] asymptomatic lacunar infarcts are frequently present in patients with vascular dementia[90–92] (typically multiple and bilateral).[93] In two prospective studies, 11 percent and 23 percent of patients with first-ever lacunes developed vascular dementia over the following 3 years.[93,94] The estimated rate of clinically diagnosed vascular dementia in this stroke subtype has been reported as 3 to 5 percent per year.[83,94] The incidence of vascular dementia has been related to the rate of stroke recurrence; demented patients had a significantly higher rate of stroke recurrence than patients who did not develop dementia (56% vs. 17%). In addition, the presence of white matter abnormality has been found to be an independent risk factor for cognitive impairment in lacunar stroke patients.[83,95] Thus cognitive impairment is relatively common in patients who suffer symptomatic lacunes, and it is influenced by stroke recurrence and by the presence of multiple infarcts and white matter abnormalities. Therefore it seems reasonable to hypothesize that interventions that will reduce stroke recurrence may also prevent cognitive decline and vascular dementia in lacunar stroke patients.

Progression of Asymptomatic Small Artery Disease

Most lacunar infarcts are asymptomatic, and approximately 20 percent of the population aged 65 years have lacunes documented by MRI.[96] The presence of silent lacunes is a risk factor for stroke and cognitive decline.[96,97] Prospective studies showed between 10 and 50 percent new silent lacunes detected by MRI over a 3-year period,[98–100] with the rate of asymptomatic lacunes higher than the rate for symptomatic lacunes.[100] Progression of white matter abnormalities has also been reported in 40 percent of the lacunar stroke patients.[99] In summary, silent lacunes are frequent among healthy elderly individuals and are a risk factor for stroke recurrence and cognitive decline.

STROKE PREVENTION IN LACUNAR STROKES

Antiplatelet Therapy in Lacunar Stroke

Most lacunar strokes are due to disease of the small cerebral arteries and not to thrombus-related atheroma, although it is likely that the final event that leads to the vessel occlusion involves platelet aggregation and thrombus formation. Therefore it is sensible to speculate that antithrombotic agents that have been proven to prevent atherothrombotic strokes should be effective in preventing stroke recurrence and vascular dementia following lacunar stroke.

So far, there have been no stroke prevention trials focusing on this important stroke subtype. Therefore all the data concerning safety and efficacy of antiplatelet therapy in lacunar stroke patients are derived from subgroup analyses of clinical trials in which all ischemic strokes were studied together. Only five randomized clinical trials for secondary stroke prevention reported the outcomes separately in subgroups of participants with lacunar stroke as their index event.[86,101–104] The definition and diagnosis criteria of lacunar stroke vary among these studies.

In the French AICLA aspirin trial, a total of 603 patients with ischemic cerebral events were included in this double-blind study to determine whether aspirin or aspirin plus dipyridamole would reduce stroke recurrence over a 3-year period compared with placebo. Ninety-seven patients with lacunar stroke as the qualifying event were enrolled. Recurrent stroke was reduced by 69 percent ($p = 0.03$) among those with small subcortical stroke given aspirin +/− dipyridamole.[103]

The Canadian-American Ticlopidine Study (ticlopidine vs. placebo), enrolled 26 percent of participants with lacunar infarct as the qualifying event ($n = 275$). The overall risk reduction of composite outcome (stroke, myocardial infarction, and vascular death) was 30 percent (95% CI 8 to 48) in favor of ticlopidine. The relative risk reduction for the endpoint stroke and stroke death among lacunar patients assigned to ticlopidine was 50 percent per year (from 10% to 5%) with a wide confidence interval (95% CI 0.76 to 76).[104]

The Cilostazol Stroke Prevention Study conducted in Japan, randomized more than 1000 stroke patients (789 with lacunar stroke as the index event) to cilostazol or placebo within 6 months of the index event. The primary outcome was stroke recurrence; the overall risk reduction was 42 percent in favor of cilostazol. Lacunar stroke patients had a slightly superior benefit, with a risk reduction of 43 percent (95% CI 3 to 67), favoring active treatment.[101]

A fourth trial, the Chinese Acute Stroke Trial (CAST), randomized more than 6000 patients with lacunar stroke as the index event to aspirin or placebo and considered stroke recurrence or death within 30 days of entry. The event rate during this short period of time was 2.6 percent in those assigned to aspirin versus 2.9 percent in the placebo group, representing a 10 percent relative risk reduction (95% CI −0.5 to 1.1).[102]

The Warfarin-Aspirin Recurrent Stroke Study (WARSS) randomized 2206 patients with noncardioembolic stroke to aspirin or oral anticoagulant with a mean follow-up of 2 years; 1237 of the enrolled patients had a lacunar infarct as index event. The outcome of stroke or death in patients with lacunar stroke was 8 percent per year on aspirin and 9 percent per year in the warfarin group, although this trend in favor of aspirin did not reach statistical significance ($p = 0.31$).[86]

Recently, the African American Aspirin Stroke Prevention Study (AAASPS) was completed. In this study 1800 African-American patients with recent noncardioembolic stroke were randomized to receive ticlopidine (500 mg per day) or aspirin (650 mg per day). Lacunar stroke was the index event in 1021 patients. The primary outcome was the constellation of recurrent stroke, myocardial infarction, or vascular death. The event rate at 2 years was 20 percent among ticlopidine-treated patients and 16 percent among those assigned to aspirin; this difference was not statistically significant (hazard ratio 1.2, 95% CI 0.94 to 1.57). Although the event rate for patients with lacunar stroke was not reported separately, based on these data aspirin is a better choice for African-American patients with recent lacunar stroke.[105]

According to WARSS, antiplatelet agents should be used instead of oral anticoagulants for stroke prevention.[86] Aspirin remains the standard initial antiplatelet agent for patients with lacunar stroke. The combination of aspirin plus dipyridamole or clopidogrel alone may be acceptable alternatives. Adding clopidogrel to aspirin for secondary stroke prevention may produce additional benefits, but there is no evidence yet to support the use of this therapy. Until the results of clinical trials are available, the recommendations for other stroke subtypes seem reasonable.[106,107]

Carotid Endarterectomy for Lacunar Stroke

The benefit of carotid endarterectomy (CEA) for stroke prevention was proven in two large randomized clinical trials.[108] In both studies lacunar stroke was uncommon and more likely associated with a milder degree of carotid stenosis. In addition, in NASCET, no relationship to plaque irregularity and ulceration was observed in patients randomized with lacunar stroke as the index event.[109] In the European study, the small number of lacunar stroke patients did not allow one to draw conclusions about the efficacy of CEA in patients with small subcortical strokes and carotid stenosis.[110] Inzitari et al.[109] in a subgroup analysis from the NASCET study found a nonsignificant benefit of CEA (relative risk reduction 53%, 95% CI −100 to 81%) for patients with lacunar stroke and severe carotid stenosis.

Based on the available data, there is insufficient evidence to routinely recommend CEA for all lacunar stroke patients with carotid stenosis. Nevertheless, for selected patients with a high degree of ipsilateral carotid stenosis ($\geq70\%$), CEA may be an alternative as long as the surgical complication risk does not exceed 6 percent.[109]

In summary, intracranial small artery disease remains understudied relative to its importance. It is a leading cause of neurological disability, because it causes lacunar stroke, white matter abnormalities, and vascular dementia. Further research in this area is needed, with randomized clinical trials focusing on populations with small subcortical strokes, the development of risk stratifications, and better assessment of the risk benefit for the use of antiplatelet agents. The Secondary Prevention of Small Subcortical Strokes (SPS3) phase III NIH-NINDS funded trial will enroll 2500 with symptomatic small subcortical strokes proven by MRI. Patients will be randomized in a factorial design to two interventions: (1) antiplatelet therapy—aspirin 325 mg per day or aspirin + clopidogrel 75 mg per day and (2) systolic targets of blood pressure control—"intensive" less than 130 mm Hg or "usual" 130 to 149 mm Hg. SPS3 aims to define the optimal intervention to prevent stroke recurrence and cognitive impairment in patients with lacunar stroke. The study started enrolling patients in May 2003; recruitment will be over a period of 3 years, with an additional 1.5 years of follow-up. The SPS3 study is the first trial for secondary stroke prevention focusing on patients with lacunar stroke.

Acknowledgment

This work was supported in part by a research grant from the National Institute of Neurological Disorders and Stroke: 2R01 NS 38529-04A1.

References

1. Fisher CM. A lacunar stroke. The dysarthria-clumsy hand syndrome. Neurology 1967;17:614–617.
2. Fisher CM. Pure sensory stroke involving face, arm, and leg. Neurology 1965;15:76–80.
3. Fisher CM. Lacunes: small, deep cerebral infarcts. Neurology 1965;15:774–784.
4. Fisher CM, Curry HB. Pure motor hemiplegia of vascular origin. Arch Neurol 1965;13:30–44.

5. Chamorro A, Sacco RL, Mohr JP, et al. Clinical-computed tomographic correlations of lacunar infarction in the Stroke Data Bank. Stroke 1991;22:175–181.
6. Kolominsky-Rabas PL, Weber M, Gefeller O, et al. Epidemiology of ischemic stroke subtypes according to TOAST criteria. Incidence, recurrence, and long-term survival in ischemic stroke subtypes: a population-based study. Stroke 2001;32:2735–2740.
7. Wolfe CDA, Rudd AG, Howard R, et al. Incidence and case fatality rates of stroke subtypes in a multiethnic population: the South London Stroke Register. J Neurol Neurosurg Psychiatry 2002; 72:211–216.
8. Boon A, Lodder J, Heuts-van Raak L, et al. Silent brain infarcts in 755 consecutive patients with a first-ever supratentorial ischemic stroke. Stroke 1994;25:2384–2390.
9. Bamford JM, Sandercock P, Jones L, et al. The natural history of lacunar infarction: the Oxfordshire Community Stroke Project. Stroke 1987;18:545–551.
10. Yip PK, Jeng JS, Lee TK, et al. Subtypes of ischemic stroke. A hospital-based stroke registry in Taiwan (SCAN-IV). Stroke 1997;28:2507–2512.
11. Rothrock JF, Lyden PD, Brody ML. Analysis of ischemic stroke in an urban southern California population. Arch Intern Med 1993;153:619–624.
12. Mohr JP, Caplan LR, Melski JW, et al. The Harvard Cooperative Stroke Registry: a prospective registry. Neurology 1978;28:754–762.
13. Bogousslavsky J, Van Melle G, Regli F. The Lausanne Stroke Registry: analysis of 1,000 consecutive patients with first stroke. For the Lausanne Stroke Registry Group. Stroke 1988;19:1083–1092.
14. Hartmann A, Rundek T, Mast H, et al. Mortality and causes of death after first ischemic stroke: the Northern Manhattan Stroke Study. Neurology 2001;57:2000–2005.
15. Boiten J, Lodder J. Prognosis for survival, handicap and recurrence of stroke in lacunar and superficial stroke. Cerebrovasc Dis 1993;3:221–226.
16. Ross G, Petrovitch H, White L, et al. Characterization of risk factors for vascular dementia: The Honolulu-Asia aging Study. Neurology 1999;53(2):337–343.
17. Tatemichi TK, Desmond D, Paik M, et al. Clinical determinants of dementia related to stroke. Ann Neurol 1993;33:568–575.
18. Fisher CM. Lacunar strokes and infarcts: a review. Neurology 1982;32:871–876.
19. Fisher CM. Thalamic pure sensory stroke: a pathologic study. Neurology 1978;28:1141–1144.
20. Boiten J, Rothwell PM, Slattery J, et al. Frequency and degree of carotid stenosis in small centrum ovale infarcts as compared to lacunar infarcts. Cerebrovasc Dis 1996;7:138–143.
21. Gan R, Sacco RL, Kargman DE, et al. Testing the validity of the lacunar hypothesis: the Northern Manhattan Stroke Study experience. Neurology 1997;48:1204–1211.
22. Wong KS, Gao S, Chan YL, et al. Mechanisms of acute cerebral infarction in patients with middle cerebral artery stenosis: a diffusion-weighted imaging and microemboli monitoring study. Ann Neurol 2002;52:74–81.
23. Young ME, Au R, Seshadri S, et al. White matter hyperintensity volume is associated with decreased executive functioning and attention: the Framingham Study (abstract). Neurology 2001;56(suppl 3).
24. Caplan L. Intracranial branch atheromatous disease: a neglected, understudied, and underused concept. Neurology 1989;39:1246–1250.
25. del Ser T, Bermejo F, Portera A, et al. Vascular dementia. A clinicopathological study. J Neurol Sci 1990;96:1–17.
26. Babikian V, Ropper AH. Binswanger's disease: a review. Stroke 1987;18:2–12.
27. Boiten J, Lodder J, Kessels F. Two clinically distinct lacunar infarct entities? A hypothesis. Stroke 1993;24:652–656.
28. Benavente O, Palacio S, Kesava P, et al. White matter abnormalities in lacunar stroke patients (abstract). Stroke 2001;32:28.
29. Benavente O, Eliasziw M, Streifler J, et al. Prognosis of lacunar stroke patients in association with leukoaraiosis (abstract). Stroke 2001;32:366.
30. Benavente O, Hart RG, Palacio S, et al. Secondary Prevention of Small Subcortical Strokes (SPS3) pilot trial: final results (abstract). Stroke 2003;34:238.
31. Schoneville W, Tuhrim S, Singer M, et al. Diffusion-weighted MRI in acute lacunar syndromes: a clinical-radiological correlation study. Stroke 1999;30:2066–2069.
32. Lindgren A, Staaf G, Geiger B, et al. Clinical lacunar syndromes as predictors of lacunar infarcts. A comparison of acute clinical lacunar syndromes and findings on diffusion-weighted MRI. Acta Neurol Scand 2000;101:128–134.
33. Fisher CM. Lacunar infarcts—a review. Cerebrovasc Dis 1991;1:311–320.
34. Fisher CM. Capsular infarcts. The underlying vascular lesions. Arch Neurol 1979;36(22):65–73.
35. Arboix A, Marti-Vilalta JL, Garcia JH. Clinical study of 227 patients with lacunar infarcts. Stroke 1990;21:842–847.

36. Foulkes MA, Wolf PA, Price TP, et al. The Stroke Data Bank: design, methods, and baseline characteristics. Stroke 1988;19:547–554.
37. Richter RW, Brust JC, Bruun B, et al. Frequency and course of pure motor hemiparesis: a clinical study. Stroke 1977;8:58–60.
38. Rascol A, Clanet M, Manelfe C, et al. Pure motor hemiplegia: CT study of 30 cases. Stroke 1982; 13:11–17.
39. Reimers J, de Wytt C, Seneviratne B. Lacunar infarction: a 12 month study. Clin Exp Neurol 1987; 24:28–32.
40. Misra UK, Kalita J. Putaminal haemorrhage leading to pure motor hemiplegia. Acta Neurol Scand 1995;91:283–286.
41. Donnan GA, Tress BM, Bladin PF. A prospective study of lacunar infarction using computerized tomography. Neurology 1982;32:49–56.
42. Hommel M, Besson G, Le Bas JF, et al. Prospective study of lacunar infarction using magnetic resonance imaging. Stroke 1990;21:546–554.
43. Kim JS. Pure sensory stroke. Clinical-radiological correlates of 21 cases. Stroke 1992;23:983–987.
44. Arboix A, Marti-Vilalta JL. Lacunar syndromes not due to lacunar infarcts. Cerebrovasc Dis 1992; 2:287–292.
45. Huang CY, Woo E, Yu YL, et al. When is sensorimotor stroke a lacunar syndrome? J Neurol Neurosurg Psychiatry 1987;50:720–726.
46. Perman GP, Racy A. Homolateral ataxia and crural paresis: case report. Neurology 1980; 30:1013–1015.
47. Fisher CM, Cole M. Homolateral ataxia and crural paresis. A vascular syndrome. J Neurol Neurosurg Psychiatry 1965;28:48.
48. Fisher CM. Ataxic hemiparesis. A pathologic study. Arch Neurol 1978;35:126–128.
49. Huang CY, Lui FS. Ataxic-hemiparesis, localization and clinical features. Stroke 1984;15:363–366.
50. Melamed E, Korn-Lubetzki I, Reches A, et al. Hemiballismus: detection of focal hemorrhage in subthalamic nucleus by CT scan. Ann Neurol 1978;4:582.
51. Janssens E, Mounier-Vehier F, Hamon M, et al. Small subcortical infarcts and primary subcortical haemorrhages may have different risk factors. J Neurol 1995;242:425–429.
52. Fisher CM. The arterial lesions underlying lacunes. Acta Neuropathol (Berlin) 1969;12:1–15.
53. Collins R, Peto R, MacMahon SW. Blood pressure, stroke and coronary heart disease. Part 2. Lancet 1990;335:827–838.
54. Lammie AG, Brannan F. Nonhypertensive cerebral small-vessel disease. Stroke 1997;28: 2222–2229.
55. Lodder J, Bamford JM. Are hypertension or cardiac embolism likely causes of lacunar infarction? Stroke 1990;21:375–381.
56. Mast H, Thompson AJ, Lee SH, et al. Hypertension and diabetes mellitus as determinants of multiple lacunar infarcts. Stroke 1995;26:30–33.
57. Sacco SE, Whisnant JP, Broderick JP, et al. Epidemiological characteristics of lacunar infarcts in a population. Stroke 1991;22:1236–1241.
58. Boiten J, Luijckx GJ, Kessels F, et al. Risk factors for lacunes. Neurology 1996;47:1109–1110.
59. Gandolfo C, Caponnetto C, Del Sette M, et al. Risk factors in lacunar syndromes: a case-control study. Acta Neurol Scand 1988;77:22–26.
60. You R, McNeil JJ, O'Malley HM, et al. Risk factors for lacunar infarction syndromes. Neurology 1995;45:1483–1487.
61. Dozono K, Ishii N, Nishihara Y, et al. An autopsy study of the incidence of lacunes in relation to age, hypertension, and arteriosclerosis. Stroke 1991;22:993–996.
62. Tuszynski MH, Petito CK, Levy DE. Risk factors and clinical manifestations of pathologically verified lacunar infarctions. Stroke 1989;20:990–999.
63. Boiten J, Lodder J. Lacunar infarcts. Pathogenesis and validity of the clinical syndromes. Stroke 1991;22:1374–1378.
64. Toni D, Iweins F, von Kummer R, et al. Identification of lacunar infarcts before thrombolysis in the ECASS I study. Neurology 2000;54:684–688.
65. Stapf C, Hofmeister C, Hartmann A, et al. Predictive value of clinical lacunar syndromes for lacunar infarcts on magnetic resonance brain imaging. Acta Neurol Scand 2000;101:13–18.
66. Singer MB, Chong J, Lu D, et al. Diffusion-weighted MRI in acute subcortical infarction. Stroke 1998;29:133–136.
67. Lai PH, Li JY, Chang CY, et al. Sensitivity of diffusion-weighted magnetic resonance imaging in the diagnosis of acute lacunar infarcts. J Formos Med Assoc 2001;100:370–376.
68. Horowitz DR, Tuhrim S, Weinberger JM, et al. Mechanisms in lacunar infarction. Stroke 1992; 23:325–327.

69. Millikan C, Futrell N. The fallacy of the lacune hypothesis. Stroke 1990;21:1251–1257.
70. Van Damme H, Demoulin JC, Limet R. Lacunar infarctions and carotid artery disease. Lancet 1991;337:1361–1362.
71. Tejada J, Diez-Tejedor E, Hernandez-Echebarria L, et al. Does a relationship exist between carotid stenosis and lacunar infarction? Stroke 2003;34:1404–1409.
72. Tejada J, Diez-Tejedor E, Hernandez L, et al. [Carotid stenosis and lacunar infarct]. Rev Neurol 1999;29:110–116.
73. Tegler CH, Shi F, Morgan T. Carotid stenosis in lacunar stroke. Stroke 1992;23:437–438.
74. Mead GE, Lewis SC, Wardlaw JM, et al. Severe ipsilateral carotid stenosis and middle cerebral artery disease in lacunar ischaemic stroke: innocent bystanders? J Neurol 2002;249:266–271.
75. Norrving B, Cronqvist S. Clinical and radiologic features of lacunar versus nonlacunar minor stroke. Stroke 1989;20:59–64.
76. Kappelle LJ, Koudstaal PJ, van Gijn J, et al. Carotid angiography in patients with lacunar infarction. A prospective study. Stroke 1988;19:1093–1096.
77. Arboix A, Padilla I, Massons J, et al. Clinical study of 222 patients with pure motor stroke. J Neurol Neurosurg Psychiatry 2001;71:239–242.
78. Mead GE, Lewis SC, Wardlaw JM, et al. Should computed tomography appearance of lacunar stroke influence patient management? J Neurol Neurosurg Psychiatry 1999;67:682–684.
79. Moncayo J, Devuyst G, Van Melle G, et al. Coexisting causes of ischemic stroke. Arch Neurol 2000;57:1139–1144.
80. Landi G, Cella E, Boccardi E, et al. Lacunar versus non-lacunar infarcts: pathogenetic and prognostic differences. J Neurol Neurosurg Psychiatry 1992;55:441–445.
81. Brainini M, Seiser A, Czvitkovits B, et al. Stroke subtype is an age-independent predictor of first-year survival. Neuroepidemiology 1992;11:190–195.
82. Clavier I, Hommell M, Besson G, et al. Long-term prognosis of symptomatic lacunar infarcts. Stroke 1994;25:2005–2009.
83. Miyao S, Takano A, Teramoto J, et al. Leukoaraiosis in relation to prognosis for patients with lacunar infarction. Stroke 1992;23:1434–1438.
84. Petty GW, Brown RDJ, Whisnant JP, et al. Ischemic stroke subtypes: a population-based study of functional outcome, survival, and recurrence. Stroke 2000;31:1062–1068.
85. Salgado AV, Ferro JM, Gouveia-Oliveira A. Long-term prognosis of first-ever lacunar stroke. Stroke 1996;27:661–666.
86. Mohr JP, Thompson JLP, Lazar RM, et al. A comparison of warfarin and aspirin for the prevention of recurrent ischemic stroke. N Engl J Med 2001;345:1444–1451.
87. Benavente O, Hart RG, Palacio S, et al. Stroke recurrence, cognitive impairment and white matter abnormalities are frequent in Hispanic Americans with lacunar stroke. Cerebrovasc Dis 2002;13(suppl 3):1–100.
88. de Jong G, Kessels F, Lodder J. Two types of lacunar infarcts: further arguments from a study on prognosis. Stroke 2002;33:2072–6.
89. Snowdon DA, Greiner LH, Mortimer JA. Brain infarction and the clinical expression of Alzheimer disease. The Nun Study. JAMA 1997;277:813–817.
90. Esiri MM, Wilcock GK, Morris JH. Neuropathological assessment of the lesions of significance in vascular dementia. J Neurol Neurosurg Psychiatry 1997;63:749–753.
91. Erkinjuntti T, Haltia M, Palo J, et al. Accuracy of the clinical diagnosis of vascular dementia: a prospective and post-mortem neuropathological study. J Neurol Neurosurg Psychiatry 1988;51:1037–1044.
92. Meyer JS, McClintic KL, Rogers RL. Aetiological considerations and risk factors for multi-infarct dementia. J Neurol Neurosurg Psychiatry 1988;51:1489–1497.
93. Loeb C, Gandolfo C, Bino G. Intellectual impairment and cerebral lesions in multiple cerebral infarcts. A clinical-computed tomography study. Stroke 1988;19:816–820.
94. Samuelsson M, Soderfelt B, Olsson GB. Functional outcome in patients with lacunar infarction. Stroke 1996;27:842–846.
95. van Swieten JC, Staal S, Kappelle J, et al. Are white matter lesions directly associated with cognitive impairment in patients with lacunar infarcts? J Neurol 1996;243:196–200.
96. Longstreth WT, Bernick C, Manolio TA, et al. Lacunar infarcts defined by magnetic resonance imaging of 3660 elderly people: the Cardiovascular Health Study. Arch Neurol 1998;55:1217–1225.
97. Vermeer SE, Den Heijer T, Koudstaal PJ, et al. Incidence and risk factors of silent brain infarcts in the population-based Rotterdam scan study. Stroke 2003;34:392–396.
98. Samuelsson M, Lindell D, Olsson GB. Lacunar infarcts: a 1-year clinical and MRI follow-up study. Cerebrovasc Dis 1994;3:221–226.

99. van Zagten M, Boiten J, Kessels F, et al. Significant progression of white matter lesions and small deep (lacunar) infarcts in patients with stroke. Arch Neurol 1996;53:650–655.

100. Yamamoto Y, Akiguchi I, Oiwa K, et al. Adverse effect of nighttime blood pressure on the outcome of lacunar infarct patients. Stroke 1998;29:570–576.

101. Gotoh F, Tohgi H, Hirai S, et al. Cilostazol Stroke Prevention Study: a placebo-controlled double-blind trial for secondary prevention of cerebral infarction. J Stroke Cerebrovasc Dis 2000; 9:147–157.

102. Chinese Acute Stroke Trial. CAST: randomised placebo-controlled trial of early aspirin use in 20,000 patients with acute ischaemic stroke. Lancet 1997;349:1641–1649.

103. Bousser MG, Eschwege E, Haguenau M, et al. "AICLA" controlled trial of aspirin and dipyridamole in the secondary prevention of athero-thrombotic cerebral ischemia. Stroke 1983;14:5–14.

104. Gent M, Blakeley JA, Easton D. The Canadian American Ticlopidine Study (CATS) in thromboembolic stroke. Lancet 1989;1:1215–1220.

105. Gorelick PB, Richardson D, Kelly M, et al. Aspirin and ticlopidine for prevention of recurrent stroke in black patients: a randomized trial. JAMA 2003;289:2947–2957.

106. Albers GW, Amarenco P, Easton D, et al. Antithrombotic and thrombolytic therapy for ischemic stroke. Chest 2001;119(suppl):300–320.

107. Collaborative meta-analysis of randomised trials of antiplatelet therapy for prevention of death, myocardial infarction, and stroke in high risk patients. Antithrombotic Trialists' Collaboration. BMJ 2002;324:71–86.

108. Rothwell PM, Eliasziw M, Gutnikov SA, et al. Analysis of pooled data from the randomised controlled trials of endarterectomy for symptomatic carotid stenosis. Lancet 2003;361:107–116.

109. Inzitari D, Eliasziw M, Sharp B, et al. Risk factors and outcome of patients with carotid stenosis presenting with lacunar stroke. Neurology 2000;54:660–666.

110. Boiten J, Rothwell PM, Slattery J, et al. Ischaemic lacunar stroke in the European Carotid Surgery Trial. Cerebrovasc Dis 1996;6:281–287.

111. Vivo R, Korv J, Roose M. First year results of the third stroke registry in Tartu (abstract). Cerebrovasc Dis 2003;16(suppl):1.

8
Unusual Causes of Stroke

Serge A. Blecic and Julien Bogousslavsky

Uncommon causes of stroke are a heterogeneous group of diseases. They may be the initial manifestation of other systemic diseases. Overall these forms of stroke are rare and represent less than 1 percent of the total admissions to a stroke unit. However, they are more common in younger stroke patients and must be considered in this population.

On the basis of the clinical presentation we divide these diseases into two main groups:

1. Unusual systemic disorders leading to stroke
2. Unusual cerebral angiopathies predisposing to stroke

UNUSUAL SYSTEMIC DISORDERS LEADING TO STROKE

These nonhereditary systemic disorders constitute a heterogeneous group of syndromes characterized by stroke resulting from an involvement of arteries generally in the absence of atherosclerosis and without inflammation. They are rare causes of stroke, and most of these pathologies are sporadic. Their frequencies can vary between 1 in 5000 to 1 in 200,000 patients. They involve the skin, the ear, or the eyes and rarely involve all the sensory organs.

Nonhereditary Systemic Disorders with Skin Involvement

Malignant Atrophic Papulosis: Kohlmeier-Degos Disease

The first case of malignant atrophic papulosis (MAP) was reported by Kohlmeier[1] in 1941; he attributed the cause of skin lesions and gastrointestinal perforations occurring in a young man to a form of thromboangiitis obliterans.

In 1942, Degos[2] examined another patient with the same symptoms and suggested it could be a different entity, which he named "papulosquamous dermatitis." Six years later, after the patient's autopsy, the term *malignant atrophic papulosis* was established. [3]

MAP is a rare and clinically distinctive vasculopathy characterized mainly by cutaneous features with frequent gastrointestinal involvement. All major organ systems can be affected,[3] but skin eruption is a constant and pathognomonic sign.[4] The condition is usually lethal, although some patients may have a benign form.[5,6] MAP occurs mainly in young adults, but sometimes it develops in childhood.[7,8]

The first symptom is general weakness, which evolves over many years.[4-6,8-22] All organ systems can be involved. In all cases clinical manifestations are the consequence of multifocal infarction. Death occurs mainly after gastrointestinal perforations or central nervous system (CNS) involvement.[3,4,10] Although this entity is easily recognizable after clinical examination or after anatomicopathological study, the cause is unknown and the treatment remains uncertain.

Dermatological involvement is constant and virtually pathognomonic of MAP, but it may be absent in the early stage.[4] Cutaneous lesions of MAP are scattered and whitish or skin colored. They may be erythematosus papules with central atrophy showing a porcelain-like appearance and disseminated on the trunk and limbs with a size varying from 2 to 5 mm (Figure 8.1). The eruption is always asymptomatic and evolves within a few days to a lesion with central atrophy and a flattened center, sharply surrounded by an erythematosus peripheral circle (Figure 8.2). In some aspects, this eruption can resemble, especially in the early stages, the dermatological findings in systemic lupus erythematosus (SLE).[11,23]

Gastrointestinal lesions are pathognomonic of MAP and in most of the cases are the cause of death.[2-4] The first gastrointestinal symptoms are often insidious

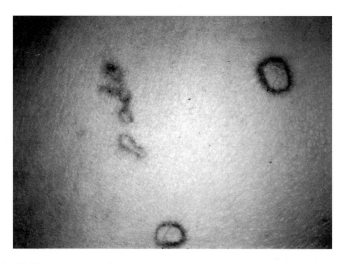

Figure 8.1   Kohlmeier-Degos disease. Cutaneous lesions of malignant atrophic papulosis (MAP) on trunk and arm in a 35-year-old woman.

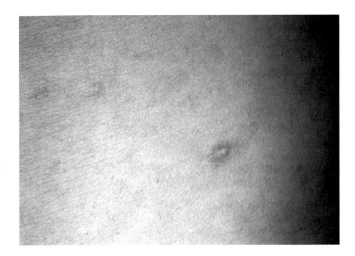

Figure 8.2   Kohlmeier-Degos disease. Papules with central atrophy showing porcelain appearance, surrounded by an erythematosus peripheral circle, disseminated on the trunk.

but after some time anorexia, diarrhea, and diffuse abdominal pain present.[1-4] Often the symptoms worsen and lead to intestinal obstruction and hemorrhage related to perforations with peritonitis.[1-4] The gastrointestinal diagnosis can easily be made by endoscopy or by laparoscopy, which reveals a lesion similar, but larger, than those observed on the skin. More rarely, perforations can be limited within the seromuscular wall.[24] Because the consequences of gastrointestinal involvement are usually severe, Casparie et al[12] emphasize the importance of routinely performing endoscopy in MAP to detect silent or early perforation, even in patients without gastrointestinal complaints.

Neurological manifestations of MAP are mainly due to CNS involvement, but a few cases of peripheral neuropathy have been reported. They can be the first manifestation of MAP, and they may precede skin or other systemic manifestations by many years, especially in children.[8,13] Neurological signs include mental dysfunction, motor and sensory deficits, ophthalmoplegia, and cranial nerve dysfunction. The neurological abnormalities are the result of multifocal infarctions or hemorrhages located in the CNS or peripheral nerves, resulting from involvement of small- or medium-size arteries or cerebral veins.[10] Peripheral neuropathies are rarely encountered and result from demyelination.[7] In 1983, Label et al[25] studied a patient with MAP who developed a polyradiculopathy with elevated cerebrospinal fluid (CSF) protein and hypoglycorrhachia, which was attributed after autopsy to multifocal infarctions and necrosis of CNS and peripheral nerves sheaths. They suggested that MAP should be added to the list of conditions that cause polyradiculopathy.

Ophthalmological symptoms are common. They were reported in 35 of 105 patients. They consist of involvement of the eye structures such as the conjunctiva, sclera, retina, choroid, uvea, eyelids, pupils, and optic tracts.[9,14,16] There are anecdotal reports of intrathoracic,[19] bladder,[21] and heart involvement[14] as well. MAP is an occlusive endarteropathy with involvement of small- and medium-size arteries and veins. The appearance of the vascular lesions is similar regardless of the tissues affected and has been classified as a proliferative vasculopathy.[2–4,18] Using refined microscopy, the lesions are characterized by intimal proliferation in the absence of an inflammatory reaction.[26] This process is confined to the intima of the vessels and always spares the media.[27]

Molenaar et al[28] identified three stages of lesion—early, intermediate, and late—that can coexist. Early lesions consist of cellular proliferation and edema of the intima with evidence for immune complex deposition; thrombosis is found occasionally and can be attributed to a secondary phenomenon. The intermediate stage is characterized by a decrease of edema and a proliferation of smooth muscle.[29,30] The late lesions consist of a cellular intimal sclerosis with hyalinization and narrowing or obliteration of the vascular lumen.[28] Although inflammation is often absent, it can sometimes be found in the early stages.[27] In the other stages, the lack of inflammatory cells helps to differentiate Degos disease from other forms of vasculitis.[26]

Electron microscopy confirms the presence of intimal proliferation with vacuolization and edema,[26] and intraluminal paramyxovirus-like inclusions are often identified in the basal surfaces of the endothelial cells. The nature of these inclusions remains controversial. They are probably nonspecific manifestations.[31]

The cause of MAP remains unknown. Several hypotheses have been proposed, but none has been confirmed. The congenital hypothesis was proposed after the observations of several cases occurring in the same family. In one report, six relatives presented clinical features of MAP.[32] In another report, a mother and her daughter were both affected.[5] In the two reports, an autosomal dominant mode of inheritance was proposed but never confirmed. An autoimmune mechanism has been proposed because the dermatological lesions observed in SLE are in some aspects similar to those found in MAP.[11,20,33] This hypothesis was supported by the presence of antiphospholipid antibodies in a case of MAP.[34,35] These interesting findings should be confirmed by other analyses in future patients. However, the lack of inflammatory cells is a strong argument against the autoimmune hypothesis. A viral cause was suspected after observation of virus-like particles in endothelial cells. These findings were not confirmed, and intracytoplasmic particles resembling paramyxovirus have subsequently been found to be the result of cellular degeneration.[31,36]

No treatment is known to be effective. Because an autoimmune process has been suspected, immunosuppressive therapy was proposed, but the benefit has not been established yet.[34,37] For symptomatic arterial occlusion, antifibrinolytic agents have been proposed, but there is no evidence of benefit.[33] In the acute phase, Degos proposed anticoagulation with heparin to avoid artery occlusion.[4] Reports concerning the use of antiplatelet therapy are inconsistent. Several reports did not show evidence of a beneficial effect,[36,38] whereas Drucker[39] showed a benefit in a patient who had abnormalities of platelet adhesiveness and aggregation. During several months of treatment the patient was free of complications, but the patient worsened when treatment was discontinued.[39–41] However, this observation must be tempered by the fact that coagulation abnormalities are not a common feature in MAP.[39–43] Surgery is commonly proposed when there is intestinal perforation.[38,40]

Sneddon Syndrome

Sneddon syndrome is defined by the presence of livedo racemosa and ischemic strokes. Some believe that arterial hypertension is a component of this syndrome.[44,45] Livedo racemosa is always present in patients with Sneddon syndrome. It is a cutaneous lesion characterized by a reddish-purple network found on the trunk and on the extremities (Figure 8.3). In contrast to the other form of livedo (named reticularis) livedo racemosa is an incomplete network found essentially in adults, whereas livedo reticularis is found mainly in children and disappears when the skin is heated. Although livedo racemosa is always found in Sneddon syndrome, it is also often seen in other autoimmune diseases such as SLE, dermatomyositis, polyarteritis nodosa, cryoglobulinemia, rheumatoid arthritis, temporal arteritis; other conditions such as neoplasia and hematological disorders; and other neurological pathologies such as Parkinson disease.[34,44–51]

The livedo is often present several years before the onset of neurological symptoms; the range varies from 1 to 35 years and the median time is 10 years. It is often present at the time that the neurological event occurs. Several reports indicated that Sneddon syndrome occurs more often in women. The sex ratio is 2:1.[34,44–51]

Infarctions in the carotid artery territory are the most frequent neurological manifestations. Recurrence is frequent and could lead to severe neurological disability or vascular dementia.

Histological studies reveal a perivascular lymphocytic infiltration of the arterial wall of the skin arteries (see Figure 8.4).[36,37] Analysis of normal skin can also disclose reduction of the lumen of arterioles resulting from proliferation of smooth muscle of the lamina elastica interna. These arteriolar changes occur in the absence of an inflammatory process.[45]

Currently, the cause of Sneddon syndrome remains unknown. Often, arterial hypertension, cigarette smoking, and use of oral contraceptives are found in association with the syndrome, but the relationship between these very common

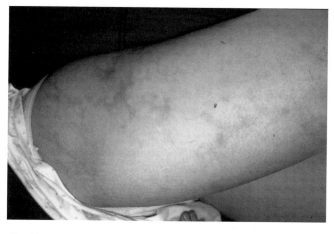

Figure 8.3   Sneddon syndrome. Livedo racemosa formed by a reddish purple network on a 25-year-old woman's right arm.

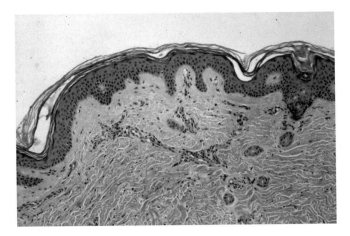

Figure 8.4   Sneddon syndrome. Skin biopsy showing lymphocytic infiltration of the media of a middle-size artery.

risk factors and the disease is not yet clearly established.[45,52–54] An autoimmune hypothesis has been proposed because Sneddon syndrome is often accompanied by antiphospholipid antibodies.[34,46–51] The primary antiphospholipid antibody syndrome includes fetal loss, peripheral venous thrombosis, thrombocytopenia, cerebrovascular events, and the presence of antiphospholipid antibodies such as anticardiolipin antibodies and lupus anticoagulant.[34,46–51,55,56] Several reports have shown that patients with livedo racemosa and ischemic stroke have high titers of antiphospholipid antibodies. A recent study of Kalashnikova et al showed that nearly 50 percent of their patients with presumed Sneddon syndrome had high titers of antiphospholipid antibodies.[34,46–51,57]

Probably two different entities coexist. The first includes patients with livedo racemosa, ischemic stroke, and the presence of antiphospholipid antibodies, who would belong to the group with primary antiphospholipid antibody syndrome.[58] The other patients, with livedo racemosa, ischemic stroke, and absence of antiphospholipid antibodies, constitute an idiopathic entity—Sneddon syndrome. In this latter group, differential diagnosis includes diseases such as endarteritis obliterans, Takayasu arteriopathy, or Divry-Van Bogaert syndrome.[59,60] Other possible causes of Sneddon syndrome such as coagulation abnormalities should be ruled out.

Currently, treatment of Sneddon syndrome consists of antiplatelet therapy. When there are recurrent neurological events, some physicians prescribe anticoagulants. Immunosuppression with cyclophosphamide 2 mg/kg daily with prednisone 1mg/kg per day may be recommended. However, the lack of an inflammatory component is a strong rationale to reject this treatment strategy.[61]

Diffuse Meningocerebral Angiomatosis and Leukoencephalopathy: Divry-Van Bogaert Syndrome

Diffuse meningocerebral angiomatosis and leukoencephalopathy is a congenital recessive disease, which involves adults and children.[59,62] This syndrome was first described in 1946 by Divry and Van Bogaert, who examined three brothers who had livedo reticularis and who gradually developed dementia, seizures, and pyramidal signs that occurred in all approximately 15 years after the diagnosis.[59] Autopsy performed at this time disclosed leptomeningeal angiopathy and brain infarcts. Demyelination was also present.[59]

Two forms can be distinguished. The adult form includes skin lesions and neurological disorders.[59] The skin findings consist of the presence of a diffuse symmetrical livedo reticularis, which can increase at the onset of neurological problems. Skin biopsies disclose increased dermal capillaries with focal loss of zonulae occludens between endothelial cells.[59] Neurological disorders include seizures, dementia, and motor disturbances. Among these symptoms, dementia is the most frequent manifestation.[59,62] The motor disturbances are related to the presence of the brain infarcts. Generally death occurs between 10 and 15 years after the onset of neurological symptoms.[59,62] In the infantile form, the onset of symptoms occurs after the age of 3 years.[59] In one patient, a poliomyelitis vaccination was the presumptive cause.[62] This form includes skin anomalies and neurological disorders. In contrast to the adult form, skin lesions can be absent but when present they do not differ from the adult form.[59,62] The neurological signs include seizures and neuropsychomotor involvement. The duration of the disease is shorter in adults, and death occurs generally within 24 months after onset of neurological signs.[59]

Neuropathological abnormalities are brain infarcts, demyelination of white matter, and cerebromeningeal angiomatosis, which is the most constant and pathognomonic finding of this disease.[59,62] Diffuse meningocerebral angiomatosis is a large corticomeningeal network with vascular congestion and multiple vessel occlusions. Microscopic examination shows fibrotic changes of the vascular walls with fatty degeneration and amyloid deposits. These abnormalities lead to diffuse cerebral infarctions in the gray and white matter. In addition, demyelination of the central white matter is observed in practically all the cases and consists of axonal and oligodendrocytic loss with astrogliosis.[59,62] These abnormalities occur mostly predominant around the vessels.

Epidermal Nevus Syndrome

The epidermal nevus syndrome is a sporadic neurocutaneous disorder that consists of epidermal nevi and congenital anomalies involving all major organs. The brain is often involved.[63–65] Two entities are commonly described: the classical form that consists of epidermal nevi and brain infarctions, and the second (often called the neurological variant) that consists of hemimegalencephaly, gyral malformation, mental retardation, seizures, and facial hemihypertrophy.[63–65] One half of the 70 patients previously described had the hemimegalencephaly variant.[64]

Neurological manifestations result from infarcts due to blood vessel dysplasia. Clinically, the epidermal nevus syndrome is found in young patients and in newborns.[63] In all patients, the diagnosis is confirmed by angiography that demonstrates vascular dysplasia consisting of segmental beading and dilatation of cerebral arteries. An increase of the vascularity in the capillary field and widening of the posterior portion of the superior sagittal sinus is often noted.[64] Less often, angiography shows fusiform aneurysms and dilation of the cavernous part of the carotid arteries.[64]

Association of Atrial Myxoma-Lentiginosis and Stroke

Facial lentiginosis associated with atrial myxoma is a rare cause of stroke.[66,67] The frequency of atrial myxoma is approximately 1 in 100,000 in autopsy series. A congenital dominant autosomal form has been described in patients with the association of lentiginosis and myxoma.[66,67]

In 1966, Forney et al[67] described an entity that combines facial lentiginosis, mitral insufficiency, myxoma, deafness, and bone abnormalities. Several patients were reported, and in all instances cerebral infarction was probably due to cardiac embolism. Embryologically, it is probably an involvement of the mesodermic structures. Although this syndrome is rare, its congenital origin leads to study of family members who could also have cardiac tumors and neoplastic conversion of skin lesions.[66]

Eosinophil-Induced Neurotoxicity and Cerebral Infarction

Hypereosinophilia is usually a secondary process in response to allergic and parasitic diseases.[68–70] Although there are beneficial effects on the primary disease, eosinophils can exert nonspecific toxic effects with concomitant damage to tissues. Both the central and peripheral nervous system are often involved by this undesirable toxicity.[68–70] According to Weaver and colleagues[70] who described a patient with cerebral involvement resulting from hypereosinophilic syndrome, the mechanisms of eosinophil-induced neuronal damage are multiple (Table 8.1).

The neurotoxic potential of eosinophil proteins must also be considered. Three basic proteins have been isolated: medial basic protein (MBP), eosinophil cationic protein (ECP), and eosinophil-derived neurotoxin (EDN). Release of MBP can damage endothelial cells and can be the cause of thrombosis and secondary artery-to-artery emboli. ECP can potentiate a hypercoagulable state and contribute to thrombotic tendency. EDN has a direct toxic action on neuronal tissue and on myelinated axons.[68–70]

The three major clinical manifestations of eosinophil-induced neurotoxicity are axonal peripheral neuropathy, dementia, and stroke.[68–70] Cerebral infarction is secondary to mainly MBP-mediated endothelial damage and ECP-mediated

Table 8.1   Mechanisms of eosinophil-induced neurotoxicity

Direct neural tissue infiltration

Damage related to eosinophil function, either by direct cytotoxicity or by antibody-dependent cellular cytotoxicity

Damage related to eosinophil products, either by secretion into neurons or by secretion of intracytoplasmic granules contained in the circulation, with subsequent damage to neural tissue

Embolic cerebral infarction related either to thrombus or generalized hypercoagulable state

Nervous system damage secondary to eosinophil mediated action in remote organ systems[50]

hypercoagulability and eosinophil-mediated cardiopathy. The patient reported by Weaver et al[70] initially had a left occipital cerebral infarction followed 3 months later by a right parietal cerebral infarction. Dementia developed 1 year later, and neurophysiological study showed a polyneuropathy.

Management consists of the treatment of the underlying cause of the hypereosinophilia and may also include prednisone or hydroxyurea. Concerning embolic cerebral infarctions, Weaver et al[70] favored anticoagulation over antiplatelet therapy.

Kawasaki Syndrome

The mucocutaneous lymph node syndrome was first described by Kawasaki in 1967, and it is considered as an acute febrile exanthematous disease.[71] The first description by Kawasaki[71] described its evolution in several Japanese children, who had a syndrome associated with fever and maculopapular skin involvement. Kawasaki syndrome is found almost exclusively in children and more rarely in young adults.[71–73]

The main features of the disease are involvement of the skin and all mucous membranes.[71] The course of the disease usually follows the same pattern. Practically all patients have fever at onset, followed within the first 3 days by a squamous skin eruption (see Figure 8.5), generalized erythema with peeling exanthema, conjunctivitis, and generalized lymphadenopathy, all signs that mimic those encountered in scarlet fever.[71] The skin of the trunk is more often affected than other areas. Following these symptoms, systemic involvement can occur, essentially resulting from multiple artery involvement. Both progressive vascular occlusion and formation of aneurysms may occur. Most patients have spontaneous lesion regression, but some can suffer stroke, subarachnoid hemorrhage, or myocardial infarction.

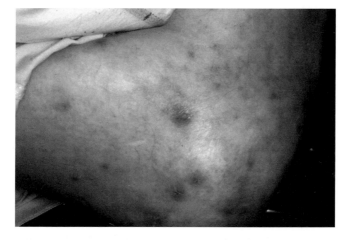

Figure 8.5 Kawasaki disease. Papular eruption on the elbow of a 12-year-old boy with Kawasaki disease.

Neurological signs include mental dysfunction, motor and sensory deficits, ophthalmoplegia, and cranial nerve dysfunction. The neurological abnormalities result from multifocal infarctions or hemorrhages located in the CNS. The mechanism by which stroke may occur is twofold. It can be the consequence of in situ middle- or small-size cerebral artery thrombosis or of emboli arising from a cardiac source, such as cardiac akinesis or atrial fibrillation after recent myocardial infarction.[74] Asymptomatic cerebral infarction has been reported in patients with only skin and mucous membrane involvement and in those with cardiac dysfunction resulting from coronary artery occlusion.

Kawasaki disease can affect all organs because it has been regarded as a panarteritis with involvement of medium- and small-size arteries. Large-artery involvement is exceptional; only one author reported a case of carotid involvement.[75] Kawasaki disease has been classified as a proliferative vasculopathy, and the lesions are characterized by intimal proliferation in the absence of an inflammatory reaction. Angiitis of coronary arteries is the most frequent finding, but cerebral arteries can also be affected. Pathologically there is involvement of both the intima and media.[74–77] Early lesions consist of intima cellular proliferation accompanied by slight edema without evidence for immune complex deposition. The second stage is marked by aneurysmal formation resulting from rupture of both the intimal and medial layers. The third stage is an occlusive endarteriolopathy, associated with an increase in platelet aggregation and adhesiveness. The late lesions consist of an acellular intimal sclerosis with hyalinization and narrowing or obliteration of the vascular lumen. Mild inflammation can sometimes be found in the early stages. Examination of eye, mouth mucous membranes, or skin lesions do not provide evidence of the presence of bacterial or viral inclusions. An autoimmune mechanism has been proposed, but the lack of increase in antibody level and the absence of lymphocytic infiltration do not support this hypothesis.[74–77]

The etiological basis of this disease remains unknown. Consequently, no treatment is known to be successful. An increase in platelet aggregation and adhesiveness has been suggested as the cause of secondary vascular occlusions; therefore antiplatelet therapy might be useful.[74–77] However, reports concerning the use of antiplatelet therapy are inconsistent and should be carefully considered because these patients are at risk of brain hemorrhage—one of the major mechanisms of the disease is aneurysm development.[7]

Nonhereditary Systemic Disorders with Eye Involvement

Eale Disease

First described in 1882, Eale disease is rare and idiopathic and encountered mainly in young men. It is an idiopathic type of retinal perivascular disorder characterized by frequent recurrent retinal and vitreous hemorrhages.[78,79] More rarely, small- and medium-size arteries of the CNS can be involved and a noninflammatory perivascular infiltrative disorder may lead to arterial occlusions.[80–82] Other organ systems can be involved, such as the gastrointestinal tract or spinal cord.[80–84]

Pathologically, there is involvement of medium- and small-size arteries with infiltration of the media by normal lymphocytes but without other inflammatory cells.[80–84] However in 1992, Sen et al[81] studied 27 patients with peripheral retinal vasculitis resulting from Eale disease. There was an increased serum α-1 acid glycoprotein level in both moderate and severe forms of Eale disease, which suggested that this entity could have an immune-mediated origin.

Current treatment consists of anticoagulation or antiplatelet therapy, but following the observations of Sen et al[81] immunosuppressive therapy should be considered in patients with moderate and severe forms of Eale disease.

Acute Posterior Multifocal Placoid Pigment Epitheliopathy

Acute posterior multifocal placoid pigment epitheliopathy (APMPPE) was first described by Gass in 1968.[85] The disease is characterized by a sudden bilateral blurring of vision associated with multifocal yellowish-white placoid lesions of the retinal pigmented epithelium.[85,86] The acute onset of blurred vision in a young adult with typical lesions in the posterior retinal pole is characteristic of APMPPE.[85] Patients with APMPPE are between 15 and 40 years; both sexes are affected, and the disease is observed in different races.[86–88]

The primary lesion affects the small choroidal arterioles, leading to ischemia of the retinal pigmented epithelium.[85] APMPPE may follow a viral-like illness of the respiratory or digestive tracts. In one patient, an adenovirus type 5 infection was found. The virus was isolated from throat swab, and the antibody titer was elevated in the serum.[79] The visual form is the most common form.[89,90] Persistent scotomas have been described, but the visual outcome is generally good. The ocular involvement may be complicated by episcleritis and keratitis, iridocyclitis, and retinal vasculitis.[89–93]

In addition to the eyes, the CNS often involved.[89–100] Neurological manifestations include severe headache, neck stiffness, and stroke. Cerebral vasculitis is also a complication of APMPPE, occurring either simultaneously or after the ocular signs.[87,95,96,100] In addition, several observations indicate that APMPPE may be a manifestation of an autoimmune disease such as erythema nodosum, thyroiditis, Crohn disease, giant cell arteritis, or acute nephritis.[86,89,92,93,95,98,99] Often, aseptic meningitis can precede the blurring of vision.[89] CSF analysis shows a lymphocytic pleocytosis and elevated protein levels. Rarely, oligoclonal bands are present in the CSF.[88–90,92] The pathogenesis of APMPPE remains unknown. Lyness and Bird[91] have speculated that hypersensitivity to tetracycline, sulfamethoxazole, and trimethoprim may precipitate the disorder.

Treatment with steroids is followed by rapid improvement of neurological signs.[86,89] Recurrences are not rare,[90,97] and cerebral infarction has developed after steroid doses have been reduced. Long-term immunosuppression with azathioprine is sometimes recommended, but data are insufficient to accept this treatment as standard therapy.[87,94]

Nonhereditary Systemic Disorders with Eye and Ear Involvement

Retinocochleocerebral Arteriolopathy

Retinocochleocerebral arteriolopathy is a diffuse encephalopathy with retinal vascular occlusions, hearing loss, and absence of systemic disease that was first described by Susac et al in 1979 in two women with psychiatric symptoms.[101] Both had retinal artery occlusions and hearing loss.[101] There were cognitive manifestations such as progressive memory loss and abulia. Blindness was the consequence of multiple retinal artery occlusions.

Bogousslavsky et al[102] described several patients with this syndrome. Laboratory tests were unremarkable; however, in a few patients there was a slight increase of the sedimentation rate, the presence of low titer antinuclear antibodies, and an increase of CSF protein content. Generally, angiography discloses segmental narrowing and involvement of small pial and cortical vessels. In one case, biopsy showed "healed angiitis."

Bogousslavsky's patients also had anomalies of T-cell lymphocyte helpers and suppressors, which led to administration of immunosuppressive therapy. One patient improved under this treatment, but another worsened.[102] Currently, steroid therapy is recommended in the acute phase, but a benefit from prolonged immunosuppressive therapy is not yet established.[103]

RARE CEREBRAL ANGIOPATHIES PREDISPOSING TO STROKE

The conditions described in this chapter represent a heterogeneous group of vasculopathies. These diseases are very rare and are estimated to account for between 1 in 50,000 and 1 in 350,000 strokes. Therefore their contribution to the absolute numbers of stroke is small. They are divided into sporadic and hereditary arteriopathies.

Sporadic Angiopathies

Arterial Dissection

Artery dissection, although categorized as an "unusual" or "other" cause of stroke, is neither a rare cause of stroke nor a "special syndrome" by itself. Although uncommon in the overall population, dissection represents the second most common cause of stroke in patients younger than 45 years and may be the foremost cause in very young adults.[104–108] Dissection is often the consequence of a traumatic injury, an atherosclerotic process, or more rarely a connective tissue disorder.[105–114] The incidence of dissection remains unknown, with an estimation for internal carotid dissection in a community-based study of 2.6 in 100,000 individuals per year; vertebral artery dissection occurred at a rate that was about one third of that rate. Extracranial dissection is far more frequent than intracranial dissection, and, in the overall population, single vessel dissection is the rule, with multiple dissections representing less than 10 percent of the observations. The site of predilection for carotid dissection is the distal part, just in front of the second cervical vertebra, where the artery is very close to the bone. The vertebral artery is most often found dissected in the distal extracranial segment at the atlas loop before entering the dura (V3 segment). Dissection occurs by a fissure and a rupture within the arterial wall leading to an intramural hematoma. The clinical consequences are broad including local symptoms such as shoulder pain, ipsilateral facial pain, headache, Horner syndrome, and stroke resulting from either artery-to-artery embolism or local artery occlusion.[106–108,111–115]

The pathogenesis of dissection remains undetermined. Although the cause seems obvious in severe direct trauma of a cervical artery with fracture of the cervical spine, dissection often occurs in otherwise healthy adults without risk factors for stroke. In such individuals, a mild physical stress, such as sudden head movement during sporting activities, cough, or another seemingly trivial trauma is often reported. Prior chiropractic manipulation of the neck has also been implicated as cause or contributor to "spontaneous" dissection. Because most dissections occur without history of trauma, an underlying arteriopathy has often been postulated. In such conditions, dissections are often multiple, and young adults are often affected.[105–107,110,111,116]

Pathologically, structural aberrations of the arterial walls and abnormal connective tissue components in the surrounding extracellular matrix leading to a weakness of the vessel wall have been proposed in these patients. Histopathological examinations of tissue specimens of affected arteries can show specific anomalies in relation with a variety of syndromes such as known heritable connective tissue disorders, fibromuscular dysplasia (FMD), and other structural and anatomical variants (including some of the other inherited disorders described later). Dissections may be diagnosed by magnetic resonance angiography (MRA), computed tomography (CT) angiography, or conventional angiography, but ultrasound-based techniques lack both sensitivity and specificity.

Treatment of arterial dissection is somewhat controversial. Options include anticoagulation, antiplatelet therapy, angioplasty with or without stenting, surgery, or conservative observation without specific medical or surgical therapy. Early anticoagulation with heparin or low-molecular-weight heparin is widely recommended at the time of diagnosis, although this aggressive approach is seldom needed for long-term prevention of subsequent stroke.

Fibromuscular Dysplasia

FMD is an arteriopathy occurring predominantly in white women. The most common age of diagnosis is between 30 to 50 years. It is the most often recognized arterial dysplasia, representing approximately 1 percent of autopsy and angiography series.[117] The renal, splanchnic, and cervico-cranial arteries are most commonly involved, with the disease having a preference for middle-size vessels. FMD is preferentially located in the distal two thirds of the renal arteries and segments of the distal extracranial vertebral and carotid arteries adjacent to the second cervical vertebra.[117–120] Occasionally, the cavernous part of the carotid arteries and the arteries of the circle of Willis may be involved.

Pathologically, the medial layer is most commonly affected, but all layers of the arterial wall can be involved.[117,118] The pathological process consists of fibrodysplasia of smooth muscles leading to the formation of rings of fibrous tissue and smooth muscle; these rings alternate with areas of medial thickening and destruction of the elastic layer, leading to alternate narrowing and widening of the arterial lumen (see Figure 8.6). Occasionally, the intimal region is involved, causing proliferation of fibrous cells resulting in a narrowing of the

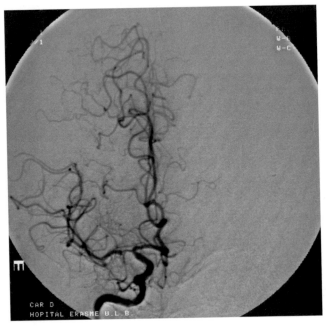

Figure 8.6   Fibromuscular dysplasia. Multiple segmental artery narrowings in a 45-year-old woman with arterial hypertension and fibromuscular dysplasia.

lumen. This less common type of FMD is mainly found in children and young adults.[117,118]

The typical appearance of FMD on angiography consists of alternating zones of widening and narrowing of the arterial lumen leading to the classical "string of beads" (see Figure 8.7) or "stack of coins" pattern.[117–124] Less frequent features are tubular stenosis, a diverticular appearance, or aneurysmal dilatation. Diagnosis is practically always made by angiography but it can be confirmed by duplex imaging of the extracranial carotid and vertebral arteries or transcranial Doppler.[121,123] MRA can also be used.[121,123,125,126] The use of MRA may avoid the need for conventional arteriography in patients suspected of having FMD after duplex examination, although the noninvasive tests all lack specificity for this diagnosis.

The mechanism by which FMD causes stroke is unclear. Although the relationship between stroke and FMD remains questionable,[117,118,125] the following mechanisms have been proposed: (1) artery-to-artery emboli, (2) local thrombosis, (3) emboli arising from a diverticulum, or (4) emboli arising from a pseudo-aneurysmal sac. A frequent cause of stroke in FMD patients is spontaneous artery dissection.[124,127–129] The association of atherosclerosis and FMD is common, but it is uncertain how much the primary condition favors the development of atheromatous disease.[117,124,126–129] The prevalence of cigarette smoking and the use of contraceptive therapy has been proposed to explain the female predominance.[117]

Currently, there are no well-established long-term treatment strategies for FMD. Antiplatelet therapy has been proposed.[117,124,126–129] Anticoagulants are

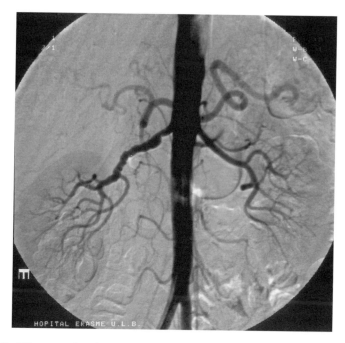

Figure 8.7   Fibromuscular dysplasia. Typical "string of beads" appearance and arterial stenosis of right renal artery in the patient shown in Figure 8.6. Arterial hypertension was attributed to the renal artery stenosis.

not recommended because of the risk of bleeding in the presence of cerebral aneurysms. Several surgical procedures have been proposed but thromboendarterectomy should only be considered when there is symptomatic carotid artery stenosis. Some endovascular specialists recommend angioplasty when the carotid or vertebral arteries are involved. This procedure, however, should be proposed with caution because it may cause arterial dissection, a known complication of FMD.[117,124,126–129]

Primitive Arteries

In the very early stages of human embryonic life, various anastomotic channels exist between the carotid and vertebrobasilar systems. They are normally present during the early stages of life and disappear when the embryo is approximately 12 to 14 mm long.[130,131] These anastomotic channels are known as the persistent primitive trigeminal, hypoglossal, otic, and proatlantal arteries.[130,132] Occasionally, some of these channels fail to regress and they persist in adult life.[130,131,133]

Occlusion of these arteries, when they persist, can lead to cerebral infarction. In 1993, Bahsi et al[133] described the case of a 55-year-old woman admitted to the hospital with loss of consciousness because of bilateral mesencephalic and thalamic infarctions. She was identified with multiple strokes located in cerebral areas supplied by the basilar artery (top-of-the-basilar syndrome). Other rare cases of ischemic stroke in the carotid territory have also been described after occlusion of the persistent trigeminal artery, a collateral of the basilar artery that reaches the internal carotid artery near the base of the skull. Anastomotic vessel occlusions are caused by either cerebral emboli or more often local thrombosis.[132,133]

Cerebral Aneurysms

Ischemic strokes secondary to subarachnoid hemorrhage result mainly from vasospasm of the major cerebral arteries. However, other mechanisms such as aneurysmal embolism may occur when aneurysmal sacs are greater than 25 mm.[117,134–136] In the presence of these giant cerebral aneurysms, emboli may arise from the sac. This is rare but must be considered in patients with this condition in whom no other cause of stroke has been identified.

The first observation was made in 1968 by Taptas and Katsiotis[135] who reported a patient who had a stroke after a subarachnoid hemorrhage and in whom angiography did not demonstrate vasospasm. A subsequent follow-up revealed that stroke was the consequence of an aneurysmal-to-artery embolus.

Four criteria have been proposed to define this mechanism of stroke: (1) the presence of transient ischemic attacks (TIAs) or ischemic stroke, (2) the presence of a thrombus in the aneurysmal sac, (3) the absence of other sources of embolism, and (4) the absence of vasospasm (determined by cerebral angiography).[137] Currently, the best noninvasive techniques for diagnosis are magnetic resonance imaging (MRI), which can image thrombosed aneurysms, and transcranial Doppler, which can provide information about the presence of associated vasospasm.[132,135,136,138] Histologically, there is a good correlation between the size of the aneurysm sac and the incidence of saccular thrombosis. The larger the aneurysm the greater the risk of an intra-aneurysmal thrombus.[132,135,136,138]

Cerebral aneurysms are treated by surgery. The surgical dissection must be precise to avoid secondary emboli. In patients for whom surgery is not an option, anticoagulants may be considered to avoid thrombus formation, but these treatments may promote fatal subarachnoid hemorrhages.

Radiation-Induced Angiopathy

The adverse effects of radiation on blood vessels have been known since the end of the 19th century. Arteries, both extracranial and intracranial, and veins have been shown to be involved.[139–141] Radiation-induced arteriopathy is a result of therapeutic irradiation of neck tumors such as lymphomas and thyroid tumors or intracranial tumors such as optic tract gliomas.

Pathologically, arterial lesions caused by radiation have been studied in both animal and human models. In animal models, Lambrechts and de Boer[141] showed that a 5-Gray radiation dose induces extensive changes in small- and middle-size arteries in hypercholesterolemic rabbits.[139,141] These changes are (1) penetration of fat into the arterial walls, (2) deposition of lipophages, (3) formation of atherosclerotic plaques in the intima, and (4) structural changes in the elastic fibers. Radiation primarily affects the endothelial cells, and the changes seems to be exacerbated by elevated cholesterol levels, which activate lysosomal enzymes and favor infiltration of lipid droplets beneath the endothe-lium.[142] Further studies using electron microscopy have demonstrated extensive changes in the endothelium. Adventitial lesions are caused by involvement of the vasa vasorum.[140]

Extrapolation to human arteries is difficult, but autopsy examinations have disclosed vacuolization and thickening of the intima, changes in the elastic fibers, and degeneration of the endothelial cells by the same process seen in animal models.[140,141] Electron microscopy has disclosed swelling and detach-ment of endothelial cells with a splitting of the basement membrane and subin-timal foam cells, which closely resemble circulating lipid-laden macrophages (leading to the production of atherosclerotic-like lesions). Subintimal foam cells in middle- and small-size vessels are a diagnostic feature of radiation therapy.[140,141] Large vessels such as the carotid or vertebral arteries are less affected by radiation therapy. However, there have been some reports of rupture of the internal carotid artery after subclavian radiation. Autopsy studies have disclosed intimal necrosis, infiltration of leukocytes, and fragmentation of elastic fibers. In addition, Glick[142] demonstrated an accumulation of fat-laden macrophages in the arterial media with atheromatous proliferation and calcification of the intima. A few studies have reported the effect of radiation therapy in large intracranial arteries with the same pathological process being demonstrated.

Clinically, the adverse effects of such therapy can be observed between 1 week to several decades after radiation. Very early manifestations are rare and generally due to skin necrosis and infection of surgical wounds. Delayed complications are more frequent and occur from 6 months to 10 years (median of 2 years) after treatment. Cerebral angiography often discloses arterial steno-sis within the radiated area (see Figure 12.1). The interval from the time of irradiation to symptomatic cerebrovascular events is directly related to the size of the irradiated arteries—the larger the vessel the longer the time interval.[142]

Kinking, Coiling, Hypoplasia, and Dolichoectasia of the Cervical Arteries

Kinking or coiling of the cervical and cerebral arteries can be observed in both the carotid and vertebral systems. The origin of these anomalies is probably congenital. In most patients, kinking has been discovered after angiography, but Doppler ultrasonography with frequency analysis and B-mode imaging can also be used for diagnosis when the cervical arteries are involved (see Figure 12.2). Kinking or coiling rarely induces symptoms or occlusive disease but may induce TIA or stroke in the case of permanent head rotation during a surgical procedure. In 1992, Brachlow et al[143] reported the incidence of a fatal intra-operative cerebral ischemia caused by kinking of the internal carotid arteries. However, in stroke patients these conditions are rarely related to cerebro-vascular event.[143,144]

Congenital hypoplasia is a rare condition. It is defined by segmental narrow-ing of the carotid or vertebral artery, practically always associated with intracranial aneurysm, anomalies of the circle of Willis vessels, or intracranial-extracranial physiological bypass. Angiography has disclosed a sudden narrowing of the internal carotid artery just after the primitive division. Carotid hypoplasia is difficult to differentiate from carotid dissection, but in hypoplasia a small carotid canal is a clue to a diagnosis of hypoplasia rather than dissection.[143,144]

Dolichoectasia of cervical and cerebral arteries consists of segmental narrowing, widening, and lengthening of arteries of both the vertebrobasilar and carotid systems. Arteries of all sizes can be affected, alone or in combination with others. Histologically, there is a thinning of the arterial wall, resulting from a rarefaction of the elastic layer, which is associated with a transformation of the media, and a fibrous tissue is observed. Atherosclerosis is the consequence but not the cause of these changes and can be observed in such arteries. Other vascular malformations can be present such as cerebral saccular aneurysm, aortic aneurysms, or carotid hypoplasia.[117,143,144] Individuals between the ages of 50 to 60 years are more often affected, and a male predominance has been observed. The consequence of this process can be cerebral infarction resulting from arterial emboli or occlusion of small arteries. Cranial nerve compression at the base of the skull can be the consequence of a dolichoectatic artery as well. Subarachnoidal hemorrhages are rare but can occur if the dolichoectatic artery ruptures.[117,143,144] The diagnosis is often made with a routine CT scan or MRI and may be confirmed by angiography, which discloses lengthening and tortuosity of the artery.

Reversible Vasoconstriction

Reversible cerebral angiopathy is characterized by the presence of multiple reversible segmental arterial narrowings.[145] The existence of this condition and its relationship with neurological deficit is a matter of debate.[145,146] Two forms have currently been identified. The first form is a consequence of the use of sympathomimetic drugs such as ergot derivatives, crack-cocaine abuse, or methylamphetamine administration.[145–147] The second form is idiopathic, the so-called Call syndrome or postpartum cerebral angiopathy.[145–149] In this form, vasoconstriction is spontaneous and occurs predominantly in adults without associated risk factors for stroke. It is more common in women, especially in the puerperium or at menopause, and is often accompanied by a history of migraine.[145–150]

The pathophysiology and cause of reversible angiopathy is focal arterial vasoconstriction. Reversible cerebral angiopathy has also been recognized following subarachnoid hemorrhage resulting from a ruptured saccular aneurysm or caused by surgical manipulation.

In all patients, neurological deficits are always preceded by high-intensity headaches, nausea, and vomiting, mimicking the symptoms found in classical migraine or subarachnoid hemorrhage.[145–150] Less often, patients can have epileptic seizures at onset. Often, neurological deficit is transient, lasting from 7 days to 6 months, but a few patients remain severely handicapped or die. Cerebral hemorrhage can occur, presumably related to reperfusion, and in some patients brain edema may be present.

The classical pattern on cerebral angiography is the presence of multiple narrowings of the arteries arising from the circle of Willis (see Figure 12.3), which generally disappear within a few days or several months after onset. Transcranial Doppler can be useful for the follow-up and the assessment of vasospasm. CSF examination is often normal, although occasionally a mild pleocytosis may be noted.[145–150]

The pathological process involved remains unclear, although severe acute arterial hypertension at onset has been proposed as the cause of an inappropriate arterial vasoconstriction in several cases.[28,29] Because there is uncertainty regarding the pathology, there is no specific treatment for the acute phase of the disease, except symptomatic treatment for headache, nausea, and vomiting.[145–150]

Endovascular Lymphoma

Also named angiotrophic large cell lymphoma or malignant angioendotheliomatosis, endovascular lymphoma causes a rare arteriopathy, which is virtually always lethal. It has a predilection for small- and middle-size vessels, mainly of the lung, but can involve all organs such as the CNS, lymphatic system, skin, spleen, and bone marrow.[151,152] Small- and middle-size vessels, either arteries or veins, are exclusively involved in endovascular proliferation leading to widening, narrowing, and vessel occlusions with extravasation of tumor cells.[153] Neoplastic large lymphoid cells are confined to the intravascular compartment and create, in the lung, a pattern akin to cellular interstitial pneumonia.[154] Genotypic and immunohistochemical studies and an atypical cytology with frequent involvement of the CNS confirm its inclusion within the group of pulmonary lymphomas. Immunohistochemical studies always disclose an endothelial infiltration of B lymphocytes with a positive reaction for CD-20, CD-45, and CD-75 IgG antibodies.[153,154] T-lymphocyte infiltration has been reported only in rare cases.

About 1 in 5000 ischemic strokes are a consequence of this rare arteriopathy. At presentation, patients demonstrate fever, dyspnea, cough, hypoxemia, and signs of CNS involvement such as paresis and obtundation. Brain CT scan or MRI disclose small subcortical infarctions. Chest x-ray film reveals bilateral fine linear infiltrates. The prognosis is extremely poor, although sporadic response to steroids has been observed.[151–154]

Moyamoya Syndrome

The first clinical description of this disease was reported in Japan by Takeuchi[155] in 1957. They reported a case of a 27-year-old man who had bilateral cerebral infarcts resulting from bilateral hypoplasia of the internal carotid artery. The term *moyamoya* means puffy, obscure, or vague, which represents the smoky presentation of the vascular network found in these patients.[156] Most patients with moyamoya are found in Asia, especially Japan. However, isolated cases have sporadically been reported from all over the world.

With the increasing recognition of this disease, Goto et al[156] recommended several criteria that could be used for diagnosis. These are (1) stenosis or occlusion of the distal intracranial portion of the internal carotid artery, the basilar trunk, or the proximal portion of the middle and anterior cerebral arteries and (2) the presence of an abnormal smoky vascular network, which is often bilateral.[157–160] Obviously all known causes of occlusion of the terminal portion of the internal carotid artery (e.g., cardiac emboli, arteriosclerosis, vasculitis, or brain tumor) must be excluded.[157–159,161,162] The annual incidence rate is estimated at 0.1 per 100,000 persons.[157–159,161–163] It affects children most often with a peak incidence at the age of 6 years.[157,158]

There are various clinical presentations that include: (1) repeated TIAs, observed mainly at the onset of the disease; (2) ischemic strokes (seen in most patients); (3) intracranial hemorrhage, probably resulting from an increase in blood pressure in the small perforators or the anastomotic network caused by occlusion of middle-size arteries; and (4) partial or generalized seizures.[156–159,161–164] Several other conditions can be associated with this disease, such as bilateral renal artery stenosis, arterial hypertension, diabetes mellitus, and multiple intracranial or systemic aneurysms.[156–159,161–164]

The cause of this syndrome remains unknown. A hereditary origin has been proposed because of the similarity of angiographic findings found in embryonic brain vessels in which the constitution of vascular wall muscle layers are often asymmetrical. This is also supported by an interfamilial coexistence with other congenital conditions such as von Recklinghausen neurofibromatosis, sickle cell anemia, and Down syndrome.[165] A congenital form occurs in about 10 percent of cases. Consequently, Fukuyama at al[164] have proposed a multifactorial mode of inheritance. Moyamoya also has been considered to be an acquired disease. In 1968, Suzuki et al implicated an autoimmune process because of the frequent association with upper respiratory tract infection.[157,158] However, in patients with moyamoya, an immune complex has not, as yet, been identified. Other conditions can favor the development of a moyamoya network, but in most cases this is a consequence of occlusion of carotid or middle or anterior cerebral arteries.[159,161,162]

Cerebral angiography remains the best diagnostic technique for moyamoya. Bilateral occlusions or, less often, stenosis of the cavernous region of the internal carotid artery in association with a puffy arteriolar network at the base of the skull are commonly identified.[155,159,161,162,166,167] This network depends on several collateral anastomoses, such as leptomeningeal anastomosis with the anterior and the posterior vascular systems, intradural anastomosis, and anastomosis of external carotid or ophthalmic arteries with anterior cerebral arteries. This pattern can evolve and anastomoses can increase or vanish. Currently, MRA allows a good estimation of the vascular network in patients suspected of having moyamoya. In addition, a combination of classical MRI and MRA allows a better definition of both the collateral network and the presence of potential small infarcts in the deep perforator artery territories. Cerebral blood flow studies using either single-photon emission computed tomography (SPECT), stable xenon-enhanced CT, or positron emission tomography (PET) are used to estimate the potential changes of regional cerebral blood flow in patients with moyamoya. PET, in particular, has the advantage of measuring cerebral blood flow and also the metabolism of oxygen, which can be an important indicator in patients considered for surgery.[155,158,167] In moyamoya patients, all of these techniques confirm a chronic low perfusion with a severe impairment of the vascular response to hypercapnia. This, however, is more marked in the forms affecting adults than those affecting children.[155,158,166,167] Other investigations such as electroencephalography can show nonspecific abnormalities. Currently, brain CT scans are not very helpful clinically.

Pathologically, stenosis or occlusion has been observed in the terminal portion of the carotid artery, the basilar trunk, and the proximal portion of the middle or anterior cerebral arteries.[161] Histologically, both the elastic lamina and media are involved. The elastic lamina is often duplicated, and the media is usually attenuated. There is generally an absence of inflammatory changes.[163] Arteries of the anastomotic network are also involved. In most patients, these arteries are dilated with intimal thickening, multiple stenoses, and, often, thrombosis of the distal portion.

Treatment of moyamoya disease depends on the pattern of symptoms that are displayed. Anticoagulation or antiplatelet therapies are usually used for stroke prevention.[49] Surgical therapy has been proposed by some, the aim being the establishment of collateral circulation to prevent further brain ischemia. Several techniques have previously been suggested: (1) cervical sympathectomy with ganglionectomy and sympathectomy of the carotid wall,[137,158] (2) direct reconstructive surgery of the cerebral arteries with or without encephalo-myo-synangiosis (this is effectively the application of temporal muscle on brain cortex to divert blood flow from the external carotid into the internal carotid system),[168,169] (3) superficial temporal-middle cerebral artery bypass,[170,171] and (4) transplantation of the omentum over the dura to increase the collateral network.[167,170–172] Most of these surgical techniques, particularly sympathectomy, have been abandoned, and their value regarding improvement of outcome is not yet known.[167,170–172]

Congential Angiopathies

This group of angiopathies is mainly represented by the congenital cutaneovascular syndromes, which have in common the presence of cutaneous abnormalities associated with cerebrovascular malformations secondary leading to arterial occlusions and intracerebral hemorrhages. Multiple aneurysms or arteriovenous malformations can also be seen. Often, the cutaneous abnormality is often present at the time of birth and constitutes a clue in the setting for congenital cutaneovascular syndromes.

Sturge-Weber Syndrome: Encephalo-facial Angiomatosis

The frequency of Sturge-Weber syndrome is estimated to be 1 in 5000 to 1 in 10,000 births. In the classical form, patients have facial nevi (see Figure 8.8) also called "port wine" lesions. Normally, the facial nevus is limited to the fifth cranial nerve distribution. The cutaneous lesion is often unilateral but can rarely involve the whole face and can extend to the trunk and extremities.[173] There is no evidence that the facial lesion is directly associated with intracranial abnormalities, but most of the patients who had intracranial vascular abnormalities have cutaneous lesions of the upper face, especially with involvement of the eyelid.[174] Sturge-Weber syndrome can also be present without the facial lesion in some cases.[173,174]

The clinical manifestations of the Sturge-Weber syndrome are due to the presence of vascular malformations. The most frequent symptom is epilepsy, which generally begins early in life.[173,175,176] Epileptic seizures can be accompanied by focal neurological signs such as hemiparesis, hemianopia, aphasia, and other cognitive and behavioral abnormalities, for which the suspected mechanism is localized cerebral hypoxia. Leptomeningeal, intracerebral,

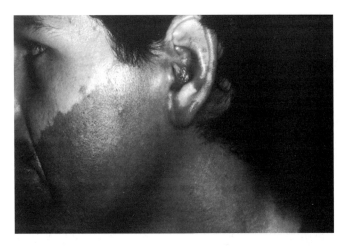

Figure 8.8   Sturge-Weber syndrome. Facial angioma.

cerebellar, and spinal cord angiomas can also be present; in these patients neurological manifestations could be the consequence of either epileptic seizures or venous or arterial occlusions.[173,175–178] Although intracerebral hemorrhages are relatively rare, subarachnoidal hemorrhages are frequent and result from leptomeningeal vessel rupture.

The diagnosis of Sturge-Weber syndrome is usually easy because of the presence of port wine angiomas (see Figure 8.9), often accompanied by ocular involvement such as cataract or glaucoma. However, because not all patients with facial nevi have brain involvement, it is necessary to perform complementary investigations to detect the patients who are at risk for cerebrovascular complications.[179–182] MRI and MRA are excellent for the detection of vascular malformations and can also be useful for evaluation of leptomeningeal or intracerebral angiomas.[183–189] Because the radiographic hallmark of Sturge-Weber syndrome is the presence of cerebral calcifications close to the leptomeningeal angioma, brain CT can be helpful for the detection of brain involvement in a newly diagnosed Sturge-Weber syndrome.[183,184] However, this investigation is only a first step and should be completed by MR examinations. Other techniques such as electroencephalogram, which characteristically shows asymmetrical slower frequency in the affected area, and positron emission tomography, which can show either hypometabolism or hypermetabolism of the affected area, provide little clinically useful information.[190] Currently, conventional arteriography should be necessary only in patients considered for surgery.

Pathologically, brain and leptomeningeal vessel calcifications are the most prominent findings. Neuronal loss and gliosis are often found and attributed to ischemic changes resulting from epileptic seizure. Microscopic examination of brain vessels discloses calcifications in the different arterial layers. Examination of leptomeningeal vessels shows hyalinization and subendothelial proliferations of arterial walls.[191,192]

Treatment of Sturge-Weber syndrome consists first in control of seizures. In case of refractory seizures, hemispherectomy has been recommended early in the life, first to improve seizure control and second to promote intellectual

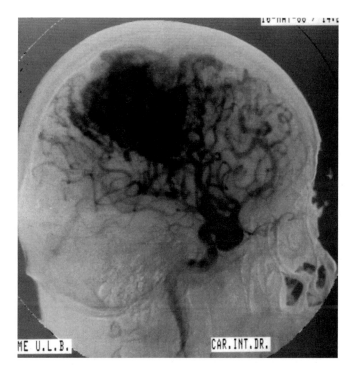

Figure 8.9 Sturge-Weber syndrome. Arteriovenous angioma in a 19-year-old man with Sturge-Weber syndrome.

development.[192,193] Prophylactic treatment with antiplatelet therapy has been proposed based on the concept that progressive deterioration could be a consequence of occlusive disease.

Ehlers-Danlos Syndrome

Ehlers-Danlos syndrome is a heterogeneous disorder characterized by joint hypermobility, skin hyperextensibility and fragility of connective tissues, and hyperelasticity of the skin. Roughly, eleven types of collagen anomalies have now been described.[194,195]

Ehlers-Danlos syndrome was first described in 1668 by Job van Mekren, who had observed a young man with extraordinary elasticity of the skin. Ehlers-Danlos syndrome is a congenital disease resulting from different base mutations in the gene for different types of collagen.[194,195] The most frequent manifestation of Ehlers-Danlos syndrome is attributed to the type IV, which results from abnormality of collagen type III. Because Ehlers-Danlos syndrome is a collagen disease, most of the neurological complications are due to arterial malformations.[196,197] The most frequent findings are intracranial aneurysms, carotid-cavernous fistula, and aortic and carotid dissections.[195–198] Cerebrovascular complications, mainly carotid or large-vessel dissections, are the most feared complications of this disorder. For this reason, angiography in these patients should be avoided or performed with extreme caution. All other organs can be involved, such as eyes, heart, kidneys, gut, and skin.[199–203]

Pathologically, Ehlers-Danlos syndrome type IV is caused by mutation in the gene for lysyl hydroxylase, which is the enzyme catalyzing the metabolism of hydroxylysine in collagen and in other proteins with collagen-like amino acid sequences.[204–210] Clinically, the diagnosis is made by fibroblast culture, which discloses a decrease in the proportion of type III collagen.

Angiokeratoma Corporis Diffusum: Fabry Disease

Angiokeratoma corporis diffusum or Fabry disease is an congenital X-linked disease characterized by abnormality of lysosomal storage and accumulation of ceramidetrihexoside caused by reduced activity of the enzyme α-galactosidase A.[211,212] The gene encoding for this enzyme is mapped to the chromosome X in position q22.[213] Because the disease is linked to the X chromosome, a complete penetrance in males is observed.

Clinically, the earliest symptoms of Fabry disease generally begin in the first decade of life and consist of dysesthesia of the extremities.[212] They always precede skin eruption, characterized by dark red papules of approximately 1 to 2 mm diameter (Figure 8.10). Generally, they are found on the trunk, scrotum, and on the proximal limbs. They can be rarely observed on the face and distal parts of the limbs[211,212,214] and may occur in clusters. Other organs can be involved, such as the eyes, with abnormalities in retinal vessels or the presence of cataracts. Later in the life, renal failure is observed and is due to nephroangiosclerosis.

Neurological complications are frequent and due either to vascular occlusions or more rarely brain hemorrhage.[196,199] Vascular occlusions are due to involvement of small and medium-size arteries by glycolipid accumulation in the elastic and in smooth muscle layers. This process leads to progressive occlusion of the vascular lumen.[215] Hemorrhages, particularly in the brain, can

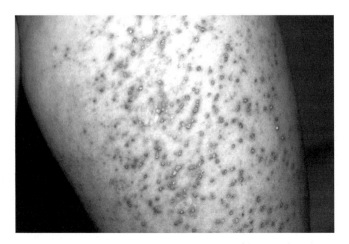

Figure 8.10 Fabry disease. Skin eruption in a patient with Fabry disease.

be the consequence of arterial hypertension, often seen in patients with renal failure, but also resulting from involvement of small and medium-size arteries because of accumulation of glycolipids. Currently, diagnosis of angiokeratoma corporis diffusum is made by the characteristic skin lesions, measurement of α-galactosidase A activity in leukocytes and fibroblasts, and blood dosage of ceramidetrihexoside. Genetic testing confirms the diagnosis.[213,215] Currently, treatment is symptomatic and consists of antiplatelet therapy, treatment of renal failure, and treatment for arterial hypertension. Experimental infusion of α-galactosidase A has not yet proved beneficial. Plasmapheresis to reduce the plasma level of ceramidetrihexoside does not improved the clinical findings.[213,215]

Hereditary Hemorrhagic Telangiectasia: Osler-Weber-Rendu Disease

Osler-Weber-Rendu disease or hereditary hemorrhagic telangiectasia (HHT) is an autosomal dominant disease, characterized by telangiectasia disseminated on the skin and nasal and visceral areas associated with recurrent hemorrhages. The most common feature is recurrent epistaxis.[216,217] Some patients can have hepatic encephalopathy resulting from multiple liver telangiectasia. Cerebrovascular events are mainly due to the presence of multiple intracranial arterial and venous malformations but also to extracranial mechanisms such as aneurysm to artery emboli. In 1983, Fisher et al[217] reported the case of a patient with HHT and recurrent right-sided paresis resulting from multiple emboli arising from a carotid-ophthalmic aneurysm. Other authors reported patients with pulmonary arteriovenous fistulas and paradoxical emboli and even air emboli in bronchovascular fistulas.[218,219] Other organs can also be involved such as the heart, gut, and urogenital system.

Treatment consists of antiplatelet therapy.[151,201–205] Anticoagulants are not recommended in these patients because of the risk of aneurysm rupture. Surgical therapy is considered only in patients with stroke resulting from emboli arising from cerebral aneurysm.[122]

Grönblad-Strandberg Syndrome: "Pseudoxanthoma Elasticum"

First described by Grönblad[220] in 1932, pseudoxanthoma elasticum is a congenital system disease involving elastic and connective tissues. The cause of this disease is an inborn anomaly of mucopolysaccharide metabolism, leading to calcifications of collagen and elastic fibers.

Phenotypically, patients can have small stature, mental retardation, and sex-developmental retardation with adrenogenital syndrome.[221] Several different systems can be impaired, but ocular and skin involvement are the most frequent. Ocular involvement consists of choroidal lesions with exudative macular degeneration and angioid streaks (see Figures 8.11 and 8.12).[222] Microscopically, the streaks are found in Bruch membrane with a choroidal capillary proliferation in the subretinal space. Skin lesions are yellowish and efflorescent, resulting from an increase of elastic fibers, and have calcifications. The appearance of this pattern has suggested the name *pseudoxanthoma elasticum.*[222] Several other organs can be involved such as the cardiovascular system and endocrine system (often thyroid function impairment).

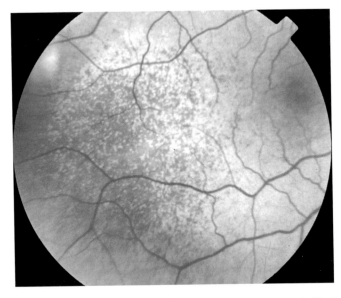

Figure 8.11   Pseudoxanthoma elasticum (Grönblad-Strandberg disease). Typical "orange peel" aspect of the retina in a young patient with carotid artery dissection resulting from pseudoxanthoma elasticum.

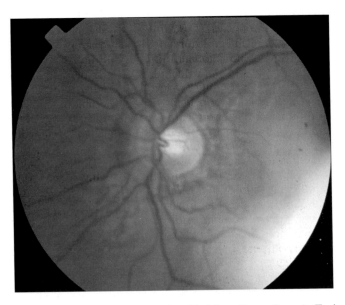

Figure 8.12   Pseudoxanthoma elasticum (Grönblad-Strandberg disease). Typical angioid streaks in a young patient with carotid artery dissection resulting from pseudoxanthoma elasticum.

Neurological symptoms are the consequence of multiple cerebral infarctions, mostly resulting from small-vessel disease, but arterial dissections can also be found. Pathologically, this process involved the elastic layer of large and medium-size arteries, leading to disruption of the elastic layer and either artery-to-artery emboli, dissection, or occlusion.

von Recklinghausen Neurofibromatosis

von Recklinghausen neurofibromatosis is a congenital disease that can involve any organ system. Currently two forms are distinguished. Type I, related to a chromosome 17 anomaly, is characterized by the presence of hyperpigmented patches of skin café au lait macules, axillary freckles, Lisch nodules, sphenoid wing dysplasia, and peripheral nerve tumors. Type II, related to a chromosome 22 anomaly, meets some criteria seen in type I and is characterized by the presence of acoustic neurinoma, often bilateral.[223,224] Both forms can be accompanied by vascular abnormalities, involving mainly the splanchnic and renal arteries.

Involvement of cerebral arteries is uncommon. It consists of occlusions of the distal part of the internal carotid arteries or of the proximal part of the anterior circulation arising from the circle of Willis, accompanied by a moyamoya collateral network.[225] Cerebral aneurysm can occur alone or be accompanied by occlusions. Currently, only about 44 cases of cerebral arterial involvement have been reported. In most cases, occlusions alone were found. In addition most of the patients had arterial hypertension, probably resulting from renal artery involvement. Histologically, arterial lesions consists of diffuse hyperplasia of the intimal layer producing luminal stenosis and intimal hyperplasia with fragmentation and reduplication of the elastic layer of the intrapetrosal segment of the internal carotid artery or of the proximal part of the anterior and middle cerebral arteries.[225,226]

Marfan Syndrome

Marfan syndrome is an inherited, autosomal dominant disorder that affects the skeletal, ocular, cardiovascular, and central nervous systems. There is extreme variability in clinical expression and some patients can have all systems involved, whereas others can have only one organ impaired. Its frequency varies from 1 in 10,000 to 1 in 50,000.[227,228]

Clinical manifestations are the consequence of involvement of eyes, arteries and veins, and the skeleton. Cardiovascular impairment is the most frequent finding in Marfan syndrome.[229,230] Involvement of large arteries such as the aorta and carotid arteries is the rule and the cause of death. Dissection of the proximal part of the aorta and of the primitive carotid arteries are the most life-threatening events. Heart involvement is not rare and consists of valvular abnormalities such as mitral and aortic insufficiency. Involvement of medium- and small-size arteries is exceptional, and, in Marfan syndrome, cerebral infarctions result from artery-to-artery emboli or carotid occlusion rather than from distal local thrombosis.[229,230]

Ocular manifestations are frequent. They result from anomalies of the connective tissue, which is the support of the different parts of the eye. Dislocation or subluxation of the lens is often observed. They occur in approximately 80 percent of the patients with Marfan syndrome and are preceded by iridodesis, a slight tremor of the iris. Clinical consequences can include glaucoma, uveitis, and cataracts. Skeletal anomalies consist of increased length of bones, and most of the patients are tall. Disproportion of the different parts of the body is characteristic of the syndrome and generally the inferior part of the body (pubic bone to feet) is taller than the upper part (pubis to head). Fingers are extremely long and constitute the so-called arachnodactily syndrome. Hyperlaxity of joints, especially of the wrist and fingers, is also a major finding. Finally, the hard palate is abnormal and has an arch-like form.

Pathologically, Marfan syndrome results from defects in the connective tissue protein fibrillin. The disease has been associated with mutations in the fibrillin gene, which is mapped to the chromosome 7.[229,231] Fibrillin is a component of microfibrils, structures found in the extracellular matrices of most tissues that lead to the formation of elastin. The appearance of microfibrils in the matrix produced by fibroblasts of patients with Marfan syndrome is different than normal cells;[232–234] involvement of the media is observed with dislocation of the elastic layer. Treatment of patients with Marfan syndrome remains symptomatic.

References

1. Kolhmeier WW. Multiple Hautnekrausen bei thrombangiitis obliterans. Arch Klin Exp Dermatol 1941;181:783–792.
2. Degos R, Delort J, Tricot R. Dermatite papulosquameuse atrophiante. Bull Soc Fr Dermatol Syphiligr 1942;49:148–150.
3. Degos RD, Tricot R. Papulose atrophiante maligne (syndrome cutanéo- intestinal mortel). Bull Mem Soc MedHop Paris 1948;64:803–806.
4. Degos R. Malignant atrophic papulosis. Br J Dermatol 1979;100:21–23.
5. Moulin GB, Franc D, Pierson MP. Papulose atrophiante de Degos familiale (mère-fille). Ann Dermatol Vénéréol 1984;111:149–155.
6. Shimazu SI, Kokubu A, Sugimoto S, et al. Long term survival in malignant atrophic papulosis: a case report and review of the Japanese literature. Nippon Geka Gakkai Zasshi 1988;89:1748–1751.
7. Horner FM, Stumpf GJ, Oseroff DA, et al. Malignant atrophic papulosis (Kohlmeier-Degos disease) in childhood. Neurology 1976;26:317–321.
8. Barabino AP, Gatti F, Colotto R, et al. An atypical paediatric case of malignant atrophic papulosis (Kohlmeier-Degos disease). Eur J Pediatr 1990;149:457–458.
9. Sibillat MA, Charpentier MF, Offret P, et al. Papulose atrophiante maligne (maladie de Degos): revue clinique a propos d' un cas. J FR Ophthalmol 1986;9:299–304.
10. Dastur DS, Shroff BS, Schroff HJ. CNS involvement in malignant atrophic papulosis (Kohlmeier-Degos disease): vasculopathy and coagulopathy. J Neurol Neurosurg Psychiatry 1981;44:156–160.
11. Doutre MB, Bioulac C, Busquet P, et al. Skin lesion resembling malignant atrophic papulosis in lupus erythematosus. Dermatologica 1987;182:45–46.
12. Casparie MM, van Huystee JW, Kneppelhout BE, et al. Endoscopic and histopathologic features of Degos' disease. Endoscopy 1991;23:231–233.
13. Rosemberg S, Lopes MB, Sotto MN, Graudenz MS. Childhood Degos disease with prominent neurological symptoms: report of a clinicopathological case. J Child Neurol 1988;3:43–46.
14. Sotrel A, Lacson AG, Huff KR. Childhood Kohlmeier-Degos disease with atypical skin lesions. Neurology 1983;33:1146–1151.
15. Muller SA, Landry M. Malignant atrophic papulosis (Degos disease). A report of two cases with clinical and histological studies. Arch Dermatol 1976;112:357–363.
16. Lee DA, Su WP, Liesegang TJ. Ophthalmic changes of Degos' disease (malignant atrophic papulosis). Ophthalmology 1984;91:295–299.
17. Magrinat G, Kerwin KS, Gabriel DA. The clinical manifestations of Degos' syndrome. Arch Pathol Lab Med 1989;113:354–362.

18. Hull RD, Raskob GE, Pineo GF, et al. Subcutaneous low-molecular-weight heparin compared with continuous intravenous heparin in the treatment of proximal-vein thrombosis. N Engl J Med 1992;326:975–982.
19. Pierce RN, Smith GJ. Intrathoracic manifestations of Degos' disease (malignant atrophic papulosis): Report of one case with a review of the literature. Chest 1978;73:79–84.
20. Requena L, Farina C, Barat A. Degos disease in a patient with acquired immunodeficiency syndrome. J Am Acad Dermatol 1998;38(5 Pt 2):852–856.
21. Lomholt G, Hjorth N, Fischerman K. Lethal peritonitis from Degos' disease (malignant atrophic papulosis): Report of one case with a review of the literature. Acta Chir Scand 1968;134:495–501.
22. Snow JL, Muller SA. Degos syndrome: malignant atrophic papulosis. Semin Dermatol 1995;14:99–105.
23. Yoshikawa H, Maruta T, Yokoji H, et al. Degos' disease: radiological and immunological aspects. Acta Neurol Scand 1996;94:353–356.
24. Fruhwirth J, Mischinger HJ, Werkgartner G, et al. Kohlmeier-Degos's disease with primary intestinal manifestation. Scand J Gastroenterol 1997;32:1066–1070.
25. Label LS, Tandan R, Albers JW. Myelomalacia and hypoglycorrhachia in malignant atrophic papulosis. Neurology 1983;33:936–939.
26. Su WP, Schroeter AL, Lee DA, et al. Clinical and histological findings in Degos' syndrome (malignant atrophic papulosis). Cutis 1985;35:131–138.
27. Demitsu T, Nakajima K, Okuyama R, Tadaki T. Malignant atrophic papulosis (Degos' syndrome). Int J Dermatol 1992;31:99–102.
28. Molenaar WM, Rosman JB, Donker AJ, Houthoff HJ. The pathology and pathogenesis of malignant atrophic papulosis (Degos' disease). Pathol Res Pract 1987;182:98–106.
29. Bulengo-Ransby SM, Burns MK, Taylor WB, et al. Peristomal atrophic papules. Degos' disease (malignant atrophic papulosis). Arch Dermatol 1992;128:256–257, 259–260.
30. Burrow JN, Blumbergs PC, Iyer PV, et al. Kohlmeier-Degos disease: a multisystem vasculopathy with progressive cerebral infarction. Aust N Z J Med 1991;21:49–51.
31. Bioulac P, Doutre MS, Beylot C. La papulose atrophiante maligne de Degos. Etude ultrastructurale d' un nouveau cas. Ann Anat Pathol Paris 1980;25:111–124.
32. Kisch LS, Bruynzeel DP. Six cases of malignant atrophic papulosis (Degos' disease) occurring in one family. Br J Dermatol 1984;111:469–471.
33. Black MM, Hudson PM. Atrophie blanche lesions closely resembling malignant atrophic papulosis (Degos' disease) in systemic lupus erythematosus. Br J Dermatol 1976;95:649–652.
34. Asherson R, Cevera R. Antiphospholipid syndrome. J Invest Dermatol 1993;100:21–27.
35. Englert HJ, Hawkes CH, Boey ML, et al. Degos' disease: association with anticardiolipin antibodies and the lupus anticoagulant. BMJ (Clin Res Ed) 1984;289:576.
36. Stahl DT, Hou-Jensen K. Malignant atrophic papulosis. Treatment with aspirin and dipyridamole. Arch Dermatol 1978;114:1687–1689.
37. Powell J, Bordea C, Wojnarowska F, et al. Benign familial Degos disease worsening during immuno-suppression. Br J Dermatol 1999;141:524–527.
38. Pallesen RM, Rasmussen NR. Malignant atrophic papulosis (Degos syndrome). Acta Chir Scand 1979;145:279–283.
39. Tribble KA, Jorrizo ME, Sanchez JL, et al. Malignant atrophic papulosis: absence of circulating immune complexes or vasculitis. J Am Acad Dermatol 1986;15:365–369.
40. McFarland HR, Wood WG, Drowns BV, Meneses AC. Papulosis atrophicans maligna (Kohlmeier-Degos disease) a disseminated occlusive vasculopathy. Ann Neurol 1978;3:388–392.
41. Drucker C. Malignant atrophic papulosis: response to antiplatelet therapy. Dermatologica 1990; 180:90–92.
42. Howsden SM, Hodge SJ, Herndon JH, Freeman RG. Malignant atrophic papulosis of Degos. Report of a patient who failed to respond to fibrinolytic therapy. Arch Dermatol 1976;112:1582–1588.
43. Daniel F, Foix C, Gray JM, et al. Papulose atrophiante maligne avec insuffisance de la fibrinolyse sanguine. Ann Dermatol Vénéréol 1982;109:763–764.
44. Montalban J, Ordi J, Barquinero J, et al. Sneddon's syndrome and anticardiolipin antibodies. Stroke 1988;19:785–786.
45. Bruyn RP. Sneddon's syndrome. Acta Neurol Scand 1991;84:460.
46. Asherson RA, Khamashta MA. Sneddon's syndrome and primary anti-phospholipid syndrome (PAPS). Br J Dermatol 1990;122:115–116.
47. Asherson RA, Khamashta MA, Hughes GR. Sneddon's syndrome. Neurology 1989;39:1138–1139.
48. Kalashnikova LA, Korczyn AD, Shavit S, et al. Antibodies to prothrombin in patients with Sneddon's syndrome. Neurology 1999;53:223–225.
49. Kalashnikova LA, Nasonov EL, Borisenko VV, et al. Sneddon's syndrome: cardiac pathology and antiphospholipid antibodies. Clin Exp Rheumatol 1991;9:357–361.

50. Kalashnikova LA, Nasonov EL, Kushekbaeva AE, et al. Anticardiolipin antibodies in Sneddon's syndrome. Neurology 1990;40(3 Pt 1):464–467.
51. Kalashnikova LN, Stoyanovich EL, Kovalyov LZ, et al. Sneddon's syndrome and the primary antiphospholipid syndrome. Cerebrovasc Dis 1994;4:476–482.
52. Rich MW. Sneddon syndrome and dementia. Mayo Clin Proc 1999;74:1306.
53. Rehany U, Kassif Y, Rumelt S. Sneddon's syndrome: neuro-ophthalmologic manifestations in a possible autosomal recessive pattern. Neurology 1998;51(4):1185–7.
54. Parmeggiani A, Posar A, De Giorgi LB, et al. Sneddon syndrome, arylsulfatase A pseudodeficiency and impairment of cerebral white matter. Brain Dev 2000;22:390–393.
55. Stockhammer GJ, Felber SR, Aichner FT, et al. Sneddon's syndrome and antiphospholipid antibodies: clarification of a controversy by skin biopsy? Stroke 1992;23:1182–1183.
56. Stockhammer G, Felber SR, Zelger B, et al. Sneddon's syndrome: diagnosis by skin biopsy and MRI in 17 patients. Stroke 1993;24:685–690.
57. Vargas JA, Yebra M, Pascual ML, et al. Antiphospholipid antibodies and Sneddon's syndrome. Am J Med 1989;87:597.
58. Schellong SM, Weissenborn K, Niedermeyer J, et al. Classification of Sneddon's syndrome. Vasa 1997;26:215–221.
59. Van Bogaert L. Sur l' angiomatose méningée avec leucodystrophie. Wien Z Nervenheilkd Deren Grenzgeb 1967;25:131–136.
60. Wohlrab J, Fischer M, Wolter M, et al. Diagnostic impact and sensitivity of skin biopsies in Sneddon's syndrome. A report of 15 cases. Br J Dermatol 2001;145:285–288.
61. Zelger B, Sepp N, Stockhammer G, et al. Sneddon's syndrome. A long-term follow-up of 21 patients. Arch Dermatol 1993;129:437–447.
62. Vonsattel J-PG, Hedley-Whyte T. Diffuse Meningocerebral Angiomatosis and Leucoencephalopathy. In HL Klawans (ed), Handbook of Clinical Neurology. Vascular Diseases, Part III. New York: Elsevier, 1989;317–324.
63. el-Shanti H, Bell WE, Waziri MH. Epidermal nevus syndrome: subgroup with neuronal migration defects. J Child Neurol 1992;7:29–34.
64. Dobyns WB, Garg BP. Vascular abnormalities in epidermal nevus syndrome. Neurology 1991;41:276–278.
65. Pavone L, Curatolo P, Rizzor, et al. Epidermal nevus syndrome: A neurologic variant with hemimegalencephaly, gyral malformation, mental retardation, seizures, and facial hemihypertrophy. Neurology 1991;41:266–271.
66. Carney JA, Gordon H, Carpenter PC, et al. The complex of myxomas, spotty pigmentation, and endocrine overactivity. Medicine 1985;64:270–283.
67. Forney WR, Robinson SJ, Pascoe DJ. Congenital heart disease, deafness, and skeletal malformation. A new syndrome. J Pediatr 1966;68:14–26.
68. Fauci A. NIH conference: the idiopathic hypereosinophilic syndrome. Ann Intern Med 1982;97:78–81.
69. Dorfman LJ, Ransom BR, Forno LS, Kelts A. Neuropathy in the hypereosinophilic syndrome. Muscle Nerve 1983;6:291–298.
70. Weaver DF, Heffernan LP, Purdy RA, Ing VW. Eosinophil-induced neurotoxicity: axonal neuropathy, cerebral infarction, and dementia. Neurology 1988;38:144–146.
71. Kawasaki T. Mucocutaneous lymph node syndrome. Clinical observation of 50 cases. Jpn J Allerg 1967;16:178–22.
72. Lapointe JS, Nugent RA, Graeb DA, et al. Cerebral infarction and regression of widespread aneurysms in Kawasaki's disease: case report. Pediatr Radiol 1984;14:1–5.
73. Laxer RMD, H.G. Fiedmark, O. Acute hemiplegia in Kawasaki disease and infantile polyarteritis nodosa. Dev Med Child Neurol 1984;26:814–881.
74. Yonesaka ST, Matubara T, Nakada T, et al. Histopathological study on Kawasaki disease with special reference to the relation between the myocardial sequelae and regional wall motion abnormalities of the left ventricle. Jpn Circ J 1992;56:352–358.
75. Lauret P. Kawasaki disease complicated by thrombosis of the internal carotid artery. Ann Dermatol Venerol 1979;106:901–905.
76. Marcella J. Kawasaki syndrome in an adult: endomyocardial histology and ventricular function during acute and recovery phases of illness. J Am Coll Cardiol 1983;2:374–378.
77. Boespflug O, Tardieu M, Losay J, Leroy D. Hémiplégie aigue compliquant une maladie de Kawasaki. Rev Neurol 1984;140:507–509.
78. Gordon MF, Coyle PK, Golub B. Eales' disease presenting as stroke in the young adult. Ann Neurol 1988;24:264–266.
79. Gatkari S, Kamdar P, Jehangir R, et al. Pars plana in vitrectomy in vitreous haemorrhage due to Eales' disease. Indian J Ophthalmol 1992;40:35–37.

80. Weber F, Conrad B. Chronic encephalitis and Eales disease. J Neurol 1993;240:299–301.
81. Sen D, Sarin G, Ghosh A, et al. Serum apha-1 glycoprotein levels in patients with idiopathic peripheral retinal vasculitis (Eales' disease). Acta Ophthalmol Copenh 1992;70:515–517.
82. Atabay C, Erdem E, Kansu T, et al. Eales' disease with internuclear ophthalmoplegia. Ann Ophthalmol 1992;24:267–269.
83. Phamthumchinda K. Eales' disease with myelopathy. J Med Assoc Thai 1992;75:255–258.
84. Ponomis E, Triantafillidis J, Tjenaki M, et al. Report of Eales' disease and ulcerative colitis in the same patient. Am J Gastroenterol 1992;87:1531–1532.
85. Gass JMD. Acute posterior multifocal placoid pigment epitheliopathy. Arch Ophthalmol 1968; 80:177–185.
86. Deutman AF, Oosterhuis JA, Boen-Tan TN, Aan de Kerk AL. Acute posterior multifocal placoid pigment epitheliopathy. Br J Ophthalmol 1972;58:863–874.
87. Stoll G, Reiners K, Schwartz A, et al. Acute posterior multifocal placoid pigment epitheliopathy with cerebral involvement. J Neurol Neurosurg Psychiatry 1991;54:77–79.
88. Azar P Jr, Gohd RS, Waltman D, Gitter KA. Acute posterior multifocal placoid pigment epitheliopathy associated with an adenovirus type 5 infection. Am J Ophthalmol 1975;80: 1003–1005.
89. Manto M, Cordonier M, Blecic S, et al. Acute posterior multifocal placoid pigment epitheliopathy presenting as an aseptic meningitidis. Eur J Neurol 1995;2:181–183.
90. Smith CH, Savino PJ, Beck RW, et al. Acute posterior multifocal placoid pigment epitheliopathy and cerebral vasculitis. Arch Neurol 1983;40:48–50.
91. Lyness AL, Bird AC. Recurrences of acute posterior multifocal placoid pigment epitheliopathy. Am J Ophthalmol 1984;98:203–207.
92. Jacklin H. Acute posterior multifocal placoid pigment epitheliopathy and thyroiditis. Arch Ophthalmol 1977;9:393–396.
93. Holt WS, Regan CD, Trempe C. Acute posterior multifocal placoid pigment epitheliopathy. Am J Ophthalmol 1976;81:403–406.
94. Bewermeyer H, Nelles G, Huber M, et al. Pontine infarction in acute posterior multifocal placoid pigment epitheliopathy. J Neurol 1993;241:22–26.
95. Bullock JD, Fletcher RL. Cerebrospinal fluid abnormalities in acute posterior multifocal placoid pigment epithelialopathy. Am J Ophthalmol 1977;84:45–49.
96. Fishman GA, Baskin M, Jednock N. Spinal fluid pleiocytosis in acute posterior multifocal placoid pigment epitheliopathy. Ann Ophthalmol 1977;9:36.
97. Kersten DH, Lessell S, Carlow TJ. Acute posterior multifocal placoid pigment epitheliopathy and late onset meningoencephalitis. Ophthalmology 1987;94:393–396.
98. Laatikainen LT, Immonen IJ. Acute posterior multifocal placoid pigment epitheliopathy in connection with acute nephritis. Retina 1988;8:122–124.
99. Priluck IR, Buettner DM. Acute posterior multifocal placoid pigment epitheliopathy: urinary findings. Arch Ophthalmol 1981;99:1560–1652.
100. Wilson CC, Sheppard EA. Acute posterior multifocal placoid pigment epitheliopathy and cerebral vasculitis. Arch Ophthalmol 1988;106:796–800.
101. Susac JO, Hardman JM, Selhorst JB. Microangiopathy of the brain and retina. Neurology 1979;29:313–316.
102. Bogousslavsky J, Gaio JM, Caplan LR, et al. Encephalopathy, deafness and blindness in young women: a distinct retinocochleocerebral arteriolopathy? J Neurol Neurosurg Psychiatry 1989; 52:43–46.
103. Heiskala H, Somer H, Kovanen J, et al. Microangiopathy with encephalopathy, hearing loss and retinal arteriolar occlusions: two new cases. J Neurol Sci 1988;86:239–250.
104. Silverboard G, Tart R. Cerebrovascular arterial dissection in children and young adults. Semin Pediatr Neurol 2000;7:289–300.
105. Rhodes RH, Phillips S, Booth FA, et al. Dissecting hematoma of intracranial internal carotid artery in an 8-year-old girl. Can J Neurol Sci 2001;28:357–364.
106. Mokri B. Headaches in cervical artery dissections. Curr Pain Headache Rep 2002;6(3):209–216.
107. Khimenko LP, Esham HR, Ahmed W. Spontaneous internal carotid artery dissection. South Med J 2000;93:1011–1016.
108. Gonzales-Portillo F, Bruno A, Biller J. Outcome of extracranial cervicocephalic arterial dissections: a follow-up study. Neurol Res 2002;24:395–398.
109. Yamashita H, Fujikawa T, Yanai I, et al. Clinical features and treatment response of patients with major depression and silent cerebral infarction. Neuropsychobiology 2001;44(4):176–182.
110. Rothwell DM, Bondy SJ, Williams JI. Chiropractic manipulation and stroke: a population-based case-control study. Stroke 2001;32:1054–1060.

111. Prabhakar S, Bhatia R, Khandelwal N, et al. Vertebral artery dissection due to indirect neck trauma: an underrecognised entity. Neurol India 2001;49:384–390.
112. Kelkar AS, Karande S, Chaudhary V, et al. Traumatic posterior cerebral artery occlusion in a 14-month-old child. Pediatr Neurol 2002;27:147–149.
113. Duverger V, Szymszyczin P, Singland JD, et al. [Spontaneous internal carotid artery dissection]. J Mal Vasc 2000;25:276–279.
114. Chaves C, Estol C, Esnaola MM, et al. Spontaneous intracranial internal carotid artery dissection: report of 10 patients. Arch Neurol 2002;59:977–981.
115. Pniewski J, Wozniak R, Chodakowska-Zebrowska M, et al. CT angiography in the diagnosis of spontaneous extracerebral vertebral artery dissection. Folia Neuropathol 2002;40(1):33–37.
116. Schievink WI. The treatment of spontaneous carotid and vertebral artery dissections. Curr Opin Cardiol 2000;15:316–321.
117. Sandmann J, Hojer C, Bewermeyer H, et al. Die fibromuskulare dysplasie als ursache zerebrale insulte. Nervenarzt 1992;63:335–340.
118. Velkey I, Lombay B, Panczel G. Obstruction of cerebral arteries in childhood stroke. Pediatr Radiol 1992;22:386–387.
119. Watanabe S, Tanaka K, Nakayama T, Kaneko M. Fibromuscular dysplasia at the internal carotid origin: a case of carotid web. No Shinkei Geka 1993;21:449–452.
120. Josien E. Extracranial vertebral artery dissection: nine cases. J Neurol 1992;239:327–330.
121. Heiserman JE, Drayer BP, Fram EK, Keller PJ. MR angiography of cervical fibromuscular dysplasia. Am J Neuroradiol 1992;13:1454–1457.
122. Humphries JE, Frierson HF Jr, Underwood PB Jr. Vaginal telangiectasias: unusual presentation of the Osler-Weber-Rendu syndrome. Obstet Gynecol 1993;81:865–866.
123. Giller CAM, Purdy D. The transcranial Doppler appearance of acute carotid artery occlusion. Ann Neurol 1992;31:101–103.
124. Edwards JM, Zaccardi MJ, Strandness DE Jr. A preliminary study of the role of duplex scanning in defining the adequacy of patients with renal artery fibromuscular dysplasia. J Vasc Surg 1992;15:604–611.
125. Schulze HE, Ebner A, Besinger UA. Report of dissection of the internal carotid artery in three cases. Neurosurg Rev 1992;15:61–64.
126. Ashleigh RJ, Weller JM, Leggate JR. Fibromuscular hyperplasia of the internal carotid artery. A further cause of the 'moyamoya' collateral circulation. Br J Neurosurg 1992;6:269–273.
127. Bour PT, Bracard I. Aneurysms of the extracranial internal carotid artery due to fibromuscular dysplasia: results of surgical management. Ann Vasc Surg 1992;6:205–208.
128. Gatalica Z, Gibas Z, Martinez-Hernandez A. Dissecting aortic aneurysm as a complication of generalized fibromuscular dysplasia. Hum Pathol 1992;23:586–588.
129. Baumgartner RW, Waespe W. Behandelbare erkrankungen des nervensystems mit kataraktbildung. Klin Monatsbl Augenheilkd 1993;202:89–93.
130. Padget D. Designation of the embryonic intersegmental arteries in references to the vertebral artery and subclavian stem. Anat Rec 1954;119:349–56.
131. Anderson RA, Sondheimer FK. Rare carotid-vertebrobasilar anastomoses with notes on the differentiation between proatlantal and hypoglossal arteries. Neuroradiology 1976;11:113–118.
132. Lasjaunias PB. Aneurysms. Berlin: Springer-Verlag, 1987.
133. Bahsi YZ, Uysal H, Peker S, Yurdakul M. Persistent primitive proatlantal intersegmental (proatlantal artery I) results in 'top of the basilar' syndrome. Stroke 1993;24:2114–2117.
134. Parenti G, Fiori L, Marconi F. Intracranial aneurysm and cerebral embolism. Eur Neurol 1992;32:212–215.
135. Taptas JN, Katsiotis PA. Arterial embolism as a cause of hemiplegia after subarachnoidal hemorrhage from aneurysm. Prog Brain Res 1968;30:357–360.
136. Nakai H, Kawata Y, Tomabechi M, et al. Markedly dilated cervical carotid arteries in a patient with a ruptured aneurysm of the anterior communicating artery: a case report. No Shinkei Geka 1993;21:333–339.
137. Suzuki S, Inoue T, Haga S, et al. Stroke due to a fusiform aneurysm of the cervical vertebral artery: case report. Neuroradiology 1998;40:19–22.
138. Kindl R, Nigbur H, Horsch S. Das extrakranielle Aneurysma der arteria carotis interna. Eine fallbeschreibung. Vasa 1993;22:256–259.
139. Murros KE, Toole JF. The effect of radiation on carotid arteries: a review article. Arch Neurol 1989;46:449–455.
140. Levinson SA, Close MB, Ehrenfeld WK, Stoney RJ. Carotid artery occlusive disease following external cervical irradiation. Arch Surg 1973;107:395–397.

141. Lambrechts HDdB. Contributions to the study of immediate and early x-ray reactions with regard to chemoprotection: VI. X-ray induced atheromatous lesions in the arterial wall of cholesterolemic rabbits. Int J Radiol Biol 1965;9:165–174.

142. Glick B. Bilateral carotid occlusive disease. Arch Pathol Lab Med 1972;93:352–355.

143. Brachlow J, Schafer M, Oliveira H, Jantzen JP. Todlische intraoperative zerebrale ischemie infolge kinking der arteria carotis interna. Anaesthesist 1992;41:361–364.

144. Weibel JF, W. Tortuosity, coiling and kinking of the internal carotid artery: etiology and radiographic anatomy. Neurology 1965;15:7–20.

145. Kitanaka C, Tanaka J, Kuwahara M, et al. Magnetic resonance imaging study of intracranial vertebrobasilar artery dissections. Stroke 1994;25:571–575.

146. Call GK, Fleming MC, Sealfon S, et al. Reversible cerebral segmental vasoconstriction. Stroke 1988;19:1159–1170.

147. Le Coz P, Woimant F, Rougemont D, et al. Benign cerebral angiopathies and phenylpropanolamine. Rev Neurol (Paris) 1988;144:295–300.

148. Bogousslavsky JD, Regli PA. Postpartum cerebral angiopathy: reversible vasoconstriction assessed by transcranial Doppler ultrasounds. Eur Neurol 1989;29:102–106.

149. Brick J. Vanishing cerebrovascular disease of pregnancy. Neurology 1988;38:804–806.

150. Mullges W, Ringelstein EB, Leibold M. Non-invasive diagnosis of internal carotid artery dissections. J Neurol Neurosurg Psychiatry 1992;55:98–104.

151. Smadja D, Mas JL, Fallet-Bianco C, et al. Intravascular lymphomatosis (neoplastic angioendotheliosis) of the central nervous system: case report and literature review. J Neuro Oncol 1991;11:171–180.

152. Wick MR, Mills SE. Intravascular lymphomatosis: clinicopathologic features and differential diagnosis. Semin Diagn Pathol 1991;8:91–101.

153. Pretre R, Reverdin A, Kalonji T, et al. Blunt carotid artery injury: difficult therapeutic approaches for an underrecognized entity. Surgery 1994;115:375–381.

154. Delplace J, Van Blercom N, Dargent JL, et al. Accidents vasculaires cérébraux d'étiologie inhabituelle et d'évolution fatale. Ann Pathol 1995;15:219–220.

155. Takeuchi KS. Hypoplasia of the bilateral internal carotid arteries. Brain Nerve 1957;9:37–43.

156. Gotoh F. Guideline to the Diagnosis of Occlusion of the Circle of Willis. In F Gotoh (ed), Annual Report of 1978 of the Research Committee on Spontaneous Occlusion of the Circle of Willis (Moyamoya Disease). Japan: Ministry of Health and Welfare, 1979;132–134.

157. Suzuki J, Takaku A, Asahi M. Evaluation of a group of disorders showing an abnormal vascular network at the base of the brain with a high incidence among the Japanese. 2: Follow-up studies by cerebral angiography. Brain Nerve 1966;18:897–908.

158. Suzuki J, Takaku A, Kodama N, Sato S. An attempt to treat cerebrovascular 'Moyamoya' disease in children. Childs Brain 1975;1:193–206.

159. Nishimoto A, Takeuchi S. Abnormal cerebrovascular network related to the internal carotid arteries. J Neurosurg 1968;29:255–260.

160. Beyer RA, Paden P, Sobel DF, Flynn FG. Moyamoya pattern of vascular occlusion after radiotherapy for glioma of the optic chiasm. Neurology 1986;36:1173–1178.

161. Gautier JC, Hauw JJ, Awada A, et al. Artères cérébrales dolichoectasiques. Association aux anevrysmes de l'aorte abdominale. Rev Neurol (Paris) 1988;144:437–446.

162. Bruno A, Adams HP Jr, Biller J, et al. Cerebral infarction due to Moyamoya disease in young adults. Stroke 1988;19:826–833.

163. Sue DE, Brant-Zawadzki MN, Chance J. Dissection of cranial arteries in the neck: correlation of MRI and arteriography. Neuroradiology 1992;34:273–278.

164. Fukuyama YK, Osawa M. Gene Study on Occlusion of the Circle of Willis, 3rd Report. In H Handa (ed), Annual Report of 1983 of the Research Committee on Spontaneous Occlusion of the Circle of Willis (Moyamoya Disease). Japan: Ministry of Health and Welfare, 1983;16–19.

165. Fujisawa IA, Nishimura K. Moyamoya disease: MR imaging. Radiology 1987;164:103–106.

166. Taki WH, Yonekawa H. Cerebral blood volume, blood flow and oxygen utilization in moyamoya disease. J Cereb Blood Flow Metab 1988;5(suppl 1):439–445.

167. Tatemichi TK, Prohovnik I, Mohr JP. Reduced hypercapnic vasoreactivity in moyamoya disease. Neurology 1988;38:1575–1578.

168. Karasawa J, Kikuchi H, Furuse S, et al. A surgical treatment of 'moyamoya disease': encephalo-myo-synangiosis. Neurol Med Chir (Tokyo) 1977;17:29–36.

169. Krayenbuhl H. The moyamoya syndrome and the neurosurgeon. Surg Neurol 1975;4:353–360.

170. Handa H, Yonekawa Y, Suda K. Postoperative Appearance of Newly Developed LDA on CT Scan. Research on the Immune Complex. In F Gotoh (ed), Annual Report of the Research Committee on Spontaneous Occlusion of the Circle of Willis. Japan: Ministry of Health and Welfare, 1981;124–143.

171. Yonekawa Y, Yasargil MG. Brain vascularisation by transplanted omentum: a possible treatment of brain ischemia. Neurosurgery 1977;1:256–259.
172. Tokunaga Y, Ohga S, Suita S, et al. Moyamoya syndrome with spherocytosis: effect of splenectomy on strokes. Pediatr Neurol 2001;25:75–77.
173. Roach ES. Diagnosis and management of neurocutaneous syndromes. Semin Neurol 1988; 8:83–96.
174. Enjolras O, Riche MC, Merland JJ. Facial portwine stains and Sturge-Weber syndrome. Pediatrics 1985;76:48–51.
175. Liang CW, Liang KH. Sturge-Weber syndrome without facial nevus. Chin Med J Engl 1992;105:964–965.
176. Taly AB, Nagaraja D, Das S, et al. Sturge-Weber-Dimitre disease without facial nevus. Neurology 1987;37:1063–1064.
177. Mizutani T, Tanaka H, Aruga T. Multiple arteriovenous malformations located in the cerebellum, posterior fossa, spinal cord, dura, and scalp with associated port-wine stain and supratentorial venous anomaly. Neurosurgery 1992;31:137–140.
178. Kennedy C, Oranje AP, Keizer K, et al. Cutis marmorata telangiectatica congenita. Int J Dermatol 1992;31:249–252.
179. Gilliam AC, Ragge NK, Perez MI, Bolognia JL. Phakomatosis pigmentovascularis type IIb with iris mammillations. Arch Dermatol 1993;129:340–342.
180. Kurtz SN, Melamed S, Blumenthal M. Cataract and intraocular lens implantation after remote trabeculectomy for Sturge-Weber syndrome. J Cataract Refract Surg 1993;19:539–541.
181. Ruby AJ, Jampol LM, Golberg MF, et al. Choroidal neovascularization associated with choroidal hemangiomas. Arch Ophthalmol 1992;110:658–661.
182. Wilms G, Van Wijck E, Demaerel P, et al. Gyriform calcifications in tuberous sclerosis simulating the appearance of Sturge-Weber disease. AJNR Am J Neuroradiol 1992;13:295–297.
183. Marti-Bonmati LM, Mulas F. The Sturge-Weber syndrome: correlation between the clinical status and radiological CT and MRI findings. Child Nerv Syst 1993;9:107–109.
184. Lassiter HA, Bibb KW, Bertolone SJ, et al. Neonatal immune neutropenia following the administration of intravenous immune globulin. Am J Pediatr Hematol Oncol 1993;15(1):120–123.
185. Magaudda A, Dalla Bernardina B, De Marco P, et al. Bilateral occipital calcification, epilepsy and coeliac disease: clinical and neuroimaging features of a new syndrome. J Neurol Neurosurg Psychiatry 1993;56:885–889.
186. Loevner L, Quint DJ. Persistent trigeminal artery in a patient with Sturge-Weber syndrome. AJR 1992;158:872–874.
187. Campistol Plana J, Lopez Castillo J, Capdevila Cirera A, Fernandez Alvarez E. Magnetic resonance with gadolinium Sturge-Weber syndrome. Ann Esp Pediatr 1993;39:33–36.
188. Benedikt RA, Brown DC, Walker R, et al. Sturge-Weber syndrome: cranial MR imaging with Gd-DTPA. AJNR 1993;14:409–415.
189. Vogl TJ, Stemmler J, Bergman C, et al. MR and MR angiography of Sturge-Weber syndrome. AJNR 1993;14:417–425.
190. Rintahaka PJ, Chugani HT, Messa C, Phelps ME. Hemimegaencephaly: evaluation with positron emission tomography. Pediatr Neurol 1993;9:21–28.
191. Tiacci C, D'Alessandro P, Cantisani TA, et al. Epilepsy with bilateral occipital calcifications: Sturge-Weber variant or a different encephalopathy? Epilepsia 1993;34:528–539.
192. Kuster W, Happle R. Neurocutaneous disorders in children. Curr Opin Pediatr 1993;5:436–440.
193. Villemure JG, Rasmussen, T. Functional hemispherectomy in children. Neuropediatrics 1993; 23:53–55.
194. Schievink WI, Limburg M, Oorthuys JW, et al. Cerebrovascular disease in Ehlers-Danlos syndrome type IV. Stroke 1990;21:626–632.
195. Munyer TP, Margulis AR. Pseudoxanthoma elasticum with internal carotid artery aneurysm. Am J Roentgenol 1981;136:1023–1024.
196. Kivirikko KI. Collagens and their abnormalities in a wide spectrum of diseases. Ann Med 1993; 25:113–126.
197. Tucker LB. Heritable disorders of connective tissue and disability and chronic disease in childhood. Curr Opin Rheumatol 1992;4:731–740.
198. Adami PM, Rohmer P. Anévrysmes evolutifs au cours d'un syndrome d'Ehlers-Danlos de type IV. A propos d'une observation. Ann Radiol Paris 1993;2:129–133.
199. Kharsa G, Molas G, Potet F, et al. Elastomes du colon. Discussion pathogenique à propos de 7 observations. Ann Pathol 1992;12:362–366.
200. Mishra M, Chambers JB, Grahame R. Ventricular septal aneurysms in a case of Ehlers-Danlos syndrome. Int J Cardiol 1992;36:369–370.

201. Majorana AF. The orodental findings in the Ehlers-Danlos syndrome. A report of 2 clinical cases. Minerva Stomatol 1992;41(3):127–133.
202. Sato T, Ito H, Miyazaki S, et al. Megacystis and megacolon in a infant with Ehlers-Danlos syndrome. Acta Paediatr Jpn 1993;35:358–360.
203. Wertelecki W, Smith LT, Byers P. Initial observation of human dermatosparaxis: Ehlers-Danlos syndrome type VIIC. J Pediatr 1992;121:558–564.
204. Smith LT, Wertelecki W, Milstone LM, et al. Human dermatosparaxis: a form of Ehlers-Danlos syndrome that results from failure to remove the amino terminal propeptide of type I procollagen. Am J Hum Genet 1992;51:235–244.
205. Richards AJ, Ward PN, Narcisi P, et al. A single base mutation in the gene for type III collagen (COL3 A1) converts glycine 847 to glutamic acid in a family with Ehlers-Danlos syndrome type IV. An unaffected family member is mosaic for the mutation. Hum Gen 1992;89: 414–418.
206. Petty EM, Seashore MR, Braverman IM, et al. Dermatosparaxis in children. A case report and review of the newly recognized phenotype. Arch Dermatol 1993;129:1310–1315.
207. Vandenberg P. Molecular basis of heritable connective tissue disease. Biochem Med Metab Biol 1993;49(1):1–12.
208. Quentin-Hoffmann EH, Robenek B, Kresse H. Genetics defects in proteoglycans biosynthesis. Genetic defects in proteoglycans biosynthesis. Pediatr Padol 1993;28(1):37–41.
209. Johnson PH, Richards AJ, Pope FM, Hopkinson DA. A COL3 A1 glycine 1006 to glutamic acid substitution in a patient with Ehlers-Danlos syndrome type IV detected by denaturing gradient gel electrophoresis. J Inherit Metab Dis 1992;15:426–430.
210. Hautala T, Heikkinen J, Kivirikko KI, Myllyla R. A large duplication in the gene for lysyl hydroxylase accounts for the type VI variant of Ehlers-Danlos syndrome in two siblings. Genomics 1993; 15:399–404.
211. Zeluff GWC, Jackson CT. Heart attack and stroke in a young man? Think Fabry's disease. Heart Lung 1978;7:1056–1061.
212. Brady RO, Gal AE, Bradley RM, et al. Enzymatic defect in Fabry's disease; ceramidetrihexosidase deficiency. N Engl J Med 1967;276:1163–1167.
213. Vetrie D, Bentley D, Bobrow M, Harris A. Physical mapping shows close linkage between the alpha-galactosidase A gene (GLA) and the DXS178 locus. Hum Genet 1993;92:95–97.
214. Thomas P. Inherited neuropathies related to disorders of lipid metabolism. Adv Neurol 1988; 48:133–144.
215. Taaffe A. Angiokeratoma corporis diffusum: the evolution of a disease entity. Postgrad Med 1977;53:78–81.
216. Neau JP, Boissonnot L, Boutaud P, et al. Manifestations neurologiques de la maladie de Rendu-Osler-Weber. A propos de 4 observations. Rev Med Intern 1987;8:75–78.
217. Fisher M, Zito JL. Focal cerebral ischemia distal to a cerebral aneurysm in hereditary hemorrhagic telangiectasia. Stroke 1983;14:419–421.
218. Iwabuchi S, Horikoshi A, Okada S, et al. Intrapleural rupture of a pulmonary arteriovenous fistula occurring just beneath the pleura: report of a case. Surg Today 1993;23:468–470.
219. Allen SW, Whitfield JM, Clarke DR, et al. Pulmonary arteriovenous malformation in the newborn: a familial case. Pediatr Cardiol 1993;14:58–61.
220. Grönblad E. Pseudoxanthoma elasticum and changes in the eye. Acta Derm Venereol 1932; 13:417–422.
221. Carlborg UE, Grönblad B, Lund E. Vascular studies in pseudoxanthoma elasticum. Acta Med Scand 1959;166(suppl 35):1–84.
222. Fasshauer K, Reimers CD, Gnau HJ, et al. Neurological complications of Grönblad-Strandberg syndrome. J Neurol 1984;231:250–252.
223. Gilly RE, Langue N, Raveau J. Sténoses artérielles cérébrales multiples et progressives, sténose de l'artère rénale et maladie de Recklinghausen. Pédiatrie 1982;37:523–530.
224. Sobata E, Ohkuma H, Suzuki S. Cerebrovascular disorders associated with Von Recklinghausen's neurofibromatosis: a case report. Neurosurgery 1988;22:544–549.
225. Cano AR, Herraiz J, Rovira A, et al. Moya-moya syndrome. Diagnosis with angio-MRI. Arch Neurobiol Madr 1992;55(6):276–279.
226. Hashiguchi T, Maruyama I, Sonoda K, et al. Ehlers-Danlos syndrome combined with Von Recklinghausen neurofibromatosis. Intern Med 1992;31:671–673.
227. Raftopoulos C, Delecluse F, Braude P, et al. Anterior sacral meningocele and Marfan syndrome: a review. Acta Chir Belg 1993;93:1–7.
228. Bennis A, Mehadji BA, Soulami S, et al. Les manifestations cardio-vasculaires des dysplasies héréditaires du tissu conjonctif. Ann Cardiol Angeiol Paris 1993;42:173–181.

229. Foster K, Ferrell R, King-Underwood L, et al. Description of a dinucleotide repeat polymorphism in the human elastin gene and its use to confirm assignment of the gene to chromosome 7. Ann Hum Gen 1993;57:87–96.
230. Simpson IA, de Belder MA, Treasure T, et al. Cardiovascular manifestations of Marfan's syndrome: improved evaluation by transoesophageal echocardiography. Br Heart J 1993;69: 104–108.
231. Ferreira A, Fernando PM, Macedo F, Capucho R. Endocardite infecciosa. Forma de apresentacao da sindrome de Marfan. Rev Port Cardiol 1993;12:571–575.
232. Christodoulou J, Petrova-Benedict R, Robinson BH, et al. An unusual patient with the neonatal Marfan phenotype and mitochondrial complex I deficiency. Eur J Pediatr 1993;152:428–432.
233. Dietz HC, McIntosh I, Sakai LY, et al. Four novel FBN1 mutations: significance for mutant transcript level and EGF-like domain calcium binding in the pathogenesis of Marfan syndrome. Genomics 1993;17:468–475.
234. Maslen CL, Glanville RW. The molecular basis of Marfan syndrome. DNA Cell Biol 1993;12: 561–572.

9
Antithrombotic Therapy for Secondary Prevention of Ischemic Stroke

Pierre Fayad and Sanjay P. Singh

In the United States, stroke is the third leading cause of death and a leading cause of chronic disability in adults. Although major advances are being made in acutely reversing ischemic brain damage and improving outcomes, such therapy is applied to less than 5 percent of all stroke victims. These statistics reinforce the major role that stroke prevention continues to play. Because transient ischemic attacks (TIAs) and stroke are the most reliable predictors of future stroke risk, secondary prevention remains the most effective and efficient strategy for preventing stroke.

Stroke recurrence within 5 years varies between 25 and 42 percent according to different studies.[1-3] About 30 percent of stroke recurrence occurs in the first 30 days.[4] Identifying the specific risk factors within each patient and modifying the risk factors is key to cutting the risk of stroke. Because atherosclerotic plaque buildup, thrombosis, and embolism represent the main pathophysiology of stroke, antithrombotic therapy is critical for further effective reduction of that risk. This chapter discusses the mechanisms of action and the supportive evidence of the different antithrombotic agents in preventing a stroke following TIA or stroke.

MECHANISM OF THROMBUS FORMATION

Hemostasis is the physiological mechanism that maintains blood in a fluid state within the vasculature.[5] A complex balance between the plasma procoagulant and anticoagulant activities is actively maintained by cellular (i.e., platelets, endothelium) and humoral (i.e., coagulation cascade proteins) mechanisms. Dysfunction, excess, or deficiency of any of these elements may result in thrombosis. The main trigger for thrombus formation is the interaction between the extracellular matrix collagen and blood, normally prevented by an intact endothelial lining that maintains normal homeostasis.

175

Thrombosis starts with an endothelial injury that exposes the subendothelial structures to the platelets. In atherosclerotic disease, which underlies most ischemic cerebrovascular disease, a disruption of the "vulnerable plaque" triggers the thrombotic process leading to platelet aggregation. Plaque disruption results from fracture of the atherosclerotic plaque's protective fibrous cap[6] or follows the superficial erosion of the intima that uncovers thrombogenic collagen in the subendothelium. Interventions aimed at stabilizing the plaque create new opportunities for preventing cardiovascular diseases beyond, and additive to, antithrombotic agents. Approaches at stabilizing the plaque are summarized in Figure 9.1.

Platelets are enucleated blood cells (derived from bone marrow megakaryocytes) that circulate to ensure the integrity of the vascular system. Their main function resides in ensuring hemostasis by forming a platelet plug and thrombi. The platelet response develops in three successive stages starting with adhesion, activation, and finally aggregation. Once the plaque is disrupted, platelet adherence is mediated by the interaction of platelet glycoprotein Ib/IX with the subendothelial von Willebrand factor under high-shear conditions and by platelet glycoprotein Ia/IIb binding to collagen under low-shear conditions. Once platelets have adhered, pseudopod formation and spreading over the injured endothelium occurs, and the proaggregant contents of platelet granules are then released.[7]

Additional platelets are recruited into the growing thrombus through three coordinated mechanisms: (1) the modified membrane of activated platelets promotes the assembly of clotting factors on the platelet surface and amplifies the thrombin generation that activates additional platelets and triggers coagulation; (2) adenosine diphosphate (ADP) secreted from the activated platelets, which stimulates nearby platelets; and (3) activated platelets generate and

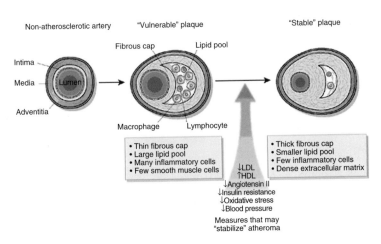

Figure 9.1   Stabilization of the plaque.
(Adapted from Libby P, Aikawa M. Stabilization of atherosclerotic plaques: new mechanisms and clinical targets. Nat Med 2002;8:1257–1262.)

release thromboxane A_2 (TXA$_2$), a potent platelet agonist that also stimulates additional platelet activation and adherence. Platelet activation conformationally activates glycoprotein IIb/IIIa (or integrin $\alpha_{IIb}\beta_3$) the platelet receptor for fibrinogen. Fibrinogen cross-links several activated platelets completing the thrombosis process with further retraction and consolidation of the clot. Clot buildup causes cerebral ischemia either by diminishing blood flow through luminal narrowing and occlusion or through fragmentation and embolization.

Coagulation, on the other hand, is initiated by blood exposure to tissue factors in the core of the ruptured plaque, injured vessel subendothelium, or the surface of activated leukocytes attracted to the damaged vessel.[8] Tissue factor binds factor VIIa with the resulting tissue factor complex activating factors IX and X. A series of subsequent steps results in the formation of the prothrombin-activating complex on the surface of the platelet consisting of factor Xa, factor Va, and calcium, generating a burst of thrombin activity. Thrombin activates platelets and factors V and VIII and converts fibrinogen to fibrin. Thrombin then binds to fibrin where it remains active.

The antithrombotic agents block one or more of the previous steps and are divided into two major groups: anticoagulants and antiplatelet agents. The anticoagulants inhibit the generation of thrombin and fibrin, and the antiplatelet agents block platelet activation and aggregation.

ORAL ANTICOAGULANTS

Coumarins

Mechanism of Action

The coumarins are the prototype of oral anticoagulants. They are vitamin K antagonists that interfere with the cyclic interconversion of vitamin K and its 2,3 epoxide. Vitamin K is a cofactor for the posttranslational carboxylation of glutamate residues to γ-carboxyglutamates on the N-terminal regions of vitamin K–dependent proteins. These coagulation factors (factors II, VII, IX, and X) require γ-carboxylation for their biological activity. Coumarins produce their anticoagulant effect by inhibiting the vitamin K conversion cycle, thereby causing hepatic production of partially carboxylated and decarboxylated proteins with reduced procoagulant activity. In addition to their anticoagulant effect, the vitamin K antagonists inhibit carboxylation of the regulatory anticoagulant proteins C and S and therefore have the potential to exert a temporary procoagulant effect.[8]

The effectiveness and usefulness of coumarins has been hindered by two major limitations: a narrow therapeutic window and a highly variable dose–response relationship. These limitations can be explained by variability in the affinity of warfarin for its hepatic receptor, changes in vitamin K content of diet, fluctuations in bioavailability, interaction with other often-used drugs, inappropriate dosage adjustments, and poor compliance. These difficulties prompted the research into newer drugs like the direct thrombin inhibitors.

Clinical Effectiveness

The use of oral anticoagulants, best represented in the United States by warfarin, has remained unchallenged for stroke prevention when a cardiac source of embolism is identified. The sources of cardiac embolism have been divided as high and low risk for embolization (Table 9.1). In most patients with high cardioembolic risk, oral anticoagulation is recommended to achieve an international normalized ratio (INR) of 2 to 3, except in cardiac tumors and infections in which it is not indicated. In most patients with atrial fibrillation, oral anticoagulation is indicated. Patients identified in the Stroke Prevention in Atrial Fibrillation trial SPAF III as having a low risk of stroke can be treated with aspirin only.[9] Patients who had a stroke with atrial fibrillation should always be treated with oral anticoagulation. For full discussions on the treatment of cardioembolic stroke, refer to Chapter 5.

The effectiveness or oral anticoagulation in preventing stroke in patients with cardiac embolism gave automatic credibility to its role in patients at risk for stroke even in patients with noncardioembolic stroke or TIA. Despite the absence of rigorous evaluations of oral anticoagulation's effectiveness and safety, oral anticoagulants became the first alternative to antiplatelet medications or a last resort when a TIA or stroke occurs in patients on antiplatelet therapy. These concepts were challenged in the past 2 decades and several large randomized trials clarified the areas in which anticoagulation is more or less effective than antiplatelet therapy. Two major randomized trials evaluated oral anticoagulation against aspirin in patients with noncardioembolic stroke: the Stroke Prevention in Reversible Ischemia Trial (SPIRIT) and the Warfarin vs. Aspirin in Recurrent Stroke Prevention (WARSS) study.

The SPIRIT study was the first serious attempt at evaluating the effectiveness of warfarin in secondary prevention of noncardioembolic stroke.[10] This was a multicenter European, mainly Dutch, randomized controlled trial in patients with noncardioembolic TIA or minor stroke enrolled within 6 months. The study compared a coumarin (phenprocoumon) to 30 milligrams of aspirin. The study was originally planned to recruit 3000 patients but was stopped after 1312

Table 9.1   Classification of cardiac sources of embolism

High Risk	Low Risk
Atrial fibrillation	Mitral valve prolapse
Mitral stenosis	Mitral annular calcification
Prosthetic mechanical valves	Patent foramen ovale
Recent MI	Atrial septal aneurysm
Left ventricular thrombus	Calcific aortic stenosis
Atrial myxoma	Mitral valve strands
Infective endocarditis	Mitral valve prolapse
Dilated cardiomyopathies	
Marantic endocarditis	

From Albers GW, Amarenco P, Easton JD, et al. Antithrombotic and thrombolytic therapy for ischemic stroke. Chest 2001;119(1 Suppl):300S–320S.

MI = myocardial infarction.

patients were enrolled when the composite primary outcome (a composite of stroke, myocardial infarction (MI), vascular death, and nonfatal major bleed) became significantly higher in the anticoagulation arm (12.5%) compared with the aspirin arm (5.4%). One half of all the major bleeds were intracranial. The trial was designed to ensure a high level of anticoagulation, which was achieved through a mean daily INR of 3.0. For every 0.5 unit rise in the INR, the risk of bleeding increased by one and one half.

The failure of higher levels of anticoagulation at preventing ischemic stroke over aspirin while significantly increasing the risk of systemic and intracranial bleeds left open the possibility that low level of anticoagulation may still be beneficial. This hypothesis supported the concept of the WARSS, a landmark study in stroke prevention that successfully used a double-blind design of anticoagulation.[11] This was a multicenter, randomized trial comparing dose-adjusted warfarin to produce an INR of 1.4 to 2.8 (the mean daily INR reached was 2.1), to that of aspirin (325 mg/day) on the composite primary endpoint of recurrent ischemic stroke or death from any cause within 2 years of follow-up. Only patients with nondisabling stroke without contraindications to receive aspirin or warfarin and without evidence of cardioembolic source and no plans for carotid endarterectomy during the follow-up period were enrolled within 30 days of the stroke onset. The study was designed to demonstrate a superiority of warfarin over aspirin and enrolled a total of 2206 patients but showed no statistically significant difference between aspirin and warfarin. Surprisingly, the primary endpoint of death or recurrent ischemic stroke was reached by 17.8 percent patients on warfarin and 16.0 percent of those on aspirin, a 10 percent trend of relative risk reduction in favor of aspirin. The lack of superiority of warfarin is not explained by an increased risk of bleeding of warfarin, because the risk of major or intracranial hemorrhage is similar in both groups, and only the risk of minor hemorrhage increased in the warfarin group.

Furthermore, the study included prospective subgroup studies that evaluated the treatment effect in patients with patent foramen ovale (PFO) (PICSS),[12] antiphospholipid antibodies (APASS), and those with fibrinogen degradation products (HAS). Surprisingly again, there was no benefit for warfarin over aspirin in any of these subgroups. There was no significant difference among those with no, small, or large PFO.[12] There was no significant difference between patients with isolated PFO and those with PFO in association with atrial septal aneurysm. A similar lack of superiority was found in patients with large-artery disease or cryptogenic stroke in which warfarin is traditionally assumed to be superior to aspirin. After such disappointing results, it is hard to justify the use of warfarin in any patient with stroke other than when a clear cardioembolic source is documented.

Direct Thrombin Inhibitors

Mechanism

The limitations of coumarins prompted the search for and development of newer anticoagulants. Direct thrombin inhibitors inactivate free thrombin and thrombin bound to fibrin, a mechanism that is largely unaffected by antiplatelet agents.

Clinical Effectiveness

Ximelagatran is the first oral direct thrombin inhibitor under phase III investigation with a fixed oral dose without the need to monitor coagulation parameters.[13] Other oral direct thrombin inhibitors are being developed or are in ongoing clinical investigations. The recently reported, but not yet published, results from the European Stroke Prevention by Oral Thrombin Inhibitor in Atrial Fibrillation (SPORTIF III) study suggest a good potential for this category of drugs and possible superiority to warfarin. SPORTIF III is an open-label, randomized, noninferiority trial, of 3407 patients with nonvalvular atrial fibrillation and one additional risk factor, randomized to ximelagatran (36 milligrams twice daily) or warfarin (dose-adjusted to an INR of 2 to 3). Patients were treated for between 12 and 26 months. Warfarin was well controlled in the study with 66 percent of INR measurements between 2.0 and 3.0. There was a statistically significant relative risk reduction of 41 percent ($p = 0.018$) for stroke and other systemic embolic events in patients treated with ximelagatran compared with warfarin. Results of the North American part of the program, SPORTIF V, which includes 3913 patients at 409 sites, are expected in late 2003. These results resurrect interest in the use and effectiveness of newer oral anticoagulants.

Safety

The risk of bleeding was not significantly different but with a lower trend in the ximelagatran arm. An increase in the liver enzyme alanine transaminase (ALT) to greater than three times the upper limit of normal was encountered in 6.5 percent of patients treated with ximelagatran, compared with 0.7 percent of patients in the warfarin group. Nearly all enzyme changes occurred within the first 6 months of treatment, were asymptomatic, and resolved with or without drug discontinuation.

ORAL PLATELET ANTAGONISTS

Oral IIb/IIIa Receptor Antagonists

The lack of warfarin superiority over aspirin in preventing stroke in most stroke patients refocused the need to develop and refine the use of antiplatelet therapy. Great hope rested on oral glycoprotein IIb/IIIa receptor antagonists that promised a powerful inhibition of the fibrinogen receptor on the platelet surface, ultimately responsible for platelet aggregation, regardless of the inciting stimulus. Indeed, intravenous IIb/IIIa antagonists in patients with acute coronary disease have been demonstrated to lower the risk of vascular events. Even in patients with acute stroke, abciximab was shown safe and well tolerated, with a potential for improving outcomes. Trials of oral glycoprotein IIb/IIIa inhibitors in patients with cardiovascular disease, however, were disappointing, with most of them stopped prematurely because of ineffectiveness or higher mortality.[14] The only trial to include secondary stroke prevention as an endpoint, Blockade of the glycoprotein IIb/IIIa Receptor to Avoid Vascular Occlusion (BRAVO) trial, was stopped early because of adverse effects.[15] The reason for these failures remains unknown. Because of the disappointment in coronary prevention, these agents never made it to testing in patients with cerebrovascular disease, resurrecting the interest in the older antiplatelet agents that remain the main pharmaceutical agents for secondary stroke prevention.

Aspirin and Aspirin Derivatives

Aspirin

Mechanism of Action

The best recognized effect of aspirin is its ability to irreversibly inhibit the enzyme cyclooxygenase (COX), blocking the prostaglandin pathway of platelet activation. In platelets this is the rate-limiting step in the synthesis of TXA_2, a powerful platelet activator. The blockage of the COX channel results from the acetylation of a strategically located serine residue, Ser 529 in the human COX-1 and Ser 516 in the human COX-2. This prevents the access of the substrate to the catalytic site of the enzyme.[16] COX-1 and COX-2 are homodines. Aspirin is 170 times more potent in inhibiting COX-1 than monocyte COX-2.[17] This includes a permanent defect in TXA_2-dependent platelet function via inhibition of COX-1. Because the production of endothelial prostacyclin (a vasodilator and platelet inhibitor) is COX-1 and COX-2 dependent, its production is inhibited to a lesser degree by aspirin, particularly at lower doses, than TXA_2, which is highly COX-1 dependent.[18]

Aspirin also inhibits COX-1 in megakaryocytes; therefore all budding platelets are dysfunctional because these enucleated cells are unable to regenerate cyclooxygenase and thus the effect of aspirin lasts for the lifespan of the platelets (~10 days). Aspirin has a half-life of 15 to 20 minutes and peak plasma levels are reached in 30 to 40 minutes. Inhibition of platelet function is evident within an hour. Enteric-coated aspirin delays the time to peak plasma level by 3 to 4 hours.

Clinical Effectiveness

The Antiplatelet Trialists Collaboration (APTC) in 2002 was a meta-analysis of 197 randomized trials of antiplatelet agents versus control and 90 randomized comparisons between antiplatelet regimens.[19] Aspirin carried an 23 percent odds reduction in vascular events (stroke, MI, and vascular death). There was no evidence to suggest that doses higher than 1000 milligrams were more effective for stroke prevention. Aspirin trials in patients with cerebrovascular disease began in the 1970s and were nearly all published before the end of 1991. The earlier trials tested the higher rheumatological doses and were smaller in size than later trials. Aspirin has been found effective in secondary stroke prevention only but not in primary prevention in which it may increase the risk of hemorrhagic stroke wiping away the potential benefits from ischemic stroke prevention.[20]

A total of 12 trials have been conducted to evaluate the efficacy of aspirin in secondary prevention of cerebrovascular and other vascular events (Table 9.2). Only four trials reported a statistically significant benefit for the primary endpoint of the study (Table 9.3). However, reductions in secondary endpoints did reach significance in some trials; the degree of benefit has varied from a nearly 50 percent reduction to an increase in risk with aspirin treatment.

Because different vascular conditions may be variably affected, the benefit of aspirin was investigated specifically in patients with cerebrovascular disease in subsequent meta-analyses (Table 9.4), each using slightly different trial selection criteria. Algra and van Gijn[34] selected placebo-controlled trials of aspirin alone in cerebrovascular patients included in the APTC meta-analysis. A more recent meta-analysis focused on the endpoint stroke and selected all trials of aspirin in patients with TIA or stroke,[35] including the second European Stroke

Table 9.2   Randomized, controlled studies of aspirin in patients with cerebrovascular disease

Study (year)	Qualifying Event	No. of Patients	Dose (mg/day)	Mean Follow-Up (mo)
AITIA (1977)[21]	Carotid territory TIA	178	1300	37
Canadian Cooperative (1978)[22]	Cerebral or retinal TIA	283[a]	1300	26
Reuther (1978)[23]	TIA, reversible ischemic neurological deficit	58	1500	24
Toulouse TIA (1982)[24]	TIA	302	900	36
Danish Cooperative (1983)[25]	Reversible cerebral or retinal ischemia of <72 hr duration	203	1000	25
AICLA (1983)[26]	Carotid or vertebrobasilar atherothrombotic TIA or stroke	402	990	36
Swedish Cooperative (1987)[27]	Minor or major stroke resulting from cerebral infarction	505	1500	24
Danish low-dose (1988)[28]	Carotid endarterectomy (97% with prior TIA or stroke)	301	50–100	25
UK-TIA (1991)[29]	TIA, minor ischemic stroke	1709	300, 1200	48
SALT (1991)[30]	TIA, minor ischemic stroke, retinal artery occlusion	1360	75	32
EAFT (1993)[31]	TIA, minor ischemic stroke	782	300	28
ESPS-2 (1996)[32]	TIA or ischemic stroke	3298	50	24

AICLA = Accidents Ischémiques Cérébraux Liés À L'athérosclérose; AITIA = Aspirin In Transient Ischemic Attack; EAFT = European Atrial Fibrillation Trial; ESPS-2 = second European Stroke Prevention Study; SALT = Swedish Aspirin Low-dose Trial; TIA = transient ischemic attack.

[a]Number of patients in aspirin and placebo groups only; total number including sulfinpyrazone-treated patients = 585.

Table 9.3   Primary endpoints and outcomes of aspirin trials in patients with cerebrovascular disease

Study (year)	Primary Endpoint	Incidence– Aspirin vs. Control	Outcome
AITIA (1977)[21]	Cerebral or retinal infarction, or death	19.4% vs. 27.1%	$p = 0.18$
Canadian Cooperative (1978)[22]	TIA, stroke, or death	Not reported	OR: 19%; $p < 0.05$[a,b]
Reuther (1978)[23]	TIA, retinal ischemia, or cerebral infarction	20.7% vs. 44.8%	$p > 0.05$ (NS)
Toulouse TIA (1982)[24]	Stroke or vascular death	<15%; same in all groups	p value not reported (NS)
Danish Cooperative (1983)[25]	Stroke or death	20.8% vs. 16.7%	$p = 0.29$ (NS)
AICLA (1983)[26]	Fatal or nonfatal cerebral infarction	10.5% vs. 18%	$p < 0.05$[a]
Swedish Cooperative (1987)[27]	Stroke or death	23% vs. 22%	p value not reported (NS)
Danish low-dose (1988)[28]	TIA, stroke, MI, vascular death	Not reported	RRR: 11% (95% CI: −38–48); $p > 0.1$
UK-TIA (1991)[29]	Major stroke, MI, or vascular death	~6%/year overall	OR: 15% (95% CI: −3–29); $p =$ NS
SALT (1991)[30]	Stroke or death	20.4% vs. 25%	RRR: 18% (95% CI: 1–33); $p = 0.02$[a]
EAFT (1993)[31]	Stroke, MI, vascular death, systemic embolism	15% vs. 19% (per year)	HR: 0.83 (95% CI: 0.65–1.05); $p = 0.12$
ESPS-2 (1996)[32]	Stroke	12.9% vs. 15.8%	RRR: 18.1%; $p = 0.013$[a]
	Death	10.9% vs. 12.3%	RRR: 10.9%; $p = 0.204$

AICLA = Accidents Ischémiques Cérébraux Liés À L'athérosclérose; AITIA = Aspirin In Transient Ischemic Attack; CI = confidence interval; EAFT = European Atrial Fibrillation Trial; ESPS-2 = second European Stroke Prevention Study; HR = hazard ratio; MI = myocardial infarction; NS = not significant; OR = odds reduction; RRR = relative risk reduction; SALT = Swedish Aspirin Low-dose Trial; TIA = transient ischemic attack.
[a]Statistically significant.
[b]Based on factorial analysis of all patients, including those treated with sulfinpyrazone or aspirin plus sulfinpyrazone.

Prevention Study-II (ESPS-2), which evaluated a very low dose 50 milligrams daily.[32] A third meta-analysis excluded trials in the settings of recent carotid endarterectomy and atrial fibrillation but included the results of ESPS-2.[36] The overall consensus from meta-analyses of trials in cerebrovascular patients is that aspirin reduces the risk of important vascular events by about 13 to 15 percent (Table 9.4).

Table 9.4 Efficacy of aspirin for prevention of vascular events in patients with cerebrovascular disease

Study (year)	No. of Trials	Endpoint	Dose Categories (mg daily)	Conclusions on Dose	Overall Aspirin Effect
Barnett (1995)[33]	8	Stroke	High: 900–1300 Low: 75–300	RRR: 11% (95% CI: −7–26) RRR: 15% (95% CI: −2–30)	Not reported
Algra (1996)[34]	10	Stroke, MI, or vascular death	High: ≤900 Med: 300 Low: ≤100	RRR: 14% (95% CI: 2–24) RRR: 9% (95% CI: −9–24) RRR: 13% (95% CI: −3–27)	RRR: 13% (95% CI: 4–21)
Johnson (1999)[35]	11	Stroke	50–1500	Regression across dose yields no linear or quadratic dose response trend	RRR: 15% (95% CI: 6–23)
Tijssen (1998)[36]	10	Stroke, MI, or vascular death	High: ≥900 Med: 300 Low: 50–75	RRR: 13% (95% CI: 2–24) RRR: 9% (95% CI: −9–24) RRR: 13% (95% CI: 3–22)	RRR: 13% (95% CI: 5–19)

CI = confidence interval; MI = myocardial infarction; RRR = relative risk reduction.

The dose of aspirin for stroke prevention has long been a topic of controversy because of inconsistent results from different trials. The earlier stroke prevention trials used the rheumatological (higher) doses of aspirin, whereas more recent studies investigated smaller doses. Only two trials, the UK-TIA and the Dutch TIA trials, directly compared two different aspirin doses.[29,37] The UK-TIA trial[29] compared the effect of aspirin 300 milligrams daily and 1200 milligrams daily against placebo in more than 2400 patients. The patients were followed for an average of 4 years. There were no differences in effectiveness between the two aspirin regimens. The Dutch TIA Trial[37] compared two dosage regimens of aspirin 30 mg/day versus 283 mg/day in 3131 patients with minor stroke or TIA. The results showed that aspirin 30 mg/day was just as effective, and there were fewer bleeding events with the lower dose. ESPS-2[32] showed that aspirin 50 mg/day was more effective than placebo in secondary stroke prevention. In addition, several meta-analyses focusing on patients enrolled into trials with stroke or TIA demonstrated a consistent similar risk reduction of stroke among low, medium, or high doses of aspirin.

This supportive evidence toward the clinical equivalency of various aspirin doses culminated with the surprising results of the Aspirin and Carotid Endarterectomy Trial (ACE).[38] The design of ACE was based on a subgroup analysis of the North American Symptomatic Carotid Endarterectomy Trial (NASCET)[39] suggesting a higher risk of stroke and death in patients on lower doses of aspirin as compared with those on higher aspirin doses. With the idea that following carotid endarterectomy there is a large thrombogenic area from the denuded media that requires higher doses of aspirin to inhibit the platelets, the trial was planned to demonstrate the superiority of higher doses of aspirin in such a setting. The ACE study compared four different doses of aspirin (1300, 650, 325, and 81 mg) that were started in 2804 patients before endarterectomy for asymptomatic or symptomatic carotid stenosis and continued for a total of 3 months. The trial was stopped early when interim analyses showed not only a lack of superiority of the higher doses but a higher risk of the combined endpoint of stroke, MI, and death when the two high doses and the two low doses were compared with each other. Furthermore, there was an increased risk of hemorrhagic stroke in the high-dose groups. The ACE trial results lend further direct support to the idea that low-dose aspirin is at least as effective as high-dose aspirin.

The confluence of all these data shifted the consensus to recommending lower doses of aspirin. The Food and Drug Administration (FDA) in 1998 changed its recommendation from high-dose aspirin for the prevention of ischemic stroke to the lower doses of 50 to 325 mg/day. Similar recommendations were echoed by the American College of Chest Physicians (ACCP).[40]

Aspirin Failure and Resistance

The concept of aspirin failure and resistance is a controversial and poorly defined one. Aspirin failure[41] has been used to define patients who suffer a recurrent stroke or TIA while on aspirin. The difficulty with this concept is that failure is expected to occur frequently because aspirin alone only reduces the risk of stroke by 15 percent on average. Failure can also be related to inaccurate diagnosis or mechanism rather than on the failure of aspirin effectiveness. Aspirin resistance[42] has been defined in patients whose in vitro platelet studies show the occurrence of platelet activation and adhesion despite the use of aspirin. In some patients increasing the dose of aspirin inhibits platelet activation. A prospective study in patients with cardiovascular disease showed that about 5 percent of patients were aspirin resistant and had a threefold increase in the risk of death, MI, and stroke as compared with those who were not resistant.[43] The debate whether such in vitro studies represent the full picture of platelet-endothelial wall interactions will remain lively for the near future.

Safety

The most notable adverse events attributable to aspirin therapy in patients with TIA or stroke are bleeding (major and minor) and gastrointestinal (GI) toxicity. A variety of bleeding complications (cerebral and GI, epistaxis, hematoma, and others) have been observed, the most dangerous being intracranial hemorrhage, which can often be fatal. To estimate the risk of hemorrhagic stroke associated with aspirin, He et al[44] analyzed data from 16 trials, most of them conducted in patients with ischemic heart disease or stroke ($N = 55,462$). Aspirin treatment (mean dose, 273 mg/day) for a mean of 37 months was associated with significant risk reduction in ischemic stroke (39 events prevented per 10,000 patients treated; $p < 0.001$). This effect was seen consistently across trials with different designs and study subgroups. These results support evidence from individual trials demonstrating that the overall benefit of aspirin in prevention of ischemic stroke is greater than the potential increase in the rate of hemorrhagic stroke. Kronmal et al[45] evaluated 5011 elderly participants in the Cardiovascular Health Study (mean age, 74 years) for a 4.2 years mean follow-up. They showed that aspirin use was associated with a fourfold increase in the risk of hemorrhagic stroke for both frequent and infrequent users compared with nonusers of the drug. Aspirin therapy may add a very low risk of hemorrhagic stroke in healthy individuals who take this agent for primary prevention.

In the ACE trial,[38] elevated rates of hemorrhagic stroke were proportional to the dose of aspirin. Intracerebral hemorrhage was highest in the high-dose aspirin groups (1.3% with 650 mg/day and 1.1% with 1300 mg/day) compared with the low-dose groups (0.6% with 81 mg/day and 0.9% with 325 mg/day). Patients undergoing endarterectomy, however, were also treated with heparin during surgery.

An analysis of the benefit-to-risk ratio of antiplatelet drugs in secondary stroke prevention was performed by Boysen [46] and included eight large stroke prevention trials. Although preventing one or two vascular events (stroke, acute MI, or vascular death) per 100 treatment-years, aspirin therapy conferred an excess risk of fatal and severe hemorrhages of 0.4 to 0.6 per 100 treatment years. This risk was substantially increased when aspirin was administered during the acute phase of stroke (0.48 fatal or severe bleeds per 100 patients in the CAST study and 0.41 in the IST study). Nevertheless, the benefit of aspirin for acute stroke remained higher than the risk (1 death or nonfatal ischemic stroke prevented per 100 treated patients).

Triflusal

Mechanism of Action

Triflusal is an antiplatelet agent structurally related to aspirin. It is a 4-trifluoromethyl derivative of salicylic acid that acts on different targets involved in platelet aggregation and vascular inflammatory processes.[47] It inhibits COX but is weaker than aspirin at inhibiting it. It inhibits phosphodiesterases and increases nitric oxide synthesis in neutrophils, resulting in increased vasodilatory potential.

Clinical Effectiveness

The effectiveness of triflusal was evaluated in the Triflusal versus Aspirin in Cerebral Infarction Prevention study (TACIP), a double-blind study that randomized 2113 patients with TIA or minor stroke within 6 months to triflusal (600 mg/day) or aspirin (325 mg/day) and followed for a mean of 30 months.[48] There was no significant difference in the primary composite outcome of stroke, MI, or vascular death between the aspirin (12.4%) or triflusal (13.1%) arms. A significant difference was found, however, in a reduced risk of cerebral hemorrhage and major systemic hemorrhage in the triflusal arm (1.9%) compared with aspirin (4%) with a *p* value of 0.004. When cerebral hemorrhage is added to the primary composite outcome of stroke, MI, and vascular death the difference between the two arms remains not significant with a higher incidence in triflusal (13.3%) compared with aspirin (12.9%). Therefore triflusal failed to show superiority to aspirin. The lower rate of hemorrhagic complications is interesting, but so far it does not justify a significant benefit over aspirin. Triflusal is currently not approved in the United States.

Thienopyridines

Mechanism of Action

Ticlopidine and clopidogrel are chemically related thienopyridine compounds, differing only by a single carboxymethyl side group in clopidogrel. Their chemical structure is distinctive from other antiplatelet agents. The release of ADP from activated platelets at the thrombosis site is a powerful platelet activator. Although their exact mechanism of interaction and effect remains unclear, the thienopyridines act as selective, noncompetitive, and irreversible binders of the ADP receptor on the platelet surface, mainly targeting the $P2Y_1$ or $P2T_{AC}$ ADP receptor subtypes and preventing activation of the platelet by ADP.[18] Their exclusive inhibition of ADP-induced platelet activation could also be represented by the following other targets of action: (1) phospholipase C and a subsequent increase in cytosolic calcium, (2) adenylate cyclase, and (3) an increase in cAMP and mobilization of the GPIIb/IIIa complex. There is suggestive evidence that the antiplatelet activity of clopidogrel and ticlopidine is mediated through their metabolites. Because of the irreversible inhibition of the ADP receptor, clopidogrel can be given once a day and the platelet function returns to normal 7 days after the last dose of clopidogrel. Newer compounds more specific for certain ADP receptor subtypes are being developed.[15]

Ticlopidine

Clinical Effectiveness

Two major trials evaluated ticlopidine in patients with cerebrovascular disease. The Canadian American Ticlopidine Study (CATS) was a randomized, double-blind, multicenter study comparing ticlopidine (250 milligrams twice daily) with placebo for the prevention of stroke, MI, or vascular death.[49] A total of 1072 patients with noncardioembolic stroke were enrolled. At the end of the study (average 24 months of follow-up) ticlopidine was associated with a 23.3 percent ($p = 0.02$) relative reduction in the risk of the primary endpoint by intention-to-treat analysis. For the secondary endpoint stroke (fatal or nonfatal), ticlopidine was associated with a 20.5 percent relative risk reduction ($p = 0.063$). The Ticlopidine Aspirin Stroke Study (TASS) was a much larger, double-blind, multicenter trial, which compared ticlopidine (250 milligrams twice daily) with aspirin (650 milligrams twice daily) in patients with recent TIA, amaurosis fugax, reversible ischemic neurological deficit, or minor stroke.[50] The relative risk reduction in stroke or death with ticlopidine was not statistically significant at 3 years, but the relative risk reduction in fatal and nonfatal stroke was significant (21%; $p = 0.024$). Ticlopidine also reduced the risk of the combined endpoint stroke, MI, or vascular death by 9 percent at 3 years, but this was not statistically significant. The 5 percent reduction in the risk of death from any cause was also not significant.

Subgroup analyses from the TASS study suggested that African-American patients benefited more from ticlopidine than white patients.[51] These findings prompted the National Institutes of Health to support a trial evaluating the efficacy of ticlopidine in African Americans exclusively (African American Antiplatelet Stroke Prevention Study [AAASPS]).[52] It showed that after 1809 patients were randomized to receive aspirin (325 milligrams twice daily) or ticlopidine (250 milligrams twice daily), ticlopidine was not superior to aspirin in reducing the primary composite endpoint of stroke, MI, and vascular death. On the contrary, there was a 10 percent relative risk reduction trend in reducing the primary endpoint in favor of aspirin that did not reach statistical significance.

Safety

Several side effects of ticlopidine are known from CATS, TASS, and postmarketing experience. The most common are diarrhea (incidence about 20% vs. 10% with placebo or aspirin), other GI effects such as dyspepsia, nausea, and pain (incidence, 7 to 14%, similar for ticlopidine and aspirin), and skin rash (incidence, 12 to 15% vs. 5 to 8% with placebo or aspirin). The occurrence of hemorrhagic events with ticlopidine is comparable to that with aspirin (9% vs. 10% in TASS). Ticlopidine is also associated with abnormal hepatic function (about 4.5% with ticlopidine vs. 1.5% with placebo in CATS) and elevated cholesterol. Of greater concern is neutropenia, which has been reported in about 2.4 percent of patients in clinical trials, necessitating biweekly blood monitoring for the first 3 months of ticlopidine therapy. The incidence of severe neutropenia (defined as a neutrophil count of $<450/mm^3$) was about 0.9 percent in TASS. Overall, severe adverse events occur in 1 to 2 percent of patients treated with ticlopidine. Thrombotic thrombocytopenic purpura (TTP), which occurs more rarely, was detected in postmarketing experience. TTP is often fatal and is difficult to anticipate, because normal platelet counts were observed within 2 weeks before onset in most of the afflicted patients. The incidence with ticlopidine is 0.02 percent with a mortality exceeding 20 percent, compared with an incidence of 0.0004 percent in the general population.[53] There is also a recent report of six cases of ticlopidine-induced lupus.[54]

Clopidogrel

Clinical Effectiveness

Clopidogrel's largest clinical evaluation was through the Clopidogrel and Aspirin Prevention in Recurrent Ischemic Events trial (CAPRIE),[55] a double-blind randomized study of aspirin (325 mg/day) or clopidogrel (75 mg/day) in 19,000 patients with either stroke, MI, or peripheral arterial disease (PAD). When all randomized patients are considered, the primary composite outcome of ischemic stroke, MI, or vascular death was 5.32 percent annually in the clopidogrel arm and 5.83 percent in the aspirin arm, with a relative risk reduction of 8.7 percent in favor of clopidogrel that was statistically significant ($p = 0.043$).

A more confusing picture is revealed when the details of the study are reviewed. When the individual groups with entry conditions of stroke or MI are considered separately, there were no significant differences between the aspirin or clopidogrel groups despite a large number of patients (>6000) enrolled with each condition. A significant 23.8 percent relative risk reduction for the composite outcome was present in the group of patients entered with PAD. The study tested positive for heterogeneity, implying that patients in different entry conditions groups (i.e., stroke, MI, or PAD) in the trial may respond differently to clopidogrel. The benefit from clopidogrel in the study was primarily carried through the benefits seen in the PAD group.

When the individual primary outcomes are considered separately, nonsignificant trends of 5.2 percent in stroke reduction and 7.6 percent for vascular death are seen in the 19,000 patients entered. MI was the only individual outcome that was significantly reduced by 19.2 percent in all patients entered. In conclusion, stroke, as an individual outcome, was not significantly reduced by clopidogrel over aspirin in primary (>12,000 patients with PAD or MI the majority of whom without prior stroke) or secondary (>6,000) prevention in the CAPRIE study.

Safety

The incidence of side effects in CAPRIE was comparable between clopidogrel and aspirin. As with ticlopidine, the most common side effects associated with clopidogrel were diarrhea (4.5% vs. 3.4%; $p < 0.05$) and rash (6% vs. 4.6%;

$p < 0.05$), although these events occurred much less frequently with clopidogrel in CAPRIE than with ticlopidine in other studies. Bleeding events occurred at similar rates with clopidogrel and aspirin (about 9.3% each), with the exception of GI bleeding, which occurred significantly more often with aspirin (2% vs. 2.7%; $p < 0.05$). Other GI events were frequently reported with both treatments but significantly more so with aspirin (15% vs. 17.6%; $p < 0.05$). Neutropenia was rare in both groups (0.26% in each), as was severe neutropenia (0.05% and 0.04% with clopidogrel and aspirin, respectively). Thus the overall safety profile of clopidogrel appears comparable to that of aspirin. Eleven cases of TTP associated with clopidogrel were identified in the postmarketing period.[56] Ten of these 11 cases occurred within the first 2 weeks of therapy. A recent report suggests that atorvastatin, when taken with clopidogrel, may antagonize the latter's antiplatelet effect, a finding that must be confirmed.[57]

Thienopyridines in Combination with Aspirin

The combination of thienopyridines with aspirin started with ticlopidine when additive effects were suggested in animal studies as well as in ex vivo platelet activation and antagonism in human studies. Several studies demonstrated either equivalence or superiority of ticlopidine and aspirin together over aspirin alone and over aspirin plus warfarin in preventing thrombotic complications of coronary stenting. Although the in vitro platelet antagonism effect of the two thienopyridines seem equivalent, there has never a clinical attempt at a direct comparison. The better safety profile of clopidogrel quickly prompted its substitution to ticlopidine in combination with aspirin, with the assumption that the effects are similar.

In addition to best standard therapy (which included aspirin in more than 95% of patients), clopidogrel was compared with placebo in a randomized study evaluating patients with acute coronary syndrome, the Clopidogrel in Unstable Angina To Prevent Recurrent Events Trial (CURE).[58] The study showed a significant decrease in the composite endpoint of MI, stroke, and vascular death, although the incidence of stroke was very small (<1.5%). Furthermore, there were significantly more patients with major bleeding in the clopidogrel and aspirin group than in the aspirin alone group (3.7% vs. 2. %; relative risk 1.38; $p = 0.001$), but there were not significantly more patients with life-threatening bleeding episodes (2.1% vs. 1.8%, $p = 0.13$) or hemorrhagic strokes. Similarly, clopidogrel showed a significant decrease of the composite endpoint of MI, stroke, and vascular death after a year when compared with placebo (along with best therapy that included aspirin in all patients) in patients undergoing elective percutaneous coronary intervention in the Clopidogrel for the Reduction of Events During Observation (CREDO).[59] Again, stroke incidence was very small (<1%) and similar in both arms but with a higher trend for major bleeds in the clopidogrel plus aspirin group. The translation of these results into stroke prevention, however, can be misleading because the risk of stroke in this cardiac group is too small to derive any conclusions, whereas the risk of serious bleeding seemed to be significantly increased.[60]

As to the equivalency between ticlopidine and clopidogrel in addition to aspirin in patients undergoing coronary stenting, a meta-analysis of randomized studies and registries comparisons of ticlopidine and clopidogrel in coronary stenting in 13,955 patients showed clopidogrel to be at least as effective as ticlopidine when added to aspirin.[61] The equivalent effectiveness between the two thienopyridines, however, appears not to have been settled yet. A recent randomized trial of 700 patients compared ticlopidine to clopidogrel in combination with aspirin after coronary stenting showed a 63 percent risk reduction of cardiovascular mortality for ticlopidine over clopidogrel.[62]

In secondary stroke prevention, the combination of ticlopidine and aspirin has not been studied. The combination of aspirin (75 mg/day) and clopidogrel (75 mg/day) is being currently compared with clopidogrel alone in the Management of Atherothrombosis with Clopidogrel in High-Risk Patients (MATCH) trial.[63] The study includes only patients who have experienced a recent stroke or TIA and are considered at high risk, defined as having a previous ischemic stroke, a previous MI, angina, symptomatic PAD, or diabetes. Patient enrollment was completed but the follow-up is continuing and the pending final results will be important to document the safety and efficacy of such a combination in patients with stroke.

Dipyridamole

Mechanism of Action

Dipyridamole is a pyrimidopyrimidine derivative from the papaverine family, which has antithrombotic properties and vasodilatory effects that are exerted on cellular (red blood cells and platelets) and vascular structures (endothelium and smooth muscle cells).[18] One of its long-recognized actions is the inhibition of phosphodiesterases that result in increased concentrations of cAMP and cGMP that act as inhibitors of platelet activation and adhesion. It additionally inhibits the uptake of adenosine by erythrocytes, thus increasing the latter's availability and effects. Adenosine stimulates platelet adenylate cyclase (resulting in increased cAMP levels) and is a powerful vasodilator. Additional potential mechanisms of action of dipyridamole have been recently identified including inhibition of fibroblast proliferation and collagen synthesis and the enhancement of nitric oxide/cGMP-mediated signaling in platelets.

The absorption of dipyridamole from instant-release formulations is variable and results in low bioavailability, thus potentially impairing reliable antithrombotic effectiveness. A new formulation with a higher dose and slower release of dipyridamole, combined with aspirin, provides a more consistent plasma level at twice-daily dosing, which is less affected by stomach acidity or concomitant medications.

Clinical Effectiveness

The ten trials comparing dipyridamole alone versus placebo showed a 23 percent odds reduction for stroke, MI, or vascular death favoring dipyridamole.[64] The combination of aspirin and dipyridamole has been compared with aspirin alone in two early small trials. The AICLA trial[26] enrolled 604 patients with cerebral ischemic events (TIA 16%, stroke 84%). They were randomized to receive placebo versus aspirin 1 g/day versus aspirin 1g/day and dipyridamole

225 mg/day. Patients were followed for 3 years. At the end of the study the number of fatal and nonfatal cerebral infarctions were 31 in the placebo group, 17 in the aspirin only group, and 18 in the aspirin and dipyridamole group. Therefore this study showed no extra benefit from adding dipyridamole to aspirin. The American-Canadian Cooperative Study group[65] enrolled 890 patients. They were randomly allocated to aspirin (325 milligrams) plus placebo or aspirin (325 milligrams) plus dipyridamole (75 milligrams) four times daily. Patients were followed for 1 to 5 years. The results did not show any benefit of adding dipyridamole to aspirin in patients with TIA.

The first European Stroke Prevention Study (ESPS)[66] was a larger study with 2500 patients randomized to receive either placebo or the combination of aspirin and dipyridamole. It showed a clear benefit for the aspirin/dipyridamole combination over placebo with a 38 percent relative reduction in the risk of fatal or nonfatal stroke. ESPS did not include an aspirin-only group. Those results prompted the reformulation of dipyridamole into a high-dose extended-release capsule combined with low-dose aspirin that had been shown to effectively inhibit platelet aggregation when administered alone, and their combined effects were additive in an ex vivo study in healthy volunteers.[67]

The ESPS-2[32] was a large, double-blind, multicenter study that, because of its 2×2 factorial design, was of sufficient statistical power to detect significant benefits of aspirin and dipyridamole, both individually and in combination. ESPS-2 evaluated a low dose of aspirin (50 milligrams daily) combined with an extended-release formulation of dipyridamole (ER-DP) administered at a higher dose (400 milligrams daily) than in previous trials. EPSP-2 randomized 6602 patients with prior stroke or TIA (77% and 23%, respectively) to one of four treatment groups: aspirin + ER-DP ($N = 1650$), aspirin alone ($N = 1649$), ER-DP alone ($N = 1654$), and placebo ($N = 1650$). Three primary endpoints were evaluated: stroke (fatal or nonfatal), stroke or death, and death from any cause. After 2 years of follow-up, relative risk reductions versus placebo for stroke were 18.1 percent ($p = 0.013$) with aspirin alone, 16.3 percent ($p = 0.039$) with ER-DP alone, and 37 percent ($p < 0.001$) with aspirin + ER-DP. Aspirin + ER-DP reduced the risk of stroke by 23.1 percent compared with aspirin alone ($p = 0.006$). Death was not significantly affected by any of the treatments, although there was a trend toward reduced mortality—risk reductions were 10.9, 7.3, and 8.5 percent with aspirin, ER-DP, and aspirin + ER-DP, respectively. The combined incidence of stroke or death was significantly reduced by each active treatment relative to placebo, largely because of the favorable impact on the incidence of stroke. Aspirin + ER-DP also reduced the risk of stroke or death compared with aspirin alone (12.9%; $p = 0.056$). Although MI was a secondary endpoint in ESPS-2, its incidence was too low to provide statistical conclusions (2.5% of all patients).

Safety

Side effects associated with aspirin and ER-DP in ESPS-2 were predictable from long-term experience with these two drugs. Common adverse events were GI symptoms (nausea, dyspepsia, gastric pain, vomiting, or diarrhea), headache, and dizziness. GI effects were associated with both drugs (30.4% with aspirin and 30.5% with ER-DP vs. 28.2% with placebo) and were somewhat increased by combining the two drugs (32.8%). Headache was associated with ER-DP treatment early in the trial, whether administered alone or in combination with aspirin (37.2% and 38.2%, respectively, vs. 32.4% with placebo and 33.1% with aspirin alone; $p = 0.001$). Bleeding was significantly more common among patients who took aspirin (placebo 4.5%, aspirin 8.2%, ER-DP 4.7%, aspirin + ER-DP 8.7%, $p = 0.001$); however, the incidence of bleeding was not increased by combining aspirin and ER-DP. Dizziness occurred most frequently in the placebo group (30.9%) and did not appear to be associated with either treatment. Except for a higher incidence of headache, much of which is transient, the safety profile of the aspirin + ER-DP combination is comparable to that of aspirin alone.

CONCLUSION

A quiet revolution has been taking place in antithrombotic therapy for stroke prevention encompassing a wider variety of options, better knowledge of mechanisms of action, cumulative evidence on effectiveness, and limitations in different conditions. Despite their proven effectiveness, antithrombotic agents remain limited in their reduction of stroke or vascular events. The failure of oral glycoprotein IIb/IIIa inhibitors and the lack of superiority of warfarin over aspirin in noncardioembolic stroke refocused the reliance on the more traditional antiplatelet agents. Different trials disappointingly demonstrated the lack of superiority of any single oral antiplatelet agent over aspirin. The diverse mechanisms of action of the available oral antiplatelet agents, however, offers the promise of additive effects when combining different agents. The combination of aspirin and ER-DP was shown to be more effective than aspirin alone at preventing stroke. Clopidogrel, which has largely replaced ticlopidine, in combination with aspirin is being tested for stroke prevention against clopidogrel alone. As antiplatelet agents are being combined, the efficacy and safety ratio for such an approach will gain more importance in clinical practice.

In the future, the recently reported effectiveness of direct thrombin inhibitors in atrial fibrillation may revive the issue of anticoagulation in stroke prevention beyond atrial fibrillation. In the meantime, antiplatelet medications are indicated in most patients for stroke prevention, in whom a cardioembolic source is not documented. Potential development of newer antithrombotic agents provides a hope for a better future in stroke prevention.[7,15]

References

1. Petty GW, Brown RD Jr, Whisnant JP, et al. Survival and recurrence after first cerebral infarction: a population-based study in Rochester, Minnesota, 1975 through 1989. Neurology 1998;50: 208–216.
2. Sacco RL, Shi T, Zamanillo MC, Kargman DE. Predictors of mortality and recurrence after hospitalized cerebral infarction in an urban community: the Northern Manhattan Stroke Study. Neurology 1994;44:626–634.
3. Hier DB, Foulkes MA, Swiontoniowski M, et al. Stroke recurrence within 2 years after ischemic infarction. Stroke 1991;22:155–161.
4. Libby P, Aikawa M. Stabilization of atherosclerotic plaques: new mechanisms and clinical targets. Nat Med 2002;8:1257–1262.

5. Rosenberg RD, Aird WC. Vascular-bed—specific hemostasis and hypercoagulable states. N Engl J Med 1999;340:1555–1564.
6. Farb A, Burke AP, Tang AL, et al. Coronary plaque erosion without rupture into a lipid core. A frequent cause of coronary thrombosis in sudden coronary death. Circulation 1996;93:1354–1363.
7. Hirsh J, Weitz JI. New antithrombotic agents. Lancet 1999;353:1431–1436.
8. Hirsh J, Dalen J, Anderson DR, et al. Oral anticoagulants: mechanism of action, clinical effectiveness, and optimal therapeutic range. Chest 2001;119(1 Suppl):8S–21S.
9. Patients with nonvalvular atrial fibrillation at low risk of stroke during treatment with aspirin: Stroke Prevention in Atrial Fibrillation III Study. The SPAF III Writing Committee for the Stroke Prevention in Atrial Fibrillation Investigators. JAMA 1998;279:1273–1277.
10. A randomized trial of anticoagulants versus aspirin after cerebral ischemia of presumed arterial origin. The Stroke Prevention in Reversible Ischemia Trial (SPIRIT) Study Group. Ann Neurol 1997;42:857–865.
11. Mohr JP, Thompson JL, Lazar RM, et al. A comparison of warfarin and aspirin for the prevention of recurrent ischemic stroke. N Engl J Med 2001;345:1444–1451.
12. Homma S, Sacco RL, Di Tullio MR, et al. Effect of medical treatment in stroke patients with patent foramen ovale: patent foramen ovale in Cryptogenic Stroke Study. Circulation 2002;105: 2625–2631.
13. Petersen P, Grind M, Adler J. Ximelagatran versus warfarin for stroke prevention in patients with nonvalvular atrial fibrillation. SPORTIF II: a dose-guiding, tolerability, and safety study. J Am Coll Cardiol 2003;41:1445–1451.
14. Chew DP, Bhatt DL, Sapp S, et al. Increased mortality with oral platelet glycoprotein IIb/IIIa antagonists: a meta-analysis of phase III multicenter randomized trials. Circulation 2001;103:201–206.
15. Bhatt DL, Topol EJ. Scientific and therapeutic advances in antiplatelet therapy. Nat Rev Drug Discov 2003;2:15–28.
16. Vane JR, Bakhle YS, Botting RM. Cyclooxygenases 1 and 2. Annu Rev Pharmacol Toxicol 1998; 38:97–120.
17. Burch JW, Stanford N, Majerus PW. Inhibition of platelet prostaglandin synthetase by oral aspirin. J Clin Invest 1978;61:314–319.
18. Patrono C, Coller B, Dalen JE, et al. Platelet-active drugs: the relationships among dose, effectiveness, and side effects. Chest 2001;119(1 Suppl):39S–63S.
19. Collaborative meta-analysis of randomised trials of antiplatelet therapy for prevention of death, myocardial infarction, and stroke in high risk patients. BMJ 2002;324:71–86.
20. Hart RG, Halperin JL, McBride R, et al. Aspirin for the primary prevention of stroke and other major vascular events: meta-analysis and hypotheses. Arch Neurol 2000;57:326–332.
21. Fields WS, Lemak NA, Frankowski RF, et al. Controlled trial of aspirin in cerebral ischemia. Stroke 1977;8:301–314.
22. A randomized trial of aspirin and sulfinpyrazone in threatened stroke. The Canadian Cooperative Study Group. N Engl J Med 1978;299:53–59.
23. Reuther R, Dorndorf W. Aspirin in Patients with Cerebral Ischemia and Normal Angiograms or Nonsurgical Lesions: The Results of a Double-Blind Trial. In K Breddin, W Dorndorf, D Loew, et al. (eds), Acetylsalicylic Acid in Cerebral Ischemia and Coronary Heart Disease: IV. Colfarit-Symposion, Berlin, 30.9.–1.10., 1977. Stuttgart, Germany: Schattauer Verlag, 1978;97–106.
24. Guiraud-Chaumeil B, Rascol A, David J, et al. Prévention des récidives des accidents vasculaires cérébraux ischémiques par les anti-agrégants plaquettaires: résultats d'un essai thérapeutique contrôlé de 3 ans. Rev Neurol (Paris) 1982;138:367–385.
25. Sorensen PS, Pedersen H, Marquardsen J, et al. Acetylsalicylic acid in the prevention of stroke in patients with reversible cerebral ischemic attacks. A Danish cooperative study. Stroke 1983; 14:15–22.
26. Bousser MG, Eschwege E, Haguenau M, et al. "AICLA" controlled trial of aspirin and dipyridamole in the secondary prevention of athero-thrombotic cerebral ischemia. Stroke 1983;14:5–14.
27. High-dose acetylsalicylic acid after cerebral infarction. A Swedish Cooperative Study. Stroke 1987; 18:325–334.
28. Boysen G, Sorensen PS, Juhler M, et al. Danish very-low-dose aspirin after carotid endarterectomy trial. Stroke 1988;19:1211–1215.
29. Farrell B, Godwin J, Richards S, et al. The United Kingdom transient ischaemic attack (UK-TIA) aspirin trial: final results. J Neurol Neurosurg Psychiatry 1991;54:1044–1054.
30. Swedish Aspirin Low-Dose Trial (SALT) of 75 mg aspirin as secondary prophylaxis after cerebrovascular ischaemic events. The SALT Collaborative Group. Lancet 1991;338:1345–1349.
31. Secondary prevention in non-rheumatic atrial fibrillation after transient ischaemic attack or minor stroke. EAFT (European Atrial Fibrillation Trial) Study Group. Lancet 1993;342:1255–1262.

32. Diener HC, Cunha L, Forbes C, et al. European Stroke Prevention Study. 2. Dipyridamole and acetylsalicylic acid in the secondary prevention of stroke. J Neurol Sci 1996;143:1–13.
33. Barnett HJ, Eliasziw M, Meldrum HE. Drugs and surgery in the prevention of ischemic stroke. N Engl J Med 1995;332:238–248.
34. Algra A, van Gijn J. Aspirin at any dose above 30 mg offers only modest protection after cerebral ischaemia. J Neurol Neurosurg Psychiatry 1996;60:197–199.
35. Johnson ES, Lanes SF, Wentworth CE III, et al. A metaregression analysis of the dose-response effect of aspirin on stroke. Arch Intern Med 1999;159:1248–1253.
36. Tijssen JG. Low-dose and high-dose acetylsalicylic acid, with and without dipyridamole: a review of clinical trial results. Neurology 1998;51(3 Suppl 3):S15–16.
37. The Dutch TIA trial: protective effects of low-dose aspirin and atenolol in patients with transient ischemic attacks or nondisabling stroke. The Dutch TIA Study Group. Stroke 1988;19: 512–517.
38. Taylor DW, Barnett HJ, Haynes RB, et al. Low-dose and high-dose acetylsalicylic acid for patients undergoing carotid endarterectomy: a randomised controlled trial. ASA and Carotid Endarterectomy (ACE) Trial Collaborators. Lancet 1999;353:2179–2184.
39. Barnett HJ, Taylor DW, Eliasziw M, et al. Benefit of carotid endarterectomy in patients with symptomatic moderate or severe stenosis. North American Symptomatic Carotid Endarterectomy Trial Collaborators. N Engl J Med 1998;339:1415–1425.
40. Albers GW, Amarenco P, Easton JD, et al. Antithrombotic and thrombolytic therapy for ischemic stroke. Chest 2001;119(1 Suppl):300S–320S.
41. Bornstein NM, Karepov VG, Aronovich BD, et al. Failure of aspirin treatment after stroke. Stroke 1994;25:275–277.
42. Helgason CM, Bolin KM, Hoff JA, et al. Development of aspirin resistance in persons with previous ischemic stroke. Stroke 1994;25:2331–2336.
43. Gum PA, Kottke-Marchant K, Welsh PA, et al. A prospective, blinded determination of the natural history of aspirin resistance among stable patients with cardiovascular disease. J Am Coll Cardiol 2003;41:961–965.
44. He J, Whelton PK, Vu B, Klag MJ. Aspirin and risk of hemorrhagic stroke: a meta-analysis of randomized controlled trials. JAMA 1998;280:1930–1935.
45. Kronmal RA, Hart RG, Manolio TA, et al. Aspirin use and incident stroke in the cardiovascular health study. CHS Collaborative Research Group. Stroke 1998;29:887–894.
46. Boysen G. Bleeding complications in secondary stroke prevention by antiplatelet therapy: a benefit-risk analysis. J Intern Med 1999;246:239–245.
47. McNeely W, Goa KL. Triflusal. Drugs 1998;55:823–833; discussion 834–825.
48. Matias-Guiu J, Ferro JM, Alvarez-Sabin J, et al. Comparison of triflusal and aspirin for prevention of vascular events in patients after cerebral infarction: the TACIP Study: a randomized, double-blind, multicenter trial. Stroke 2003;34:840–848.
49. Gent M, Blakely JA, Easton JD, et al. The Canadian American Ticlopidine Study (CATS) in thromboembolic stroke. Lancet 1989;1:1215–1220.
50. Hass WK, Easton JD, Adams HP Jr, et al. A randomized trial comparing ticlopidine hydrochloride with aspirin for the prevention of stroke in high-risk patients. Ticlopidine Aspirin Stroke Study Group. N Engl J Med 1989;321:501–507.
51. Weisberg LA. The efficacy and safety of ticlopidine and aspirin in non-whites: analysis of a patient subgroup from the Ticlopidine Aspirin Stroke Study. Neurology 1993;43:27–31.
52. Gorelick PB, Richardson D, Kelly M, et al. Aspirin and ticlopidine for prevention of recurrent stroke in black patients: a randomized trial. JAMA 2003;289:2947–2957.
53. Bennett CL, Davidson CJ, Raisch DW, et al. Thrombotic thrombocytopenic purpura associated with ticlopidine in the setting of coronary artery stents and stroke prevention. Arch Intern Med 1999; 159:2524–2528.
54. Spiera RF, Berman RS, Werner AJ, et al. Ticlopidine-induced lupus: a report of 4 cases. Arch Intern Med 2002;162:2240–2243.
55. A randomised, blinded, trial of clopidogrel versus aspirin in patients at risk of ischaemic events (CAPRIE). CAPRIE Steering Committee. Lancet 1996;348:1329–1339.
56. Bennett CL, Connors JM, Carwile JM, et al. Thrombotic thrombocytopenic purpura associated with clopidogrel. N Engl J Med 2000;342:1773–1777.
57. Lau WC, Waskell LA, Watkins PB, et al. Atorvastatin reduces the ability of clopidogrel to inhibit platelet aggregation: a new drug-drug interaction. Circulation 2003;107:32–37.
58. Yusuf S, Zhao F, Mehta SR, et al. Effects of clopidogrel in addition to aspirin in patients with acute coronary syndromes without ST-segment elevation. N Engl J Med 2001;345: 494–502.

59. Steinhubl SR, Berger PB, Mann JT III, et al. Early and sustained dual oral antiplatelet therapy following percutaneous coronary intervention: a randomized controlled trial. JAMA 2002;288: 2411–2420.
60. Albers GW, Amarenco P. Combination therapy with clopidogrel and aspirin: can the CURE results be extrapolated to cerebrovascular patients? Stroke 2001;32:2948–2949.
61. Bhatt DL, Bertrand ME, Berger PB, et al. Meta-analysis of randomized and registry comparisons of ticlopidine with clopidogrel after stenting. J Am Coll Cardiol 2002;39:9–14.
62. Mueller C, Roskamm H, Neumann FJ, et al. A randomized comparison of clopidogrel and aspirin versus ticlopidine and aspirin after the placement of coronary artery stents. J Am Coll Cardiol 2003;41:969–973.
63. Hacke W. From CURE to MATCH: ADP receptor antagonists as the treatment of choice for high-risk atherothrombotic patients. Cerebrovasc Dis 2002;13(Suppl 1):22–26.
64. Wilterdink JL, Easton JD. Dipyridamole plus aspirin in cerebrovascular disease. Arch Neurol 1999;56:1087–1092.
65. Persantine aspirin trial in cerebral ischemia—Part III: risk factors for stroke. The American-Canadian Co-Operative Study Group. Stroke 1986;17:12–18.
66. European Stroke Prevention Study. ESPS Group. Stroke 1990;21:1122–1130.
67. Muller TH. Inhibition of thrombus formation by low-dose acetylsalicylic acid, dipyridamole, and their combination in a model of platelet-vessel wall interaction. Neurology 2001;57(5 Suppl 2): S8–S11.

10
Risk Factor Modification for Secondary Prevention

Sean Ruland

There is estimated to be more than 700,000 new and recurrent strokes in the United States annually.[1] It is difficult to accurately estimate the percentage of recurrent strokes given that many initial ischemic events may be silent or of low severity and go unreported. It is also estimated that the annual incidence of transient ischemic attack (TIA) is 200,000 to 500,000.[2] Furthermore, advances in neuroimaging techniques have revealed that most patients having transient neurological symptoms lasting longer than 1 hour but less than the traditional definition of 24 hours have radiographic evidence of brain infarction.[3] This has prompted the TIA Working Group to call for redefining the duration of TIA to less than 1 hour. In any case, these events should be viewed as a warning sign.

A history of a previous stroke or TIA is an independent risk for stroke recurrence. The recurrent risk of stroke after a first stroke has been reported to be 5 to 14 percent in the first year and 25 to 40 percent over the first 5 years.[4] In a randomized controlled clinical trial in Europe of antiplatelet therapy for secondary stroke prevention, the risk of recurrent stroke was 15.2 percent with the placebo over 24 months.[5] It is not known whether having a second or third stroke confers additional risk. Following a TIA, the early risk of stroke is substantial. In an observational study in northern California, the risk of stroke in 1707 patients presenting to the emergency department with the diagnosis of TIA was 10.5 percent in the next 90 days. One half of these events occurred within the next 2 days. In addition, age older than 60 years, diabetes mellitus (DM), duration of episode of more than 10 minutes, and associated motor or speech impairment were independent predictors of risk for subsequent stroke.[6] The occurrence of a stroke or TIA warrants an expeditious workup for cause; treatment with antithrombotic medication or revascularization, as appropriate; and adherence to a strategy to control vascular risk factors.

Over the years, the understanding of vascular risk factors has grown. Observational epidemiological studies have provided the impetus for clinical trials of risk factor control strategies that have yielded significant reductions in the risk of first stroke and cardiovascular events. Unfortunately, despite these successful strategies, rates of risk factor awareness, treatment, and control are poor.[7]

Until recently, risk factor control for the prevention of recurrent stroke was not well studied. Management strategies were either adopted from primary prevention trials or discounted perhaps because of therapeutic nihilism. During the past decade new information has become available regarding control of risk factors in reducing the rate of recurrent stroke. This chapter clarifies management of risk factors in secondary prevention and discusses practical strategies for risk factor control.

HYPERTENSION

The sixth report of the Joint National Committee (JNC VI) defines hypertension as a blood pressure greater than 140/90 mm Hg[8] (Table 10.1). Hypertension is associated with a relative risk of 3.0 to 5.0 for stroke.[9] The Third National Health and Nutrition Examination Survey (NHANES III), conducted in the United States from 1988 to 1991, reported the prevalence of hypertension to be 32.4 percent in non-Hispanic blacks, 23.3 percent in non-Hispanic whites, and 22.6 percent in Mexican-Americans. Hypertension is under-recognized because various cohort studies have reported rates of previously undiagnosed hypertension in the 16 to 26 percent range. Similarly, rates of treatment vary from 56 to 84 percent and rates of control to published guidelines vary from 28 to 55 percent.[10–16]

For years, controversy surrounded the issue of blood pressure control after incident stroke. There was not only a lack of proven benefit but also a concern about potential safety issues in patients with cerebrovascular disease. It remains accepted that one should avoid precipitously lowering blood pressure in the acute stages of cerebral ischemia when the potentially viable penumbra with autoregulatory compromise hangs in the balance. In addition, acute blood pressure lowering should be avoided in patients with a high-grade stenosis in large- or medium-size cerebral arteries with poor collateral compensation leading to a state of misery perfusion. However, newer data have led to a paradigm shift in favor of long-term blood pressure control.

Several relatively small exploratory analyses of clinical trial data showed a trend in favor of blood pressure lowering for recurrent stroke prevention.[17–20]

Table 10.1   JNC VI blood pressure categories

Optimal	<120/80 mm Hg
Normal	<130/85 mm Hg
High-normal	130–139/85–89 mm Hg
Hypertension	
Stage 1	140–159/90–99 mm Hg
Stage 2	160–179/100–109 mm Hg
Stage 3	>180/>110 mm Hg

Adapted from the Sixth Report of the Joint National Committee on Hypertension (JNC VI). Arch Intern Med 1997;157:2413–2446.

However, the Perindopril Protection Against Recurrent Stroke Study (PROGRESS) was a randomized, placebo-controlled, clinical trial of a perindopril-based blood pressure–lowering regimen that enrolled more than 6000 subjects with a previous stroke or TIA.[21] Use of the diuretic indapamide was allowed at the discretion of the treating physician. The overall blood pressure–lowering effect was an average of 9.0/4.0 mm Hg, which translated into a 28 percent relative risk reduction for recurrent stroke. The subgroup of subjects that received both perindopril and indapamide had an average blood pressure reduction of 12.3/5.0 mm Hg and a 43 percent relative reduction for recurrent stroke.

Other trials in primary prevention have shown reductions in stroke for beta blockers, diuretics, calcium channel blockers, and angiotensin-converting enzyme (ACE) inhibitors in both younger and elderly subjects including those with isolated systolic hypertension.[22–24] However, there may be advantages to the use of selective tissue-ACE inhibitors.

ACE inhibitors affect the renin-angiotensin (AT)-aldosterone system. Renin is released by the kidneys in response to a depletion of sodium and water.[25] It cleaves hepatically produced angiotensinogen to AT I. ACE is the enzyme that catalyzes the conversion of AT I to AT II. AT II is a vasoactive agent that causes vasoconstriction within the vascular beds of the kidneys and systemic circulation, renal sodium reabsorption, and adrenal secretion of aldosterone. Aldosterone further promotes renal sodium reabsorption. Most ACE is confined to tissue within the vascular wall and only about 10 percent is within the serum.

Inhibition of tissue-ACE has been shown to improve compliance in both cardiac and vascular tissue[26–30] (Table 10.2). This may lead to a benefit independent of the blood pressure–lowering effect. For example, the Heart Outcomes Prevention Evaluation (HOPE) Study showed a reduction in cardiovascular events and stroke with minimal blood pressure reduction (3/2 mm Hg) for 9297 randomized high-risk subjects treated with the tissue-ACE inhibitor ramipril versus placebo.[31]

For the purpose of defining the goal for blood pressure maintenance, the JNC VI considers a previous stroke as evidence of target organ damage (TOD)[8] (Table 10.3). The JNC VI recommends the goal blood pressure for patients with TOD to be less than 130/85 mm Hg. Specific recommendations concerning indications for lifestyle modification, particular antihypertensive agents in

Table 10.2   Cardiovascular effects of ACE inhibitors

Improve vascular compliance
Interstitial collagen regression
Improve coronary reserve
Normalize left ventricular hypertrophy
Reduce vascular smooth muscle proliferation
Augment fibrinolysis
Reduce propensity for atherosclerotic plaque rupture
Decrease development of atherosclerosis

Data taken from references 26–30.

ACE = angiotensin-converting enzyme.

Table 10.3   JNC VI target organ damage

Heart diseases
    Left ventricular hypertrophy
    Angina/history of myocardial infarction
    History coronary revascularization
Stroke or transient ischemic attack
Nephropathy
Peripheral arterial disease
Hypertensive retinopathy

Adapted from the Sixth Report of the Joint National Committee on
Hypertension (JNC VI). Arch Intern Med 1997;157:2413–2446.

special populations, and other circumstances are beyond the scope of this chapter. It is recommended that the JNC VI guidelines are followed for tailoring therapy.

In addition, encouraging patients to participate in their blood pressure management may improve compliance and enhance care. It may be beneficial to have patients self-monitor their blood pressure and maintain logs for presentation at office visits. This may provide further insight into the effect of treatment and need for additional treatment.

DIABETES

The hallmark of DM is persistent hyperglycemia. It has been estimated to increase the risk of stroke by 1.5 to 3.0 times.[9] The prevalence of DM was 6.6 percent in NHANES I, and approximately one half of cases were previously undiagnosed. In addition, the prevalence increased with age and was 17.7 percent in 65 to 74 year olds.[32] Furthermore, in clinical trials of stroke prevention, the percentage with baseline DM ranged from 5 to 31 percent (mean 17.1%) in those studies enrolling predominantly non–African-American subjects and 39.1 percent in a trial of exclusively African-American subjects.[33]

Glycemic control is well known to decrease the incidence of microvascular complications associated with DM such as retinopathy, nephropathy, and neuropathy. However, evidence supporting a reduction in the incidence of macrovascular complications such as stroke and coronary artery disease has not been shown definitively.

Elevated serum glucose at the time of presentation of stroke has been associated with higher mortality and morbidity and early stroke recurrence rates compared with those with euglycemia in nonlacunar stroke patients.[34,35] This may be a reflection of secondary cerebral injury resulting from acidosis from the anaerobic metabolism of glucose to lactate in areas with compromised cerebral blood flow. Despite the known benefits of glycemic control, a report of diabetic patients examined in a stroke clinic has shown persistent hyperglycemia after up to 2 years of follow-up.[15] Glycemic management strategies should adhere to the clinical practice recommendations of the American Diabetes Association.[36]

HYPERLIPIDEMIA

Over the past several decades, increased awareness of hyperlipidemia has been reported.[37–39] However, rates of control remain poor. In survivors of myocardial infarction and stroke who participated in NHANES III, elevated cholesterol was previously diagnosed in 32 percent but was adequately controlled in only 49 percent.[7]

The role of hyperlipidemia is not as well-defined for stroke as it is for coronary artery disease. Several factors need to be considered in the failure to establish this relationship. Stroke is a heterogeneous disease characterized by several subtypes. Specific subtypes may be variably susceptible to particular risk factors including lipids. For example, patients with atheromatous carotid artery disease may be more affected by elevated blood lipids than those with cardioembolic stroke or stroke of unknown cause. Few studies have accounted for this factor. Furthermore, middle-age subjects were enrolled by many of the studies to evaluate coronary heart disease as a primary endpoint. The relationship between stroke and lipids in these studies may have been limited because stroke incidence is known to rise 10 to 20 years later than that of coronary heart disease.[40] For example, a study of 6352 Hawaiian Japanese men compared the incidence of thromboembolic stroke between patients 60 to 74 and 51 to 59 years old. An approximately 2.5 times higher incidence was seen in the older group. In addition, a linear relationship between total cholesterol levels and stroke incidence was observed.[41] A case-control study of men and women, mean age 64.6 years, showed a relationship between atherothrombotic stroke or TIA and elevated total cholesterol, low-density lipoprotein (LDL), triglycerides, and low high-density lipoprotein (HDL) levels.[42]

Clinical trials of the HMG CoA reductase inhibitor (statin) class of lipid-lowering agents have shown reductions in stroke outcomes among patients with coronary artery disease. The Scandinavian Simvastatin Survival Study (4S) showed a 30 percent relative risk reduction ($p < 0.00001$) of cerebral ischemic events among 4444 subjects with a history of coronary heart disease or angina, mean total cholesterol of 263 mg/dL, and mean age of 59 years who were treated with simvastatin compared with placebo.[43] The Cholesterol and Recurrent Events (CARE) trial showed a 31 percent relative risk reduction ($p = 0.03$) of stroke in 4159 subjects with a history of myocardial infarction, mean total cholesterol level 209 mg/dL, mean LDL level 139 mg/dL, and mean age of 59 years treated with pravastatin compared with placebo.[44] Similarly, a 23 percent relative risk reduction ($p = 0.02$) of ischemic stroke was seen in the Long-term Intervention with Pravastatin in Ischemic Disease (LIPID) study in subjects treated with pravastatin compared with placebo.[45]

Statin therapy has been shown to reduce stroke in individual trials and meta-analyses for patients with a broad range of baseline characteristics.[46–48] The Medical Research Council and British Heart Foundation Heart Protection Study enrolled more than 20,500 subjects and included those with normal baseline cholesterol levels.[49] One half had a prior stroke or TIA. Subjects were randomized in a 2×2 factorial design to receive simvastatin 40 mg, antioxidant vitamins, or matching placebo and followed for up to 5 years. A preliminary report showed a 27 percent relative risk reduction for stroke in those patients treated with simvastatin versus matching placebo. There was no lower limit of baseline total cholesterol level below which a benefit was not seen.

No positive or negative effects were shown for treatment with antioxidant vitamins.

No benefit for stroke prevention has been shown for alternative means of cholesterol lowering. Strategies have included diet, medication, and surgery.[50,51] However, these trials lacked homogeneity for stroke subtype and enrolled primarily middle-aged subjects.

Why have the statin agents been successful for stroke prevention when other cholesterol lowering strategies have failed and why have they been effective in patients with normal baseline cholesterol levels not necessarily predictive of an increased risk? Statin agents have shown a rapid therapeutic response for reducing stroke and cardiovascular events following administration in clinical trials. In addition, the magnitude of the outcome reductions are greater than would be predicted by models of lipid-lowering therapy alone. This suggests effects that go beyond cholesterol lowering. Therefore, other therapeutic mechanisms have been proposed[52,53] (Table 10.4).

Statins inhibit HMG-CoA reductase, the enzyme responsible for the rate-limiting step of cholesterol production in the liver. This leads to upregulation of receptors for LDL on hepatocytes and removes LDL from the circulation. LDL is an important component in the lipid core of an atherosclerotic plaque. In its oxidized form, LDL is a promoter of the atherosclerotic process.

The core of an atherosclerotic plaque is composed of lipid, lipid-laden macrophages (foam cells), T lymphocytes, smooth muscle, and collagen. It is bound by a thin fibrous cap. The macrophages produce matrix metalloproteinases capable of fibrous cap degradation. The T lymphocytes release cytokines that inhibit smooth muscle proliferation and collagen production within the fibrous cap. Unstable plaques are prone to rupture, hemorrhage, and thrombosis.

Oxidized LDL stimulates protease activation within endothelial cells causing apoptosis. It also triggers macrophages to engulf LDL, transforming them into foam cells. Macrophages and T lymphocytes enhance leukocyte attachment to the endothelium by inducing expression of adhesion molecules. Through inhibition of nitric oxide synthase, oxidized LDL impairs vasomotor reactivity and enhances platelet aggregation.[54]

Statins have been shown to decrease lipid content, oxidation, inflammation, matrix metalloproteinase, and apoptosis while increasing collagen and tissue inhibitor of metalloproteinase in carotid plaques taken from 11 patients who were treated with pravastatin 40 mg for a mean of 3 months before endarterectomy compared with 13 controls.[54] C-reactive protein, a marker of inflammation, was shown to be reduced in subjects randomly selected from the CARE trial who were treated with pravastatin 40 mg daily.[55]

Table 10.4　Nonlipid-lowering mechanisms of HMG-CoA reductase inhibitors

Stabilize atherosclerotic plaque
Anti-inflammation
Improved vasomotor reactivity
Antithrombotic

Adapted from Hess DC, Demchuk AM, Brass LM, Yatsu FM. HMG-CoA reductase inhibitors (statins): a promising approach to stroke prevention. Neurology 2000;54:790–796.

Improved cerebral vasomotor reactivity has been shown with transcranial Doppler ultrasound following the administration of acetazolamide in patients treated with pravastatin 20 mg daily for 2 months.[56] The mechanism is thought to be mediated by upregulation of endothelial nitric oxide synthase expression. In addition, atorvastatin has been shown to decrease platelet activation in animal models.[57,58]

Although the American Heart Association recommends treatment of abnormal blood lipids in patients with a previous stroke and TIA who have a history of coronary artery disease,[59] there is increasing evidence that statin use may be beneficial in other high-risk individuals. The National Cholesterol Education Program Adult Treatment Panel (NCEP ATP) III defines the LDL goal in high-risk individuals to be less than 100 mg/dL, less than or equal to 150 mg/dL for triglycerides, and considers HDL a risk factor if less than 40 mg/dL.[60] The NCEP ATP III defines high risk as those individuals with coronary heart disease, symptomatic carotid artery disease, peripheral arterial disease, DM, or abdominal aortic aneurysm.

HORMONE REPLACEMENT THERAPY

The incidence of stroke in women is less than in men in the premenopausal years. It increases postmenopausally, doubling every 10 years to equal that of men. Subsequently, more women suffer mortality from stroke because they live longer.[4] The delay in the rise of stroke incidence suggests a protective effect of estrogen against stroke. Estrogen has been shown to have antioxidant properties, to enhance production of vasoactive substances such as nitric oxide and prostaglandin, and to have a favorable effect on cholesterol profile.[61] However, more recently, the use of hormone replacement therapy in the prevention of cardiovascular disease and stroke has become controversial.

In the Heart and Estrogen/Progestin Replacement Study (HERS II), 2763 postmenopausal women with a history of coronary artery disease and mean age of 67 years were randomized to treatment with conjugated estrogen 0.625 mg daily plus medroxyprogesterone acetate 2.5 mg daily or placebo.[62] They were followed for a mean of 6.8 years. No significant reduction in cardiovascular outcome including stroke was demonstrated. In addition, twice the rate of venous thromboembolism was reported.[63]

In the largest randomized controlled clinical trial of postmenopausal hormone replacement therapy, the Women's Health Initiative enrolled 16,608 women with a mean age of 63 years.[64] They were randomized to treatment with conjugated equine estrogen 0.625 mg plus medroxyprogesterone acetate 2.5 mg daily or placebo. After a mean follow-up of 5.2 years, there were 29 percent more coronary heart disease outcomes, 41 percent more strokes, and more than twice the rate of venous thromboembolism.

The Women's Estrogen for Stroke Trial enrolled 664 postmenopausal women with a history of stroke or TIA within 90 days.[65] They were randomized to receive blind treatment with 17-beta estradiol 1 mg daily or placebo. After a mean follow-up of 2.8 years, there was no difference in stroke, death, or nonfatal stroke rates for those in the treatment group compared with the controls.

The evidence does not support a benefit from hormone replacement therapy with estrogen or the combination of estrogen and progestin for stroke or cardiovascular disease prevention. In addition, possible harmful effect exists such as venous thromboembolism. Therefore, hormone replacement therapy should not be employed in the prevention of recurrent stroke and possibly should be avoided in patients with a history of cardiovascular disease or stroke.

CIGARETTE SMOKING

Cigarette smoking is an established risk factor for stroke. The relative risk is nearly double for ischemic stroke and nearly triple for subarachnoid hemorrhage compared with that of nonsmokers. Furthermore, there is a continuous relationship between number of daily cigarettes smoked and risk of stroke.[66–68] Cigarettes may contribute to stroke risk by predisposing to atheroma formation,[69] increasing circulating fibrinogen,[70] enhancing platelet aggregation,[71] and causing arterial vasoconstriction.[72]

Smoking cessation has been shown to lead to a reduction in stroke risk similar to that of nonsmokers within 2 to 4 years.[66,68] Despite this, the ability to affect behavioral change has proven difficult. A prospective study in the United Kingdom of 151 smokers who survived to their 1-year follow-up showed that only 41 percent had ceased smoking.[73] Similarly, a stroke prevention clinic in Canada reported only 11 percent of smokers with a previous ischemic stroke or TIA had successfully quit by 12-month follow-up.[74]

A smoking cessation strategy should be a mandatory component of any risk factor management program. A report from the Cochrane Tobacco Addiction Review group suggested that even brief advice from health care professionals could increase the cessation rate by 69 percent.[75] Clinical practice guidelines from the United States Public Health Service state that patients should not only be counseled about the benefits of smoking cessation but also offered resources such as nicotine replacement and bupropion when appropriate.[76] A randomized clinical trial of treatment with a nicotine patch, bupropion hydrochloride, and bupropion hydrochloride and a nicotine patch for 9 weeks compared with placebo showed the odds ratio for abstinence at 12 months to be 0.84 (0.6 to 1.8), 2.3 (1.4 to 3.9), and 3.0 (1.8 to 4.9), respectively.[77] Anxiolytics have been found ineffective and the effectiveness of aversion therapy, mecamylamine, acupuncture, hypnotherapy, and exercise is unknown.[75]

ALCOHOL CONSUMPTION

There has been conflicting evidence about the association between alcohol consumption and stroke risk. Methodological barriers such as stroke subtype heterogeneity, differing risk across different populations (e.g., age, gender, race, and ethnicity), and validation of patient self-reporting of alcohol consumption may have obscured a relationship. However, a review of 62 epidemiological studies of moderate alcohol consumption and risk of stroke has suggested a J-shaped relationship predominantly notable in whites.[78] This relationship has been confirmed in a more recent meta-analysis that showed a 64 percent increase in the relative risk of total stroke for consumption of more than 60 g of alcohol per day; a 17 percent and 20 percent decrease in the relative risk of total and ischemic stroke, respectively, for consumption of less than 12 g per day; and a 28 percent reduction in the relative risk of ischemic stroke for consumption of 12 to 24 g per day.[79]

Heavy alcohol consumption can adversely affect the risk of stroke by multiple mechanisms. It has been associated with elevation in blood pressure, increased risk of coronary heart disease, cardiac arrhythmias, large-artery atherosclerosis, alteration in lipid profiles, reduction of cerebral blood flow, and changes in hematocrit and hemostasis.[77] Binge-drinking has been associated with a higher risk of cardioembolic, atheroembolic, and cryptogenic stroke.[80] It also has been shown to enhance platelet activation.[81] However, favorable effects of light-to-moderate alcohol consumption include an increase in HDL fraction and plasminogen activation.

To reduce the risk of ischemic and hemorrhagic stroke, patients should be advised to abstain from binge-drinking. Supportive resources such as abuse counseling should be provided for those with chronic alcohol abuse. Patients need not be discouraged from light-to-moderate alcohol consumption of two or fewer drinks daily because this may be protective from ischemic stroke. Because the addictive potential of alcohol is well known and because the predictability for abuse in an individual may not be known, patients should not be encouraged to engage in regular light-to-moderate alcohol consumption for its protective effect if they currently do not.

HYPERHOMOCYSTEINEMIA

Homocysteine is an amino acid intermediate in the metabolic pathway of dietary methionine. It can be reconverted back to methionine by methionine synthase or catalyzed to cysteine by cystathionine beta-synthase. Methionine synthase utilizes methyl-tetrahydrofolate as a substrate and cobalamin (vitamin B_{12}) as a cofactor. The methyl-tetrahydrofolate is produced from the reduction of dietary folate by methylene tetrahydrofolate reductase. Cystathionine beta-synthase utilizes pyridoxine (vitamin B_6) as a cofactor. Elevated serum homocysteine has been associated with coronary heart disease and stroke.[82–86] Although elevated homocysteine has been associated with several hematological changes favoring a procoagulant state,[87] its primary effect is likely to be atherogenic.[88]

Lowering of the serum homocysteine concentration has been successfully accomplished through B vitamin supplementation.[82,89,90] Whether or not this strategy equates to a reduction in stroke is not known although it has been shown to reduce the restenosis rate following percutaneous coronary intervention.[90] The Vitamin Intervention for Stroke Prevention (VISP) and Vitamins to Prevent Stroke (VITATOPS) studies are ongoing randomized clinical trials testing the hypothesis that supplementation with a combination of folic acid, vitamin B_{12}, and vitamin B_6 prevents recurrent stroke.[91,92]

PHYSICAL INACTIVITY

Physical inactivity has been shown to have an inverse relationship with cardiovascular disease and stroke.[93,94] In addition, exercise may have beneficial effects on other vascular risk factors such as cholesterol, blood pressure, and body mass index.

Physical activity has been shown to reduce the relative risk of death resulting from stroke by nearly one half. This association has been seen for both men and women across a broad range of ages.[95,96] Furthermore, a reduction in the risk of recurrent stroke was associated with higher levels of physical activity in the Northern Manhattan Stroke Study for patients that had an increase of left ventricular mass at baseline.[97]

Does the type of exercise make a difference? The Women's Health Initiative observed 73,743 women age 50 to 79 years for up to 5.9 years. No significant difference in risk reduction was seen comparing walking with vigorous exercise.[98] All patients who are physically capable and medically cleared should be advised to engage in a regular regimen of moderate physical exercise of 30 to 45 minutes daily.

Since the submission of this chapter for publication, new guidelines for the diagnosis, treatment, and classification of blood pressure have been published by the JNC VII group.

References

1. American Heart Association 1999 Heart and Stroke Statistical Update. Dallas, TX: American Heart Association, 1998.
2. Johnston SC. Transient ischemic attack. N Engl J Med 2002;347:1687–1692.
3. Albers GW, Caplan LR, Easton JD, et al. Transient ischemic attack—proposal for a new definition. N Engl J Med 2002;347:1713–1716.
4. Sacco RL, Benjamin EJ, Broderick JP, et al. Risk factors. Stroke 1997;28:1507–1517.
5. Diener HC, Cunha L, Forbes C, et al. European Stroke Prevention Study 2: dipyridamole and acetylsalicylic acid in the secondary prevention of stroke. J Neurol Sci 1996;143:1–13.
6. Johnston SC, Gress DR, Browner WS, Sidney S. Short-term prognosis after emergency department diagnosis of TIA. JAMA 2000;284:2901–2906.
7. Qureshi AI, Suri MFK, Guterman LR, Hopkins LN. Ineffective secondary prevention of cardiovascular events in the US population: report from the Third National Health and Nutrition Examination Survey. Arch Intern Med 2001;161:1621–1628.
8. The Sixth Report of the Joint National Committee on Hypertension (JNC VI). Arch Intern Med 1997;157:2413–2446.
9. Sacco RL. Ischemic Stroke. In PB Gorelick, M Alter (eds), Handbook of Neuroepidemiology. New York: Marcel Dekker, 1994;77–119.
10. Burt VL, Whelton P, Roccella EJ, et al. Prevalence of hypertension in the US adult population: results from the Third National Health and Nutrition Examination Survey, 1988-1991. Hypertension 1995;25:305–313.
11. Burt VL, Cutler JA, Higgins M, et al. Trends in the prevalence, awareness, treatment, and control of hypertension in the adult US population: data from the Health Examination Surveys, 1960-1991. Hypertension 1995;26:60–69.
12. Bone LR, Hill MN, Stallings R, et al. Community health survey in an urban African-American neighborhood: distribution and correlates of elevated blood pressure. Ethn Dis 2000;10:87–95.
13. Freeman V, Rotimi C, Cooper R. Hypertension prevalence, awareness, treatment, and control among African Americans in the 1990's: estimates from the Maywood Cardiovascular Survey. Am J Prev Med 1996;12:177–185.
14. Kernan WN, Viscoli CM, Brass LM, et al. Blood pressure exceeding national guidelines among women after stroke. Stroke 2000;31:415–419.
15. Joseph LN, Babikian VL, Allen NC, Winter MR. Risk factor modification in stroke prevention: the experience of a stroke clinic. Stroke 1999;30:16–20.

16. Nieto FJ, Alonso J, Chambless LE, et al. Population awareness and control of hypertension and hypercholesterolemia: the Atherosclerosis Risk in Communities Study. Arch Intern Med 1995;155:677–684.
17. Carter AB. Hypotensive therapy in stroke survivors. Lancet 1970; 1:485–489.
18. Hypertension-Stroke Cooperative Study Group. Effect of antihypertensive treatment on stroke recurrence. JAMA 1974;229:409–418.
19. Dutch TIA Trial Study Group. Trial of secondary prevention with atenolol after transient ischaemic attack or non-disabling ischaemic stroke. Stroke 1993;24:543–548.
20. Eriksson S, Olofsson BO, Wester PO for the TEST Study Group. Atenolol in secondary prevention after stroke. Cerebr Vasc Dis 1995;5:21–25.
21. PROGRESS Collaborative Group. Randomised trial of a perindopril-based blood-pressure-lowering regimen among 6105 individuals with previous stroke or transient ischaemic attack. Lancet 2001;358:1033–1041.
22. Psaty BM, Smith N, Siscovick DS, et al. Health outcomes associated with antihypertensive therapies used as first-line agents: a systemic review and meta-analysis. JAMA 1997;277:739–745.
23. Staessen JA, Fagard R, Thijs L, et al. Randomised double-blind comparison of placebo and active treatment for older patients with isolated systolic hypertension. The Systolic Hypertension in Europe (Syst-Eur) Trial Investigators. Lancet 1997;350:757–764.
24. SHEP Cooperative Research Group. Prevention of stroke by antihypertensive drug treatment in older persons with isolated systolic hypertension: final results of the Systolic Hypertension in the Elderly Program (SHEP). JAMA 1991;265:3255–3264.
25. Weber KT. Aldosterone in congestive heart failure. N Engl J Med 2001;345:1689–1697.
26. Cohn JN. ACE inhibition and vascular remodeling of resistance vessels. Vascular compliance and cardiovascular implications. Heart Dis 2000;2:S2–S6.
27. Schwartzkopff B, Beh M, Mundhenke M, Strauer BE. Repair of coronary arterioles after treatment with perindopril in hypertensive heart disease. Hypertension 2000;36:220–225.
28. Sihn I, Schroeder AP, Aalkjaer C, et al. Normalization of structural cardiovascular changes during antihypertensive treatment with a regimen based on the ACE-inhibitor perindopril. Blood Pressure 1995;4:241–248.
29. Thybo NIK, Stephens N, Cooper A, et al. Effect of antihypertensive treatment on small arteries of patients with previously untreated essential hypertension. Hypertension 1995;25(part I):475–478.
30. Walters MR, Bolster A, Dyker AG, Lees KR. Effect of perindopril on cerebral and renal perfusion in stroke patients with carotid disease. Stroke 2001;32:473–478.
31. The Heart Outcomes Prevention Evaluation Study Investigators. Effects of an angiotensin-converting-enzyme inhibitor, ramipril, on cardiovascular events in high-risk patients. N Engl J Med 2000;342:145–153.
32. Harris MI, Hadden WC, Knowler WC, Bennett PH. Prevalence of diabetes and impaired glucose tolerance and plasma glucose levels in U.S. population aged 20-74 yr. Diabetes 1987;36:523–534.
33. Ford Lynch G, Leurgans S, Raman R, et al. A comparison of stroke risk factors in patients enrolled in stroke prevention trials: a report from the African American Antiplatelet Stroke Prevention Study (AAASPS). J Natl Med Assoc 2001;93:79–86.
34. Sacco RL, Shi T, Zamanillo MC, Kargman DE. Predictors of mortality and recurrence after hospitalized cerebral infarction in an urban community: the Northern Manhattan Stroke Study. Neurology 1994;44:626–634.
35. Bruno A, Biller J, Adams HP Jr, et al. Acute blood glucose level and outcome from ischemic stroke. Trial of ORG 10172 in Acute Stroke Treatment (TOAST) Investigators. Neurology 1999;52:280–284.
36. American Diabetes Association. Standards of medical care for patients with diabetes mellitus. Diabetes Care 2002;25:213–229.
37. Sempos CT, Cleeman JI, Carroll MD, et al. Prevalence of high blood cholesterol among US adults: an update based on guidelines from the second report of the National Cholesterol Education Program Adult Treatment Panel. JAMA 1993;269:3009–3014.
38. Pieper RM, Arnett DK, McGovern PG, et al. Trends in cholesterol knowledge and screening and hypercholesterolemia awareness and treatment, 1980-1992: The Minnesota Heart Survey. Arch Intern Med 1997;157:2326–2332.
39. Szklo M, Chambless LE, Folsom AR, et al. Trends in plasma cholesterol levels in the Athero-sclerosis Risk in Communities (ARIC) Study. Prev Med 2000;30:252–259.
40. Amarenco P. Hypercholesterolemia, lipid-lowering agents, and the risk for brain infarction. Neurology 2001;57(5 suppl 2):S35–S44.
41. Benfante R, Katsukhiko Y, Hwang L, et al. Elevated serum cholesterol is a risk factor for both coronary heart disease and thromboembolic stroke in Hawaiian Japanese men: implications of shared risk. Stroke 1994;25:814–820.

42. Hachinski V, Graffagnino C, Beaudry M, et al. Lipids and stroke: a paradox resolved. Arch Neurol 1996;53:303–308.
43. Scandinavian Simvastatin Survival Study Group. Randomised trial of cholesterol lowering in 4444 patients with coronary heart disease: the Scandinavian Simvastatin Survival Study (4S). Lancet 1994;344:1383–1389.
44. Sacks FM, Pfeffer MA, Moye LA, et al. The effect of pravastatin on coronary events after myocardial infarction in patients with average cholesterol levels. N Engl J Med 1996;335:1001–1009.
45. White HD, Simes RJ, Anderson NE, et al. Pravastatin therapy and the risk of stroke. N Engl J Med 2000;343:317–326.
46. Di Mascio R, Marchioli R, Tognoni G. Cholesterol reduction and stroke occurrence: an overview of randomized clinical trials. Cerebrovasc Dis 2000;10:85–92.
47. Hebert PR, Gaziano JM, Chan KS, Hennekens CH. Cholesterol lowering with statin drugs, risk of stroke, and total mortality: an overview of randomized trials. JAMA 1997;278:313–321.
48. Blauw GJ, Lagaay AM, Smelt AH, Westendorp RG. Stroke, statins, and cholesterol: a meta-analysis of randomized, placebo-controlled, double-blind trials with HMG-CoA reductase inhibitors. Stroke 1997;28:946–950.
49. Heart Protection Study Collaborative Group. MRC/BHF heart protection study of cholesterol lowering with Simvastatin in 20,536 high-risk individuals: a randomised placebo-controlled trial. Lancet 2002;360:7–22.
50. Atkins D, Psaty BM, Koepsell TD, et al. Cholesterol reduction and the risk for stroke in men: a meta-analysis of randomized, controlled trials. Ann Intern Med 1993;119:136–145.
51. Hebert PR, Gaziano M, Hennekens CH. An overview of trials of cholesterol lowering and risk of stroke. Arch Intern Med 1995;155:50–55.
52. Hess DC, Demchuk AM, Brass LM, Yatsu FM. HMG-CoA reductase inhibitors (statins): a promising approach to stroke prevention. Neurology 2000;54:790–796.
53. Rosenson RS, Tangney CC. Antiatherothrombotic properties of statins: implications for cardiovascular event reduction. JAMA 1998;279:1643–1650.
54. Crisby M, Nordin-Fredriksson G, Shah PK, et al. Pravastatin treatment increases collagen content and decreases lipid content, inflammation, metalloproteinases, and cell death in human carotid plaques: implications for plaque stabilization. Circulation 2001;103:926–933.
55. Ridker PM, Rifai N, Pfeffer MA, et al. Inflammation, pravastatin, and the risk of coronary events after myocardial infarction in patients with average cholesterol levels. Cholesterol and Recurrent Events (CARE) Investigators. Circulation 1998;98:839–844.
56. Sterzer P, Meintzschel F, Rosler A, et al. Pravastatin improves cerebral vasomotor reactivity in patients with subcortical small-vessel disease. Stroke 2001;32:2817–2820.
57. Laufs U, Gertz K, Huang P, et al. Atorvastatin upregulates type III nitric oxide synthase in thrombocytes, decreases platelet activation, and protects from cerebral ischemia in normocholesterolemic mice. Stroke 2000;31:2437–2449.
58. Alfon J, Royo T, Garcia-Moll X, Badimon L. Platelet deposition on eroded vessel walls at a stenotic shear rate is inhibited by lipid-lowering treatment with atorvastatin. Arterioscler Thromb Vasc Biol 1999;19:1812–1817.
59. Wolf PA, Clagett GP, Easton JD, et al. Preventing ischemic stroke in patients with prior stroke and transient ischemic attack: a statement for healthcare professionals from the Stroke Council of the American Heart Association. Stroke 1999;30:1991–1994.
60. Executive Summary of the Third Report of the National Cholesterol Education Program (NCEP) Expert Panel on Detection, Evaluation, and Treatment of High Blood Cholesterol in Adults (Adult Treatment Panel III). JAMA 2001;285:2486–2497.
61. Mendelsohn ME, Karas RH. Mechanisms of disease: the protective effects of estrogen on the cardiovascular system. N Engl J Med 1999;340:1801–1811.
62. Grady D, Herrington D, Bittner V, et al. Cardiovascular disease outcomes during 6.8 years of hormone therapy: Heart and Estrogen/Progestin Replacement Study follow-up (HERS II). JAMA 2002;288:49–57.
63. Hulley S, Furberg C, Barrett-Connor E, et al. Noncardiovascular disease outcomes during 6.8 years of hormone therapy: Heart and Estrogen/Progestin Replacement Study follow-up (HERS II). JAMA 2002;288:58–66.
64. Writing Group for the Women's Health Initiative Investigators. Risks and benefits of estrogen plus progestin in healthy postmenopausal women: principal results from the Women's Health Initiative Randomized Controlled Trial. JAMA 2002;288:321–333.
65. Viscoli CM, Brass LM, Kernan WN, et al. A clinical trial of estrogen-replacement therapy after ischemic stroke. N Engl J Med 2001;345:1243–1249.

66. Wolf PA, D'Agostino RB, Kannel WB, et al. Cigarette smoking as a risk factor for stroke: the Framingham Study. JAMA 1988;259:1025–1029.
67. Shinton R, Beevers G. Meta-analysis of relation between cigarette smoking and stroke. BMJ 1989;298:789–794.
68. Kawachi I, Colditz GA, Stampfer MJ, et al. Smoking cessation and decreased risk of stroke in women. JAMA 1993;269:232–236.
69. Gill JS, Shipley MJ, Tsementzis SA, et al. Cigarette smoking: a risk factor for hemorrhagic and nonhemorrhagic stroke. Arch Intern Med 1989;149:2053–2057.
70. Kannel WB, D'Agostino RB, Belanger AL. Fibrinogen, cigarette smoking and risk of cardiovascular disease: insights from the Framingham Study. Am Heart J 1987;113:1006–1010.
71. Levine PH. An acute effect of cigarette smoking on platelet function: a possible link between smoking and arterial thrombosis. Circulation 1973;48:619–623.
72. Rogers RL, Meyer JS, Judd BW, Mortel KF. Abstention from cigarette smoking improves cerebral perfusion among elderly chronic smokers. JAMA 1985;253:2970–2974.
73. Redfern J, McKevitt C, Dundas R, et al. Behavioral risk factor prevalence and lifestyle change after stroke: a prospective study. Stroke 2000;31:1877–1881.
74. Mouradian MS, Majumdar SR, Senthilselan A, et al. How well are hypertension, hyperlipidemia, diabetes, and smoking managed after a stroke or transient ischemic attack? Stroke 2002;33: 1656–1659.
75. Lancaster T, Stead L, Silagy C, Sowden A for the Cochrane Tobacco Addiction Review Group. Effectiveness of interventions to help people stop smoking: findings from the Cochrane Library. BMJ 2000;321:355–358.
76. The Tobacco Use and Dependence Clinical Practice Guideline Panes, Staff, and Consortium Representatives. A clinical practice guideline for treating tobacco use and dependence: a US Public Health Service Report. JAMA 2000;283:3244–3254.
77. Jorenby DE, Leischow SJ, Nides MA, et al. A controlled trial of sustained-release bupropion, a nicotine patch, or both for smoking cessation. N Engl J Med 1999;340:685–691.
78. Camargo CA Jr. Moderate alcohol consumption and stroke: the epidemiologic evidence. Stroke 1989;20:1611–1626.
79. Reynolds K, Lewis BL, Nolen JD, et al. Alcohol consumption and risk of stroke: a meta-analysis. JAMA 2003;289:579–588.
80. Hillbom M, Numminen H, Juvela S. Recent heavy drinking of alcohol and embolic stroke. Stroke 1999;30:2307–2312.
81. Numminen H, Syrjala M, Benthin G, et al. The effect of acute ingestion of a large dose of alcohol on the hemostatic system and its circadian variation. Stroke 2000;31:1269–1273.
82. Malinow MR. Plasma homocysteine: a risk factor for arterial occlusive diseases. J Nutr 1996;126(S4):1238S–1243S.
83. Stampfer MJ, Malinow MR, Willett WC, et al. A prospective study of plasma homocysteine and risk of myocardial infarction in US physicians. JAMA 1992;268:877–881.
84. Morris MS, Jacques PF, Rosenberg IH, et al. Serum total homocysteine concentration is related to self-reported heart attack or stroke history among men and women in the NHANES III. J Nutr 2000;130:3073–3076.
85. Perry IJ, Refsum H, Morris RW, et al. Prospective study of serum total homocysteine concentration and risk of Stroke in middle-aged British men. Lancet 1995;346:1395–1398.
86. Bots ML, Launer LJ, Lindemans J, et al. Homocysteine and short-term risk of myocardial infarction and stroke in the elderly: the Rotterdam Study. Arch Intern Med 1999;159:38–44.
87. Kristensen B, Malm J, Nilsson TK, et al. Hyperhomocysteinemia and hypofibrinolysis in young adults with ischemic stroke. Stroke 1999;30:974–980.
88. Eikelboom JW, Hankey GJ, Anand SS, et al. Association between high homocysteine and ischemic stroke due to large- and small-artery disease but not other etiologic subtypes of ischemic stroke. Stroke 2000;31:1069–1075.
89. Boushey CJ, Beresford SA, Omenn GS, Motulsky AG. A quantitative assessment of plasma homo-cysteine as a risk factor for vascular disease. Probable benefits of increasing folic acid intakes. JAMA 1995;274:1049–1057.
90. Schnyder G, Roffi M, Flammer Y, et al. Effect of homocysteine-lowering therapy with folic acid, vitamin B12, and vitamin B6 on clinical outcome after percutaneous coronary intervention. The Swiss Heart Study: a randomized controlled trial. JAMA 2002;288:973–979.
91. The VITATOPS Trial Study Group. The VITATOPS (Vitamins to Prevent Stroke) Trial: rationale and design of an international, large, simple, randomised trial of homocysteine-lowering multivitamin therapy in patients with recent transient ischaemic attack or stroke. Cerebrovasc Dis 2002;13:120–126.

92. Spence JD, Howard VJ, Chambless LE, et al. Vitamin Intervention for Stroke Prevention (VISP) Trial: rationale and design. Neuroepidemiology 2001;20:16–25.
93. Kohl HW. Physical activity and cardiovascular disease: evidence for a dose response. Med Sci Sports Exerc 2001;33(suppl 6):S472–483.
94. Wannamethee SG, Shaper AG. Physical activity and the prevention of stroke. J Cardiovasc Risk 1999;6:213–216.
95. Ellekjaer H, Holmen J, Ellekjaer E, Vatten L. Physical activity and stroke mortality in women: ten-year follow-up of the Nord-Trondelag Health Survey, 1984-1986. Stroke 2000;31:14–18.
96. Lee CD, Blair SN. Cardiorespiratory fitness and stroke mortality in men. Med Sci Sports Exerc 2002;34:592–595.
97. Rodriguez CJ, Sacco RL, Sciacca RR, et al. Physical activity attenuates the effect of increased left ventricular mass on the risk of ischemic stroke: the Northern Manhattan Stroke Study. J Am Coll Cardiol 2002;39:1482–1488.
98. Manson JE, Greenland P, LaCroix AZ, et al. Walking compared with vigorous exercise for the prevention of cardiovascular events in women. N Engl J Med 2002;347:716–725.

11
Rapid Clinical Evaluation

Chelsea S. Kidwell and Jeffrey L. Saver

Minutes matter in the acute stroke patient. In all but the most exceptional case, threatened tissue is no longer salvageable much beyond 6 hours after symptom onset. Prompt, efficient clinical evaluation is essential to deliver acute therapies effectively. An expansive and exquisitely detailed clinical evaluation is inappropriate in the acute setting. Instead, the evaluation of the acute stroke patient is an urgent and iterative process. Succeeding caretakers and providers in the healthcare system—dispatchers, ambulance personnel, emergency department (ED) nurses, emergency physicians, neurologists, and others—perform rapid evaluations of increasing detail. At each stage, the examiner first elicits the key elements of the history and examination needed to guide pressing triage decisions and then returns serially to the bedside to gather additional information to complete the clinical picture.

THE STROKE CHAIN OF SURVIVAL AND RECOVERY

The "stroke chain of survival and recovery" is a useful framework for conceptualizing integrated prehospital and ED acute stroke care, including clinical evaluation.[1,2] The "seven Ds" in the stroke chain of survival or recovery are as follows (Figure 11.1): (1) detection of the onset of stroke signs and symptoms; (2) dispatch through activation of the emergency medical service (EMS) system and prompt EMS response; (3) delivery of the victim to the receiving hospital while providing appropriate prehospital assessment and care and prearrival notification; (4) door—ED triage; (5) data—ED evaluation, including head computed tomography (CT) scan; (6) decision about potential therapies; and (7) drug therapy.[1] To be successful, each link in the chain must function efficiently. The first five steps in this chain compose the early clinical evaluation of the stroke patient.

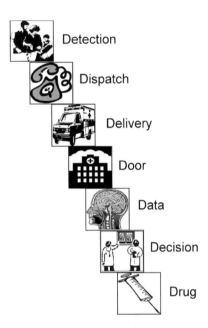

Figure 11.1   Stroke chain of survival: the seven Ds.

DETECTION OF THE ONSET OF STROKE SIGNS AND SYMPTOMS

The first "D" in the stroke chain of survival or recovery is detection of stroke signs and symptoms by the patient, a family member, friend, or other bystander. Detection not only requires awareness of the signs and symptoms of stroke but also requires an understanding of the urgency for rapid medical attention and the importance of activating the 911 system. The first and most crucial evaluation of the acute stroke patient is made by the patient himself or herself or someone with them, recognizing a possible stroke in progress and rapidly activating the emergency medical system.

However, most studies performed to date demonstrate that members of the public in general, and stroke patients in particular, have suboptimal knowledge about stroke.[3–5] Kothari et al[6] interviewed 163 possible stroke patients admitted to the ED and found that 39 percent did not know a single sign or symptom of a stroke. Williams et al[7] interviewed 67 stroke patients and found that only 25 percent correctly interpreted their symptoms.

The American Stroke Association and the National Stroke Association have identified five cardinal warning signs of a possible stroke in progress of which adults should be aware: (1) sudden weakness or numbness of the face, arm, or leg, especially on one side of the body; (2) sudden confusion, trouble speaking, or understanding; (3) sudden trouble seeing in one or both eyes; (4) sudden trouble walking, dizziness, loss of balance, or incoordination; and (5) sudden severe headache with no known cause (Table 11.1). Of these, weakness on one side of the body is the single most important sign to emphasize. All individuals

Table 11.1   Stroke warning signs*

Sudden weakness, especially on one side of the body
Sudden trouble speaking
Sudden trouble with vision
Sudden dizziness, walking difficulty
Sudden severe headache

*If you or someone with you has one or more of these signs, don't delay! Call 911 immediately!

at risk for stroke and their family members, indeed all adults, should be instructed in these warning signs.

The importance of activating the 911 system when a stroke warning sign is observed cannot be overemphasized.[6,8–10] Any other type of first contact merely leads to needless delay. In one study of 1159 patients, median time from onset to ED arrival was 1 hour 24 minutes when the patient's first contact was the 911 system, versus 3 hours 32 minutes when the patient first called the receiving hospital and 4 hours 30 minutes when the patient first called their primary physician.[8] In another study, among 163 acute stroke patients, those transported to hospital by 911 were far more likely to arrive within 3 hours versus those transported by private vehicle (47% vs. 19%, $p = 0.001$).[6]

The urgency of stroke symptoms and the importance of calling 911 should be stressed not only with individuals at risk for stroke but also with all adults. Strokes may cause aphasia and deprive a patient of the ability to communicate or produce anosognosia and deprive the patient of the ability to appreciate a deficit. The responsibility for early activation of the EMS system then falls on friends, family, workplace colleagues, and bystanders who happen to be on scene. Among 617 stroke patients, transport by 911 was more likely to occur if on-scene observers (family, friends, coworkers), rather than the patient, first identified that the patient was having worrisome symptoms.[11]

Both small- and large-scale campaigns have been undertaken to educate the public about stroke. In the prethrombolytic era, Alberts et al[12] demonstrated that a community public education program could improve presentation within 24 hours from 42 to 86 percent. In the thrombolytic era, Dornan et al[13] performed a baseline survey of stroke knowledge followed by a public stroke education campaign. Following the campaign, they found a significant increase in public knowledge of stroke warning signs (ability to name one stroke warning sign increased from 57% to 78%). Women were found to be more knowledgeable about stroke at baseline and more likely to improve knowledge with education. Other groups have also demonstrated that targeted stroke education programs are successful in increasing the public's knowledge of stroke risk factors, particularly in the elderly.[14]

The National Stroke Association Clinical Trials Accelerated Program found that centers provided with the tools for a public education program were more successful in enrolling patients in acute stroke trials.[15] In the National Institute of Neurological Disorders and Stroke (NINDS) tissue plasminogen activator (t-PA) trials, study coordinators used a variety of educational techniques to increase public awareness about stroke. Anecdotal observations suggested a trend toward improved stroke awareness and all participating centers were successful in recruiting substantial numbers of patients within narrow treatment time windows.[16,17]

Over the last several years, large-scale public stroke education programs have been sponsored by the National Stroke Association, the American Heart/Stroke Association, and the National Institutes of Health. These programs emphasize recognition of stroke warning signs and stroke risk factors and the critical message that stroke is a medical emergency, a "brain attack," and that the 911 system should be activated if a stroke is suspected. The effect of these national educational programs is not yet clear and simply increasing stroke awareness and knowledge may not necessarily change behavior and decrease delays to presentation. Although several large-scale educational programs have been effective in changing behavior in the past (50% reduction in smoking in United States, increased use of seatbelts, increased use of condoms with acquired immunodeficiency syndrome [AIDS] education),[18] educational campaigns geared to earlier response to chest pain have been largely unsuccessful at decreasing delays to seeking medical care with median time to arrival remaining at 3 hours after symptom onset.[19,20]

DISPATCH

The second "D" in the stroke chain of survival is dispatch through activation of the EMS system and prompt EMS response. EMS systems expand emergency medical care into the community, including prehospital management for acute stroke victims. The role of the EMS includes rapid identification of acute stroke patients, expeditious transport to a definitive care facility, and prearrival notification of the receiving hospital, enabling activation of the stroke team and preparation of a neuroimaging scanner.

Once a 911 call is placed, the dispatcher becomes the first medical contact for the patient. Enhanced 911 call systems that automatically display the caller's address have been adopted in many communities and are of particular benefit for stroke patients who are dysarthric or aphasic. The dispatcher assesses the type and nature of the complaint and based on this information makes the decision regarding dispatch priority and level of expertise (e.g., ALS [advanced life support] or BLS [basic life support]), decisions that will influence hospital arrival time. Many communities have recently adopted specific stroke run codes that dispatch stroke patients at highest levels of urgency, equivalent to patients with acute myocardial infarction or trauma, but this practice is not yet universal.

The general medical supervision, training, and expertise among dispatchers vary from one community to another. In a study of 61 "911" calls for patients with a final diagnosis of stroke in San Francisco, Porteous, Corry, and Smith[21] found that the dispatch code was "CVA (cerebrovascular accident)" in only 31 percent of calls and that most (59%) ambulances were dispatched at low priority.[21] Even when the caller used the word "stroke," only half of these cases were dispatched as such.

EMS systems are increasingly using formal structured query algorithms to help dispatchers identify acute stroke patients by phone conversations with patients and on-scene witnesses.[22] Although the stroke recognition algorithms employed in these protocols have not yet been prospectively validated, it is likely that these formal instruments aid in dispatcher recognition and response to stroke.

In addition to identifying potential stroke calls, dispatchers may play an important role in optimizing rapid transport by instructing the caller before vehicle arrival to confirm time of onset, prepare for transport, collect medical records, and collect medications.

DELIVERY

The third "D" in the stroke chain of survival is delivery of the patient to the receiving hospital while providing appropriate prehospital assessment and evaluation. For the stroke patient, optimal delivery requires (1) accurate stroke recognition by prehospital personnel, (2) accurate rating of stroke severity by prehospital personnel, (3) appropriate in-field treatment, (4) prearrival notification of the receiving hospital, and (5) rapid patient transport. Current and emerging activities of prehospital personnel in acute stroke care include initiating appropriate supportive treatments in the field (start of intravenous [IV] line and fluid support, administration of supplemental oxygen if needed); avoiding potentially detrimental treatments (overaggressive blood pressure reduction); radio alerting the receiving hospital of the imminent arrival of an acute stroke patient, allowing the stroke team to be mobilized and neuroimaging suites to be readied; diverting acute stroke patients to dedicated stroke critical care centers; and administering neuroprotective agents in the field.[23–26]

Stroke Knowledge

The specific training in stroke received by prehospital personnel varies widely among communities. In a recent nationwide multiple choice survey of paramedics and advanced emergency medical technicians (EMTs), although most EMS providers were knowledgeable about the symptoms of stroke, they were often unaware of the therapeutic time window for thrombolysis and the recommended avoidance of blood pressure reduction in the acute stroke setting.[27] These findings suggest a need for a standardized stroke curriculum for prehospital personnel.

Stroke Identification

As the first medical personnel to physically encounter acute stroke patients, paramedics and EMTs are in a unique position to expedite and optimize stroke care. However, prehospital personnel can only be effective in stroke care if they are able to reliably identify patients likely to be experiencing acute stroke. Several studies have demonstrated that accuracy of stroke identification by prehospital personnel is modest and variable across communities, when a formal stroke recognition instrument is not employed. In different communities, sensitivity for stroke recognition by prehospital personnel ranged widely but typically fell in the 60 to 80 percent range, and positive predictive values were suboptimal, in the 60 to 75 percent range.[28–31] These results in part reflect variations in stroke educational programs provided to prehospital personnel. Until recently, stroke recognition and management was not emphasized in prehospital training curriculums.

It is important to recognize that identifying stroke in the field is a challenging task, because prehospital personnel encounter many more stroke mimic than true stroke patients, including patients with alcohol and drug intoxication, postictal hemiparesis, hypoglycemia or other metabolic encephalopathies, and other nonstroke causes of acute neurological deficits. In one study, true stroke cases accounted for only 3 percent of all paramedic runs, and stroke mimics outnumbered true strokes by more than 10 to 1.[32] Accordingly, training programs aimed at improving stroke recognition in the field must emphasize not only recognition of neurological deficits (to improve sensitivity) but also exclusion of stroke mimics (to improve specificity). Simply treating all neurological deficit patients as possible stroke patients would risk "burn-out" of in-hospital stroke teams activated by prearrival notification, diversion of many nonstroke patients to stroke critical care centers, and exposure of nonstroke patients to neuroprotective agents in the field.

Several structured diagnostic evaluation instruments have been designed specifically to aid paramedics and EMTs in identifying acute stroke patients in the field. Prospective field testing has validated two instruments, the Los Angeles Prehospital Stroke Screen (LAPSS) and the Face Arm Speech Test (FAST), and suggested that paramedic performance in stroke recognition improves substantially when they are routinely employed.[33,34] International emergency cardiovascular care guidelines formulated by the American Heart Association, the European Resuscitation Council, and other international organizations to guide prehospital care worldwide incorporate two instruments, the LAPSS and the Cincinnati Prehospital Stroke Scale (CPSS) as recommended options for stroke identification.[35]

Los Angeles Prehospital Stroke Screen

The LAPSS was designed not only to identify acute stroke patients by examination but also to exclude likely stroke mimics by history and glucose testing and to provide critical information required for the rapid evaluation and triage of acute stroke patients.[33] The LAPSS (Figure 11.2) is a one-page instrument that takes 1 to 3 minutes to perform and consists of four history items, a blood glucose measure, and three motor examination items. The four history items and serum glucose item exclude potential stroke mimics (history of seizure, hyperglycemia or hypoglycemia, patients wheelchair bound or bedridden with baseline deficits, younger-than-typical stroke population) or patients unlikely to qualify for acute stroke interventions or trials (onset >24 hours, wheelchair bound or bedridden at baseline). The instrument is designed to emphasize not only sensitivity but also specificity and positive predictive value to identify the best candidates for prearrival activation of the stroke team and, in the future, in-field neuroprotective treatment.[32]

The examination, intended to identify the most obvious and common types of stroke, tests for unilateral face, arm, and/or hand weakness. The examination

LOS ANGELES PREHOSPITAL STROKE SCREEN (LAPSS)

A. Patient name _____   _____
                                 Last   First

B. Information/history from:
  ☐ Patient
  ☐ Family member _____   Phone: _____
  ☐ Other _____

C. Last known time patient was at baseline or deficit free and awake:
  Military time: _____
  Date: _____

SCREENING CRITERIA

	Yes	No	Unknown
1. Age > 45	☐	☐	☐
2. History of seizures or epilepsy absent	☐	☐	☐
3. Symptom duration less than 12 hours	☐	☐	☐
4. At baseline, patient is not wheelchair bound or bedridden	☐	☐	☐
5. Blood glucose between 60 and 400	☐	☐	☐

6. Exam: Look for obvious asymmetry

	Normal	Right	Left
Facial smile/grimace:	☐	☐ Droop	☐ Droop
Grip:	☐	☐ Weak grip ☐ No grip	☐ Weak grip ☐ No grip
Arm strength:	☐	☐ Drifts down ☐ Falls rapidly	☐ Drifts down ☐ Falls rapidly

	Yes	No
On exam, patient has primarily unilateral (not bilateral) weakness:	☐	☐
Items 4, 5, 6, 7, 8, 9 all YES's (or unknown) → LAPSS screening criteria met:	☐	☐

Figure 11.2   Los Angeles Prehospital Stroke Screen (LAPSS).

focuses solely on motor deficits for several reasons: (1) 80 to 90 percent of stroke patients have unilateral motor weakness, (2) motor weakness is a major determinant of long-term disability, (3) health personnel from a broad range of training backgrounds can easily and reliably perform testing for motor weakness, (4) acute stroke patients who are free of any motor weakness are both uncommon and generally not in need of aggressive acute stroke interventions, and (5) other candidate neurological items for a prehospital neurological screening examination, such as visual field deficit, oculomotor disturbance, and language impairment, were felt to have liabilities of poor reproducibility, lack of specificity, excessive complexity, and/or reliance on the patient and examiner sharing the same language.

In a prospective validation study, paramedics performed LAPSS screening in the field on 1198 consecutive transports. Paramedic performance employing the LAPSS demonstrated sensitivity of 91 percent and positive predictive value of 86 percent. The positive predictive value improved to 97 percent after correction of documentation errors.[33] In a pilot trial of neuroprotective therapy administered by paramedics in the field to 20 acute stroke patients, the LAPSS demonstrated 95 percent sensitivity, 100 percent specificity, and 100 percent positive predictive value.[36] The LAPSS has been widely adopted and has been successfully employed for prearrival notification of receiving hospitals, diversion of patients to acute stroke critical care centers, and enrollment of patients in a trial of prehospital initiation of experimental neuroprotective stroke therapy.[23,26]

Cincinnati Prehospital Stroke Screen and the Face Arm Speech Test

The CPSS (initially called the Out-of-Hospital National Institutes of Health Stroke Scale) is a three-item examination designed to aid prehospital personnel in identifying acute stroke patients (Figure 11.3). Kothari et al[37] derived the scale by analyzing National Institutes of Health Stroke Scale (NIHSS) findings recorded by physicians in an ED on 74 patients with acute ischemic stroke and 225 nonstroke patients. The three components of the NIHSS found to be the most discriminating predictors of stroke were facial palsy, arm motor testing, and dysarthria. The investigators modified the third item to combine dysarthria and aphasia into a single item called best language. In a subsequent report, physician versus paramedic/EMT use of the scale was compared on 171 patients examined by physicians while the paramedics/EMTs watched, and all recorded findings. Good correlation was noted between prehospital providers and physicians on arm weakness but only fair correlation for facial droop and speech.[38] No prospective, in-the-field validation study for the CPSS has yet been reported, but performance is likely to be analogous to that of the similar FAST instrument.

The FAST was developed by Harbison et al and modeled closely on the CPSS. Like the CPSS, it is a three-item examination with components testing facial weakness, arm drift, and speech disturbance. It differs from the CPSS in that speech disturbance is rated based on paramedic assessment during normal conversation with the patient rather than patient formal repetition of a single test sentence. In a prospective, field study in which paramedic-identified stroke patients were diverted to a stroke critical care center, paramedics employing the FAST demonstrated a positive predictive value of 79 percent in the identification of stroke.[34]

CINCINNATI PREHOSPITAL STROKE SCALE	
Facial droop	**Have patient smile or show teeth**
Normal	Both sides move equally
Abnormal	One side does not move as well
Arm drift	**Patient closes eyes and holds both arms out**
Normal	Both sides move equally or no movement at all
Abnormal	One side does not move as well or drifts downward
Speech	**Have patient say, "You can't teach an old dog new tricks"**
Normal	Patient uses correct words without slurring
Abnormal	Slurs words, uses inappropriate words, or is unable to speak

Any or one or more abnormal finding is suggestive of acute stroke.

Figure 11.3 Cincinnati Prehospital Stroke Scale.

Mobile Telemedicine Field Recognition of Stroke

A promising complementary approach to paramedic identification for field recognition of stroke is to employ mobile telemedicine, with transmission of video, audio, and physiological monitoring data from the rescue vehicle to a computer workstation at the receiving hospital staffed by a physician or nurse. An integrated mobile telecommunications system called TeleBAT has been pioneered by stroke investigators at the University of Maryland and uses wireless digital cellular communication.[39] While en-route to the ED, an ambulance installed televideo system provides a hospital neurologist with real-time visual access to a patient's neurological examination and transmission of vital signs. Prospective studies using the TeleBAT system are underway. Although the initial TeleBAT system required a high cost technology infrastructure, rapid evolution of commercial cellular transmission network technology suggests that off the shelf video-cell phone systems may soon permit this general strategy to be widely adopted.

Rating Stroke Severity in the Field

Quantitative rating of stroke severity by paramedics in the field is a desirable practice, in addition to accurate discrimination of stroke versus nonstroke patients.

A simple measure of prehospital stroke severity permits receiving hospitals to preliminarily determine the urgency of care required for patients called in from the field, allows regional systems to select for diversion patients with deficit severities most likely to benefit from comprehensive care, and provides critical pretreatment baseline data in prehospital trials of neuroprotective therapy.

The NIHSS is the most widely employed in-hospital instrument to rate stroke severity in the United States. Paramedics can be trained to apply the full NIHSS successfully.[40] However, the comparatively lengthy, 5- to 10-minute duration of a standard NIHSS examination makes this approach impractical for field evaluation. Tirschwell et al[41] have developed a shortened NIHSS for prehospital use, comprised of the five items that were most predictive of long-term outcome in a clinical trial dataset: left leg strength, right leg strength, best gaze, visual fields, and best language. The shortened NIHSS is a promising instrument that awaits prospective, field validation.

The Los Angeles Motor Scale (LAMS) is a prehospital stroke severity instrument that was constructed by assigning point values to LAPSS items of facial weakness, arm strength, and grip to yield a total 0 to 5 scale (Figure 11.4). Retrospective studies suggest that this simple three-item severity inventory predicts functional outcomes with accuracy nearly comparable to that of the full NIHSS and exhibits good interrater and intrarater reliability.[42,43] Use of the LAMS scoring of the LAPSS is a highly expeditious approach to identification of stroke patients and assessment of stroke severity in the field, obviating the need for paramedic performance of separate stroke recognition and stroke severity rating examinations.

Treatment in the Field

The primary role of EMS is to ensure that a patient is medically stable and transported to a medical facility for definitive care. Prehospital personnel should obtain a rapid history including past medical history and current medications,

LOS ANGELES MOTOR SCALE (LAMS)				
	Normal	Right	Left	Total
Facial smile/grimace	☐ (0)	☐ Droop (1)	☐ Droop (1)	
Grip	☐ (0)	☐ Weak grip (1) ☐ No grip (2)	☐ Weak grip (1) ☐ No grip (2)	
Arm strength	☐ (0)	☐ Drifts down (1) ☐ Falls rapidly (2)	☐ Drifts down (1) ☐ Falls rapidly (2)	
			TOTAL Score	

Figure 11.4   Los Angeles Motor Scale (LAMS).

perform an abbreviated examination, and deliver treatment with emphasis on stabilizing airway, breathing, and circulation (the ABCs).[44] Many EMS systems have developed standing field protocols specific for stroke. Although these protocols vary from one community to another, in-field stroke treatments typically include obtaining a serum glucose measure and correcting severe hypoglycemia if detected, administering supplemental oxygen, and placing a peripheral IV line. Field protocols should also emphasize the importance of rapid transport, encouraging prehospital personnel to employ a strategy of "scoop and go" rather than lingering on scene to acquire nonessential historical information. Duldner et al[45] reported that implementation of a formal out-of-hospital stroke protocol improved evaluation and management of patients, with increased initiation of IV access, pulse oximetry, and blood glucose measures.

In the future, paramedics may deliver neuroprotective agents in the field to stabilize the ischemic penumbra and preserve threatened tissue until definitive revascularization can be achieved by in-hospital treatment. In a pilot trial, paramedic initiation of the experimental neuroprotective agent magnesium sulfate in stroke patients in the ambulance was demonstrated to be feasible and safe and to markedly accelerate therapy start compared with initiation only after hospital arrival.[26]

Hospital Notification and Transport

Prehospital personnel may help minimize delays by notifying the receiving hospital from the field that a stroke patient is being transported. This allows the receiving hospital to clear and ready a CT (or magnetic resonance [MR]) scanner, call in radiological technicians if needed, and activate the stroke team in advance. No studies have been conducted with stroke patients to determine the timesaving of using this approach. However, in the analogous setting of patients with acute myocardial infarction, significant reductions in time to treatment (from 130 minutes to 81 minutes) with thrombolytic agents were achieved by prehospital transmission of the electrocardiogram and prenotification to the receiving hospital.[46]

After the patient is evaluated and stabilized in the field, stroke patients should be rapidly transported to the ED. Upgrading potential thrombolytic candidates to a higher priority (more rapid level of transport) decreases both transport and ED triage delays. Decisions regarding whether to employ lights and siren when transporting stroke patients must be made with care, balancing clinical gains against the increased risk of traffic accidents. Accordingly, decisions regarding lights and siren transport for stroke patients are best made by individual EMS systems, based on knowledge of local traffic patterns and EMS practices.

DOOR

The fourth "D" in the stroke chain of survival is "door," which stresses the role of rapid triage, evaluation, and early mobilization of resources once the patient has arrived to the ED (Figure 11.5). Historically, stroke patients were triaged in the ED as low priority, because there was little that could be done acutely

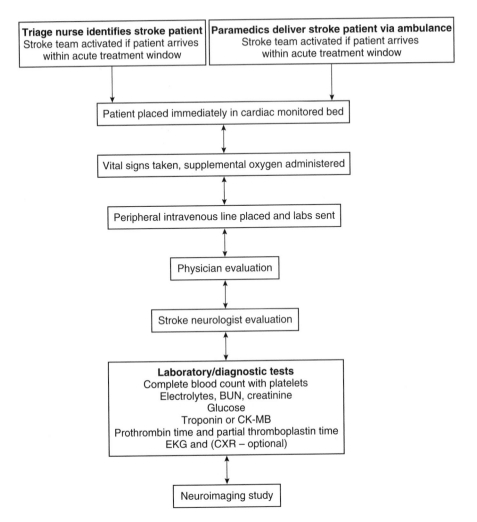

Figure 11.5 Emergency Department Stroke Patient Evaluation and Treatment. (Events often occur simultaneously.)

besides supportive care. Delays were common at many levels, including initial triage, nursing evaluation, physician evaluation, obtaining laboratory and other diagnostic tests, and evaluation by a neurologist. To change this established pattern of response and sense of therapeutic nihilism, EDs are developing comprehensive plans for rapid evaluation and treatment of the stroke patient. These plans need to include ongoing education of personnel and establishment of designated stroke teams and protocols.[47]

Optimizing the care of the acute stroke patient in the ED requires a team approach. The team concept is of established value for treatment of patients with trauma and acute myocardial infarction[48–50] and can be appropriately applied to patients with stroke to shorten delays to treatment and potentially improve patient outcome. Several groups have demonstrated that implementation of a stroke team in both academic and community hospitals does in fact decrease interval delays (e.g., reducing the interval from ED arrival to CT completion from 139 to 50 minutes).[9,51] Other groups have demonstrated that activation of a stroke team permits earlier neurological consultation and that early involvement of a neurologist (within 6 hours) lead to better patient outcome.[52,53]

Because the ED plays such a critical role in the initial evaluation and treatment of acute stroke patients in the current era of thrombolytic therapy, it has been suggested that patients only be transported to hospitals that have stroke expertise and at a minimum are capable of delivering IV t-PA in a rapid and safe manner. A conference convened by the National Institutes of Health issued a consensus statement detailing target time goals in the evaluation and management of stroke thrombolytic candidates.[54] These recommendations include (1) physician evaluation within 10 minutes of patient arrival in the ED, (2) notification of the stroke team within 15 minutes of arrival, (3) initiation of a head CT within 25 minutes of arrival, (4) interpretation of the CT scan within 45 minutes of arrival, (5) ensuring a door-to-drug (needle) time of 60 minutes from arrival in 80 percent of patients, and (6) transferring the patient to an inpatient setting within 3 hours of arrival. In addition, stroke expertise should be available within 15 minutes of hospital arrival for patients who meet thrombolytic treatment criteria and neurosurgical expertise within 2 hours. In hospitals where a neurologist is not available within 15 minutes of arrival, emergency physicians may develop stroke expertise and successfully administer t-PA.[55]

The designation of "stroke critical care centers" is increasingly being recognized as an attractive public policy response to the challenge of acute stroke care.[56,57] In this regional framework of care, similar to the trauma center model, stroke patients are diverted from the closest medical facility, if that facility is not equipped to respond to acute stroke, and routed directly to hospitals designated as stroke centers with proven capability to deliver thrombolytic therapy. Advantages of stroke center systems include ensuring minimal level of expertise in acute stroke therapies; standardization of care; availability of more sophisticated imaging technologies; formal tracking of outcomes and continuous quality improvement programs; and access to research and newly emerging interventions, including acute endovascular procedures. Disadvantages may include longer prehospital transport times, lack of availability in rural areas, and logistical and political constraints. A complementary option is to link community and rural hospitals to designated stroke centers using telemedicine, with remotely provided radiological and neurological expertise to supplement local providers.[58] Alternatively, helicopter and air rescue services may be used in remote areas to rapidly transport acute patients to stroke centers.

In Canada and Germany, and in pilot sites in the United States, implementation of stroke center regional systems has been shown to substantially improve the delivery of acute stroke care, increasing the number of patients receiving thrombolytic therapy for stroke and decreasing the frequency of treatment protocol deviations. Health care personnel in Ontario developed a Regional Acute Stroke Protocol in which all ambulance services bypass the closest hospital to deliver acute stroke patients to a single designated stroke center. Sixty percent of all acute strokes in the region were diverted to the designated stroke critical care center, and fully 22 percent of these patients were treated with IV t-PA.[59] In Houston, six hospitals were designated stroke critical care centers for ambulance diversion, paramedics were trained in a version of the LAPSS, and in-hospital acute stroke response team systems were optimized. After implementation of the stroke critical care system, the proportion of acute stroke patients taken to designated stroke centers increased from 58 to 70 percent and the proportion of stroke patients receiving IV t-PA increased from 7.4 to 10.8 percent.[60]

DATA

The fifth "D" in the chain of stroke resuscitation is the collection of data on patient arrival. The goals of the initial evaluation of a patient with acute stroke are to (1) determine whether an immediate complication is likely, (2) confirm that ischemic stroke and not a mimic is the likely cause of the focal deficit, (3) assess the reversibility of the pathology, (4) obtain clues to the likely vascular mechanism and cause, and (5) guide the selection of appropriate treatment.

The first step in the evaluation is no different than with any other critically ill patient. The ABCs should rapidly be assessed to ensure patient stability. The first priority is to initiate resuscitation if there is any airway, ventilatory, or hemodynamic compromise. Once these essential domains are assessed, and treated if necessary, the patient can be specifically evaluated for cerebral ischemia.

History

Obtaining an accurate history swiftly is an important skill in treating acute stroke patients. Often the history will need to be obtained serially. A brief 5-minute synopsis from the most cogent observer is sufficient to guide ordering of initial diagnostic and therapeutic studies. When these are underway, a more thorough history can be elicited from the patient and all other available witnesses.

Establishing the time of stroke onset is especially important because it determines the available treatment options. Information should be sought from the patient, family members, and anyone who was with the patient at the time of ictus. It may be necessary to call witnesses who did not accompany the patient to the hospital. Asking pointed questions can help witnesses more accurately pinpoint onset time. It is useful to keep television listings in the ED and ask patients what program they were watching at time of onset. Consulting the TV listings can then identify stroke onset time with precision. In perhaps one third of patients, onset cannot be specified precisely, because they awoke from sleep with their deficits or were found down and are aphasic or anosognosic, rendering them unable to communicate or unaware of the time their deficit started. For thrombolytic decision making in these circumstances, to maximize safety, the onset time is assumed to be immediately after the time the patient was last seen well, rather than the time the deficit was first observed or some intervening moment. For example, time of onset for patients who awake from sleep with new deficits is assumed to be the time they went to sleep. Consequently, the 20 percent of ischemic stroke patients who awaken from sleep with their deficit are generally not candidates for conventional thrombolytic stroke therapy.

Other essential history questions focus on ruling out stroke mimics and provisionally characterizing the stroke mechanism. Seizures, intoxications, head trauma, and acute systemic infections are inquired after. The presence of cervical trauma and neck pain may point toward a diagnosis of dissection. Headaches and nausea raise the possibility of intracerebral hemorrhage or brainstem infarction. The tempo of deficit onset is ascertained. Registry studies suggest that strokes with maximum disability at onset but without headache are most often found to be embolic, either cardiac or artery-to-artery, whereas those with a fluctuating course are more likely due to thrombosis.[61,62] A history of multiple prior transient ischemic attacks (TIAs) in the same circulation suggests an atherothrombotic mechanism. A steadily expanding deficit over 5 to 20 minutes is typical of intracerebral hemorrhage.

Inquiring about previous medical conditions also sheds light on the stroke mechanism. Patients suffering from cardiac disease, including arrhythmia, valvular disease, ventricular aneurysm, patent foramen ovale, and congestive heart failure, are prone to cardioembolic events. A history of hypertension, coronary artery disease, tobacco use, diabetes, or claudication is associated with large-vessel atherothrombosis. Hypertension and to a lesser degree tobacco use and diabetes also are often seen in lacunar infarcts.

Physical Examination

The initial physical examination should be strategic, rather than exhaustive, and need not exceed 10 minutes. The goals of the initial examination are to determine patient level of consciousness, stroke severity, stroke localization, and stroke cause.[63,64]

Careful neurovascular examination includes auscultating the heart for the presence of gallops, murmurs, or dysrhythmias. The peripheral vascular system is interrogated by palpating the radial, femoral, and pedal pulses to determine strength and regularity. The carotid artery is palpated and the neck auscultated for bruits. It should be borne in mind that cervical bruits may arise not only from stenosis of the internal carotid artery but also from stenosis of the external and common carotid artery and from hyperdynamic states.

The funduscopic examination provides a unique opportunity to visualize blood vessels directly. Signs of internal carotid artery disease include cholesterol crystals, retinal infarctions, and venous stasis retinopathy. Subretinal hemorrhages and papilledema suggest raised intracranial pressure.

Unexplained fever or nuchal rigidity raises the possibility of other diagnoses such as meningitis or other infection or subarachnoid hemorrhage. Coma is extremely uncommon in acute ischemic stroke and suggests intracerebral or subarachnoid hemorrhage or metabolic and other nonstroke processes.

The neurological examination includes rapid screening of mental state, including tests of aphasia and neglect; cranial nerve evaluation including visual field and ocular motility testing; and motor, coordination, sensory, reflex, and gait examination. The severity of deficits is a fair indication of the volume of brain at ischemic risk and of prognosis if no interventional treatment is

NIHSS		Score Total
Patient Name:	Date: Time:	_____
Source of Information: ☐ Patient Exam ☐ Other Lay Observer ☐ Verbal Report (Check all that apply) ☐ Patient ☐ Family Member Outside MD ☐ Outside Hospital Chart		

NIH Stroke Scale Item	Function	Scores	Exam
1a. Level of Consciousness (Alert, drowsy, etc.)	Alert Drowsy Stuporous (requires repeated stimuli) Comatose (reflex responses only)	0 1 2 3	___
1b. LOC Questions (Month, age)	Both correct One correct Incorrect	0 1 2	___
1c. LOC Commands (Open, close eyes, make fist, let go)	Obeys both correctly Obeys one correctly Incorrect	0 1 2	___
2. Best Gaze (Eyes open—patient follows examiner's finger or face)	Normal Partial gaze palsy Forced deviation	0 1 2	___
3. Visual (Introduce visual stimulus/threat to patient's visual field quadrants)	No loss Partial hemianopia Complete hemianopia Bilateral hemianopia	0 1 2 3	___
4. Facial Palsy (Show teeth, raise eyebrows, and squeeze eyes shut)	Normal Minor asymmetry Partial (lower face paralysis) Complete	0 1 2 3	___
5a. Motor Arm—Left (Elevate extremity 90° and score drift/movement)	No drift Drift Some effort against gravity No effort against gravity No movement Amputation, joint fusion	0 1 2 3 4 9	___
5b. Motor arm—Right (Elevate extremity 90° and score drift/movement)	No drift Drift Some effort against gravity No effort against gravity No movement Amputation, joint fusion	0 1 2 3 4 9	___
6a. Motor leg—Left (Elevate extremity 30° and score drift/movement)	No drift Drift Some effort against gravity No effort against gravity No movement Amputation, joint fusion	0 1 2 3 4 9	___

Figure 11.6   National Institute of Health Stroke Scale (NIHSS).

6b. Motor leg—Right (Elevate extremity 30° and score drift/movement)	No drift	0	
	Drift	1	
	Some effort against gravity	2	
	No effort against gravity	3	
	No movement	4	
	Amputation, joint fusion	9	___
7. Limb Ataxia (Finger–nose, heel down shin)	Absent	0	
	Present in both upper and lower	1	
	Present in both	2	___
8. Sensory (Pin prick to face, arm, trunk, and leg—compare side to side)	Normal	0	
	Partial loss	1	
	Dense loss	2	___
9. Best Language (Name items, describe a picture and read sentences)	No aphasia	0	
	Mild–moderate aphasia	1	
	Severe aphasia	2	
	Mute	3	___
10. Dysarthria (Evaluate speech clarity by patient repeating listed words)	Normal articulation	0	
	Mild–moderate slurring	1	
	Severe, nearly intelligible, or worse	2	___
11. Extinction and Inattention (Use information from prior testing to identify neglect or double simultaneous stimuli testing)	No neglect	0	
	Partial neglect	1	
	Profound neglect	2	___

Figure 11.6 (Continued).

undertaken, whereas the pattern of neurological deficits permits localization within the cerebrum and within the cerebral vasculature.

Formal Stroke Scales

Use of a formal examination scale permits reproducible quantification of stroke severity. In widest use for focal stroke is the NIHSS (Figure 11.6), which has been incorporated into formal guidelines for thrombolytic therapy decision making.[65] An efficient practice is to perform an NIHSS examination in all patients, supplemented by key additional neurological examination elements relevant to the individual patient's complaints and findings. The NIHSS is comprised of 13 items grading orientation, language, hemiattention, motor, sensory, coordination, and visual deficits and takes 5 to 10 minutes to perform. Performance of the NIHSS requires the use of a safety pin for sensory testing and special cards for speech and language testing. The NIHSS yields a total score between 0 (no measured deficit) and 42 (deep coma). Stroke severity may be broadly categorized by the NIHSS as mild (score 0 to 5), moderate (6 to 20), and severe (>20). Patients with an NIHSS greater than 20 have a higher incidence of intracerebral hemorrhage when treated with t-PA, and an NIHSS >22 is a formal caution in the Federal Drug Administration (FDA) prescribing instructions for t-PA; however, in the NINDS–t-PA trials, patients with entry NIHSS >20 had more good outcomes if treated with t-PA than placebo.

Table 11.2   The Hunt and Hess scale

Grade	Neurological status
I	Asymptomatic; or minimal headache and slight nuchal rigidity
II	Moderate to severe headache; nuchal rigidity; no neurological deficit except cranial nerve palsy
III	Drowsy; minimal neurological deficit
IV	Stuporous; moderate to severe hemiparesis; possibly early decerebrate rigidity and vegetative disturbances
V	Deep coma; decerebrate rigidity; moribund appearance

For patients with subarachnoid hemorrhage, the Hunt and Hess Scale (Table 11.2) is a useful formal severity measure of prognostic and therapeutic importance. Patients are graded on a scale from 1 (least affected) to 5 (most affected). Patients with grades 1 to 3 on arrival have a better prognosis and are candidates for early surgical clipping. Patients with grades 4 or 5 have a worse prognosis and are generally not candidates for early surgery.

Rapid Recognition of Typical Stroke Syndromes

Decision making in acute stroke care requires being able to recognize cardinal stroke syndromes rapidly. In the acute setting, examiners should not dwell on the arcana of neurological semiology. The time urgency of early therapy does not permit fine-grained localization of findings to subnuclei and fractionated tracts. The ability to recognize broad clinical patterns comprising seven key stroke syndromes suffices for all but the most unusual cases. These seven syndromes reflect ischemic strokes localized in dominant cerebral hemisphere, nondominant cerebral hemisphere, brain stem, cerebellum, lacunar (penetrating small vessel) distributions, and primary intracerebral and subarachnoid hemorrhages (Table 11.3).

After initial therapeutic decisions are made, more detailed neurological examination will elicit additional findings that permit more precise clinical localization. Characteristic stroke syndromes associated with ischemia within the distributions of distinct arterial territories of the anterior and posterior circulations are listed in Table 11.4.

Laboratory Evaluation

Table 11.5 lists recommended tests that should be ordered on all stroke patients on an emergent basis. The frequent coexistence of heart disease with ischemic stroke mandates concern in all patients for acute myocardial infarction, congestive heart failure, arrhythmias, and sudden death, dictating the need for cardiac enzymes, electrocardiography, and chest radiograph. The possibility of early aspiration and pneumonitis also supports chest radiography. Cardiac monitoring should be maintained continuously to detect intermittent atrial fibrillation. Glucose measurement is essential because hypoglycemia and hyperglycemia may mimic or exacerbate stroke deficits. Electrolyte and renal dysfunction may

Table 11.3   Seven key stroke syndromes

Syndrome	Symptoms
Left (dominant) hemisphere	Right hemiparesis
	Right hemisensory loss
	Right visual field deficit
	Left gaze preference
	Aphasia
Right (nondominant) hemisphere	Left hemiparesis
	Left hemisensory loss
	Left visual field deficit
	Right gaze preference
	Neglect for left hemispace
Brain stem	Hemiparesis or quadriparesis
	Unilateral or bilateral sensory loss
	Crossed signs (deficits on one side of face and other side of body)
	Dysconjugate gaze or gaze palsy, nystagmus
	Dysarthria or dysphagia
	Vertigo, nausea, vomiting
	Decreased level of consciousness
Cerebellum	Truncal/gait ataxia
	Limb ataxia
	Nystagmus
Lacunar (small vessel)	
Pure motor hemiparesis	Contralateral face, arm, and leg weakness
Pure sensory stroke	Face, arm, and leg numbness; paresthesias or pain
Sensorimotor stroke	Contralateral face, arm, and leg weakness and hypoesthesia
Clumsy hand/dysarthria	Dysarthria, dysphagia, facial weakness, tongue deviation, clumsy hand
Ataxic hemiparesis	Ataxia and contralateral weakness
Intracerebral hemorrhage	One of the above focal syndromes, plus
	Headache
	Neck pain, stiffness
	Nausea, vomiting
	Decreased level of consciousness
Subarachnoid hemorrhage	Abrupt headache at onset
	Neck stiffness, pain
	Decreased level of consciousness
	Cranial nerve abnormalities

also exacerbate stroke impairments. Tests of blood cell counts, platelet count, and the clotting system identify coagulation abnormalities that may have contributed to the acute stroke and that will influence urgent management.

Differential Diagnosis

Diverse nervous system diseases produce acute focal neurological deficits. Among patients with neurological complaints transported by ambulance,

Table 11.4 Territorial ischemic stroke syndromes

Cerebral artery	Symptoms
Middle cerebral artery (MCA)	Contralateral hemiparesis (face and arm weaker than leg)
	Contralateral hemisensory loss (face and arm denser than leg)
	Contralateral visual field deficit
	Dominant hemisphere
	Aphasia–global (complete MCA), Broca (superior division), or
	Wernicke (inferior division)
	Gerstmann syndrome
	Nondominant hemisphere
	Contralateral neglect
	Constructional apraxia
Anterior choroidal	Contralateral hemiparesis
	Contralateral hemisensory loss
	Contralateral visual field defect
Anterior cerebral artery	Contralateral leg paresis
	Contralateral leg hypoesthesia
	Language dysfunction (mutism, transcortical motor aphasia)
	Unilateral ideomotor apraxia, alien hand syndrome
	Primitive reflexes (paratonia, grasp)
	Abulia
Posterior cerebral artery	Contralateral homonymous hemianopsia (occipital)
	Memory loss (mesial temporal)
	Contralateral hemisensory loss (thalamus)
	Alexia without agraphia (dominant hemisphere)
Medial medullary penetrators	Contralateral hemiparesis
	Contralateral loss of vibration and position sense
	Ipsilateral cranial nerve (CN) XII palsy
Lateral medullary circumferential arteries (Wallenberg)	Contralateral loss of pain and temperature
	Ipsilateral loss of pain and temperature sensation on face
	Ipsilateral Horner syndrome
	Dysphagia and dysarthria
	Ipsilateral dysmetria
	Vertigo
	Hiccoughs
Anterior inferior cerebellar artery	Ipsilateral deafness
	Ipsilateral facial palsy and/or gaze palsy or skew deviation
	Ipsilateral facial sensory loss
	Contralateral sensory loss
Medial pontine penetrators	Contralateral hemiparesis
	Ipsilateral CN VI palsy
Lateral pontine circumferential arteries	Ipsilateral CN VIII injury with deafness or tinnitus
Midbrain penetrators	Contralateral hemiparesis
	Ipsilateral CN III palsy

Table 11.4   (Continued)

Cerebral artery	Symptoms
Superior cerebellar artery	Ipsilateral dysmetria and limb movement disorders
	Ipsilateral Horner syndrome
	Contralateral pain and temperature sensory loss
	Contralateral CN IV palsy
Distal basilar artery ("top of the basilar")	Oculomotor—Parinaud syndrome (vertical gaze paresis, lid retraction, skew deviation, impaired convergence)
	Unilateral or bilateral CN III palsy
	Pupils: small reactive pupils and ptosis (sympathetic involvement)
	Behavioral changes: delirium, somnolence, coma
	Visual field defects: hemianopia, cortical blindness, Balint syndrome
Anterior watershed	Proximal bibrachial paresis (man-in-barrel syndrome)
	Transcortical motor aphasia
Posterior watershed	Cortical blindness with macular sparing (Anton syndrome—deny deficits)
	Transcortical sensory aphasia
	Balint syndrome (simultagnosia, optic ataxia, ocular apraxia)
Lacunar syndromes	
Pure motor hemiparesis	Contralateral face, arm, and leg weakness
Pure sensory stroke	Face, arm, and leg numbness, paresthesias or pain
Sensorimotor stroke	Contralateral face, arm, and leg weakness and hypoesthesia
Clumsy hand/dysarthria	Dysarthria, dysphagia, facial weakness, tongue deviation, clumsy hand
Ataxic hemiparesis	Ataxia and contralateral weakness

nonstroke causes outnumber stroke by 10 to 1. Nonetheless, stroke is a distinctive clinical syndrome that can generally be easily discriminated from its leading mimics. Patients with focal seizures and postictal paralysis generally have a history of tonic and clonic movements ("positive" motor activity) at onset, often with a rapid march; stroke patients have weakness ("negative" motor deficits) from the start. Hypoglycemia and other toxic metabolic encephalopathies typically produce confusional states without major focal motor, sensory, or visual deficits; stroke typically produces focal elementary neurological findings. Patients with migrainous neurological deficits generally exhibit a slow march of spreading symptoms over 10 to 20 minutes and often an accompanying headache; ischemic stroke patients typically experience a maximal deficit at onset or progresses in stepwise, not smooth fashion, with no or mild headache. Neuroimaging helps to exclude the rare tumor or other fixed structural lesion masquerading as acute stroke. Integration of patient demographics, history, physical examination, screening labs, and neuroimaging almost invariably allows a secure diagnosis of stroke or stroke mimic to be rendered promptly (Table 11.6).

Table 11.5   Laboratory evaluation for patients with acute ischemic stroke

Initial tests for all patients
Electrocardiogram and initiation of continuous cardiac monitoring
Chest x-ray
Complete blood count
Platelet count
Prothrombin time
Partial thromboplastin time
Electrolytes
Blood glucose
Troponin or CK/MB
Blood urea nitrogen/creatinine
Pulse oximetry
Additional tests in select patients
Lateral cervical spine x-ray (if trauma is suspected)
Lumbar puncture (if subarachnoid hemorrhage suspected and CT negative)
Electroencephalogram (if seizure suspected)
Pregnancy test (in women of child-bearing age)
Liver function tests (if altered level of consciousness)
Arterial blood gas (if hypoxia suspected)
Urine toxicology (if substance abuse suspected)
Blood cultures and erythrocyte sedimentation rate (if endocarditis or other
  infection suspected)

CK/MB = creatine kinase MB band; CT = computed tomography.

CONCLUSION

The clinical evaluation of the acute stroke patient is now a multidisciplinary effort, crossing the boundaries of the prehospital and hospital-based setting.[44] Dispatchers, EMS providers, ED physicians, neurologists, and other providers all contribute to the serial elicitation of the clinical history and physical

Table 11.6   Leading differential diagnosis considerations in potential stroke patients

Condition	Diagnostic aids
Hypoglycemia	Low fingerstick blood glucose
Hyperglycemia	High fingerstick blood glucose
Hyponatremia/uremia	Myoclonus, chemistry panel
Toxic encephalopathy	History, toxicology screen
Postictal (Todd) paralysis	Seizure at onset, prior seizures
Migraine with aura	Headache, slow march over 10–20 min
Hypertensive encephalopathy	Severe hypertension, headache, papilledema
Trauma	History, physical exam, imaging
Subdural hematoma	Subacute onset, imaging findings
Neoplasm	Subacute onset, imaging findings
Encephalitis/meningitis	Fever, meningismus, photophobia, CSF
Transient global amnesia	Isolated anterograde memory loss
Bell palsy	Isolated, peripheral CN VII palsy
Conversion/malingering	Precipitating stressor, inconsistent examination

CN = cranial nerve; CSF = cerebrospinal fluid.

examination. The advent of interventional acute stroke therapy and the need for rapid decision making has only enhanced the importance of the bedside history and examination of the stroke patient. The clinical evaluation guides the selection and interpretation of the limited laboratory and imaging diagnostic tests that may be obtained within early treatment time windows. In the critical first hours after stroke onset, prompt syndrome recognition, severity delineation, and lesion localization will permit informed treatment choices that may improve the quality of patients' existences for the rest of their lives.

References

1. Hazinski MF. Demystifying recognition and management of stroke. Curr Emerg Cardiac Care 1996;7:8.
2. Pepe PE, Zachariah BS, Sayre MR, Floccare D. Ensuring the chain of recovery for stroke in your community. Chain of recovery writing group. Prehosp Emerg Care 1998;2:89–95.
3. Pancioli AM, Broderick J, Kothari R, et al. Public perception of stroke warning signs and knowledge of potential risk factors. JAMA 1998;279:1288–1292.
4. Barsan WG, Brott TG, Olinger CP, et al. Identification and entry of the patient with acute cerebral infarction. Ann Emerg Med 1988;17:1192–1195.
5. National Stroke Association. Stroke remains a deadly mystery to many Americans. Be Stroke Smart 1996;13:13–22.
6. Kothari R, Sauerbeck L, Jauch E, et al. Patients' awareness of stroke signs, symptoms, and risk factors. Stroke 1997;28:1871–1875.
7. Williams LS, Bruno A, Rouch D, Marriott DJ. Stroke patients' knowledge of stroke. Influence on time to presentation. Stroke 1997;28:912–915.
8. Barsan WG, Brott TG, Broderick JP, et al. Time of hospital presentation in patients with acute stroke. Arch Intern Med 1993;153:2558–2561.
9. Bratina P, Greenberg L, Pasteur W, Grotta JC. Current emergency department management of stroke in Houston, Texas. Stroke 1995;26:409–414.
10. Zweifler RM, Drinkard R, Cunningham S, et al. Implementation of a stroke code system in Mobile, Alabama. Diagnostic and therapeutic yield. Stroke 1997;28:981–983.
11. Schroeder EB, Rosamond WD, Morris DL, et al. Determinants of use of emergency medical services in a population with stroke symptoms: the second delay in accessing stroke healthcare (dash ii) study. Stroke 2000;31:2591–2596.
12. Alberts MJ, Perry A, Dawson DV, Bertels C. Effects of public and professional education on reducing the delay in presentation and referral of stroke patients. Stroke 1992;23:352–356.
13. Dornan WA, Stroink AR, Pegg EE, et al. Community stroke awareness program increases public knowledge of stroke. Stroke 1998;29:288.
14. Stern EB, Berman M, Thomas JJ, Klassen AC. Community education for stroke awareness: an efficacy study. Stroke 1999;30:720–723.
15. Todd HW. Lessons from current and previous stroke public education campaigns. Proceedings of a National Symposium on Rapid Identification and Treatment of Acute Stroke, December 1996, Bethesda, MD.
16. Barsan WG, Brott TG, Broderick JP, et al. Urgent therapy for acute stroke. Effects of a stroke trial on untreated patients. Stroke 1994;25:2132–2137.
17. Daley S, Braimah J, Sailor S, et al. Education to improve stroke awareness and emergent response. The NINDS rt-PA Stroke Study Group. J Neurosci Nurs 1997;29:393–396.
18. Maibach EW. Lessons for success in public education campaigns. Proceedings of a National Symposium on Rapid Identification and Treatment of Acute Stroke, December 1996, Bethesda, MD.
19. Ho MT, Eisenberg MS, Litwin PE, et al. Delay between onset of chest pain and seeking medical care: the effect of public education. Ann Emerg Med 1989;18:727–731.
20. Hedges JR, Feldman HA, Bittner V, et al. Impact of community intervention to reduce patient delay time on use of reperfusion therapy for acute myocardial infarction: rapid early action for coronary treatment (REACT) trial. React Study Group. Acad Emerg Med 2000;7:862–872.
21. Porteous GH, Corry MD, Smith WS. Emergency medical services dispatcher identification of stroke and transient ischemic attack. Prehosp Emerg Care 1999;3:211–216.
22. Medical Dispatch Protocol v11. Salt Lake City: National Academy of Emergency Dispatch, 2000.

23. Saver J, Kidwell C, Eckstein M, Starkman S. Emerging applications of the Los Angeles Prehospital Stroke Screen (LAPSS), a validated tool for prehospital stroke recognition. Stroke Intervent 2001;2:6–8.
24. Merino JG, Silver B, Wong E, et al. Extending tissue plasminogen activator use to community and rural stroke patients. Stroke 2002;33:141–146.
25. Harbison J, Massey A, Barnett L, et al. Rapid ambulance protocol for acute stroke. Lancet. 1999; 353:1935.
26. Saver JL, Kidwell CS, Leary MC, et al. Results of the field administration of stroke treatment—magnesium (fast-mag) pilot trial: a study of prehospital neuroprotective therapy. Stroke 2002; 33:363–364.
27. Crocco TJ, Kothari RU, Sayre MR, Liu T. A nationwide prehospital stroke survey. Prehosp Emerg Care 1999;3:201–206.
28. Smith WS, Isaacs M, Corry MD. Accuracy of paramedic identification of stroke and transient ischemic attack in the field. Prehosp Emerg Care 1998;2:170–175.
29. Hanson S, Adlis S, Weaver A, et al. Accuracy of prehospital stroke diagnosis: treatment implications (abstract). Stroke 1995;26:157.
30. Zweifler RM, York D, U TT, et al. Accuracy of paramedic diagnosis of stroke. J Stroke Cerebrovasc Dis 1998;7:446–448.
31. Kothari R, Barsan W, Brott T, et al. Frequency and accuracy of prehospital diagnosis of acute stroke. Stroke 1995;26:937–941.
32. Kidwell CS, Saver JL, Schubert GB, et al. Design and retrospective analysis of the Los Angeles Prehospital Stroke Screen (LAPSS). Prehosp Emerg Care 1998;2:267–273.
33. Kidwell CS, Starkman S, Eckstein M, et al. Identifying stroke in the field. Prospective validation of the Los Angeles Prehospital Stroke Screen (LAPSS). Stroke 2000;31:71–76.
34. Harbison J, Hossain O, Jenkinson D, et al. Diagnostic accuracy of stroke referrals from primary care, emergency room physicians, and ambulance staff using the face arm speech test. Stroke 2003;34:71–76.
35. Guidelines 2000 for cardiopulmonary resuscitation and emergency cardiovascular care. Part 7: the era of reperfusion: Section 2: acute stroke. The American Heart Association in collaboration with the International Liaison Committee on Resuscitation. Circulation 2000;102:I204–216.
36. Saver JL, Kidwell CS, Leary MC, et al. Administering neuroprotective stroke therapy in the field: the field administration of stroke treatment—magnesium (FAST-MAG) pilot trial. Stroke 2001; 33:353.
37. Kothari R, Hall K, Brott T, Broderick J. Early stroke recognition: developing an out-of-hospital NIH stroke scale. Acad Emerg Med 1997;4:986–990.
38. Kothari RU, Pancioli A, Liu T, et al. Cincinnati Prehospital Stroke Scale: reproducibility and validity. Ann Emerg Med 1999;33:373–378.
39. LaMonte MP, Xiao Y, Mackenzie CF, et al. Tele-BAT: mobile telemedicine for the brain attack team (abstract). Stroke 1998;29:312.
40. Smith WS, Corry MD, Fazackerley J, Isaacs M. Paramedic accuracy in the application of the NIH stroke scale to victims of stroke. Acad Emerg Med 1997;4:379–380.
41. Tirschwell DL, Longstreth WT Jr, Becker KJ, et al. Shortening the NIH stroke scale for use in the prehospital setting. Stroke 2002;33:2801–2806.
42. Llanes JN, Starkman S, Kidwell CS, Eckstein M. The LAPSS Motor Scale (LAMS): a new measure for characterizing stroke severity in the field (abstract). Stroke 2001;32:323.
43. Ferguson K, Kidwell CS, Starkman S, et al. Inter-rater and intra-rater reliability of the Los Angeles Motor Scale (LAMS), a prehospital measure of stroke severity (abstract). Stroke 2002;33:384.
44. Suyama J, Crocco T. Prehospital care of the stroke patient. Emerg Med Clin North Am 2002; 20:537–552.
45. Duldner JE, Burlle AM, Costello MS, et al. Effect of a stroke protocol on management of out-of-hospital stroke patients. Acad Emerg Med 1998;5:440.
46. Kereiakes DJ, Gibler WB, Martin LH, et al. Relative importance of emergency medical system transport and the prehospital electrocardiogram on reducing hospital time delay to therapy for acute myocardial infarction: a preliminary report from the cincinnati heart project. Am Heart J 1992;123:835–840.
47. McDowell FH, Brott TG, Goldstein M, et al. Stroke: the first six hours—National Stroke Association consensus statement. Stroke Clin Updates 1993;14:1–12.
48. Petrie D, Lane P, Stewart TC. An evaluation of patient outcomes comparing trauma team activated versus trauma team not activated using TRISS analysis. Trauma and Injury Severity Score. J Trauma 1996;41:870–873.
49. Driscoll PA, Vincent CA. Organizing an efficient trauma team. Injury 1992;23:107–110.

50. Markel KN, Marion SA. CQI: improving the time to thrombolytic therapy for patients with acute myocardial infarction in the emergency department. J Emerg Med 1996;14:685–689.
51. Englander EN, Morich DH, Minniti MM. Accelerating the evaluation of acute stroke patients in a community hospital. Neurology 1998;50:A114.
52. Gomez CR, Malkoff MD, Sauer CM, et al. Code stroke. An attempt to shorten inhospital therapeutic delays. Stroke 1994;25:1920–1923.
53. Davalos A, Castillo J, Martinez-Vila E. Delay in neurological attention and stroke outcome. Cerebrovascular diseases study group of the Spanish Society of Neurology. Stroke 1995;26: 2233–2237.
54. Bock BF. Response system for patients presenting with acute stroke. Proceedings of a National Symposium on Rapid Identification and Treatment of Acute Stroke, December 1996, Bethesda, MD.
55. Broderick JP. Logistics in acute stroke management. Drugs 1997;54(suppl 3):109–116.
56. Alberts MJ, Hademenos G, Latchaw RE, et al. Recommendations for the establishment of primary stroke centers. Brain attack coalition. JAMA 2000;283:3102–3109.
57. Adams R, Acker J, Alberts M, et al. Recommendations for improving the quality of care through stroke centers and systems: an examination of stroke center identification options: Multidisciplinary consensus recommendations from the advisory working group on stroke center identification options of the American Stroke Association. Stroke 2002;33:e1–7.
58. Levine SR, Gorman M. "Telestroke": the application of telemedicine for stroke. Stroke 1999; 30:464–469.
59. Riopelle RJ, Howse DC, Bolton C, et al. Regional access to acute ischemic stroke intervention. Stroke 2001;32:652–655.
60. Persse D, Hinton RC, Acker JE, et al. Templates for Organizing Stroke Triage. NINDS Symposium Proceedings: Improving the Chain of Recovery for Acute Stroke in Your Community, December 2002, Bethesda, MD.
61. Foulkes MA, Wolf PA, Price TR, et al. The stroke data bank: design, methods, and baseline characteristics. Stroke 1988;19:547–554.
62. Caplan LR, Hier DB, D'Cruz I. Cerebral embolism in the Michael Reese Stroke Registry. Stroke 1983;14:530–536.
63. Kalafut MA, Saver JL. The Acute Stroke Patient: The First Six Hours. In SN Cohen (ed), Management of Ischemic Stroke. New York: McGraw-Hill, 2000;17–52.
64. Adams HP Jr. Guidelines for the management of patients with acute ischemic stroke: a synopsis. A special writing group of the Stroke Council, American Heart Association. Heart Dis Stroke 1994; 3:407–411.
65. Brott T, Adams HP Jr, Olinger CP, et al. Measurements of acute cerebral infarction: a clinical examination scale. Stroke 1989;20:864–870.

12
Rapid Diagnostic Evaluation

David S. Liebeskind

The diagnosis of acute ischemic stroke poses a particular challenge for clinicians. Unlike other areas of medicine where the sensitivity and specificity of a diagnostic test are paramount, the diagnosis of ischemic stroke must also be established with only minimal delay. The temporal profile of cerebral ischemia and rapid onset of irreversible brain injury necessitates expedient triage and diagnosis, with prompt selection of rational treatment. These pathophysiological constraints are further complicated by the delayed presentation of most ischemic stroke patients. The clinician must prudently select from available diagnostic tools, weighing the relative advantage of the additional information provided, balanced by any potential detriment incurred by the delay to treatment. Neuroimaging techniques have recently evolved in rapid succession, with progressive refinement in anatomical detail of the brain parenchyma and cerebral vasculature, providing physiological information on cerebral perfusion and metabolism. Despite these advances and a plethora of reports detailing the role of these advanced imaging modalities in stroke diagnosis, only noncontrast computed tomography (CT) is routinely performed during the acute phase and revered as an essential diagnostic tool. Other imaging modalities and laboratory investigations are selectively used and generally lack compelling data to support their routine use. The relative vulnerability of the brain to ischemia and rapid onset of cerebral edema make imaging studies ideal for stroke diagnosis. This chapter emphasizes the dominant role of imaging studies in the diagnosis of acute ischemic stroke, highlighting the relative advantages and disadvantages of each modality. Ancillary diagnostic studies such as laboratory tests are discussed, underscoring the clinical significance of selected investigations.

COMPUTED TOMOGRAPHY

Practical Considerations

CT is the principal diagnostic modality for acute stroke evaluation. Noncontrast CT of the head is universally accepted as the initial study required for evaluation of the acute stroke patient. CT is widely available on a 24-hour basis and most clinicians caring for stroke patients have at least basic skills in interpretation of these studies. In many centers, a noncontrast CT scan is obtained immediately on patient arrival in the emergency room. Noncontrast CT is typically less expensive than magnetic resonance imaging (MRI) and imaging data do not require postprocessing. The principal risk of CT is related to the effects of radiation, although it is generally confined to the head. In the setting of acute stroke, the relative advantages of ischemic stroke diagnosis typically outweigh the risk of radiation. In pregnant women, MRI may be preferred. CT readily addresses several critical questions in the clinical care of a patient with the acute onset of a focal neurological deficit.

Brain Imaging

Intracranial hemorrhage is promptly excluded with CT as hyperdensity within the parenchyma, or subarachnoid, subdural, or epidural space. The possibility of hemorrhage in these locations may be considerable in any patient with a history of head trauma. Identification of intracranial hemorrhage on CT may be promptly followed by urgent neurosurgical consultation. Although recognition of obvious areas of bleeding like an epidural hematoma or lobar hemorrhage may be rapidly triaged, subtler forms of intracranial bleeding such as petechial hemorrhagic conversion or isolated subarachnoid hemorrhage may be difficult to ascertain on an initial noncontrast CT scan. Alteration of window width and center levels may be critical in defining areas of suspected hemorrhage as well as regions of ischemia that may appear hypodense (Figure 12.1). Dynamic alteration of these parameters is easily performed on the console of the CT scanner or on a viewing monitor with image manipulation tools. This advantage is lost if only hard film copies of the CT scan are available for review. Actual measurement of tissue density in Hounsfield units within regions of interest is also possible with dynamic image interpretation. For instance, calcification of the basal ganglia may be differentiated from petechial hemorrhagic conversion

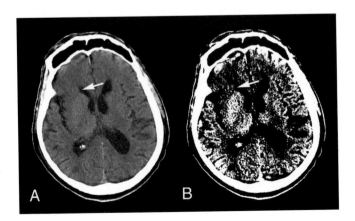

Figure 12.1 Alteration of window width and center levels on noncontrast computed tomography (CT) of an acute right middle cerebral artery stroke (**A,** standard settings; **B,** optimized settings) facilitates detection of hypodensity (*arrows*).

of an ischemic stroke on the basis of Hounsfield density measurements. Such differentiation may be critical in the triage of a potential candidate for thrombolysis or antithrombotic therapy.

CT hypodensity is the signature of cerebral ischemia, with an exquisite dependence on the duration and severity of ischemia or hypoperfusion. Although individual variation from patient to patient may exist, hypodensity typically becomes manifest within hours of ischemic onset, reflecting incipient cerebral edema. The determinants of such hypodensity are poorly understood but likely depend on perfusion thresholds and the inherent vulnerability of brain parenchyma.[1] Although hypodensity is generally accepted as a marker of irreversible injury, hypoperfusion may also manifest as regions of reversible hypodensity.[2] For practical purposes, hypodensity is usually interpreted as an evolving infarction with minimal chance of tissue viability. In the first few hours after stroke onset, either frank hypodensity or alteration of the normal CT appearance of brain architecture may indicate ischemic change. These CT changes are commonly referred to as early infarct signs. The most common early infarct signs include loss of the cortical ribbon, insular changes, sulcal effacement, blurring of the basal ganglia, and hypodensity of the caudate head, observed in 31 to 81 percent of cases.[3–5] Hypodense lesions may be easier to detect at the cortical ribbon compared with deeply situated ischemic lesions. The hyperdense middle cerebral artery sign (HMCAS) is also considered to be an "early infarct sign," yet it should be considered separately because it represents acute vascular thrombosis rather than a parenchymal marker of ischemia. All of the described early infarct signs are specific to middle cerebral artery (MCA) distribution ischemia, although similar findings may be noted in other vascular distributions (Figure 12.2). Early CT findings and other manifestations of hypodensity are accentuated by alteration of window width and center levels. In fact, the definition of CT hypodensity is determined by these settings and comparisons need to incorporate this aspect. Much attention has been devoted to the extent of CT hypodensity as a marker of outcome and hemorrhagic conversion in the setting of thrombolysis. Despite increasing use of early CT findings as markers of evolving ischemia, recent analyses have shown that they may not have an influence on patient outcome.[3,6,7] Hypodensity spanning one third of the MCA territory has been suggested as a lesion size that dichotomizes patient outcome and the risk of hemorrhagic conversion.[8] The significance of this finding, or the one-third MCA rule, has been passionately debated.[6,7] Inter-rater reliability of this finding is only modest and the extent of hypodensity is more likely to be accurately reflected by volumetric calculation of lesion size on multiple axial cuts.[8] Attempts to automate this procedure are currently under investigation.[9] Other investigators have attempted to quantify the extent of CT hypodensity in acute stroke with similar analyses with regard to outcome. Use of Alberta Stroke Program Early CT Score (ASPECTS), a standardized score for CT assessment of stroke, uses specific axial slices to estimate lesion extent (Figure 12.3).[10,11] These measurements of CT hypodensity are not applicable to posterior circulation cases, however. CT evaluation of the posterior fossa is limited by volume-averaging of bony structures and brain stem lesions are therefore more difficult to appreciate (Figure 12.4). As with most imaging procedures, artifacts may degrade the utility of CT. Numerous CT artifacts are recognized; however, streak artifacts emanating from bony structures (Figure 12.5) and partial volume averaging are most commonly encountered.

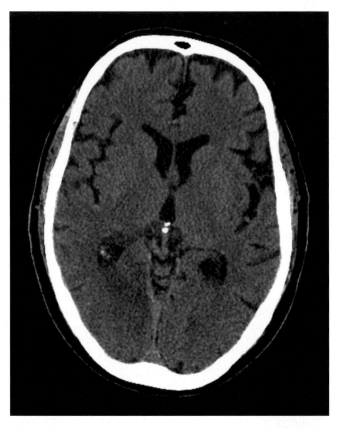

Figure 12.2   Noncontrast computed tomography (CT) reveals subtle hypodensity as an early infarct sign of a right posterior cerebral artery stroke.

The volume of an ischemic lesion is not directly correlated with clinical severity because lesions in various locations may interfere with neurological structures that differ in function. Ultimately, dysfunctional regions of brain parenchyma may not appear hypodense on CT, despite diminished perfusion to these areas. Although subtle CT findings are quite common, the detection of such findings is clearly influenced by the extent of the clinical history available at the time of image interpretation. Retrospective review of initial CT scans after further imaging or later in the hospital course often reveals subtle findings that were not initially appreciated. This dependence on the clinical history and lesion local-ization probably accounts for significant variability in the interpretation of CT scans between various specialists. Given such discrepant descriptions and vari-ability in the interpretation of CT hypodensity,[7] it is fortunate that only large and relatively obvious CT hypodensities seem to affect the clinical care of an acute stroke patient. CT cases with only subtle ischemic findings and truly normal scans often get lumped into the category of the "normal CT" that is often described in the emergency room setting. The pattern of CT hypodensity may reveal an underlying stroke cause because identification of numerous areas

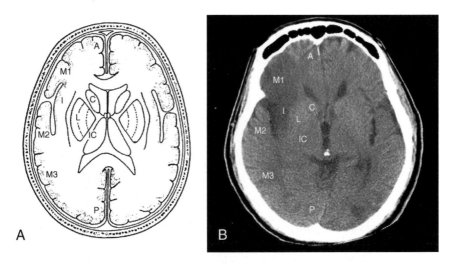

Figure 12.3 Application of the Alberta Stroke Program Early CT Score (ASPECTS) method **(A)** to an axial slice of a noncontrast computed tomography (CT) of a right middle cerebral artery stroke **(B)** yields a score of two for involvement of the M1 and I regions.

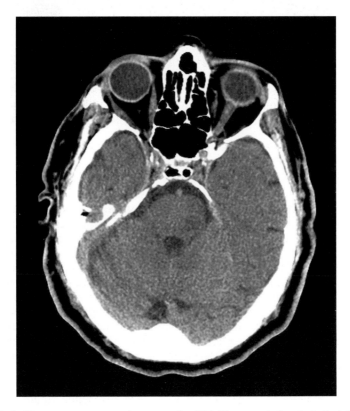

Figure 12.4 Noncontrast computed tomography (CT) illustrates ischemia in the left anterior inferior cerebellar artery distribution that may be difficult to appreciate due to adjacent bony structures.

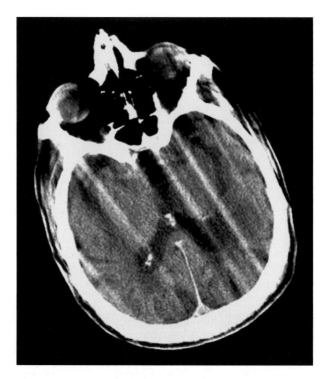

Figure 12.5 Linear streak artifacts resulting from bony structures on a noncontrast computed tomography (CT) may limit study interpretation.

of hypodensity may suggest an underlying vascular pattern, such as simultaneous anterior and MCA strokes associated with distal internal carotid artery thrombosis. There may also be variability in the degree of hypodensity, differentiating acute from subacute strokes.

The use of contrast-enhanced CT scans has waned with the advent of MRI. Although the acquisition of a contrast-enhanced CT scan may assist the diagnosis of acute ischemic stroke, the benefit of contrast enhancement is often considered to be only marginal in the general population. Adjunctive use of intravenous contrast may help demarcate regions of progressive ischemia due to breakdown of the blood-brain barrier. Prominent enhancement is typically appreciated during the subacute period. The use of intravenous contrast may actually obscure subtle regions of hypodensity, although contrast enhancement may differentiate an underlying tumor or abscess from an ischemic stroke. The principal risk of an enhanced CT scan is related to adverse contrast reactions and renal impairment, although concerns of adverse contrast effects must be balanced with the benefits of the diagnostic information in the setting of acute stroke. The likelihood of a contrast reaction and the renal status of a patient may not be rapidly assessed within minutes of acute stroke presentation, although potential complications may be readily treated on an urgent basis. Acquisition of an enhanced CT scan increases radiation exposure and expense as well, with relatively minimal diagnostic benefit. However, with the recent advent of multidetector CT scanners and advanced postprocessing software, intravenous contrast has taken a new role in the generation of CT angiographic and perfusion images. Despite the potential risks and disadvantages of contrast administration, the diagnostic benefits of CT angiography (CTA) and CT perfusion (CTP) often outweigh these factors.

Vascular Imaging

Indirect information on the status of the cerebral vasculature may be abstracted from noncontrast CT scans. Although contrast administration may define the abrupt occlusion of a vessel as a filling defect, thrombosis may increase the conspicuity of an arterial or venous structure. CT hyperdensity within a vascular structure may assist diagnosis of an arterial or venous stroke, especially when juxtaposed with a region of hypodensity. HMCAS is the most prominent example of this effect (Figure 12.6). More distal thrombosis of the MCA within the Sylvian fissure has been described as the MCA dot sign,[12] although similar hyperdensities may be appreciated in any vascular territory. The significance of

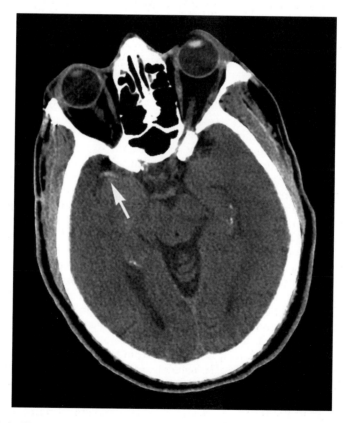

Figure 12.6 Hyperdense middle cerebral artery sign (HMCAS) (*arrow*) depicted on noncontrast computed tomography (CT).

the HMCAS is even more controversial than parenchymal early CT infarct signs and a consistent definition of the HMCAS is not routinely employed.[13,14] Distal hyperdensities such as the MCA dot sign portend a better prognosis than the HMCAS.[12] Patients affected by dehydration or increased blood viscosity resulting from other causes of an elevated hematocrit may have vessels that appear hyperdense on CT. Such diffuse vascular hyperdensity may be differentiated from the HMCAS or other hyperdense vessels associated with a vascular occlusion on the basis of Hounsfield density calculation.[14,15] Although measurement of this parameter is easily performed on the console or image viewing system, most clinicians communicate such findings based on a qualitative impression of the images. Vascular hyperdensity may also be caused by calcification in the setting of a calcific embolus, or associated with atherosclerotic large-vessel disease of the intracranial circulation. Calcification of the distal intracranial carotid arteries is a nonspecific finding, although it may point to an arterial source of thromboembolism in selected cases. When vascular hyperdensity is appreciated in the venous system, the diagnosis of cerebral venous thrombosis may be established. A delta sign, or axial impression of hyperdensity in the posterior aspect of the superior sagittal sinus, may represent thrombosis of this structure. Venous hyperdensity may be more difficult to interpret, as extensive thrombosis may cause hyperdensity of numerous venous structures. These relatively subtle examples of vascular information derived from noncontrast CT scans may be inferior to angiographic studies, but the clinician should maximally use all information provided on a given imaging study.

CTA may define the status of the arteries and veins and has rapidly expanded in clinical practice within the last several years, being implemented as newer CT scanners are updated in the community. Current CT scanners all provide the capability of performing CTA, propelling CTA as a practical imaging modality for emergent application and selection of thrombolytic candidates.[16,17] The expense of CTA is similar to an enhanced CT scan with an additional cost incurred by technical and computer analytic charges. The risks of CTA are similar to those previously described for enhanced CT studies. Postprocessing software can produce multiple renditions of vascular information, including three-dimensional (3D) images (Figure 12.7) and reformatted multiplanar two-dimensional (2D) projections. The wealth of information provided by CTA postprocessing has been offset by concerns related to the practical application of postprocessing in the real-time setting of acute stroke care. Postprocessing is performed on a neighboring computer workstation, but few clinicians are familiar with the associated image manipulation and software navigation. Even in the absence of postprocessed images, the raw or source image data provide a significant amount of vascular information because of the accurately timed opacification of large vascular structures and thin axial cuts acquired as part of the technique. Inspection of CTA source images may easily reveal large-vessel occlusion or stenosis. CTA provides fairly accurate anatomical information without the limitations of flow artifacts that plague magnetic resonance (MR) angiographic techniques. Distal vascular structures are therefore visualized better with CTA than MR angiography (MRA). Although MRA may help identify hemodynamically significant large-vessel stenoses as a result of signal dropout associated with flow artifact, CTA may estimate luminal caliber more accurately. Vascular lesions, such as stenoses, aneurysms, or arteriovenous malformations, may be delineated in detail with simultaneous depiction of

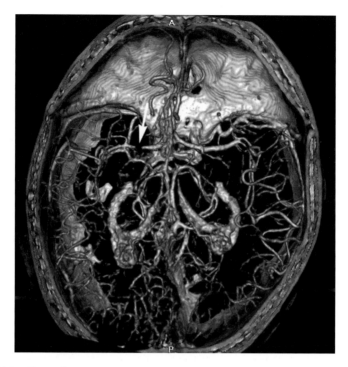

Figure 12.7 Three-dimensional (3D) postprocessed computed tomography angiography (CTA) image of middle cerebral artery occlusion (*arrow*).

adjacent vessels. The capacity of CTA to illustrate diminutive vessels at more distal aspects of the arterial tree may be useful in characterizing collateral circulatory patterns in various conditions. In acute ischemic stroke, the status of the collateral circulation may be an important determinant of outcome. This facet may help identify patients that are likely to experience subsequent neurological deterioration during the acute and early subacute phases of ischemic stroke. Such information regarding collaterals may also help guide management during this critical period. The relationship of collaterals and cerebral perfusion may help explain the clinical course of stroke patients and assist prognosis. Evaluation of extreme distal vascular structures is limited by simultaneous opacification of arterial and venous structures, making it difficult to discern patent terminal arterial branches from draining cortical veins. On the other hand, the simultaneous enhancement of venous structures makes CTA a useful technique for the diagnosis of cerebral venous thrombosis, although this application is used less frequently.

The advent of helical CT scanners also allows for contemporaneous imaging of the intracranial and extracranial cerebrovascular circulation in a rapid and noninvasive manner. This diagnostic imaging approach has been used to identify large-vessel intracranial occlusions and more proximal sources of artery-to-artery emboli within minutes of emergency room arrival.[16] CTA can depict the arterial anatomy from the aortic arch to distal cortical branches within

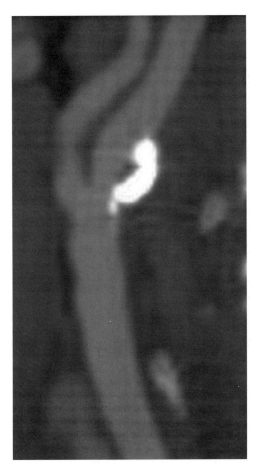

Figure 12.8 Computed tomography angiography (CTA) depiction of proximal internal carotid artery plaque with calcifications and ulceration.

seconds. This feature of CTA may be useful for planned interventional therapeutic procedures. Enhancement of the vessel lumen with CTA outlines the contour of the luminal surface, depicting ulcerations that may be associated with atherosclerotic plaque (Figure 12.8). This aspect of CTA is quite advantageous in the extracranial portion of the internal carotid artery, where plaque characteristics, including fatty deposits, may be seen in the vessel wall. Cervicocephalic arterial dissections may be identified in several vessels with only a single contrast injection. Information on the extracranial circulation may allow the clinician to plan for early revascularization of an internal carotid stenosis (see Chapter 6). Calcification is a key limitation of CTA, however, obscuring the vessel lumen in occasional cases. This limitation principally affects extracranial CTA, where accurate quantification of stenoses is important. In such cases, MRA or ultrasound may be reasonable noninvasive alternatives.

Physiological Imaging

CTP is a recent innovation that is rapidly promoting CT-based acute stroke evaluation as a significant competitor to MRI-based techniques.[16,18–20] Although CTP is not widely endorsed at present, the ability to rapidly provide perfusion information along with angiographic (CTA) and conventional CT images of the brain is an attractive feature.[16,19,21–24] The risks and expenses are identical to CTA. During CTA acquisition the contrast bolus may be divided into two injections to generate CTP images. Forty milliliters (mL) of contrast can be injected into a large vein at a rate of 4 to 10 mL per second for the perfusion scan, with various perfusion parameter maps created on a postprocessing computer workstation. CTP is based on the indicator-dilution principle of measuring tissue perfusion, where the change in signal intensity (measured in Hounsfield units) is proportional to the concentration of contrast in a given pixel. The linear relationship of contrast concentration and signal intensity allows for straightforward quantification of cerebral perfusion. Tracking the first pass of a contrast bolus within an artery allows for determination of perfusion maps. Automated software allows the user to define the arterial and venous seed points with calculation of cerebral blood volume (CBV), mean transit time (MTT), and cerebral blood flow (CBF). Recent research has established the validity of the various quantitative perfusion parameters; however, even crude estimates may be helpful in the acute setting.[19,23,24] CBV may be abnormal in ischemic regions, with prolonged MTT and diminished CBF. The predictive values of these parameters with regard to stroke outcome remain controversial; however, current investigators are employing these perfusion maps to characterize the ischemic penumbra extending outside the areas of core infarction.[22] The perfusion mismatch concept is being explored with CT in a manner similar to current multimodal MRI approaches (described later in this chapter).

Alternative CT-based perfusion approaches include xenon-CT (XeCT) scans, in which the inert gas xenon is used as a diffusible tracer. XeCT has been employed at some centers for several years, providing perfusion information in various conditions, including cases deemed too unstable for MRI. Additional hardware and support services are required for this technique and angiographic information is not acquired at the same time. Although xenon is widely available as an anesthetic agent, its use as a contrast medium is under current evaluation by the Food and Drug Administration because of reported adverse effects including mental status changes.

Multimodal CT imaging, employing CTA/CTP or XeCT, may be useful in many cases, but future research will need to address whether such an exhaustive approach is necessary or cost-effective for the general stroke population.[25]

MAGNETIC RESONANCE IMAGING

Practical Considerations

MRI revolutionized neuroimaging during the early 1980s, followed by a renaissance in stroke diagnosis during the mid-1990s with the introduction of advanced conventional pulse sequences, diffusion-weighted imaging (DWI), and perfusion-weighted imaging (PWI). MRI is widely revered as the ultimate diagnostic tool for acute stroke diagnosis, delineating ischemic injury within minutes of stroke onset and differentiating lesions that may mimic ischemia on CT.[26,27] The broad range and variability of technical parameters, including numerous pulse sequences and imaging protocols, provide vast information on the status of the ischemic brain, but the rapidly expanding technology may limit practical image interpretation and analysis by some clinicians. Knowledge of the various artifacts encountered on MRI is also an essential component of study interpretation. Cost is a significant limitation of MRI, with relatively few contraindications other than implanted metallic hardware such as a pacemaker or older aneurysm clip. Claustrophobia may be an obstacle for some patients, although it may be addressed with sedative medication. Gadolinium contrast material has an acceptable risk profile, although its use is controversial in the setting of pregnancy. MRI may rapidly detect cerebral ischemia; however, this modality is rarely used as the initial diagnostic study for acute stroke patients. Despite widespread availability of MRI in outpatient practice, it is not as accessible as CT and is even more scarce for emergency or urgent inpatient evaluation. Some centers may provide imaging time only during specific hours and others devote imaging slots preferentially to outpatient cases. Hyperacute MRI, however, is rarely employed as the critical thrombolytic decisions can be made with noncontrast CT. CT is generally preferred due to concerns regarding accurate diagnosis of subarachnoid hemorrhage. CT may also rapidly provide an alternative diagnosis in a patient with the acute onset of a focal neurological deficit, thereby obviating the need for MRI. Unstable patients in critical condition may not tolerate being isolated in the magnet and clinicians may have concerns regarding limited ability for intensive monitoring of the patient. Furthermore, obtaining an MRI in the hyperacute period may delay thrombolytic treatment, thereby decreasing its potential benefit. Acquisition time for hyperacute MRI should realistically include the time required to transport the patient to the magnet, set up monitoring for the patient, protocol the study, and obtain images. The utility of MRI is ultimately determined by the clinician's needs. Each MRI sequence provides slightly different information on the status of the brain and vascular structures. An MRI study is essentially a composite of several sequences or depictions that reflect various aspects of cerebral ischemia. Protocols may also be adapted to obtain specific sequences in various anatomical planes, depending on the area of interest and the questions being posed. Although the standard MRI protocol for acute stroke may take 20 to 45 minutes, protocols may be tailored to the most crucial sequences in 6 to 8 minutes; identifying acute ischemia with DWI, providing detailed structural assessment with fluid-attenuated inversion-recovery (FLAIR) images, and illustrating hemorrhagic components with gradient-recalled echo (GRE) or echo-planar susceptibility weighted images.[28] Hyperacute MRI may be helpful in difficult cases in which clinical localization is elusive or when seizures herald the onset of a focal deficit.[29] Outside of the hyperacute period, few clinicians oversee the acquisition of an MRI study as treatment decisions are not as pivotal and maximal information can be obtained from the interpretation of all sequences considered as a group. Furthermore, the specific temporal sequence of imaging sequences may be modified to provide additional information. Post-gadolinium FLAIR images, for example, are sensitive to blood-brain barrier disruption, producing dramatic enhancement of ischemic regions. MRI artifacts, such as

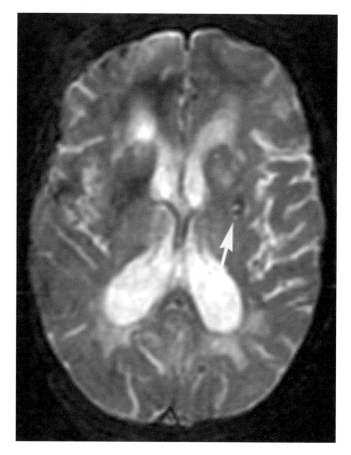

Figure 12.9 Gradient-recalled echo (GRE) image of hemosiderin deposition (*arrow*) associated with prior hemorrhage.

blooming of hemosiderin on GRE, also provide important diagnostic information (Figure 12.9).

Brain Imaging

Conventional MRI pulse sequences provide the most detailed anatomical view of the ischemic brain, largely excluding lesions or pathology that may mimic stroke symptoms and accurately characterizing the presence of intracranial hemorrhage. Although bony anatomy is best illustrated with CT, brain parenchyma in proximity to bony structures is more accurately illustrated with MRI. The posterior fossa, including the brainstem and cerebellum, are better depicted with MRI. T1-weighted images detail the structural integrity of brain parenchyma, revealing older ischemic insults with less information regarding more acute ischemic regions. Encephalomalacic areas of the brain appear

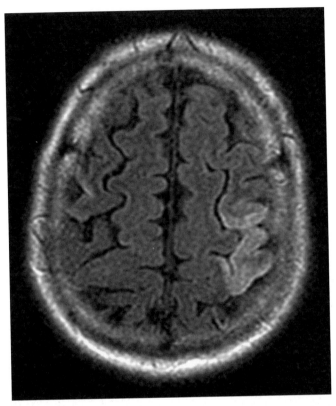

Figure 12.10   Fluid-attenuated inversion-recovery (FLAIR) sequence demonstrates hyperintensity associated with cortical infarction juxtaposed with nulling of cerebrospinal fluid (CSF) signal within the subarachnoid space.

hypointense because of destruction and resorption of parenchyma. Blurring of normal tissue interfaces may be seen in acute or subacute ischemia; however, such findings are subtle compared with similar findings on T2-weighted images. T2-weighted sequences emphasize cerebral edema because of an exquisite sensitivity for water, which appears hyperintense on these images. Ischemic cerebral edema consists of cytotoxic and vasogenic components. Cytotoxic edema develops within minutes of ischemic onset because of energy depletion of cellular membrane ion pumps with subsequent influx of water. Vasogenic edema follows several hours later when the blood barrier becomes leaky, allowing intravascular fluid to seep into the extracellular space. The intracellular or extracellular location of water cannot be determined on T2-weighted images; however, characteristic features may be apparent. Early T2-weighted changes in ischemia include findings that are analogous to CT correlates, generally depicting loss of normal architectural boundaries at the cortical level, insula, and basal ganglia. Ensuing vasogenic edema swells cortical gyri, obliterating the intervening sulci, with marked T2-hyperintensity of subcortical white matter structures. Proton-density sequences also reflect ischemic edema; however, the use of this sequence has largely been replaced by the acquisition of FLAIR images.

Table 12.1 MRI correlates of intracranial hemorrhage delineated by signal intensity on T1- and T2-weighted sequences

Phase	Time	Hemoglobin	T1	T2
Hyperacute	<24 hr	Oxyhemoglobin (intracellular)	Iso or hypo	Hyper
Acute	1–3 days	Deoxyhemoglobin (intracellular)	Iso or hypo	Hypo
Early subacute	>3 days	Methemoglobin (intracellular)	Hyper	Hypo
Late subacute	>7 days	Methemoglobin (extracellular)	Hyper	Hyper
Chronic	>14 days	Hemosiderin (extracellular)	Iso or hypo	Hypo

MRI = magnetic resonance imaging.

FLAIR images are essentially T2-weighted, with the application of an inversion pulse to null cerebrospinal fluid (CSF) signal. FLAIR is particularly sensitive to ischemic changes and has therefore become a basic component of most MRI protocols for stroke. FLAIR demonstrates regions of signal abnormality adjacent to CSF-filled spaces, such as the lateral ventricles or subarachnoid space (Figure 12.10).[30] Signal abnormalities in these areas may be difficult to ascertain on T2-weighted images because of juxtaposed hyperintensity of adjacent CSF. Conversely, T2-weighted images may be superior to FLAIR in the depiction of brain stem ischemia. GRE images are particularly sensitive to paramagnetic substances, exaggerating the presence of blood products. This blooming of hemorrhagic foci is an artifactual distortion on GRE that may be useful in detecting microhemorrhage associated with petechial hemorrhagic conversion of an ischemic infarct, cerebral amyloid angiopathy, or hypertension.[28,31,32] GRE hypointensity therefore adds to the well-known MRI correlates of intracranial hemorrhage (Table 12.1).

The administration of intravenous gadolinium further characterizes parenchymal injury associated with cerebral ischemia. Following injection of gadolinium, T1-weighted images are routinely acquired in the axial and coronal planes. Gadolinium reaches ischemic tissue as a result of early reperfusion, collateral supply, subsequent recanalization, or as part of even later repair within a zone of infarction. Ischemia or early infarcts may be imperceptible on postgadolinium T1-weighted images; however, subacute strokes manifest prominent enhancement associated with reperfusion and alteration of the normal tissue architecture (Figure 12.11). Cortical lesions typically demonstrate gyriform enhancement during the subacute period, although laminar necrosis may produce a similar appearance. Enhancement is therefore a useful marker in the age determination of an ischemic lesion.[33] Nonischemic differential diagnoses such as an abscess or neoplasm may produce enhancement in a characteristic pattern.

Although more refined conventional MRI sequences such as FLAIR have furthered stroke diagnosis, the advent of DWI radically transformed the diagnostic evaluation of stroke. DWI capitalizes on the random diffusion properties of water molecules in the brain, dichotomizing cytotoxic and vasogenic edema. Within minutes of stroke onset, cytotoxic edema leads to restricted diffusion of water molecules that are trapped in the intracellular space. Vasogenic edema manifests augmented diffusion of water molecules that are able to freely move within the fluid-laden extracellular space. Following the acquisition of images with a pair of magnetic field gradient pulses placed symmetrically around a

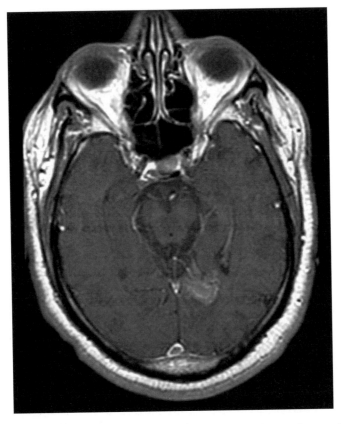

Figure 12.11   Hyperintensity on post-gadolinium T1-weighted image due to enhancement of a subacute left posterior cerebral artery stroke.

180-degree radiofrequency pulse, the diffusion of water molecules may be assessed. Variation in the time and amplitude (*b* value) of the gradient pulse influences the sensitivity of diffusion imaging.[34] Measurement at different *b* values allows for calculation of the apparent diffusion coefficient (ADC). ADC values may be used to generate ADC images that show restricted diffusion (cytotoxic edema) as hypointense lesions and elevated diffusion (vasogenic edema) as hyperintense lesions. Diffusion images, commonly referred to as DWI, reveal hyperintensity in regions with altered diffusion. These artifact-laden images have poor resolution; however, acute ischemic lesions are evident as bright spots superimposed on a darker background containing older ischemic insults. DWI is able to differentiate the age of ischemic strokes, because of the combined effects of restricted or elevated diffusion associated with cytotoxic or vasogenic edema, respectively. The temporal profile of the ADC in ischemic stroke has a characteristic course, punctuated by an early and late decline with pseudonormalization of the ADC at 9 to 14 days.[35–37] DWI was initially considered to be specific for stroke diagnosis, but subsequent observations have revealed DWI abnormalities in multiple pathological conditions.[38,39] DWI

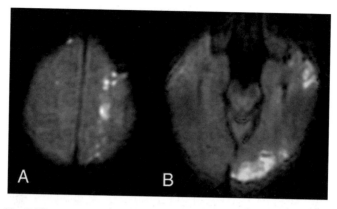

Figure 12.12   Diffusion-weighted imaging (DWI) illustrates a characteristic watershed pattern of ischemia between the middle cerebral artery and anterior cerebral artery (**A**) and between the middle cerebral artery and posterior cerebral artery (**B**).

also has several limitations that should be considered, including artifactual hyperintensity at tissue interfaces such as the temporal bone and cortical perimeter. DWI hyperintensities may also be due to "T2-shinethrough," produced by prominent T2-weighted signal abnormalities and evident as hyperintensity on the ADC maps. The presence of intracranial hemorrhage may produce heterogeneous signal abnormalities as well.[40] DWI artifactual lesions are typically symmetric, whereas ischemic lesions are more likely to be asymmetric. DWI is also not as versatile in the brain stem where lesions may be overlooked.[41,42] DWI may help determine stroke cause by illustrating characteristic patterns of infarct distribution (Figure 12.12).[29,43–45] Although DWI lesions may exhibit reversibility,[46] most DWI lesions are considered synonymous with a region of core infarction or ischemic tissue destined for infarction. Surrounding this area of core infarction, a penumbral zone may experience diminished perfusion and functional compromise with minimal or absent diffusion abnormality.[47]

Vascular Imaging

Indirect vascular information may also be abstracted from conventional MRI sequences. Correlates of the CT HMCAS may be observed on most MRI sequences, depending on the age of intraluminal thrombus and flow dynamics.[48] Intraluminal thrombosis is most apparent on T2-weighted or GRE images, whereas arterial flow abnormalities are best observed on FLAIR.[49–51] FLAIR vascular hyperintensities appear as bright serpentine structures within the subarachnoid space, most commonly within the Sylvian fissure (Figure 12.13).[50,52] These artifacts associated with diminished flow have been correlated with hypoperfusion and may be indicative of collateral flow.[50,51] FLAIR hyperintensity may also be seen in thrombosed or adjacent venous structures in the setting of venous ischemia. Indirect vascular information is critical in cervicocephalic arterial dissection, in which axial fat-saturation T1-weighted images are optimal

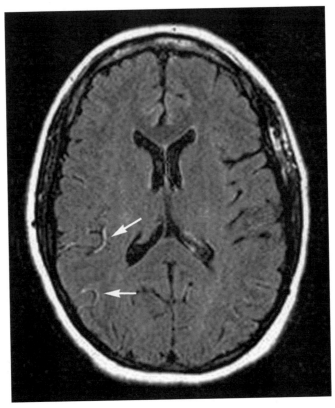

Figure 12.13 Serpentine fluid-attenuated inversion-recovery (FLAIR) vascular hyperintensities (*arrows*) associated with right middle cerebral artery ischemia.

for diagnosis (Figure 12.14). Although aneurysms and arteriovenous malformations may be evident on conventional sequences, dedicated angiographic
studies are obligatory. Identification of many indirect vascular findings may
prompt further noninvasive evaluation with MRA.

MRA can noninvasively detail the arterial and venous anatomy of the head
and neck. Similar artifactual flow gaps may be commonly seen in the supra-
clinoid portion of the internal carotid arteries. The considerable sensitivity of
MRA to flow perturbations leads to signal loss or flow gaps. These flow gaps
may be useful in detection of flow-limiting stenoses; however, quantification
of luminal compromise is unfeasible. Even when complete signal loss is not
apparent, MRA tends to overestimate luminal stenoses. Distal vascular segments beyond the proximal portions of the major arteries are poorly visualized
on MRA. Intracranial MRA is therefore insensitive in the evaluation of vasculitis or terminal branch occlusions. Magnetic resonance venography (MRV) may
employ a time-of-flight technique typically used for arterial imaging or a phase-
contrast (PC) technique that can assess flow direction within the larger venous
structures. PC MRV is advantageous for assessment of patency within the
venous sinuses, where venous drainage patterns may be altered in the setting of

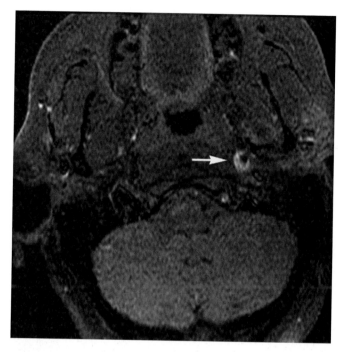

Figure 12.14   Axial fat-saturation T1-weighted image demonstrates crescent-shaped hyperintensity (*arrow*) of intramural hematoma in cervicocephalic arterial dissection.

thrombosis. MRA and MRV are particularly useful as these studies are routinely acquired in conjunction with stroke MRI; however, conventional angiography may be indicated for further characterization of a vascular occlusion, vasculopathy, or complex vascular lesion.

Contemporaneous administration of intravenous gadolinium may improve visualization, particularly in the extracranial circulation. Contrast-enhanced MRA (CE-MRA) may be superior in the depiction of carotid stenoses or arterial dissections. CE-MRA may diminish flow artifacts that cause signal dropout at the skull base on conventional MRA. Intracranial CE-MRA is rarely employed because of the complex vascular anatomy that limits appropriate timing of the contrast bolus.

Physiological Imaging

Perfusion MRI demonstrates alterations of blood flow that accompany acute ischemic stroke. Assessment of cerebral perfusion is typically conducted following the diagnosis of ischemic stroke to determine the degree of hemodynamic compromise associated with a proximal vascular lesion such as a carotid stenosis. PWI is therefore obtained with knowledge of the vascular anatomy, most commonly evaluated by MRA. The vascular anatomy is a principal determinant of cerebral hemodynamics, although the angiographic evaluation of vascular segments distal to the circle of Willis that play a vital role in collateral circulatory patterns is unreliable with MRA. PWI evaluates the existing hemodynamic state without knowledge of the exact source or route of collaterals. Arterial flow can be tracked with an intravenous injection of gadolinium or with arterial spin-labeling,[53] a technique that is entirely noninvasive. Gadolinium is relatively expensive, whereas arterial spin-labeling incurs no additional cost. Estimates of CBF may be generated from signal alteration accompanying downstream arrival of contrast or labeled bolus. Various hemodynamic measurements including time to peak (TTP), CBV, MTT, and CBF can be derived, although inherent differences in these techniques may account for variability in the derived perfusion parameters. Improved CBF maps on gadolinium-based PWI may be obtained if the component of signal alteration associated with large vessel enhancement is subtracted.[54] Continuous arterial spin-labeling may be repeated to obtain serial perfusion studies over a short time interval, more reliably reflecting the dynamic nature of CBF in acute ischemic stroke. Prediction of final infarct volume from perfusion parameters has been an elusive goal,[55] challenging investigators to identify the most reliable single parameter.[56–58] The relationship of the individual perfusion parameter abnormalities with respect to the core infarct region approximated by DWI forms the basis for the MRI mismatch concept, with the intervening region being evidence of the ischemic penumbra and the potential target of therapeutic interventions. The goal of revascularization or thrombolysis is to minimize the growth of tissue volume destined for infarction beyond the existing diffusion abnormality. Although improved antegrade blood flow through a compromised vessel may achieve this goal, augmentation of the collateral circulation may also improve outcome. Indirect evidence of collaterals may be inferred from MTT maps or delayed arterial transit effects on arterial spin-labeled MRI (Figure 12.15).[53] Such perfusion information may be useful to guide therapeutic blood pressure management beyond the acute window into the subacute phase of stroke.

ULTRASONOGRAPHY

Unlike the previously mentioned angiographic studies, including CTA and MRA, that require patient transport to the scanner, ultrasonography is portable. Transcranial Doppler (TCD) ultrasonography or carotid Duplex scans may be performed in any patient location. Although most ultrasound studies for acute stroke are generally performed with the goal of determining stroke cause some time after acute evaluation and management (see Chapter 4) these tools can be used for rapid evaluation of vascular patency in the field, office, or emergency room. TCD enables the clinician to assess the patency and hemodynamic status of the major arterial segments in both the anterior and posterior circulations. TCD is entirely noninvasive, providing immediate information regarding blood flow velocity and pulsatility. TCD is widely available and inexpensive, without a significant risk profile. Operator skills are important, however, to reliably insonate the vessels of interest. Temporal acoustic bone windows may be limited in some patients (20% to 30% of patients),[59] precluding evaluation of the anterior, posterior, and middle cerebral artery. Interpretation of TCD may also be difficult in complex cases, although rapid evaluation of a single vessel

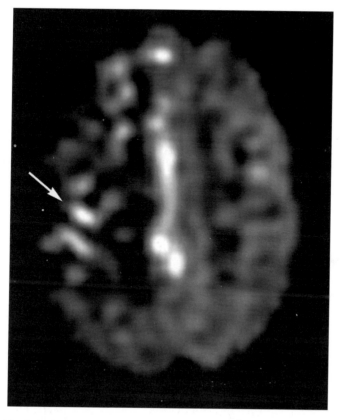

Figure 12.15 Delayed arterial transit effects on arterial spin-labeled magnetic resonance imaging (MRI) (*arrow*) resulting from prolongation of mean transit time (MTT) suggest collateral blood flow in right middle cerebral artery stroke.

with suspected thrombosis is feasible.[60] Future hardware adaptations and the approval of experimental contrast agents may expand the diagnostic potential of TCD.[60–63] Serial measurements are possible, allowing for monitoring during therapeutic interventions such as thrombolysis.[64–66] TCD may actually augment recanalization because of ultrasonic mechanical energy delivered to the clot nidus.[67] The use of TCD during thrombolysis has garnered interest in grading of vascular patency with a standardized scale.[66] The Thrombolysis in Brain Ischemia (TIBI) score has been shown to correlate with initial stroke severity and predict clinical outcome in the acute stroke setting.[68]

Duplex ultrasonography of the carotid and vertebral arteries may reveal a proximal arterial source of cerebral ischemia once a stroke diagnosis has been established. Duplex ultrasonography can be rapidly performed at the bedside, identifying an extracranial stenosis or occlusion. Ultrasonography is widely available, although this modality is a traditionally a component of the diagnostic workup for acute ischemic stroke, pursuing stroke cause rather than establishing an acute vascular diagnosis. Insonation of the vertebral arteries may be technically challenging, limiting application in posterior circulation ischemia.

CONVENTIONAL ANGIOGRAPHY—VASCULAR IMAGING AND A THERAPEUTIC OPPORTUNITY

Conventional angiography was once the principal diagnostic modality for stroke; however, diagnostic catheter-based angiography during the acute phase of ischemic stroke has largely been replaced by advanced imaging techniques. Conventional angiography is most commonly obtained for potential therapeutic interventions including thrombolysis or mechanical revascularization (see Chapters 13 and 15). Diagnostic angiography may be required to confirm a diagnosis or to better characterize a vascular anomaly; however, this is rarely pursued within the acute phase. Diagnostic angiography is available at most hospitals; however, considerable variability exists in specialty coverage and hours of availability. The invasive nature of conventional angiography is associated with a 1 to 2.5 percent risk of complications, including adverse effects of contrast. Nevertheless, conventional angiography remains the definitive modality for evaluation of the cerebral circulation. The combination of excellent spatial and temporal resolution provides detailed angiographic information, incorporating anatomical features and flow properties. Although revered as the gold standard, negative angiograms in the acute phase of ischemic stroke do not necessarily rule out embolic arterial occlusion, because negative angiography may result from recanalization associated with transient embolic occlusion or vascular occlusion within the microvasculature.[69] Advances in interventional stroke therapy including intra-arterial thrombolysis have rekindled interest in the characterization of angiographic findings during the acute phase of ischemic stroke. Relatively primitive descriptions of vessel patency have been replaced by more refined angiographic grading systems, incorporating critical information on flow dynamics including the collateral circulation.[70] These advances may further knowledge of stroke pathophysiology, without contributing practical implications for stroke diagnosis outside of the therapeutic realm.

NUCLEAR MEDICINE

Nuclear medicine studies, including single photon emission computed tomography (SPECT) and positron emission tomography (PET) have been used for many years to study cerebral ischemia. These modalities may be available for clinical application in individual cases of acute ischemic stroke, although routine use is impractical. SPECT provides relative CBF information that is analogous to currently available CT-based perfusion methods.[71–73] PET may be used to quantitatively measure metabolism and CBF.[74] PET remains the gold standard measurement tool for research purposes but is only infrequently used in clinical practice. SPECT and PET are available only at selected institutions on a limited time basis. Advance planning is also necessary to prepare radionuclides for these studies. The information obtained from these nuclear medicine studies can be approximated in the acute setting with perfusion techniques described previously in this chapter.

LABORATORY INVESTIGATIONS

Routine

The lack of a specific laboratory test or serological study for the diagnosis of acute ischemic stroke has relegated laboratory tests to an adjunctive role during the acute phase. Selected laboratory studies are obtained during the first few hours of stroke onset to assist therapeutic decisions or identify abnormalities that may require treatment as part of the supportive care of the stroke patient. A complete blood count with platelets and basic coagulation parameters, including a prothrombin time and activated partial thromboplastin time, should be obtained to guide antithrombotic or thrombolytic management. Serum glucose, electrolytes, and renal function should be assayed because such abnormalities may affect stroke outcome.[75–77] Elevations of blood glucose during acute stroke, for instance, have been associated with worse clinical outcome and a higher probability of symptomatic intracranial hemorrhage.[75–78] Cardiac enzymes may reveal myocardial ischemia that may not be suspect but is amenable to treatment. Other laboratory studies are not crucial during the acute period but serve an important role in the subsequent determination of stroke cause. An erythrocyte sedimentation rate or rapid plasma reagent study may identify a specific cause of cerebral ischemia. Although the clinician may be compelled to run a battery of blood tests during the acute period, this may rapidly increase cost and abandon a rational diagnostic strategy. An extensive hypercoagulable assessment, for instance, should only be requested in selected patients.[79,80] In contrast, condensing the diagnostic stroke workup into the acute period may lead to erroneous clinical decisions. For example, a positive anticardiolipin assay during acute stroke may not necessarily dictate a diagnosis of antiphospholipid antibody syndrome.[81] Similarly, acute determination of serum lipids or serum homocysteine may be invalid.[82] A practical guide to laboratory investigations in acute stroke is contained in Table 12.2.

Table 12.2   Laboratory investigations in acute stroke

All Cases	*Selected Cases*
Blood glucose	Pregnancy test
Complete blood count (CBC) with platelets	Hepatic function studies
Prothrombin time (PT) or international normalized ratio (INR)	Toxicology screen
	Blood alcohol level
Activated partial thromboplastin time (aPTT)	Arterial blood gas
Serum electrolytes	Cardiac enzymes
Renal function studies	Erythrocyte sedimentation rate (ESR)
	Rapid plasmin reagent (RPR)
	Hypercoagulable assays

Brain Damage and Vascular Correlates

The onset of cerebral ischemia induces numerous hemostatic alterations and biochemical changes that can be measured by serological evaluation.[81,83–98] Despite years of research, investigators have failed to establish a reliable serological marker of acute cerebral ischemia that is adequately sensitive and specific. The development of such a test would improve rapid diagnosis of acute ischemic stroke, allowing physicians to institute treatment within the shortest time interval. As a result of perpetual efforts to establish such a marker, numerous derangements have been identified in the blood.[81,83,85–99] An ideal biochemical marker would reflect ischemic change within the brain with high sensitivity and minimal invasiveness. Blood samples can be obtained in any patient location and serial measurements are feasible. Unfortunately, baseline values before stroke onset cannot be determined for use as a comparison. The clinical implications of serological abnormalities remain unclear. Uric acid elevation during acute ischemic stroke, for instance, is associated with decreased final infarct volume and improved neurological outcome, attributed to an endogenous antioxidant response.[100,101] These values, however, depend on associated co-morbidities and baseline values, and lack specificity for acute ischemic stroke. Systemic acute phase reactants may be detected,[84–86,89] but measurement of these factors does not aid stroke diagnosis. Relatively specific biochemical markers of cerebral ischemia include matrix metalloproteinases, neuron-specific enolase, myelin basic protein, S-100β protein, thrombomodulin, and tau protein, reflecting structural changes in the acute stroke period.[102–105] The use of a panel of such markers, rather than a single biochemical marker, may improve sensitivity.[98]

FUTURE DIAGNOSTIC METHODS

Advanced MRI techniques such as diffusion tensor imaging (DTI), magnetic resonance spectroscopy (MRS), and functional MRI (fMRI) may be added to current MRI protocols for ischemic stroke, providing further insight. DTI may demonstrate diffusion anisotropy and subtle changes in fiber tracts following stroke.[106,107] DTI may eventually be useful in stroke rehabilitation during the subacute and chronic phases, whereas acute DTI may be less informative because structural changes within the brain that influence this method may not yet be present. The time constraints of acute stroke evaluation may not afford lengthy testing with fMRI. Future adaptations may provide further physiological information obtained through relatively basic motor tasks during the acute phase. Multivoxel MRS may help identify metabolic signatures of the ischemic penumbra, including lactate elevation and decreased N-acetyl-aspartate, but this modality is also likely to require considerable time thereby limiting its application in acute ischemic stroke.[108] Many of these techniques, however, may not be applicable during the acute phase of ischemic stroke.

Multimodal diagnostic strategies will likely play an active role in future stroke diagnosis. Multimodal CT with CTA and CTP or XeCT may provide community centers with the ability to rapidly assess ischemic strokes.[20,109] Use of combined CT/CTA/CTP may not only rapidly determine optimal therapy but may also reduce the total cost of stroke evaluation through elimination of unnecessary tests that may be acquired during several subsequent days of hospitalization.[25] Combined approaches incorporating various modalities may also flourish. Angiography suites with dedicated MRI components or hybrid PET-CT scanners may provide correlative data improving diagnosis.

The correlation of clinical and radiographical findings in acute stroke may help stratify stroke subtypes, assist therapeutic strategies, and strengthen prognostic assessments. The combination of clinical and diagnostic data may help predict subsequent patient outcome,[110] and image-guided assessment of parenchyma, vasculature, and physiology may be developed for selected patients, extending the window of therapeutic opportunity.

References

1. Grond M, von Kummer R, Sobesky J, et al. Early x-ray hypoattenuation of brain parenchyma indicates extended critical hypoperfusion in acute stroke. Stroke 2000;31:133–139.
2. Jaillard A, Hommel M, Baird AE, et al. Significance of early CT signs in acute stroke. A CT scan-diffusion MRI study. Cerebrovasc Dis 2002;13:47–56.
3. Patel SC, Levine SR, Tilley BC, et al. Lack of clinical significance of early ischemic changes on computed tomography in acute stroke. JAMA 2001;286:2830–2838.
4. Roberts HC, Dillon WP, Furlan AJ, et al. Computed tomographic findings in patients undergoing intra-arterial thrombolysis for acute ischemic stroke due to middle cerebral artery occlusion: results from the PROACT II trial. Stroke 2002;33:1557–1565.
5. Rother J. CT and MRI in the diagnosis of acute stroke and their role in thrombolysis. Thromb Res 2001;103(suppl 1):S125–133.
6. Gilligan AK, Markus R, Read S, et al. Baseline blood pressure but not early computed tomography changes predicts major hemorrhage after streptokinase in acute ischemic stroke. Stroke 2002;33:2236–2242.
7. Dippel DW, Du Ry van Beest Holle M, van Kooten F, Koudstaal PJ. The validity and reliability of signs of early infarction on CT in acute ischaemic stroke. Neuroradiology 2000;42:629–633.
8. Kalafut MA, Schriger DL, Saver JL, Starkman S. Detection of early CT signs of >1/3 middle cerebral artery infarctions: interrater reliability and sensitivity of CT interpretation by physicians involved in acute stroke care. Stroke 2000;31:1667–1671.
9. Maldjian JA, Chalela J, Kasner SE, et al. Automated CT segmentation and analysis for acute middle cerebral artery stroke. AJNR Am J Neuroradiol 2001;22:1050–1055.
10. Pexman JH, Barber PA, Hill MD, et al. Use of the Alberta Stroke Program Early CT Score (ASPECTS) for assessing CT scans in patients with acute stroke. AJNR Am J Neuroradiol 2001;22:1534–1542.
11. Barber PA, Demchuk AM, Zhang J, Buchan AM. Validity and reliability of a quantitative computed tomography score in predicting outcome of hyperacute stroke before thrombolytic therapy. ASPECTS Study Group. Alberta Stroke Programme Early CT Score. Lancet 2000;355:1670–1674.
12. Barber PA, Demchuk AM, Hudon ME, et al. Hyperdense sylvian fissure MCA "dot" sign: a CT marker of acute ischemia. Stroke 2001;32:84–88.
13. Berge E, Nakstad PH, Sandset PM. Large middle cerebral artery infarctions and the hyperdense middle cerebral artery sign in patients with atrial fibrillation. Acta Radiol 2001;42:261–268.
14. Koo CK, Teasdale E, Muir KW. What constitutes a true hyperdense middle cerebral artery sign? Cerebrovasc Dis 2000;10:419–423.
15. Gadda D, Vannucchi L, Niccolai F, et al. CT in acute stroke: improved detection of dense intracranial arteries by varying window parameters and performing a thin-slice helical scan. Neuroradiology 2002;44:900–906.
16. Ezzeddine MA, Lev MH, McDonald CT, et al. CT angiography with whole brain perfused blood volume imaging: added clinical value in the assessment of acute stroke. Stroke 2002;33: 959–966.
17. Verro P, Tanenbaum LN, Borden NM, et al. CT angiography in acute ischemic stroke: preliminary results. Stroke 2002;33:276–278.
18. Schramm P, Schellinger PD, Fiebach JB, et al. Comparison of CT and CT angiography source images with diffusion-weighted imaging in patients with acute stroke within 6 hours after onset. Stroke 2002;33:2426–2432.

19. Lee KH, Lee SJ, Cho SJ, et al. Usefulness of triphasic perfusion computed tomography for intravenous thrombolysis with tissue-type plasminogen activator in acute ischemic stroke. Arch Neurol 2000;57:1000–1008.
20. Mayer TE, Hamann GF, Baranczyk J, et al. Dynamic CT perfusion imaging of acute stroke. AJNR Am J Neuroradiol 2000;21:1441–1449.
21. Eastwood JD, Lev MH, Azhari T, et al. CT perfusion scanning with deconvolution analysis: pilot study in patients with acute middle cerebral artery stroke. Radiology 2002;222:227–236.
22. Lev MH, Segal AZ, Farkas J, et al. Utility of perfusion-weighted CT imaging in acute middle cerebral artery stroke treated with intra-arterial thrombolysis: prediction of final infarct volume and clinical outcome. Stroke 2001;32:2021–2028.
23. Wintermark M, Thiran JP, Maeder P, et al. Simultaneous measurement of regional cerebral blood flow by perfusion CT and stable xenon CT: a validation study. AJNR Am J Neuroradiol 2001;22:905–914.
24. Lee KH, Cho SJ, Byun HS, et al. Triphasic perfusion computed tomography in acute middle cerebral artery stroke: a correlation with angiographic findings. Arch Neurol 2000;57:990–999.
25. Gleason S, Furie KL, Lev MH, et al. Potential influence of acute CT on inpatient costs in patients with ischemic stroke. Acad Radiol 2001;8:955–964.
26. Fiebach J, Jansen O, Schellinger P, et al. Comparison of CT with diffusion-weighted MRI in patients with hyperacute stroke. Neuroradiology 2001;43:628–632.
27. Fiebach JB, Schellinger PD, Jansen O, et al. CT and diffusion-weighted MR imaging in randomized order: diffusion-weighted imaging results in higher accuracy and lower interrater variability in the diagnosis of hyperacute ischemic stroke. Stroke 2002;33:2206–2210.
28. Kidwell CS, Saver JL, Villablanca JP, et al. Magnetic resonance imaging detection of microbleeds before thrombolysis: an emerging application. Stroke 2002;33:95–98.
29. Gerraty RP, Parsons MW, Barber PA, et al. Examining the lacunar hypothesis with diffusion and perfusion magnetic resonance imaging. Stroke 2002;33:2019–2024.
30. Dechambre SD, Duprez T, Grandin CB, et al. High signal in cerebrospinal fluid mimicking subarachnoid haemorrhage on FLAIR following acute stroke and intravenous contrast medium. Neuroradiology 2000;42:608–611.
31. Hermier M, Nighoghossian N, Derex L, et al. MRI of acute post-ischemic cerebral hemorrhage in stroke patients: diagnosis with T2*-weighted gradient-echo sequences. Neuroradiology 2001;43:809–815.
32. Tsushima Y, Tamura T, Unno Y, et al. Multifocal low-signal brain lesions on T2*-weighted gradient-echo imaging. Neuroradiology 2000;42:499–504.
33. Karonen JO, Partanen PL, Vanninen RL, et al. Evolution of MR contrast enhancement patterns during the first week after acute ischemic stroke. AJNR Am J Neuroradiol 2001;22:103–111.
34. Geijer B, Sundgren PC, Lindgren A, et al. The value of b required to avoid T2 shine-through from old lacunar infarcts in diffusion-weighted imaging. Neuroradiology 2001;43:511–517.
35. Fiebach JB, Jansen O, Schellinger PD, et al. Serial analysis of the apparent diffusion coefficient time course in human stroke. Neuroradiology 2002;44:294–298.
36. Huang IJ, Chen CY, Chung HW, et al. Time course of cerebral infarction in the middle cerebral arterial territory: deep watershed versus territorial subtypes on diffusion-weighted MR images. Radiology 2001;221:35–42.
37. Lansberg MG, Thijs VN, O'Brien MW, et al. Evolution of apparent diffusion coefficient, diffusion-weighted, and T2-weighted signal intensity of acute stroke. AJNR Am J Neuroradiol 2001;22:637–644.
38. Geijer B, Holtas S. Diffusion-weighted imaging of brain metastases: their potential to be misinterpreted as focal ischaemic lesions. Neuroradiology 2002;44:568–573.
39. Hinman JM, Provenzale JM. Nonischemic causes of hyperintense signals on diffusion-weighted magnetic resonance images: a pictorial essay. Can Assoc Radiol J 2000;51:351–357.
40. Kang BK, Na DG, Ryoo JW, et al. Diffusion-weighted MR imaging of intracerebral hemorrhage. Korean J Radiol 2001;2:183–191.
41. Kuker W, Weise J, Krapf H, et al. MRI characteristics of acute and subacute brainstem and thalamic infarctions: value of T2- and diffusion-weighted sequences. J Neurol 2002;249:33–42.
42. Oppenheim C, Stanescu R, Dormont D, et al. False-negative diffusion-weighted MR findings in acute ischemic stroke. AJNR Am J Neuroradiol 2000;21:1434–440.
43. Kang DW, Chu K, Ko SB, et al. Lesion patterns and mechanism of ischemia in internal carotid artery disease: a diffusion-weighted imaging study. Arch Neurol 2002;59:1577–1582.
44. Kastrup A, Schulz JB, Mader I, et al. Diffusion-weighted MRI in patients with symptomatic internal carotid artery disease. J Neurol 2002;249:1168–1174.

45. Koennecke HC, Bernarding J, Braun J, et al. Scattered brain infarct pattern on diffusion-weighted magnetic resonance imaging in patients with acute ischemic stroke. Cerebrovasc Dis 2001;11:157–163.
46. Fiehler J, Foth M, Kucinski T, et al. Severe ADC decreases do not predict irreversible tissue damage in humans. Stroke 2002;33:79–86.
47. Fiehler J, Knab R, Reichenbach JR, et al. Apparent diffusion coefficient decreases and magnetic resonance imaging perfusion parameters are associated in ischemic tissue of acute stroke patients. J Cereb Blood Flow Metab 2001;21:577–584.
48. Flacke S, Urbach H, Keller E, et al. Middle cerebral artery (MCA) susceptibility sign at susceptibility-based perfusion MR imaging: clinical importance and comparison with hyperdense MCA sign at CT. Radiology 2000;215:476–482.
49. Toyoda K, Ida M, Fukuda K. Fluid-attenuated inversion recovery intraarterial signal: an early sign of hyperacute cerebral ischemia. AJNR Am J Neuroradiol 2001;22:1021–1029.
50. Tsushima Y, Endo K. Significance of hyperintense vessels on FLAIR MRI in acute stroke. Neurology 2001;56:1248–1249.
51. Kamran S, Bates V, Bakshi R, et al. Significance of hyperintense vessels on FLAIR MRI in acute stroke. Neurology 2000;55:265–269.
52. Maeda M, Yamamoto T, Daimon S, et al. Arterial hyperintensity on fast fluid-attenuated inversion recovery images: a subtle finding for hyperacute stroke undetected by diffusion-weighted MR imaging. AJNR Am J Neuroradiol 2001;22:632–636.
53. Chalela JA, Alsop DC, Gonzalez-Atavales JB, et al. Magnetic resonance perfusion imaging in acute ischemic stroke using continuous arterial spin labeling. Stroke 2000;31:680–687.
54. Carroll TJ, Haughton VM, Rowley HA, Cordes D. Confounding effect of large vessels on MR perfusion images analyzed with independent component analysis. AJNR Am J Neuroradiol 2002;23:1007–1012.
55. Fiehler J, von Bezold M, Kucinski T, et al. Cerebral blood flow predicts lesion growth in acute stroke patients. Stroke 2002;33:2421–2425.
56. Grandin CB, Duprez TP, Smith AM, et al. Which MR-derived perfusion parameters are the best predictors of infarct growth in hyperacute stroke? Comparative study between relative and quantitative measurements. Radiology 2002;223:361–370.
57. Schaefer PW, Hunter GJ, He J, et al. Predicting cerebral ischemic infarct volume with diffusion and perfusion MR imaging. AJNR Am J Neuroradiol 2002;23:1785–1794.
58. Parsons MW, Yang Q, Barber PA, et al. Perfusion magnetic resonance imaging maps in hyperacute stroke: relative cerebral blood flow most accurately identifies tissue destined to infarct. Stroke 2001;32:1581–1587.
59. Gahn G, von Kummer R. Ultrasound in acute stroke: a review. Neuroradiology 2001;43:702–711.
60. Koga M, Kimura K, Minematsu K, Yamaguchi T. Relationship between findings of conventional and contrast-enhanced transcranial color-coded real-time sonography and angiography in patients with basilar artery occlusion. AJNR Am J Neuroradiol 2002;23:568–571.
61. Gerriets T, Goertler M, Stolz E, et al. Feasibility and validity of transcranial duplex sonography in patients with acute stroke. J Neurol Neurosurg Psychiatry 2002;73:17–20.
62. Hansberg T, Wong KS, Droste DW, et al. Effects of the ultrasound contrast-enhancing agent Levovist on the detection of intracranial arteries and stenoses in Chinese by transcranial Doppler ultrasound. Cerebrovasc Dis 2002;14:105–108.
63. Totaro R, Marini C, Sacco S, et al. Contrast-enhanced transcranial Doppler sonography in patients with acute cerebrovascular diseases. Funct Neurol 2001;16:11–16.
64. Christou I, Burgin WS, Alexandrov AV, Grotta JC. Arterial status after intravenous TPA therapy for ischaemic stroke. A need for further interventions. Int Angiol 2001;20:208–213.
65. Christou I, Felberg RA, Demchuk AM, et al. Intravenous tissue plasminogen activator and flow improvement in acute ischemic stroke patients with internal carotid artery occlusion. J Neuroimaging 2002;12:119–123.
66. El-Mitwalli A, Saad M, Christou I, et al. Clinical and sonographic patterns of tandem internal carotid artery/middle cerebral artery occlusion in tissue plasminogen activator-treated patients. Stroke 2002;33:99–102.
67. Behrens S, Spengos K, Daffertshofer M, et al. Potential use of therapeutic ultrasound in ischemic stroke treatment. Echocardiography 2001;18:259–263.
68. Demchuk AM, Burgin WS, Christou I, et al. Thrombolysis in brain ischemia (TIBI) transcranial Doppler flow grades predict clinical severity, early recovery, and mortality in patients treated with intravenous tissue plasminogen activator. Stroke 2001;32:89–93.
69. Derex L, Tomsick TA, Brott TG, et al. Outcome of stroke patients without angiographically revealed arterial occlusion within four hours of symptom onset. AJNR Am J Neuroradiol 2001;22:685–690.

70. Qureshi AI. New grading system for angiographic evaluation of arterial occlusions and recanalization response to intra-arterial thrombolysis in acute ischemic stroke. Neurosurgery 2002;50: 1405–1414; discussion 1414–1415.
71. Iseda T, Nakano S, Yano T, et al. Time-threshold curve determined by single photon emission CT in patients with acute middle cerebral artery occlusion. AJNR Am J Neuroradiol 2002;23: 572–576.
72. Barthel H, Hesse S, Dannenberg C, et al. Prospective value of perfusion and X-ray attenuation imaging with single-photon emission and transmission computed tomography in acute cerebral ischemia. Stroke 2001;32:1588–1597.
73. Marchal G, Bouvard G, Iglesias S, et al. Predictive value of (99m)Tc-HMPAO-SPECT for neurological outcome/recovery at the acute stage of stroke. Cerebrovasc Dis 2000;10:8–17.
74. Heiss WD. Imaging the ischemic penumbra and treatment effects by PET. Keio J Med 2001;50:249–256.
75. Els T, Klisch J, Orszagh M, et al. Hyperglycemia in patients with focal cerebral ischemia after intravenous thrombolysis: influence on clinical outcome and infarct size. Cerebrovasc Dis 2002;13:89–94.
76. Parsons MW, Barber PA, Desmond PM, et al. Acute hyperglycemia adversely affects stroke outcome: a magnetic resonance imaging and spectroscopy study. Ann Neurol 2002;52: 20–28.
77. Capes SE, Hunt D, Malmberg K, et al. Stress hyperglycemia and prognosis of stroke in nondiabetic and diabetic patients: a systematic overview. Stroke 2001;32:2426–2432.
78. Bruno A, Levine SR, Frankel MR, et al. Admission glucose level and clinical outcomes in the NINDS rt-PA Stroke Trial. Neurology 2002;59:669–674.
79. Bushnell CD, Siddiqi Z, Goldstein LB. Improving patient selection for coagulopathy testing in the setting of acute ischemic stroke. Neurology 2001;57:1333–1335.
80. Bushnell C, Siddiqi Z, Morgenlander JC, Goldstein LB. Use of specialized coagulation testing in the evaluation of patients with acute ischemic stroke. Neurology 2001;56:624–627.
81. Berge E, Friis P, Sandset PM. Hemostatic activation in acute ischemic stroke. Thromb Res 2001;101:13–21.
82. Howard VJ, Sides EG, Newman GC, et al. Changes in plasma homocyst(e)ine in the acute phase after stroke. Stroke 2002;33:473–478.
83. Gariballa SE, Hutchin TP, Sinclair AJ. Antioxidant capacity after acute ischaemic stroke. Q J Med 2002;95:685–690.
84. Grau AJ, Reis A, Buggle F, et al. Monocyte function and plasma levels of interleukin-8 in acute ischemic stroke. J Neurol Sci 2001;192:41–47.
85. Ilzecka J, Stelmasiak Z. Increased serum levels of endogenous protectant secretory leukocyte protease inhibitor in acute ischemic stroke patients. Cerebrovasc Dis 2002;13:38–42.
86. Kouwenhoven M, Carlstrom C, Ozenci V, Link H. Matrix metalloproteinase and cytokine profiles in monocytes over the course of stroke. J Clin Immunol 2001;21:365–375.
87. Kozuka K, Kohriyama T, Nomura E, et al. Endothelial markers and adhesion molecules in acute ischemic stroke—sequential change and differences in stroke subtype. Atherosclerosis 2002;161:161–168.
88. Lip GY, Blann AD, Farooqi IS, et al. Abnormal haemorheology, endothelial function and thrombogenesis in relation to hypertension in acute (ictus <12 h) stroke patients: the West Birmingham Stroke Project. Blood Coagul Fibrinolysis 2001;12:307–315.
89. Lip GY, Blann AD, Farooqi IS, et al. Sequential alterations in haemorheology, endothelial dysfunction, platelet activation and thrombogenesis in relation to prognosis following acute stroke: The West Birmingham Stroke Project. Blood Coagul Fibrinolysis 2002;13:339–347.
90. Matsumori A, Takano H, Obata JE, et al. Circulating hepatocyte growth factor as a diagnostic marker of thrombus formation in patients with cerebral infarction. Circ J 2002;66:216–218.
91. McConnell JP, Cheryk LA, Durocher A, et al. Urinary 11-dehydro-thromboxane B(2) and coagulation activation markers measured within 24 h of human acute ischemic stroke. Neurosci Lett 2001;313:88–92.
92. Perini F, Morra M, Alecci M, et al. Temporal profile of serum anti-inflammatory and pro-inflammatory interleukins in acute ischemic stroke patients. Neurol Sci 2001;22:289–296.
93. Polidori MC, Cherubini A, Stahl W, et al. Plasma carotenoid and malondialdehyde levels in ischemic stroke patients: relationship to early outcome. Free Radic Res 2002;36:265–268.
94. Turaj W, Slowik A, Wyrwicz-Petkow U, et al. The prognostic significance of microalbuminuria in non-diabetic acute stroke patients. Med Sci Monit 2001;7:989–994.
95. Zaremba J, Losy J. sPECAM-1 in serum and CSF of acute ischaemic stroke patients. Acta Neurol Scand 2002;106:292–298.

96. Dahl T, Kontny F, Slagsvold CE, et al. Lipoprotein(a), other lipoproteins and hemostatic profiles in patients with ischemic stroke: the relation to cardiogenic embolism. Cerebrovasc Dis 2000;10:110–117.
97. Haapaniemi E, Tatlisumak T, Soinne L, et al. Plasminogen activator inhibitor-1 in patients with ischemic stroke. Acta Neurochir Suppl 2000;76:277–278.
98. Hill MD, Jackowski G, Bayer N, et al. Biochemical markers in acute ischemic stroke. CMAJ 2000;162:1139–1140.
99. Christensen H, Boysen G. Blood glucose increases early after stroke onset: a study on serial measurements of blood glucose in acute stroke. Eur J Neurol 2002;9:297–301.
100. Chamorro A, Obach V, Cervera A, et al. Prognostic significance of uric acid serum concentration in patients with acute ischemic stroke. Stroke 2002;33:1048–1052.
101. Waring WS. Uric acid: an important antioxidant in acute ischaemic stroke. Q J Med 2002;95:691–693.
102. Bitsch A, Horn C, Kemmling Y, et al. Serum tau protein level as a marker of axonal damage in acute ischemic stroke. Eur Neurol 2002;47:45–51.
103. Hesse C, Rosengren L, Vanmechelen E, et al. Cerebrospinal fluid markers for Alzheimer's disease evaluated after acute ischemic stroke. J Alzheimers Dis 2000;2:199–206.
104. Oh SH, Lee JG, Na SJ, et al. The effect of initial serum neuron-specific enolase level on clinical outcome in acute carotid artery territory infarction. Yonsei Med J 2002;43:357–362.
105. Montaner J, Alvarez-Sabin J, Molina C, et al. Matrix metalloproteinase expression after human cardioembolic stroke: temporal profile and relation to neurological impairment. Stroke 2001;32:1759–1766.
106. Green HA, Pena A, Price CJ, et al. Increased anisotropy in acute stroke: a possible explanation. Stroke 2002;33:1517–1521.
107. Mukherjee P, Bahn MM, McKinstry RC, et al. Differences between gray matter and white matter water diffusion in stroke: diffusion-tensor MR imaging in 12 patients. Radiology 2000; 215:211–220.
108. Wild JM, Wardlaw JM, Marshall I, Warlow CP. N-acetylaspartate distribution in proton spectroscopic images of ischemic stroke: relationship to infarct appearance on T2-weighted magnetic resonance imaging. Stroke 2000;31:3008–3014.
109. Kilpatrick MM, Yonas H, Goldstein S, et al. CT-based assessment of acute stroke: CT, CT angiography, and xenon-enhanced CT cerebral blood flow. Stroke 2001;32:2543–2549.
110. Johnston KC, Wagner DP, Haley EC Jr, Connors AF Jr. Combined clinical and imaging information as an early stroke outcome measure. Stroke 2002;33:466–472.

13
Thrombolytic Therapies

Fahmi M. Al-Senani and James C. Grotta

INTRAVENOUS THROMBOLYSIS

The proper use of intravenous (IV) recombinant tissue plasminogen activator (rt-PA) significantly prevents disability and increases the likelihood of independence after suffering an ischemic stroke. The idea of achieving arterial recanalization by using intravenously administered lytic therapy for the treatment of acute ischemic stroke has been around since the 1950s.[1] Success, however, did not occur until the use of modern more clot-selective lytic drugs and study design emphasizing careful patient selection, particularly early therapy. To date eight large-scaled IV thrombolysis trials have been reported (Table 13.1); five using IV rt-PA[2–5] and three[6–8] using streptokinase. All three streptokinase trials were stopped prematurely for safety concerns. Ten-day mortality rates for patients that received streptokinase were much higher (34 to 36%) than for those who received placebo (18 to 20%). Most deaths were secondary to intracranial hemorrhage (ICH).

Despite higher bleeding and mortality rates with streptokinase, several important observations were made in the streptokinase trials that suggested possible benefit for lytic therapy if the safety issue could be solved. In the survivors of the Multicenter Acute Stroke Trial-Europe Study Group (MAST-E) Trial there was a trend toward less severe disability at 6 months in the streptokinase group, indicating a possible benefit for thrombolysis. In the Multicenter Acute Stroke Trial-Italy (MAST-I) patients treated with streptokinase within 3 hours tended to fare better than those who received placebo. Although the streptokinase + aspirin (ASA) group had a higher 6-month fatality rate; they had the lowest rate of disability at 6 months. In the Australian Streptokinase (ASK) Trial, patients treated with streptokinase within 3 hours trended toward a more favorable outcome than those who received placebo, or those that received streptokinase after 3 hours. These results indicated a possible benefit for thrombolysis and a better response if thrombolysis was started earlier.

Table 13.1   Thrombolysis trials in acute ischemic stroke

Trial	Thrombolytic/Dose	Time Window	Mean Time to Treatment
NINDS part I[2]	rt-PA 0.9 mg/kg	<3 hr	119 min
NINDS part II[2]	rt-PA 0.9 mg/kg	<3 hr	119 min
ECASS 1[3]	rt-PA 1.1 mg/kg	<6 hr	264 min
ECASS 2[4]	rt-PA 0.9 mg/kg	<6 hr	NA
ATLANTIS[5]	rt-PA 0.9 mg/kg	3–5 hr*	268 min
MAST-E[6]	Streptokinase 1.5 million units	<6 hr	270 min
MAST-I[7]	Streptokinase 1.5 million units	<6 hr	NA
ASK[8]	Streptokinase 1.5 million units	<4 hr	208 min

ASK = Australian Streptokinase; ATLANTIS = Alteplase Thrombolytic for Acute Noninterventional Therapy in Ischemic Stroke; ECASS = European Cooperative Acute Stroke Study; MAST-E = Multicenter Acute Stroke Trial-Europe Study Group; MAST-I: Multicenter Acute Stroke Trial-Italy; NA = not applicable; NINDS = National Institute of Neurological Disorders and Stroke; rt-PA = recombinant tissue plasminogen activator.
*Initially 0–6 hr.

All five IV rt-PA trials were multicentered, randomized, placebo-controlled, and double-blinded. Only the National Institute of Neurological Disorders and Stroke (NINDS) Trials were unequivocally positive. One was stopped prematurely after futility analysis showed no benefit of rt-PA (Alteplase Thrombolysis for Acute Noninterventional Therapy in Ischemic Stroke [ATLANTIS]).

In the European Cooperative Acute Stroke Study (ECASS) Trials, patients were enrolled within 6 hours of symptoms. Exclusion criteria included massive strokes or computed tomography (CT) scan evidence of hemorrhage or major infarction involving one third or greater of the middle cerebral artery (MCA) territory. In ECASS 1,[3] 90-day mortality was greater in the rt-PA group (22%) than the placebo group (16%). However, when all patients that had "protocol violations" (these composed 17% of the study population) were excluded (and only the *target population* was studied) this difference became nonsignificant (19% vs. 15%). The was no difference in the modified Rankin Score (mRS) and the Scandinavian Stroke Scale between rt-PA and placebo groups in the intention-to-treat (ITT) analysis, but a significant improvement was seen in the target population. These findings indicated that strict adherence to study guidelines is imperative and this has been confirmed in all subsequent trials and postmarketing experience. On post hoc analysis, those treated with rt-PA within 3 hours were more likely to be independent than those who received placebo (46% vs. 21%), again indicating the great importance of early treatment.

In ECASS 2,[4] in which 80 percent of patients were treated in the 3 to 6 hour time window, a nonsignificant 3.7 percent absolute risk reduction was noted in those who received rt-PA (40.3% vs. 36.6%). Post hoc analysis using other clinical endpoints revealed an 8.3 percent absolute risk reduction in favor of those treated with rt-PA.

The ATLANTIS Trial,[5] which was originally a 0 to 6 hour trial, was modified midway through the trial. The 0 to 3 hour and later the 5- to 6-hour time periods were removed because of safety concerns and publication of the NINDS trial. Later the trial was discontinued after interim futility analysis indicated that the number of patients planned for the 3- to 5-hour time window would be insufficient to demonstrate benefit for rt-PA.

The NINDS part 1 and 2 Trials[2] were similar in inclusion and exclusion criteria. They differed only in their primary and secondary outcomes. They were later combined and results were stratified according to the length of time until treatment with rt-PA. The NINDS Trials differed from the ECASS Trials in two important aspects: All patients were treated within 3 hours (half 0 to 90 minutes and half 91 to 180 minutes poststroke symptom onset), and hemorrhage was the only CT scan exclusionary finding. The dose was 0.9 mg/kg (maximum 90 mg) given as a 10 percent bolus over 1 minute and 90 percent infused over 1 hour. Antiplatelets and anticoagulant were withheld for 24 hours after treatment. In part 1, the primary objective was to detect "early improvement," defined as complete resolution of neurological symptoms or an improvement in the National Institutes of Health Stroke Scale (NIHSS) by 4 points at 24 hours. In part 2, the primary objective was to measure functional outcome at 3 months.

In part 1, no difference was detected in the primary outcome at 24 hours. However, when part 1 and 2 studies were combined in post hoc analysis, an improvement was seen in median 24-hour NIHSS, in favor of the rt-PA treated patients; this was seen in both the 0 to 90 minute and 91 to 180 minute treatment intervals. In part 2 all functional 3-month outcome scales were significantly better in the rt-PA treated patients (Table 13.2). There was a 12 percent absolute increase in the number of patients with minimal or no disability at 3 months and a 32 percent relative risk reduction. In other words if 100 patients were treated with rt-PA and 100 with placebo, 12 more patients would be independent at 3 months. The number-needed-to-treat was 8.3.

The likelihood of a favorable outcome was significantly associated with earlier treatment. When adjusted for baseline NIHSS, patients treated at 60 minutes after symptoms were four times more likely to have a favorable outcome, whereas those treated 2 hours after symptom onset were about twice as likely to have a favorable outcome, compared with those that received placebo (Figure 13.1).[9]

Table 13.2 NINDS part 2

	% With a Favorable Outcome				
	rt-PA	Placebo	Odds Ratio	Relative Risk	p Value
Barthel index	50	38	1.6	1.3	0.026
Modified Rankin scale	39	26	1.7	1.5	0.019
Glasgow outcome scale	44	32	1.6	1.4	0.025
NIHSS	31	20	1.7	1.5	0.033

NIHSS = National Institutes of Health Stroke Scale; NINDS = National Institute of Neurological Disorders and Stroke; rtPA = recombinant tissue plasminogen activator.

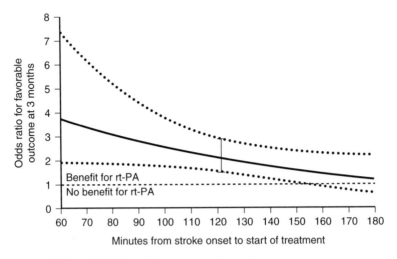

Figure 13.1   Odds ratio for favorable outcome at 3 months.

There was no significant difference in 3-month mortality between the treated and placebo groups (17% vs. 21%). Patients with small-vessel, large-vessel, and cardioembolic strokes that were treated with rt-PA all had better outcomes at 3 months compared with placebo-treated patients. Symptomatic hemorrhage occurred in 6.4 percent in the rt-PA group, compared with 0.6 percent in the placebo group. Patients with symptomatic hemorrhage were more likely to have higher NIHSS (median 20 vs. 14). Also patients with CT scan signs of early mass effect, hypodensity, and edema were 7.8 times more likely to develop symptomatic ICH.[10]

One might ask why only the NINDS trials showed such a positive result, whereas other thrombolytic trials were unsuccessful. The main reasons included restriction of patients to a shorter time window from symptom onset, a lower rt-PA dose, and strict adherence to all inclusion and exclusion criteria (Table 13.3). Adherence to these criteria remains essential for the safe and effective use of rt-PA in clinical practice.

Adherence to the 3-Hour Time Window

Obtaining the correct time-of-onset of symptoms is extremely important. Common pitfalls include assuming the time-of-onset of symptoms, in a patient who awakens with symptoms, as the time when he or she awakens; ischemia could have started immediately after a patient went to sleep. Thus the time the patient was *last seen normal* should be used as the time-of-onset of symptoms. Another difficult scenario is the patient with fluctuating symptoms; our common practice is to ascertain whether or not the patient's symptoms resolved completely between episodes. If symptoms resolved completely, the time-of-onset is defined by the onset of the latest (most recent) attack.

Table 13.3 Eligibility criteria for treatment of acute ischemic stroke with intravenous rt-PA

Inclusion criteria
Ischemic stroke onset time <3 hr (symptom onset to bolus time)
A deficit measurable on the NIHSS
No evidence of hemorrhage on CT scan

Exclusion criteria
Stroke or serious head trauma within 3 mo
Major surgery within 14 days
History of ICH
SBP >185 mm Hg or DBP >110 mm Hg, or aggressive lowering of BP to meet these limits
Rapidly improving or minor symptoms
Symptoms suggestive of SAH
GI or GU hemorrhage within 21 days
Arterial puncture within 7 days that is noncompressible
Seizure at the onset of stroke
Elevated PTT for patients on heparin
PT >15 sec
Platelet count <100,000/mm^2
Glucose <50 or >400 mg/dL

BP = blood pressure; CT = computed tomography; DBP = diastolic blood pressure; GI = gastrointestinal; GU = genitourinary; ICH = intracranial hemorrhage; NIHSS = National Institutes of Health Stroke Scale; PT = prothrombin time; PTT = partial thromboplastin time; SAH = syndrome of inappropriate secretion of antidiuretic hormone; SBP = systolic blood pressure.

Correct rt-PA Dose

Data from all the IV rt-PA trials and rt-PA dose escalation trials[11,12] have shown that stroke patients given rt-PA at a dose of 0.9 mg/kg are less likely to have ICH than those given a higher dose. In the dose escalation trials, higher doses were calculated on a mg/m^2 basis to decrease the total dose received by obese patients. These were later converted to a mg/kg dose with a maximum dose of 90 mg.

Strict Adherence to All Inclusion and Exclusion Criteria

Seventeen percent of patients entered into ECASS 1[3] should not have been randomized because of protocol violations. The mortality rate for protocol violators was 33 percent compared with only 15 percent for those treated with rt-PA who did not have protocol violation. Results from the rt-PA Stroke Survey[13] and the Calgary experience[14] have shown that rates of symptomatic ICH were as low as 4 and 5 percent, respectively. However, when protocol deviations occurred, symptomatic ICH rates increased to 11 and 27 percent, respectively. These results from postmarketing studies highlight the need for meticulous attention to detail when using thrombolytics. Using a checklist at the patient's bedside is helpful and may avoid overlooking important inclusion and exclusion criteria or emergent management issues (Table 13.4) such as blood pressure and rt-PA dosage.

Table 13.4   Treatment and management

Patient arrives in emergency department
Rapid triage (vital signs, glucose fingerstick, focused history and examination, NIHSS)
Place 2 IV lines and send blood to lab for stat Hct, platelet count, glucose, (and PT/PTT if the patient has recently received heparin or coumadin)
ECG
Place Foley catheter if needed
Emergent noncontrast CT scan to rule out ICH
Decision to treat (review all inclusion/exclusion criteria)
Discuss potential benefits and risks with patient and/or family
Administer rt-PA 0.9 mg/kg (max 90 mg)
Give 10% bolus over 1 minute and 90% infusion over 1 hr
Hold anticoagulant and antiplatelets for 24 hr
Always keep BP <185/110 mm Hg (labetalol, nicardipine)
Avoid unnecessary IV sticks or arterial lines for 24 hr
No urinary catheter insertion for 30 min after rt-PA infusion
No NG tubes for 24 hr
Admit patient to stroke unit or ICU for neurological and vital sign monitoring

BP = blood pressure; CT = computed tomography; ECG = electrocardiogram; Hct = hematocrit; ICU = intensive care unit; ICH = intracranial hemorrhage; IV = intravenous; NG = nasogastric; NIHSS = National Institutes of Health Stroke Scale; rt-PA = recombinant tissue plasminogen activator.

Although it is important to adhere to published guidelines when using IV rt-PA, there are several misperceptions that often lead to exclusion of appropriate patients. The most common is to exclude patients at either end of the stroke severity spectrum. An example is those patients with high NIHSS score or early ischemic changes on the CT scan. Although it is true that such patients have suffered severe strokes and usually do poorly whether or not they are treated, patients with early ischemic changes on CT but who fulfill all other criteria also benefit from IV rt-PA,[15] as do patients with high NIHSS scores.[16] Another situation in which appropriate patients are often excluded is when the stroke is mild. There were no NIHSS score cutoffs in the NINDS trial. Patients with low NIHSS scores were eligible and were often included. Recent studies have shown that a substantial portion of such patients deteriorate and do poorly without treatment.[17] A good rule of thumb is that regardless of the NIHSS score, if the deficit is severe enough to be disabling if it persisted, it is severe enough to benefit from treatment.

Translating the Trial Results to Clinical Practice

Evidence from the NINDS Trials that rt-PA is beneficial in acute ischemic stroke has not only placed rt-PA on the pharmacy's shelf for the emergent treatment of acute ischemic stroke but, more importantly, has established that patients can be identified in the field, transported by ambulance, triaged, have appropriate radiological and hematological workup, and be given IV rt-PA within 3 hours. This paradigm shift in the treatment of acute ischemic stroke has given local ambulance services, emergency medical staffs, radiologists, neurologists, and hospitals the responsibility to develop acute stroke treatment protocols for their individual communities. Only with cooperation of all involved specialties can the treatment of acute stroke be optimized. Education of all staff involved in the care of stroke patients is of paramount importance. Educational efforts directed at medical staff will increase the percentage of patients treated with rt-PA.[18] The study centers involved in the NINDS rt-PA Trial have published their experience in developing a systematic approach to acute stroke.[19] In our experience, a nurse practitioner's involvement in education and all aspects of stroke patient care is very valuable.

Accessibility of patients to treatment centers is of prime importance. In the United States only 1 to 2 percent of stroke patients are currently treated with IV rt-PA.[20] The development of a citywide stroke dispatch system has resulted in higher treatment rates. The designation of a stroke center and the development of a stroke triage system in Cologne, Germany has resulted in an increase in rt-PA treated patients from 1 to 5 percent,[21] and other experienced centers in the United States report treatment rates as high as 15 percent of all ischemic stroke patients.[22] A close relationship must be developed and fostered between designated stroke centers and the local ambulance services. More information regarding the rapid identification and treatment of acute ischemic stroke has been published by the NINDS.[23]

Real-World Experience with IV rt-PA–Phase IV Trials

In the controlled environment of a university or teaching hospital, and under tight scrutiny of a clinical trial, clinical outcomes are expected to be better than in a real-world setting. Many have questioned the reproducibility of thrombolysis trials in community hospitals.

Three community-based rt-PA observational studies have been reported.[24–26] The three phase IV trials adopted the NINDS criteria for treating patients with rt-PA. Although they had similar methodologies, caution must be taken when comparing clinical trials. The three phase IV trials did not have a control group; many of the centers taking part in these studies had vast experience in acute stroke care, and clinical outcomes are also expected to improve over time (NINDS patients were treated from 1991 to 1994, Canadian Activase for Stroke Effectiveness Study [CASES] from 1999 to 2002, Standard Treatment with Alteplase to Reverse Stroke [STARS] from 1997 to 1998, and Cologne from 1996 to 1998). Results are summarized in Table 13.5.

Many who question the safety of IV rt-PA often cite the Cleveland area experience[20] as proof that rt-PA cannot be given outside the realms of a stroke center. This survey was a retrospective analysis and less reliable than prospectively collected data.[24–26] Cases were collected from 29 different hospitals with stroke treatment rates ranging from 0 to 6 percent. Protocol violations occurred in 50 percent of those treated, and hemorrhage rates were 15.7 percent. The American Academy of Emergency Medicine published a Position Statement for the use of IV rt-PA for acute ischemic stroke. They stated that IV rt-PA for acute ischemic stroke cannot yet be classified as "standard of care."[27] A more practical statement was published by the Canadian Association of Emergency Physicians, with certain recommendations (Table 13.6) aimed at preventing protocol violations and the use of rt-PA by inexperienced physicians.[28]

Table 13.5 Results of phase IV postmarketing rt-PA trials

	Median Baseline NIHSS	Mean Time to Treatment (min)	Protocol Violations (%)	Mortality at 90 days (%)	Symptomatic ICH (%)	NIHSS 0–1 at 3 mo	Barthel 95–100 at 3 mo	Rankin 0–1 at 3 mo
NINDS placebo[2]	14	120	?	21	0.6	20	38	26
NINDS rt-PA[2]	14	120	?	17	6.4	31	50	39
Cologne[24]	12	124	2	12	5	42	53	40
STARS*[25]	13	164	32.6	13	3.3	NA	NA	35
CASES[26]	14	NA	10	22	4	31	NA	NA

CASES = Canadian Activase for Strjie Effectiveness Study; ICH = intracranial hemorrhage; NIHSS = National Institutes of Health Stroke Scale; NINDS = National Institute of Neurological Disorders and Stroke; rt-PA = recombinant tissue plasminogen activator; STARS = Standard Treatment with Alteplase to Reverse Stroke.

*30 day assessments.

Table 13.6 Recommendations of the Canadian Association of Emergency Physicians

Recommendation #1: Only radiologists or neurologists with demonstrated expertise in neuroradiology should provide interpretation of CT scans of the head used for the purpose of deciding whether to administer thrombolytic agents to stroke patients.
Recommendation #2: Stroke thrombolysis should be limited to centers with appropriate neurological and neuroimaging resources that are capable of administering this therapy within 3 hours. In such centers, emergency physicians should identify potential candidates, initiate low risk interventions and facilitate prompt CT scanning. They should not be the primary decision makers concerning the administration of thrombolytic agents to stroke patients. Neurologists should be directly involved before the administration of thrombolytic therapy.
Recommendation #3: Administration of thrombolytic agents to stroke patients should be carried out only in the setting of an approved research protocol or a formal clinical practice protocol. These protocols should adhere to the NINDS eligibility criteria. All data on adherence to protocols and patient outcomes should be collated in a central Canadian registry for the purposes of tracking the safety and efficacy of this intervention.

CT = computed tomography; NINDS = National Institute of Neurological Disorders and Stroke.

In summary, patients given IV rt-PA according to NINDS criteria fare much better than those that are not treated. However, adherence to these criteria requires careful evaluation preferably by physicians experienced in the management of stroke patients.

INTRA-ARTERIAL THROMBOLYSIS

The idea of performing an emergency angiogram and instilling a thrombolytic (and/or mechanical thrombolysis) is very fascinating and exciting. The ability to navigate a catheter to a diseased vessel, visualize the offending thrombus or embolus, and dissolve it with local thrombolytics is feasible and is commonly employed in many tertiary medical centers. Although many consider this approach still experimental, most experienced acute stroke teams have witnessed dramatic clinical improvement associated with successful intra-arterial (IA) thrombolysis, and clinical trials have suggested effectiveness in the treatment of carefully selected patients with acute ischemic stroke within 6 hours of symptom onset.

The major benefit of IV thrombolysis over IA therapy is the ability to start treatment very fast and the ability to deliver the treatment in centers that have CT capability but no endovascular expertise. IA therapy takes longer and requires an experienced endovascular team. Potential benefits of IA thrombolysis include actual visualization of the offending clot; detailed delineation of the intracranial circulation, especially the extent of collateral circulation (giving the treating physician an immediate, detailed description of the pathophysiology); use of smaller doses of thrombolytics; and the ability to assess the success and extent of thrombolysis (all of which can aid the treating physician in the subsequent care of the patient, in regard to hemodynamic management, anticoagulation, etc.). Furthermore, in patients with larger clots that are less likely to lyse after IV rt-PA, the IA approach provides the ability to alter the dose of thrombolytics or use mechanical dislocation of the clot, if necessary. Larger clots located in the internal carotid artery (ICA), basilar artery, and proximal intracranial arteries may not lyse with standard doses of IV rt-PA, and the IA approach may be the best means for achieving rapid recanalization in these patients in particular.

Although many of these aspects of acute IA therapy seem theoretically viable, the IA approach remains experimental and is not readily accessible to many stroke victims. Primary IA thrombolysis, "bridging" IV plus IA thrombolysis, or IV plus "rescue" IA thrombolytic techniques have been studied.

Primary Intra-arterial Thrombolysis Trials

Two randomized, placebo-controlled, multicentered trials of IA thrombolysis have been performed: Prolyse in Acute Cerebral Thromboembolism (PROACT) I and II.[29,30] PROACT I assessed the safety and recanalization rates of IA prourokinase (proUK) for MCA strokes within 6 hours of symptom onset. Patients had to have occlusions of the M1 or M2 segments of the MCA. A standard dose of proUK and IV heparin was given. Recanalization rates with proUK were 58 percent and only 14 percent with placebo at 120 minutes. Symptomatic hemorrhage rates were 15 percent in the proUK group versus 7 percent in the placebo group. The hemorrhage rate was significantly related to the dose of heparin used; thus the heparin doses were lowered during the trial.

In PROACT II,[30] an open-labeled, clinical efficacy trial, patients with MCA stroke were randomized 2:1 to proUK plus IV heparin versus IV heparin alone. Patients had a mean NIHSS of 17, and a mean symptom onset-to-treatment time of 5.3 hours. At 90 days, 40 percent of the proUK and 25 percent of the control patients ($p = 0.043$) had a modified Rankin score of 2 or less (normal to slight disability, but independent). Recanalization rates were 66 percent in the proUK group and 18 percent in the control group. Symptomatic ICH occurred in 10 percent of the proUK and 2 percent of the control patients. Mortality rates were similar. One finding in PROACT II was that only a small proportion of acute stroke patients met clinical and arteriographic criteria for IA treatment.

Intravenous Bridging Plus Intra-arterial Thrombolysis

Although recanalization rates are probably higher with IA compared with IV thrombolysis,[31] an unfortunate drawback of IA thrombolysis is the time delay from the decision to treat with IA thrombolytics until the IA infusion actually begins. It usually takes 70 to 120 minutes from acquisition of a CT scan until the IA thrombolytic infusion begins,[32] because of time delays involving mobilization of the angiography team. Patients who seem to be appropriate candidates for IA thrombolysis may be treated with IV rt-PA, with the intention that the IV rt-PA will start acting on the clot by the time the interventional team is organized and IA thrombolysis is started. Two sequential trials that addressed this issue were the Emergency Management of Stroke (EMS) Bridging Trial,[33] and Interventional Management of Stroke (IMS).[34]

In the EMS Trial[33] patients either received IV rt-PA and IA rt-PA (IV/IA) *or* IV placebo and IA rt-PA (placebo/IA) to assess the potential benefit of IV rt-PA before IA therapy. The IV rt-PA dose was 0.6 mg/kg in the EMS trial, 10 percent bolus, and then 30-minute infusion. Thirty-five patients were enrolled, 17 received both IV/IA rt-PA and 18 received placebo/IA rt-PA. Recanalization rates were higher in the IV/IA group compared with the placebo/IA group (Thrombolysis in Myocardial Ischemia [TIMI] 3 flow at 2 hours, 54% vs. 10%). There was no difference in the clinical outcomes in the two groups. Mortality was greater in the IV/IA group (5 vs. 1); the overall low number of deaths, and the incidence of non-thrombolysis–related deaths in the IV/IA group, makes interpreting causative mortality rates problematic. One patient in the IV/IA group died of an aortic dissection (that was the cause of his stroke), another died of breast cancer on day 87, and a third died from an acute MI after pulling out his femoral sheath and hemorrhaging. Symptomatic ICH occurred in 0 percent and 5.5 percent at 24 hours, and in 11.8 percent and 5.5 percent at 72 hours (in the IV/IA and placebo/IA groups, respectively). The authors stated that the combined treatment regimen is feasible and safe. Clinical outcomes could not be reliably determined because of small treatment numbers and the unbalanced randomization, with larger strokes assigned to the IV/IA group and more adverse events unrelated to treatment occurring in the IV/IA group.

Preliminary results of the larger, non-placebo–controlled, IMS Trial[34] are promising. Patients with MCA ischemic strokes with NIHSS of 10 or greater were treated with IV rt-PA (0.6 mg/kg), sent for an emergent angiogram, and given rt-PA intra-arterially if a clot was visualized. For patients with initial NIHSS of 10 or greater, 29 percent of patients treated in the IMS Trial had a Rankin score of 0 to 1 at 90 days, compared with 17 percent of the IV placebo patients in the NINDS trial. A time versus outcome effect was seen within the patients in the IMS Trial; those treated within 2 hours fared better than those treated after 2 hours. Time intervals to treatment were very good, with IA rt-PA given at approximately 3½ hours (Table 13.7). Symptomatic intracerebral hemorrhage rates were 6 percent in the IMS Trial, a rate that is acceptable with thrombolysis of large ischemic strokes.

A word of caution should be noted when comparing end points of different trials: There are inherent differences between the IV/IA trials (which generally include more severe strokes, with larger clot burdens) and IV only trials (which usually include less severe strokes), and thus comparing the results or complication rates of these different trials is erroneous. Another interesting observation has been made in the placebo arm of the ECASS I and II Trials; a good outcome was observed in 29 percent in part I and 37 percent in part II. Thus comparing trials may be dangerous, even if they are done only a few years apart and by the same investigators.

Table 13.7 IMS trial intervals

Onset to IV rt-PA	140 min
Onset to angiogram	183 min
Onset to IA rt-PA	212 min

IA = intra-arterial; IMS = Interventional Management of Stroke; IV = intravenous; rt-PA = recombinant tissue plasminogen activator.

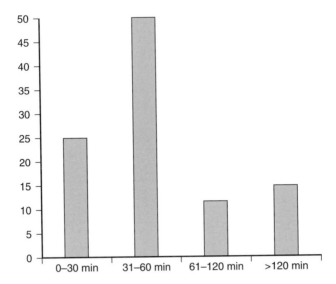

Figure 13.2 Recanalization rates after IV rt-PA.
(Reprinted with permission from Endo S, Kuwayama N, Hirashima Y, et al. Results of urgent thrombolysis in patients with major stroke and atherothrombotic occlusion of the cervical internal carotid artery. Am J Neuroradiol 1998;19:1169–1175.)

Intravenous Plus Rescue Intra-arterial Thrombolysis

A significant subgroup of patients with large-vessel ischemic lesions given IV thrombolytics do not recanalize, probably because the clot burden is too great, and the concentration of thrombolytics is too low to dissolve the clot before significant brain infarction occurs. Recanalization with IV rt-PA generally occurs 30 to 60 minutes after bolus (see Figure 13.2).[35] Furthermore, about 25 percent of those who recanalize will re-occlude. Three months after IV rt-PA, patients who recanalize fare better than those who do not (Figure 13.3); at 3 months

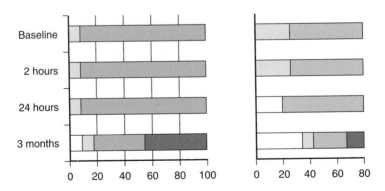

Figure 13.3 Outcomes correlated with recanalization.
(Reprinted with permission from Alexandrov AV, Grotta JC. Arterial reocclusion in stroke patients treated with intravenous tissue plasminogen activator. Neurology 2002;59:862–867.)

Table 13.8   IA retevase protocol for ischemic stroke

Dilute 1 unit in 5 cc NS
Infuse 1 cc/min
Repeat angiogram at 10, 20, 25, and 30 min, then every 5–10 min
Max dose:
  8 units/vessel
  10 units/2 vessels
  6 units w/IV tPA
Use of mechanical disruption is allowed
Give heparin 2000 units bolus, then 450 units/hr for duration of procedure

IA = intra-arterial; IV = intravenous; NS = normal saline.

approximately 50 percent of those who recanalize have a modified Rankin score of 0 to 1, compared with less than 10 percent of those who do not recanalize.[36]

Because of the possible added benefit of IA therapy to achieve lysis and prevent re-occlusion, in some centers certain patients receive rescue IA thrombolysis, in which patients are offered IA therapy in addition to conventional IV rt-PA. In our institution, we inform and mobilize the angiography team for all acute stroke patients with NIHSS greater than 10, because NIHSS scores above 10 are associated with a >90 percent probability of visualizing a clot on initial angiography. In most cases, patients will receive full dose IV rt-PA. We will consider adjunctive IA therapy as long as there is the potential to reach the clot with a catheter within 5 hours of symptom onset and the CT scan does not show advanced ischemic changes. We have adopted an IA protocol similar to that used by Qureshi et al[37] (Table 13.8).

The availability of emergent transcranial Doppler (TCD) ultrasound is a valuable tool that can add a great deal of information in the acute setting, particularly for selecting patients for such rescue IA therapy. Neurological changes can be correlated with the flow status in the responsible vessel. If symptoms and TCD signals do not improve within 30 minutes, the patient may be eligible for emergent rescue IA thrombolysis.

More recently, mechanical thrombolysis, including balloon angioplasty, has been used to dislodge clot distally and to increase the surface area of the clot, thus giving thrombolytic drugs more surface area to lyse.[38] Retevase is used intra-arterially because faster recanalization rates have been documented in the coronary literature and in our own anecdotal experience. Retevase is given distal to, in, and proximal to the clot itself. Many other endovascular techniques and thrombolytics are under study, including external (TCD) and IA ultrasound, IA lasers, mechanical snares, and other mechanical devices. Unfortunately, currently no head-to-head analysis of different techniques or combination of techniques and thrombolytics has been published to guide treatment selection.

CONCLUSION

IV and probably IA thrombolysis provide the medical community and their patients the first real opportunity to improve outcome after stroke beyond what can be achieved by good nursing care and rehabilitation. The success of the

NINDS studies in particular provide hope that other therapies based on achieving early restoration of perfusion will be successful, particularly if they increase the speed, completeness, and safety of achieving arterial recanalization. However, to use this treatment effectively and safely, it is critical to treat patients urgently and to adhere to established treatment guidelines.

References

1. Sussman BJ, Fitch TS. Thrombolysis with fibrinolysin in cerebral arterial occlusion. JAMA 1958;167:1705–1709.
2. The National Institute of Neurological Disorders and Stroke (NINDS). rt-PA Stroke Study Group: tissue plasminogen activator for acute ischemic stroke. N Engl J Med 1995;333:1581–1587.
3. Hacke W, Kaste M, Fieschi C, et al. Intravenous thrombolysis with recombinant tissue plasminogen activator for acute hemispheric stroke: the European Cooperative Acute Stroke Study (ECASS). JAMA 1995;274:1017–1025.
4. Hacke W, Kaste M, Fieschi C, et al. Randomised double-blind placebo-controlled trial of thrombolytic therapy with intravenous alteplase in acute ischemic stroke (ECASS II). Lancet 1998;352:1245–1251.
5. Clark WM, Wissman S, Albers G, et al. Recombinant tissue-type plasminogen activator (Alteplase) for ischemic stroke 3 to 5 hours after symptom onset. The ATLANTIS Study: a randomized controlled trial. Alteplase thrombolysis for acute noninterventional therapy in ischemic stroke. JAMA 1999;282:2019–2026.
6. The Multicenter Acute Stroke Trial-Europe Study Group (MAST-E). Thrombolytic therapy with streptokinase in acute ischemic stroke. N Engl J Med 1996;335:145–150.
7. Multicenter Acute Stroke Trial-Italy (MAST-I) Group. Randomized controlled trial of streptokinase, aspirin, and combination of both in treatment of acute ischaemic stroke. Lancet 1995; 346:1509–1514.
8. Donnan GA, Davis SM, Chambers BR, et al. Streptokinase for acute ischemic stroke with relationship to time of administration: Australian Streptokinase (ASK) Trial Study Group. JAMA 1996;276:961–966.
9. Marler JR, Tilley BC, Lu M, et al. Early stroke treatment associated with better outcome: The NINDS rt-PA Stroke Study. Neurology 2000;55:1649–1655.
10. The NINDS rt-PA Stroke Study Group. Intracerebral hemorrhage after intravenous t-PA therapy for ischemic stroke. Stroke 1997;28:2109–2118.
11. Brott TG, Haley EC, Levy DE, et al. Urgent therapy for stroke part I. Pilot study of tissue plasminogen activator administered within 90 minutes. Stroke 1992;23:632–640.
12. Haley EC, Levy DE, Brott TG, et al. Urgent therapy for stroke part II. Pilot study of tissue plasminogen activator administered 91-180 minutes from onset. Stroke 1992;23: 641–645.
13. Tanne D, Bates VE, Verro P, et al. Initial clinical experience with IV tissue plasminogen activator for acute ischemic stroke: a multicenter survey. The t-PA Stroke Survey Group. Neurology 1999;53:424–427.
14. Buchan AM, Barbar PA, Newcommon N, et al. Effectiveness of t-PA in acute ischemic stroke: outcome relates to appropriateness. Neurology 2000;54:679–684.
15. Patel SC, Levine Sr, Tilley BC, et al. Lack of clinical significance of early ischemic changes on computed tomography in acute stroke. JAMA 2001;286:2830–2838.
16. The NINDS t-PA Stroke Study Group. Generalized efficacy of t-PA for acute stroke. Stroke 1997;28:2119–2125.
17. Barber PA, Zhang J, Demchuk AM, et al. Why are stroke patients excluded from TPA therapy? Neurology 2001;56:1015–1020.
18. Morgenstern LB, Straub L, Chan W, et al. Improving delivery of acute stroke therapy: the TLL Temple Foundation Stroke Project. Stroke 2002;33:160–166.
19. The National Institute of Neurological Disorders and Stroke (NINDS) rt-PA Stroke Study Group. A systems approach to immediate evaluation and management of hyperacute stroke experience at eight centers and implications for community practice and patient care. Stroke 1997;28: 1530–1540.
20. Katzan IL, Furlan AJ, Lloyd LE, et al. Use of tissue-type plasminogen activator for acute ischemic stroke. The Cleveland Area Experience. JAMA 2000;283:1151–1158.

21. Grond M, Stenzel C, Schmulling S, et al. Early intravenous thrombolysis for acute ischemic stroke in community based approach. Stroke 1998;29:1544–1549.
22. Grotta JC, Burgin WS, El-Mitwalli A, et al. Intravenous tissue-type plasminogen activator therapy for ischemic stroke: Houston experience 1996-2000. Arch Neurol 2001;58:2009–2013.
23. Marler JR, Jones PW, Emr M. Proceedings of a National Symposium on Rapid Identification and Treatment of Acute Stroke. Bethesda, Md: The National Institute of Neurological Disorders and Stroke, National Institute of Health, 1997 (http://www.ninds.nih.gov/health_and_medical/stroke_proceedings/titlepage.htm).
24. Schmulling S, Grond M, Rudolf J, et al. One year follow up in acute stroke patients treated with rt-PA in clinical routine. Stroke 2000;31:1552–1554.
25. Hill D, Woolfendeu A, Teal PA, et al. Intravenous alteplase for stroke: the Canadian experience. Stroke Intervent 2000;2:3–8.
26. Albers GW, Bates VE, Clark W, et al. Intravenous tissue-type plasminogen activator for treatment of acute stroke: the Standard Treatment with Alteplase to Reverse Stroke (STARS) Study. JAMA 2000;283:1145–1150.
27. The Work Group on Thrombolytic Therapy in Stroke. Position statement on the use of intravenous thrombolytic therapy in the treatment of stroke (www.aaem.org/positionstatements/thrombolytic-therapy.shtml).
28. The CAEP Committee on Thrombolytic Therapy for Acute Ischemic Stroke. Position statement on thrombolytic therapy for acute ischemic stroke. CJEM 2001;3:8–14.
29. del Zoppo GJ, Higashida RT, Furlan AJ, et al. PROACT: A phase II randomized trial of recombinant pro-urokinase by direct arterial delivery in acute middle cerebral artery stroke. PROACT Investigators. Prolyse in Acute Cerebral Thromboembolism. Stroke; 1998;29:4–11.
30. Furlan A, Higashida RT, Wechsler L, et al. Intra-arterial prourokinase for acute ischemic stroke. The PROACT II study: a randomized controlled trial. Prolyse in Acute Cerebral Thromboembolism. JAMA 1999;282:2003–2011.
31. Endo S, Kuwayama N, Hirashima Y, et al. Results of urgent thrombolysis in patients with major stroke and atherothrombotic occlusion of the cervical internal carotid artery. Am J Neuroradiol 1998;19:1169–1175.
32. Kalafut MA, Saver JL. The Acute Stroke Patient: The First Six Hours. In SN Cohen (ed), Management of Ischemic Stroke. New York: McGraw-Hill, 2000;17–52.
33. Lewandowski CA, Frankel M, Tomsick TA. Combined intravenous and intra-arterial r-TPA versus intra-arterial therapy of acute ischemic stroke. Emergency Management of Stroke (EMS) Bridging Trial. Stroke 1999;30:2598–2605.
34. Broderick J for the IMS Study Investigators. The Interventional Management of Stroke (IMS) Study: Preliminary Results. Presented at the 7th International Symposium in Thrombolysis and Acute Stroke Therapy, May 27, 2002, Lyon, France.
35. Christou I, Alexandrov AV, Burgin WS, et al. Timing of recanalization after tissue plasminogen activator therapy determined by transcranial Doppler correlates with clinical recovery from ischemic stroke. Stroke 2000;31:1812–1816.
36. Alexandrov AV, Grotta JC. Arterial reocclusion in stroke patients treated with intravenous tissue plasminogen activator. Neurology 2002;59:862–867.
37. Qureshi AI, Siddiqui AM, Suri MF, et al. Aggressive mechanical clot disruption and low-dose intra-arterial third-generation thrombolytic agent for ischemic stroke: a prospective study. Neurosurgery 2002;51:1319–1329.
38. Song JK, Cacayorin ED, Campbell MS, et al. Intracranial balloon angioplasty of acute terminal internal carotid artery occlusions. AJNR 2002;23:1308–1312.

14
Antithrombotic Therapy for Acute Ischemic Stroke

Brett L. Cucchiara and Scott E. Kasner

The rationale for use of antithrombotic therapy in acute cerebrovascular ischemia is multifaceted (1) to prevent recurrent thrombosis in recanalized vessels, (2) to halt thrombus propagation in partially occluded and collateral vessels, (3) to prevent recurrent embolization, (4) to prevent noncerebral thrombotic complications (i.e., deep venous thrombosis, pulmonary emboli, myocardial infarction [MI]), and (5) possibly to augment the body's intrinsic fibrinolytic mechanisms. The various available antithrombotic therapies target different steps in the coagulation pathway, and this heterogeneity of mechanism of action may have implications for their effectiveness at achieving the these goals and their risk of causing untoward side effects, primarily bleeding (Table 14.1).

Most acute antithrombotic therapies were initially developed for or tested in patients with coronary syndromes, and a large body of data has proven the benefit of a number of these agents in this population. However, important differences between cerebral and coronary ischemia exist, and extrapolation from trials in one disease process to the other, although intuitively appealing, has significant limitations. One such difference is that the mechanisms of vascular occlusion in ischemic stroke are heterogeneous. For instance, vascular occlusion resulting from a cardiac embolus rich in fibrin and erythrocytes is distinct from thrombus formation at the site of an unstable atherosclerotic plaque, which is distinct from lacunar infarction resulting from lipohyalinosis. In contrast, acute coronary syndromes are consistently due to a single mechanism: rupture of an atherosclerotic plaque and superimposed local thrombus formation. A second major difference is that the risk of hemorrhagic complications, in particular intracranial hemorrhage (ICH), appears to be much higher in stroke patients. This is most clearly illustrated by the rate of ICH following use of intravenous (IV) tissue plasminogen activator (t-PA) (<1% in patients with MI compared with >6% in patients with stroke) but applies consistently to all antithrombotic therapies to a greater or lesser degree. Possible explanations for

Table 14.1 Currently available antithrombotic agents with potential use in acute ischemic stroke

Oral antiplatelet agents	Heparins
Aspirin	Unfractionated heparin
Ticlopidine	Low-molecular-weight heparins
Clopidogrel	Dalteparin
Dipyridamole	Enoxaparin
Glycoprotein IIb/IIIa inhibitors	Tinzaparin
Abciximab	Heparinoids
Tirofiban	Danaparoid
Eptifibatide	Direct thrombin inhibitors
	Argatroban
	Bivalirudin
	Lepirudin

this difference in hemorrhage risk include a greater prevalence of hypertension and underlying chronic ischemic brain injury in stroke patients, early cerebral edema and breakdown of the blood-brain barrier as a consequence of acute cerebral infarction, and the generally older age of stroke patients.

ORAL ANTIPLATELET AGENTS

Aspirin

Aspirin irreversibly inhibits cyclooxygenase, thus blocking production of thromboxane A_2, an important promoter of platelet activation. The antiplatelet effect of aspirin occurs within 1 hour of oral administration and, being irreversible, persists for the entire platelet life span. Evidence supporting a beneficial effect of aspirin in patients with acute stroke comes primarily from two very large, randomized trials and one much smaller trial.

1. International Stroke Trial (IST)
   IST randomized 19,435 patients with acute ischemic stroke to receive aspirin 300 mg daily or to avoid aspirin.[1] This trial was performed simultaneously with an analysis of acute heparin therapy (described later), so half of the patients also received one of two doses of subcutaneous (SQ) heparin. Investigators were not blinded to treatment assignment. Therapy was initiated within 48 hours of symptom onset and continued for 14 days or until hospital discharge. Aspirin reduced the risk of recurrent ischemic stroke from 3.9 percent to 2.8 percent ($p < 0.05$). There was a nonsignificant (NS) reduction in 14-day mortality favoring aspirin (9.0% vs. 9.4%, NS). There was no significant increase in the rate of intracerebral hemorrhage in patients treated with aspirin (0.9% vs. 0.8%, NS). The combined endpoint of death or nonfatal stroke was reduced from 12.4 percent to 11.3 percent ($p < 0.05$). At 6 months, there was a trend toward a lower percentage of aspirin-treated

patients being dead or dependent (62.2% vs. 63.5%, $p = 0.07$, a difference of 13 per 1000). Overall, aspirin use offered a small but significant benefit when started within the first 48 hours after stroke onset.

2. Chinese Acute Stroke Trial (CAST)

In CAST, 21,106 patients with acute ischemic stroke were given either aspirin 160 mg daily or placebo within 48 hours after the onset of symptoms. Treatment was continued for 4 weeks or until hospital discharge, whichever came first.[2] Aspirin reduced the risk of recurrent ischemic stroke from 2.1 percent to 1.6 percent ($p = 0.01$) and mortality from 3.9 percent to 3.3 percent ($p = 0.04$). There was a small, NS increased risk of hemorrhagic stroke in patients who received aspirin (1.1% vs. 0.9%, NS). The combined endpoint of death or nonfatal stroke was reduced from 5.9 percent to 5.3 percent ($p = 0.03$), and the proportion of patients dead or dependent was reduced from 31.6 percent to 30.5 percent ($p = 0.08$), comparable to the results seen in IST.

3. CAST + IST meta-analysis

A prospectively planned meta-analysis of the individual patient data from CAST and IST focused on events occurring during the treatment period (4 weeks in CAST, 2 weeks in IST) has been performed. This showed a reduction in recurrent ischemic stroke of 7 per 1000 (1.6% vs. 2.3%, $p < 0.000001$) and a reduction in death without further stroke of 4 per 1000 (5.0% vs. 5.4%, $p = 0.05$). An increase in hemorrhagic stroke or transformation of 2 per 1000 was also identified (1.0% vs. 0.9%, $p = 0.07$). Overall, aspirin therapy resulted in a net decrease in the overall risk of further stroke or death in the hospital of 9 per 1000 (8.2% vs. 9.1%, $p = 0.001$). The treatment effect was similar in all subgroups analyzed with no differential effectiveness by age, sex, level of consciousness, atrial fibrillation, computed tomography (CT) findings, blood pressure, stroke subtype, or concomitant heparin use.[3]

4. Multicentre Acute Stroke Trial-Italy (MAST-I)

In MAST-I, patients were randomized to streptokinase, aspirin, the combination of streptokinase and aspirin, or neither. Treatment with aspirin was started within 6 hours of symptom onset and continued for 10 days. A comparison of the aspirin alone group ($n = 153$) with the group that received placebo only ($n = 156$) showed a small benefit in favor of aspirin, but this was not statistically significant. Specifically, the 10-day case fatality rate was 10 percent in the aspirin group and 13 percent in the placebo group, and the 6 month composite outcome of case fatality or disability was 61 percent versus 68 percent in favor of aspirin. No significant increased risk of ICH was observed with aspirin therapy. It must be emphasized that the sample size in MAST-I was very small, none of the findings were statistically significant, and the placebo group received no aspirin for the first 10 days following stroke onset.[4]

Effect of Time to Treatment on Aspirin Efficacy

Although both CAST and IST enrolled patients within 48 hours of stroke onset, a significant number of patients were treated in the hyperacute period. Combining the two studies, about 1700 patients were randomized in <3 hours, and almost 3900 patients randomized within 3 to 6 hours of symptom onset. A prespecified combined analysis of the CAST and IST data showed a relatively consistent treatment effect size regardless of time to treatment.[3] On the basis of the available evidence, therefore, the beneficial effect of aspirin in acute stroke does not appear to be critically time dependent, unlike thrombolytic therapy.

Efficacy of Aspirin in Acute Stroke Compared with Myocardial Infarction

The benefit of early aspirin therapy in patients with acute stroke may be less robust than that seen in acute MI. The International Study of Infarct Survival 2 (ISIS-2) Trial randomized 17,187 patients within 24 hours of suspected acute MI to four arms in a fashion similar to MAST-I.[5] A comparison of the aspirin-only to the placebo-only arms showed a substantial, highly significant mortality reduction at 5 weeks in favor of aspirin (9.4% vs. 11.8%, $p < 0.00001$), as well as a reduction in nonfatal recurrent MI (1.0% vs. 2.0%, $p < 0.00001$) and non-fatal stroke (0.3% vs. 0.6%, $p < 0.01$). There was no excess of intracranial or systemic hemorrhage in the aspirin group. ISIS-2 showed that treatment of 1000 patients with acute MI with aspirin would prevent 25 deaths and 10 to 15 nonfatal recurrent vascular events (MI or stroke) at 5 weeks. Thus aspirin treatment in the setting of MI resulted in a decrease of 35 to 40 per 1000 in the overall risk of recurrent MI, stroke, or death. This is roughly four times the benefit seen with aspirin therapy in acute stroke in the pooled analysis of CAST and IST.

This may be partially due to a greater mortality rate following MI than stroke, providing greater statistical power to confirm efficacy. Arguing against this explanation, however, is the fact that the mortality rate in IST (9.0% to 9.4%) at 14 days was comparable to the 5-week mortality rate in ISIS-2 (9.4% to 11.8%).

Safety of Aspirin in Patients with Intracranial Hemorrhage

In CAST, patients could be randomized without a CT scan provided the patient was not comatose and the investigator was *reasonably certain* that hemorrhagic stroke could be excluded. Similar inclusion criteria were used in IST. A pre-specified combined analysis of the patients in both CAST and IST who had ICH and were inadvertently randomized ($n = 773$) did not show evidence of benefit or harm with aspirin treatment. The frequency of further stroke or death (within 4 weeks in CAST, 2 weeks in IST) was 16 percent in the aspirin group and 18 percent in the placebo group.[3] Longer term outcome data available for the 597 patients with hemorrhage enrolled in IST similarly showed no clear benefit or harm with aspirin (dead or dependent at 6 months: 76% aspirin vs. 82% placebo.)

It must be recognized that the population of patients with ICH inadvertently treated with aspirin in IST and CAST was not equivalent to a population of unselected patients with ICH seen in routine clinical practice. If prerandomization CT scanning could not be performed in CAST or IST, investigators used clinical judgment (history, physical examination, and risk factor profile) to select patients unlikely to have ICH. Of the 8889 patients randomized before CT, only 773 (8.7%) were subsequently determined to have an ICH, suggesting that investigators were remarkably accurate at making this determination. Most likely, patients with ICH enrolled in CAST and IST had small hemorrhages and/or an atypical presentation. It seems unwise to interpret the results of IST and CAST as a blanket endorsement of the safety of aspirin in patients with ICH.

Other Antiplatelet Agents/Combination Oral Antiplatelet Therapy

There is little data regarding the use of antiplatelet agents other than aspirin (i.e., dipyridamole, a phosphodiesterase inhibitor, and ticlopidine and clopidogrel, adenosine diphosphate [ADP] receptor blockers) in the treatment of patients with acute stroke. Data on combination aspirin and clopidogrel therapy in patients with acute coronary syndromes may have some potential relevance but have important limitations. The Clopidogrel in Unstable Angina to Prevent Recurrent Events (CURE) trial randomized 12,563 patients with unstable angina or non-Q wave MI to combination therapy with aspirin and clopidogrel versus aspirin alone. Treatment was begun within 24 hours of symptom onset.[6] Clopidogrel was given as a 300-mg loading dose, because several days are required to achieve maximal platelet inhibition when started at the usual daily dose of 75 mg/day. The primary outcome (cardiovascular death, MI, and stroke) occurred in 11.4 percent of patients on aspirin versus 9.3 percent of those receiving combination therapy, a 20 percent relative risk reduction ($p < 0.001$). However, a 1.0 percent increase (2.7% aspirin, 3.7% aspirin plus clopidogrel, $p = 0.001$) in major hemorrhage in the combination therapy group was identified. Application of the CURE trial results to acute stroke patients is inappropriate given that stroke patients have a higher risk of ICH complicating antithrombotic therapies and may have a differential response to antithrombotic agents compared with patients with coronary ischemia.[7] The increased risk of hemorrhage seen in CURE must be considered a strong cautionary note given the previously noted distinctions between acute coronary syndromes and acute ischemic stroke.

Practical Implications

Aspirin 160 to 300 mg/day started within 48 hours of ischemic stroke is of modest but significant benefit and should be administered early to most ischemic stroke patients (Table 14.2 and Figure 14.1). No particular subgroup of patients has been shown to receive greater or lesser benefit from aspirin. Because there does not appear to be any advantage to hyperacute treatment with aspirin, we do not advocate immediate aspirin therapy until CT scanning can be performed to rule out ICH, provided such facilities are available within a reasonable time frame. For the aspirin-allergic patient, it appears reasonable to treat acutely with clopidogrel. In this situation, clopidogrel should probably be given initially as a loading dose of 300 mg/day, followed by the usual 75 mg daily dose. Combinations of antiplatelet drugs cannot be recommended in the acute setting at this time.

Table 14.2   Effect of various therapies for treatment of acute stroke

Agent	Trial	Outcome	Effect
Aspirin	IST	Hemorrhagic stroke at 2 wk	Harm of 1 per 1000 (NS)
		Death or nonfatal stroke at 2 wk	Benefit of 11 per 1000 ($p < 0.05$)
		Dead or dependent at 6 mo	Benefit of 13 per 1000 ($p = 0.07$)
	CAST	Hemorrhagic stroke at 2 wk	Harm of 2 per 1000 (NS)
		Death or nonfatal stroke at 1 mo	Benefit of 7 per 1000 ($p = 0.03$)
		Dead or dependent at 1 mo	Benefit of 11 per 1000 ($p = 0.08$)
Heparin (any dose)	IST	Recurrent ischemic stroke at 2 wk	Benefit of 9 per 1000 ($p < 0.01$)
		Hemorrhagic stroke at 2 wk	Harm of 8 per 1000 ($p < 0.00001$)
		Major extracranial hemorrhage	Harm of 9 per 1000 ($p < 0.00001$)
		Pulmonary embolism	Benefit of 3 per 1000 ($p < 0.05$)
		Death or nonfatal stroke at 2 wk	Benefit of 4 per 1000 (NS)
		Dead or dependent at 6 mo	No effect (0 per 1000, NS)
Heparin 5000 U bid	IST	Recurrent ischemic stroke at 2 wk	Benefit of 12 per 1000 ($p < 0.001$)
		Hemorrhagic stroke at 2 wk	Harm of 3 per 1000 ($p < 0.05$)
		Major extracranial hemorrhage	Harm of 2 per 1000 (NS)
		Pulmonary embolism	Benefit of 12 per 1000 (NS)
		Death or nonfatal stroke at 2 wk	Benefit of 12 per 1000 ($p < 0.05$)
		Dead or dependent at 6 mo	Harm of 2 per 1000 (NS)

CAST = Chinese Acute Stroke Trial; IST = International Stroke Trial; NS = nonsignificant.

HEPARINS

Both unfractionated heparin (UFH) and low-molecular-weight heparins (LMWH) bind the serine protease inhibitor antithrombin III and dramatically accelerate its inhibitory binding effect on thrombin and factor Xa. This neutralization accounts for their anticoagulant effects. LMWH and UFH differ in their relative inhibition of thrombin and factor Xa, with LMWH more potently inhibiting factor Xa. Because factor Xa plays a role early in the coagulation cascade, it is thought that this "upstream" inhibition may have a greater antithrombotic effect by attenuating the amplification loops that occur with subsequent stages of coagulation activation. Clinical trials in patients with acute coronary syndromes have provided some evidence to suggest greater efficacy for LMWH (particularly enoxaparin) over UFH, although this has not been universal.[8–10] There may be a slightly greater risk of hemorrhagic complications with LMWH compared with UFH in this population.[11] Practical advantages of LMWH over UFH include simpler dosing regimens (SQ vs. IV, once or twice daily with fixed doses vs. continuous dose-adjusted infusion) without the need for laboratory monitoring.

Unfractionated Heparin

Heparin Trials in the Pre-Computed Tomography Era

Early trials of anticoagulation in acute stroke did not suggest a benefit for UFH therapy, with the possible exception of patients with progressing stroke.[12–14]

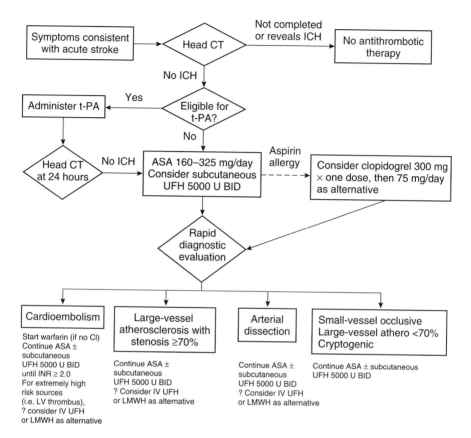

Figure 14.1 Flow chart: a practical approach to decisions about acute antithrombotic therapy. ASA = aspirin/acetylsalicylic acid; CI = contraindication; ICH = intracerebral hemorrhage; LMWH = low-molecular-weight heparins/heparinoids; LV = left ventricle; t-PA = tissue plasminogen activator; UFH = unfractionated heparin.

Interpretation of these studies is limited by design flaws, performance before reliable diagnosis of ICH with CT, and use of older heparin dosing regimens.

Cerebral Embolism Study Group

The Cerebral Embolism Study Group (CESG) randomized 45 patients with cardioembolic ischemic stroke to dose-adjusted IV heparin (partial thromboplastin time [PTT] 1.5 to 2.5 times baseline) or placebo for 10 days.[15] Treatment was started within 48 hours of stroke onset. Of the 21 patients in the placebo group, 2 experienced recurrent embolization and 2 developed delayed hemorrhagic infarction, compared with none of the 24 patients treated with heparin. Limitations of this study include the small sample size and the avoidance of all antithrombotic therapy (i.e., aspirin, low-dose SQ heparin) in the placebo group. Nevertheless, many authors have recommended use of IV heparin in patients with cardioembolic stroke based on these findings.

Acute Partial Stroke

In 1986, Duke et al[16] reported the results of a double-blind randomized study of IV dose-adjusted heparin in 225 patients with acute stroke. This remains the largest randomized trial of IV dose-adjusted heparin performed to date. The study enrolled patients with noncardioembolic "partial" completed stroke within 48 hours of symptom onset, and treatment was continued for 7 days. Partial stroke was defined as motor weakness such that the combined flexor strength of the proximal muscle groups on the paretic side added up to at least 5 on the United Kingdom's Medical Research Council scale (this would be roughly equivalent to a National Institutes of Health Stroke Scale [NIHSS] total motor score, as measured by items 5 and 6, of ≤4). No difference was seen between the placebo and heparin groups in terms of degree of neurological change; stroke progression over 7 days; or functional level at 7 days, 3 months, or 1 year after treatment. A significantly greater number of heparin-treated patients died within the year after stroke, but because these deaths occurred 3 to 12 months after stroke onset it seems unlikely this was related to treatment.

International Stroke Trial

IST was the first major multicenter, randomized trial to evaluate heparin in acute ischemic stroke.[1] This study enrolled 19,435 patients within 48 hours of stroke onset and made no specific requirements regarding stroke etiology, vascular distribution, or likelihood of progression at baseline. Patients received either 12,500 U SQ heparin twice daily or 5000 U twice daily or were assigned to "avoid heparin" for a course of 14 days or until hospital discharge, if sooner. This trial was performed simultaneously with an analysis of acute aspirin therapy (described previously), so half the patients also received aspirin. The rate of recurrent ischemic stroke at 14 days in the patients allocated heparin (either dose) was significantly reduced (2.9% vs. 3.8%), but the rate of hemorrhagic stroke was increased equivalently (1.2% vs. 0.4%). There was no difference in death or nonfatal recurrent stroke at 14 days between the heparin and no heparin groups (11.7% vs. 12.0%), and no difference in number dead or dependent at 6 months (62.9% for both groups). Treatment with heparin resulted in a 9 per 1000 excess of transfused or fatal extracranial bleeding. There was no subgroup of patients that appeared to receive special benefit or harm from heparin treatment. Notably, this included more than 3000 patients with atrial fibrillation and more than 2000 patients with posterior-circulation stroke.

   The risk of hemorrhagic complications was substantially greater with high-dose (12,500 U twice daily) compared to low-dose (5000 U twice daily) heparin. High-dose versus low-dose heparin was associated with a greater rate of transfused or fatal extracranial hemorrhage (2.0% vs. 0.6%), hemorrhagic stroke (1.8% vs. 0.7%), and death or nonfatal stroke at 14 days (12.6% vs. 10.8%, $p = 0.007$).

   When compared with the avoid heparin group, high-dose heparin was associated with a NS increase of 5 per 1000 in early death or recurrent stroke and a strongly significant increase of 16 per 1000 in transfused or fatal extracranial bleeds. In contrast, low-dose heparin was associated with a significant reduction of 12 per 1000 in early death or recurrent stroke without a significant excess of major extracranial hemorrhage.

Comparison of the patients who received both aspirin and low-dose SQ heparin to those receiving aspirin alone did suggest a possible benefit to combination therapy, with a reduction in early death (8.0% vs. 9.3%), early recurrent stroke or ICH (2.8% vs. 3.7%), and little increased risk of major extracranial hemorrhage. This seemingly promising trend is tempered by the fact that the observations were based on subgroup analysis, and the favorable effect of combination therapy was no longer apparent at 6 months.

Low-Molecular-Weight Heparins or Heparinoids

At present, there have been six large, randomized trials of LMWH/heparinoids in the treatment of acute stroke. Overall, these trials have not provided evidence of benefit in the treatment of patients with acute stroke and have confirmed an increased risk of both ICH and systemic bleeding with LMWH/heparinoid therapy (Table 14.3).

1. Fraxaparine in Ischemic Stroke Study (FISS)

   FISS randomized 312 patients to one of three treatments, all given subcutaneously: high-dose nadroparin, low-dose nadroparin, or placebo.[17] Patients were enrolled within 48 hours of symptom onset and received study medication for 10 days. All patients came from one of four hospitals in Hong Kong, a factor that may be important to consider given previously established differences in prevalence of certain stroke mechanisms (i.e., intracranial atherosclerosis) in Asian compared with Caucasian populations. A significant reduction in the percentage of patients dead or dependent at 6 months was found with nadroparin compared with placebo (45% dead or dependent in high-dose nadroparin group, 52% in low-dose nadroparin group, and 65% in the placebo group, $p = 0.005$ for trend). Suprisingly, this difference in outcome at 6 months was not identified at 10 days, nor was it significant ($p = 0.12$) at 3 months.

Table 14.3 Risk of hemorrhagic complications in low-molecular-weight heparin/heparinoid trials

Trial	N (total)	Intracranial Hemorrhage (%)		Major Extracranial Hemorrhage (%)	
		Control[a]	Drug	Control[a]	Drug
FISS	306	0	0	4.8	4.0–5.9
FISS-bis	766	2.8	3.7–6.1	?	?
TOAST	1266	0.9	2.9	1.1	3.9
HAEST	449	1.8	2.8	1.8	5.8
TAIST	1484	0.2	0.6–1.4	0.4	0.4–0.8

FISS = Fraxaparine in Ischemic Stroke Study; HAEST = Heparin in Acute Embolic Stroke Trial; TOAST = Trial of ORG 10172 in Acute Stroke Treatment.

[a]Control = placebo in FISS, FISS-bis, TOAST; aspirin in HAEST, TAIST.

2. FISS-bis

   This follow-up study to FISS was designed to confirm the efficacy of nadroparin in a larger sample.[18] Design was similar to FISS, except that treatment was begun within 24 hours of symptom onset. A total of 767 patients were randomized. There was no significant difference in the number of patients dead or disabled between the three groups. Nadroparin was associated with a lower incidence of pulmonary emboli but a higher frequency of hemorrhage, including ICH (symptomatic ICH rate 2.8% placebo; 3.7% low-dose nadroparin; 6.1% high-dose nadroparin).

3. Trial of ORG 10172 (Danaparoid) in Acute Stroke Treatment (TOAST)

   TOAST randomized 1281 patients within 24 hours of stroke onset to treatment with dose-adjusted IV danaparoid or placebo.[19] There was a trend toward better outcomes in the danaparoid group at 7 days; however, at 3 months there was no significant difference in outcomes between the groups (favorable outcome in 75.2% of danaparoid treated patients and 73.7% of placebo patients, $p = 0.49$). Hemorrhagic complications were more common in the danaparoid group, including symptomatic ICH (2.3% danaparoid, 0.8% placebo, $p = 0.05$). An analysis based on stroke subtype suggested a possible benefit in patients with large-vessel atherosclerosis (>50% stenosis). This finding is discussed later.

4. Heparin in Acute Embolic Stroke Trial (HAEST)

   HAEST randomized 449 patients with acute ischemic stroke and atrial fibrillation to either dalteparin or aspirin within 30 hours of stroke onset.[20] HAEST is unique among heparin trials in that, by including only patients with atrial fibrillation, a population of stroke patients with a homogenous stroke mechanism was evaluated. During the initial 2 weeks following randomization, recurrent ischemic stroke occurred in 8.5 percent of the dalteparin group and 7.5 percent of the aspirin group (odds ratio [OR] 1.13; 95% confidence interval [CI] 0.57 to 2.24). The percentage of patients with cerebral hemorrhage, stroke progression, and death was similar in both groups. No significant difference in functional outcomes or death was seen at 2 weeks or 3 months after enrollment.

5. Therapy of Patients with Acute Stroke (TOPAS)

   The TOPAS trial randomized 404 patients to one of four doses of certoparin within 12 hours of stroke onset, and therefore had the shortest time window of any anticoagulation trial.[21] There was no placebo group in this trial. There was no difference between the groups in the proportion of patients achieving a favorable outcome (Barthel index >90 points) at 3 months or in the percentage of patients with recurrent stroke or transient ischemic attack (TIA) within 6 months. Major hemorrhagic complications were more frequent in the highest dose group. Given the lack of a placebo group, TOPAS can only be considered to provide evidence for a lack of benefit for higher versus lower doses of LMWH but does not exclude the possibility of an advantage of LMWH over placebo.

6. Tinzaparin in Acute Ischemic Stroke Trial (TAIST)

   The TAIST Trial randomized 1486 patients to high-dose tinzaparin, medium-dose tinzaparin, or aspirin within 48 hours of stroke onset. Treatment was continued for up to 10 days.[22] The percentage of patients independent at 6 months was similar for all three treatment groups (41.5% high-dose tinzaparin, 42.4% medium-dose tinzaparin, and 42.5% aspirin). Mortality, disability, and measures of neurological deterioration were also similar among treatment groups. A significantly higher rate of ICH was seen with high-dose tinzaparin compared with aspirin (1.4% vs. 0.2%; OR 7.15, 95% CI 1.10 to 163), but there were fewer patients with symptomatic deep venous thrombosis (DVT) in the tinzaparin group (0% vs. 1.8%). Analysis of predefined subgroups (stroke mechanism, posterior vs. anterior circulation, and treatment within or after 24 hours) revealed no particular group in which a significant benefit to tinzaparin was evident.

Is There a Subgroup of Patients Who Might Benefit from Heparin?

Large-Vessel Stenosis or Occlusion

Given the heterogeneous pathophysiology of stroke, it is plausible that a particular therapy might be beneficial only in stroke resulting from certain mechanisms. The proven efficacy of heparin and LMWH in the treatment of acute coronary syndromes provides theoretical grounds to suggest that such benefit might be most likely to occur in patients with stroke resulting from large-vessel stenosis, the stroke mechanism most analogous to the mechanisms of vascular occlusion that occur in MI. Indeed, post hoc analysis of the TOAST trial suggested a therapeutic benefit of danaparoid in patients with >50 percent internal carotid artery stenosis or occlusion. In this subgroup, a favorable outcome was seen at 3 months in 68.3 percent of the danaparoid-treated patients compared with 53.2 percent of those receiving placebo ($p = 0.02$). A similar treatment effect was seen at 7 days.[23] It has also been suggested that the positive findings in the initial FISS trial might be explained by a high prevalence of intracranial stenosis in the exclusively Asian population enrolled, in contrast to all the subsequent LMWH trials that were negative but generally enrolled patients of a different ethnic or racial background. In contrast to these reports, the TAIST trial did not find any evidence of benefit in the subgroup of patients with stroke resulting from large-artery disease.[22] As acute neuroimaging evolves, it may be practical to rapidly identify acute stroke patients with large-vessel stenosis and therefore tailor therapy to the particular mechanism causing cerebral ischemia. Whether heparins might be of use in such a paradigm awaits further study.

Cardioembolism

Early reports from the Cerebral Embolism Study Group suggested a possible benefit to acute anticoagulation in patients with cardioembolic stroke. Although intuitively sensible, large trials have not confirmed this benefit. Indeed, the HAEST trial, which exclusively enrolled patients with atrial fibrillation, showed no benefit to dalteparin compared with aspirin.[20] Similarly, subgroup analysis of more than 3000 patients with atrial fibrillation in the IST trial showed no benefit for heparin.[1] Analysis of the subgroup of patients with cardioembolic stroke in the TOAST trial ($n = 266$) showed no benefit to treatment with danaparoid.[19] Some authors have suggested that there may be particular sources of cardioembolism (such as atrial fibrillation with identifiable mural thrombus) that place patients at such high risk of recurrent ischemic events that anticoagulation is warranted.[24] At present, this remains speculative.

Dissection

Despite the lack of any definitive trials, many experts continue to recommend the use of heparin in patients with carotid or vertebral dissection. The mural hematoma present in arterial dissection may function as a proximal embolic source or as a site of progressive thrombosis leading to vessel occlusion, suggesting a beneficial role for anticoagulants. Patients with dissection may be younger and less likely to have preceding structural brain injury and/or hypertension and thus may be at lower risk of hemorrhagic complications. In a study of 28 consecutive patients with dissection of the internal carotid artery, Molina et al[25] demonstrated that microembolic signals on transcranial Doppler monitoring were associated with recurrent ischemic events and that these signals were markedly reduced with therapeutic levels of heparin but not with subtherapeutic levels. A Cochrane Database systematic review of reported case series (no randomized trials have been performed) concluded that there was no significant difference in odds of death or disability with treatment with antiplatelet agents compared with anticoagulants.[26] However, analysis of the recurrent stroke rate alone suggested a possible benefit for anticoagulant therapy, with a rate of recurrent stroke (both ischemic and hemorrhagic) of 3.4 percent with no therapy, 4.2 percent with antiplatelet therapy, and 1.5 percent with anticoagulation. It must be emphasized that these data are markedly limited given their nonrandomized nature.

Transient Ischemic Attack

In patients with recent or multiple TIAs, the risk of cerebral infarction appears to be highest in the period immediately following the transient events, particularly during the first 48 hours.[27] To minimize this risk, many neurologists consider the use of heparin appropriate while the underlying cause is investigated. However, no clinical data have proven heparin to be an effective therapy in patients with recent TIA. Early studies in the pre-CT area suggested a reduction in recurrent TIA and stroke but an increase in hemorrhagic stroke in patients treated with anticoagulation.[12,13] A population-based retrospective study evaluated the effect of heparin in patients with recent (<30 days) TIA.[28] No significant differences were observed in the risk of death, stroke, or recurrent TIA between the 102 patients treated with heparin and the 187 patients who did not receive heparin. In a small randomized study, heparin was compared with aspirin (1300 mg/day) in 55 patients with recent TIA.[29] Recurrent TIA occurred in equal proportions during an average treatment period of 5.5 days, but infarction was more common in the aspirin group. The study sample size was too small for meaningful statistical analysis. Crescendo TIA, in which multiple TIAs occur during a brief period with increasing duration or severity of deficit, is a particularly ominous situation. While conflicting data obscure the role of heparin in this situation, its use is prevalent.[30,31]

Progressing Stroke

The potential benefit of heparin in progressing stroke, or stroke-in-evolution, is unclear. No universal definition exists for stroke-in-evolution, so interpretation of the conflicting literature is nearly impossible.[32–34] Several different mechanisms may contribute to acute worsening of the neurological deficit, including propagation of thrombus, recurrent embolism, cerebral edema, hemorrhagic transformation, toxic-metabolic factors, and delayed neuronal death or apoptosis. Heparin would only be expected to have a favorable effect on the first two of these mechanisms. The earliest trials of heparin for progressing stroke were performed during the pre-CT era and had numerous design flaws but suggested that heparin was beneficial.[12–14,35] More recent but still uncontrolled studies have challenged the value of heparin in this setting, with one report demonstrating that up to half of the patients continued to deteriorate despite early heparin treatment.[32,36] Some studies have suggested that progression is a more common complication of stroke in the vertebrobasilar system than the carotid territory, although it remains uncertain whether heparin actually has a different effect in each vascular distribution.[31,37]

Effect of Time to Treatment on Heparin Efficacy

A prespecified secondary analysis of the results of IST considered the effect of time to treatment on outcome. Although all patients in IST were enrolled within 48 hours of stroke onset, 3141 patients were randomized within 6 hours and 7225 within 12 hours.[1] There was no evidence of better outcome with earlier treatment.

A small consecutive case series of patients with stroke and atrial fibrillation treated with heparin suggested a greater likelihood of complete recovery with early (<6 hours) as opposed to late (6 to 48 hours) heparinization.[38] Patients were treated with either IV or high-dose SQ heparin aimed at achieving an activated partial thromboplastin time (aPTT) of 1.5 to 2.0 times normal. This study was small ($n = 231$) and not randomized or blinded, and, because it was a case series, it cannot account for other possible advantages of early hospital care.

In contrast, a meta-analysis of trials of LMWH in stroke actually suggested a possible advantage to *later* treatment (>24 hours after stroke onset), possibly resulting from an increased risk of ICH with early therapy.[39] This hypothesis was supported by subsequent data from TAIST, in which an increased occurrence of ICH was seen with earlier administration of tinzaparin.[22]

Practical Implications

Overall, there is little evidence to support routine use of dose-adjusted IV or high-dose SQ UFH, or full-dose LMWH in acute stroke patients. Although heparin may reduce the risk of recurrent ischemic stroke, this reduction is counterbalanced by an increase in risk of ICH. There may be a benefit (and does not appear to be significant risk) to low-dose SQ heparin (5000 U twice daily) given for a short time (<14 days), possibly in combination with aspirin. After the initial evaluation to determine stroke mechanism, there may be some role for anticoagulation in a minority of patients (Figure 14.1). Patient subgroups for which some limited data and expert opinion suggest possible benefit to heparins, and for which further study is necessary, include those with large-vessel stenosis, arterial dissection, or TIA. In contrast, acute anticoagulation of patients with stroke resulting from atrial fibrillation has been clearly shown to be of no benefit.

If Used, How Should Heparin Be Given?

UFH can be administered by the IV or SQ route, by infusion or by repeated doses, titrated to a therapeutic level by the PTT or given as a fixed dose. Many institutions employ heparin-dosing protocols to standardize such therapy, and a weight-based nomogram for IV heparin dosing specifically in patients with TIA or stroke has been reported and validated.[40] In terms of safely achieving a therapeutic PTT, fixed-dose SQ heparin administration appears to compare favorably to dose-adjusted IV administration. One report found that the percentage of patients achieving a therapeutic PTT (defined as PTT 1.5 to 2 times control) at 24 hours was 43 percent with a fixed dose of 12,500 units of SQ heparin given every 12 hours compared with 49 percent with a dose-adjusted IV heparin infusion started at 1000 IU/hour, and excessive PTT levels were seen in 14 percent of the patients treated with fixed-dose SQ compared with 33 percent of those treated with IV dose-adjusted heparin.[38]

Elevated blood pressure, elevated PTT, large infarct size, increasing patient age, prolonged duration of therapy, and use of bolus dosing have all been implicated as risk factors for hemorrhage associated with heparin therapy but only on the basis of limited evidence.[38,41] If use of acute anticoagulation is considered, extreme caution should be used in patients with these risk factors, and rigorous monitoring and regulation of PTT levels should be undertaken.

EMERGING ANTITHROMBOTIC THERAPIES

Glycoprotein IIb/IIIa Inhibitors

Glycoprotein IIb/IIIa (GIIb/IIIa) inhibitors function as antiplatelet agents by binding directly to the GIIb/IIIa receptor on the platelet membrane, blocking fibrinogen-platelet binding and platelet aggregation. In contrast to aspirin, GIIb/IIIa inhibitors not only decrease platelet aggregation but also reduce the rate of tissue factor initiated thrombin generation in vitro.[42] This finding supports an additional beneficial role in the setting of acute vascular thrombosis. Available GIIb/IIIa inhibitors include abciximab, eptifibatide, and tirofiban.

A number of case reports and small case series have suggested utility of the GIIb/IIIa inhibitors in treatment of acute stroke, either alone or in combination with thrombolytic therapy.[43-45] Two small series with retrospective controls have suggested a benefit, both in terms of recanalization and clinical outcome, to IV eptifibatide combined with intra-arterial (IA) t-PA compared with IA t-PA alone[46] and to IV abciximab + IA urokinase compared with IA urokinase alone.[47] The small number of patients included and the nonrandomized nature of these trials demands caution in their interpretation, but the results appear promising.

Two preliminary randomized, controlled safety studies of abciximab in patients with acute stroke have been performed. In the first, 74 patients were enrolled within 24 hours of acute ischemic stroke (54 received one of four doses of abciximab, 20 received placebo.) There were no cases of major symptomatic ICH in either group, and a trend toward a better outcome in the abciximab group was observed.[48] In the subsequent Abciximab in Emergent Stroke Treatment Trial (AbESTT), which has been presented only in abstract form, 400 patients were randomly assigned to receive either abciximab (0.25 mg/kg bolus followed by 0.125 µg/kg/min infusion for 12 hours) or placebo within 6 hours of symptom onset.[49] Forty-nine percent of patients treated with active drug had excellent recovery (defined as a modified Rankin score of 0 or 1) compared with 40 percent of those given placebo (OR 1.41, 95% CI 0.95 to 2.10). Furthermore, 46 percent treated with abciximab had essentially no residual neurological deficit (defined by an NIHSS score of 0 or 1) compared with only 34 percent of those given placebo (OR 1.65, 95% CI 1.10 to 2.48). Similar trends were observed with other outcome measures suggesting a consistent benefit of abciximab. The likelihood of a good outcome was higher among those patients treated with abciximab within 5 hours of stroke onset. Unfortunately, patients with severe strokes (NIHSS >14) did not appear to benefit from active treatment. Symptomatic intracerebral hemorrhage occurred after abciximab treatment in 3.6 percent of patients but in only 1 percent of placebo-treated patients. This difference was not statistically significant, probably due to issues of statistical power. Based on these results, a pivotal phase III trial is planned to assess the role of abciximab in acute stroke. Although abciximab is available in the United States for use in cardiac disease, it cannot be recommend for use in acute ischemic stroke until further research is completed.

Direct Thrombin Inhibitors

The major role of thrombin is to convert fibrinogen to fibrin, but thrombin also acts through a number of feedback mechanisms to amplify the coagulation response by directly activating coagulation factors, platelets, and fibrinolysis inhibitors.[50] Unlike the heparins, which exert their anticoagulant effects by binding the cofactor antithrombin, direct thrombin inhibitors may block all the major procoagulant effects of thrombin without an intermediary factor. Further, clot-bound thrombin, which appears to be relatively protected from heparin-stimulated antithrombin III–mediated inhibition, may be more effectively blocked by direct thrombin inhibitors.[51]

Despite these theoretical advantages, initial trials of direct thrombin inhibitors in patients with acute coronary syndromes have been disappointing, with no clear evidence for greater efficacy compared with IV heparin and a possible increased rate of bleeding.[52–57]

Argatroban, an intravenously administered direct thrombin inhibitor approved for use as an anticoagulant in patients with heparin-induced thrombocytopenia, has undergone preliminary testing in patients with acute stroke. In an initial multicenter pilot trial, 119 patients were randomized to either argatroban or placebo. Treatment was started relatively late, with roughly half the patients treated more than 48 hours after symptom onset. Clinical outcome was assessed with a nonstandard rating of global improvement. At 1 month, 54 percent of the patients treated with argatroban were noted to have significant improvement compared with 24 percent of the placebo group ($p < 0.01$). There was no excess of ICH in the argatroban group.[58]

In a subsequent, multicenter randomized trial involving 176 patients randomized to receive IV argatroban (high or low dose) or placebo within 12 hours of stroke symptom onset, there were no differences in clinical outcome among the treatment allocation groups. Symptomatic ICH occurred in 3 of 59 (5.1%) patients given high-dose argatroban, 2 of 58 (3.4%) given low-dose argatroban, and 0 of 54 (0%) given placebo. These apparent differences among groups were not statistically significant ($p = 0.18$).[59] At present, argatroban cannot be recommended for routine use in patients with acute ischemic stroke. However, this drug may have a role in stroke patients who also suffer from heparin-induced thrombocytopenia.

Ancrod

Derived from Malaysian pit viper venom, ancrod is a defibrinogenating agent that splits fibrinopeptide A from fibrinogen, depleting the substrate required for thrombus formation. Decreasing fibrinogen also decreases blood viscosity, which may have favorable effects on the cerebral circulation. Preliminary small, randomized trials suggested that use of ancrod was safe in ischemic stroke, and one double-blind study of 132 patients treated within 6 hours suggested a benefit to ancrod treatment compared with placebo.[60–62] A much larger trial, The Stroke Treatment with Ancrod Trial (STAT), randomized 500 patients within 3 hours of symptom onset to either ancrod or placebo.[63] The ancrod infusion rate was adjusted based on measured fibrinogen levels. The percentage of patients reaching favorable functional status, defined as a Barthel index ≥ 95, at 90 days was greater (42.2% vs. 34.4%, $p = 0.04$), and the percentage of severely disabled patients was lower in the ancrod treated group (11.8% vs. 19.8%, $p = 0.01$). Symptomatic ICH was more frequent with ancrod treatment (5.2% vs. 2.0%, $p = 0.06$). In contrast to the positive results of STAT, the European Stroke Treatment with Ancrod Trial (ESTAT) was terminated after enrollment of 1222 patients when a preplanned interim analysis showed that the probability of benefit from ancrod was too low to justify continuation of the trial.[64] In addition, 90-day mortality (although not total mortality) was higher in the ancrod treated group. ESTAT differed from STAT in that patients were enrolled within 6 hours, as opposed to 3 hours, of symptom onset.

CONCLUSION

There is clear evidence of a modest but significant benefit for early aspirin therapy in patients with acute stroke (Table 14.2). Low-dose SQ heparin, possibly given in combination with aspirin, may be beneficial, although this is not clearly established. There is little evidence to support routine use of full-dose heparin,

LMWH, or heparinoids in unselected patients with acute stroke. Whether certain subgroups of patients, such as those with large-vessel stenosis or arterial dissection, might benefit from anticoagulation remains unknown. Ongoing studies will help define the role of newer antithrombotic therapies such as the GIIb/IIIa inhibitors and the direct thrombin inhibitors.

References

1. International Stroke Trial Collaborative Group. The International Stroke Trial (IST): a randomised trial of aspirin, heparin, both, or neither among 19435 patients with acute ischaemic stroke. Lancet 1997;349:1569–1581.
2. CAST (Chinese Acute Stroke Trial) Collaborative Group. CAST: randomised placebo-controlled trial of early aspirin use in 20,000 patients with acute ischaemic stroke. Lancet 1997;349:1641–1649.
3. Chen ZM, Sandercock P, Pan HC, et al. Indications for early aspirin use in acute ischemic stroke: a combined analysis of 40,000 randomized patients from the Chinese acute stroke trial and the international stroke trial. On behalf of the CAST and IST collaborative groups. Stroke 2000; 31:1240–1249.
4. Multicentre Acute Stroke Trial—Italy (MAST-I) Group. Randomised controlled trial of streptokinase, aspirin, and combination of both in treatment of acute ischemic stroke. Lancet 1995; 346:1509–1514.
5. ISIS-2 (Second International Study of Infarct Survival) Collaborative Group. Randomised trial of intravenous streptokinase, oral aspirin, both, or neither among 17,187 cases of suspected acute myocardial infarction: ISIS-2. Lancet 1988;2:349–360.
6. The Clopidogrel in Unstable Angina to Prevent Recurrent Events Trial Investigators. Effects of clopidogrel in addition to aspirin in patients with acute coronary syndromes without ST-segment elevation. N Engl J Med 2001;345:494–502.
7. Albers GW, Amarenco P. Combination therapy with clopidogrel and aspirin: can the CURE results be extrapolated to cerebrovascular patients? Stroke 2001;32:2948–2949.
8. Klein W, Buchwald A, Hillis SE, et al. Comparison of low-molecular-weight heparin with unfractionated heparin acutely and with placebo for 6 weeks in the management of unstable coronary artery disease. Fragmin in Unstable Coronary Artery Disease Study (FRIC). Circulation 1997;96:61–68.
9. Comparison of two treatment durations (6 days and 14 days) of a low molecular weight heparin with a 6-day treatment of unfractionated heparin in the initial management of unstable angina or non-Q-wave myocardial infarction: FRAX.I.S. (FRAxiparine in Ischaemic Syndrome). Eur Heart J 1999;20:1553–1562.
10. Antman EM, Cohen M, Radley D, et al. Assessment of the treatment effect of enoxaparin for unstable angina/non-Q-wave myocardial infarction. TIMI 11B-ESSENCE meta-analysis. Circulation 1999;100:1602–1608.
11. Wong GCMD, Giugliano RPMDSM, Antman EMMD. Use of low-molecular-weight heparins in the management of acute coronary artery syndromes and percutaneous coronary intervention. JAMA 2003;289:331–342.
12. Baker RN, Broward JA, Fang HC, et al. Anticoagulant therapy in cerebral infarction. Report on cooperative study. Neurology 1962;12:823–835.
13. Fisher CM. Anticoagulant therapy in cerebral thrombosis and cerebral embolism: a national cooperative study, interim report. Neurology 1961;11(part 2):119–131.
14. Carter AB. Anticoagulant treatment in progressing stroke. Br Med J 1961;2:70–73.
15. Cerebral Embolism Study Group. Immediate anticoagulation of embolic stroke: a randomized trial. Stroke 1983;14:668–676.
16. Duke RJ, Bloch RF, Turpie AGG, et al. Intravenous heparin for the prevention of stroke progression in acute partial stable stroke: a randomized controlled trial. Ann Intern Med 1986;105:825–828.
17. Kay R, Wong KS, Yu YL, et al. Low-molecular-weight heparin for the treatment of acute ischemic stroke. N Engl J Med 1995;333:1588–1593.
18. Hommel M for the FISS bis Investigators Group. Fraxiparine in Ischemic Stroke Study (FISS bis). Cerebrovasc Dis 1998;8(suppl 4):19.
19. The Publications Committee for the Trial of ORG 10172 in Acute Stroke Treatment (TOAST) Investigators. Low molecular weight heparinoid, ORG 10172 (danaparoid), and outcome after acute ischemic stroke: a randomized controlled trial. JAMA 1998;279:1265–1272.

20. Berge E, Abdelnoor M, Nakstad PH, Sandset PM. Low molecular-weight heparin versus aspirin in patients with acute ischaemic stroke and atrial fibrillation: a double-blind randomised study. HAEST Study Group. Heparin in Acute Embolic Stroke Trial. Lancet 2000;355:1205–1210.
21. Diener HC, Ringelstein EB, von Kummer R, et al. Treatment of acute ischemic stroke with the low-molecular-weight heparin certoparin: results of the TOPAS trial. Therapy of Patients With Acute Stroke (TOPAS) Investigators. Stroke 2001;32:22–29.
22. Bath PM, Lindenstrom E, Boysen G, et al. Tinzaparin in acute ischaemic stroke (TAIST): a randomised aspirin-controlled trial. Lancet 2001;358:702–710.
23. Adams HP Jr, Bendixen BH, Leira E, et al. Antithrombotic treatment of ischemic stroke among patients with occlusion or severe stenosis of the internal carotid artery: a report of the Trial of Org 10172 in Acute Stroke Treatment (TOAST). Neurology 1999;53:122–125.
24. Moonis M, Fisher M. Considering the role of heparin and low-molecular-weight heparins in acute ischemic stroke. Stroke 2002;33:1927–1933.
25. Molina CA, Alvarez-Sabin J, Schonewille W, et al. Cerebral microembolism in acute spontaneous internal carotid artery dissection. Neurology 2000;55:1738–1741.
26. Lyrer P, Engelter S. Antithrombotic drugs for carotid artery dissection. Cochrane Database Syst Rev 2000(4):CD000255.
27. Johnston SC, Gress DR, Browner WS, Sidney S. Short-term prognosis after emergency department diagnosis of TIA. JAMA 2000;284:2901–2906.
28. Keith DS, Phillips SJ, Whisnant JP, et al. Heparin therapy for recent transient focal cerebral ischemia. Mayo Clin Proc 1987;62:1101–1106.
29. Biller J, Bruno A, Adams HP Jr, et al. A randomized trial of aspirin or heparin in hospitalized patients with recent transient ischemic attacks. A pilot study. Stroke 1989;20:441–447.
30. Nehler MR, Moneta GL, McConnell DB, et al. Anticoagulation followed by elective carotid surgery in patients with repetitive transient ischemic attacks and high-grade carotid stenosis. Arch Surg 1993;128:1117–1123.
31. Putnam SF, Adams HP. Usefulness of heparin in initial management of patients with recent transient ischemic attacks. Arch Neurol 1985;42:960–962.
32. Haley EC, Kassell NF, Torner JC. Failure of heparin to prevent progression in progressing ischemic infarction. Stroke 1988;19:10–14.
33. Gautier JC. Stroke-in-progression. Stroke 1985;16:729–733.
34. Irino T, Watanabe M, Nishide M, et al. Angiographical analysis of acute cerebral infarction followed by "cascade"-like deterioration of minor neurological deficits. What is progressing stroke? Stroke 1983;14:363–368.
35. Millikan CH, McDowell FH. Treatment of progressing stroke. Stroke 1981;12:397–409.
36. Ramirez-Lassepas M, Quinones MR, Nino HH. Treatment of acute ischemic stroke. Open trial with continuous intravenous heparinization. Arch Neurol 1986;43:386–390.
37. Biller J, Bruno A, Adams HP, et al. A randomized trial of aspirin or heparin in hospitalized patients with recent transient ischemic attacks. A pilot study. Stroke 1989;20:441–447.
38. Chamorro A, Vila N, Ascaso C, Blanc R. Heparin in acute stroke with atrial fibrillation: clinical relevance of very early treatment. Arch Neurol 1999;56:1098–1102.
39. Bath PM, Iddenden R, Bath FJ. Low-molecular-weight heparins and heparinoids in acute ischemic stroke: a meta-analysis of randomized controlled trials. Stroke 2000;31:1770–1778.
40. Toth C, Voll C. Validation of a weight-based nomogram for the use of intravenous heparin in transient ischemic attack or stroke. Stroke 2002;33:670–674.
41. Cerebral Embolism Study Group. Immediate anticoagulation of embolic stroke: brain hemorrhage and management options. Stroke 1984;15:779–789.
42. Butenas S, Cawthern KM, van't Veer C, et al. Antiplatelet agents in tissue factor-induced blood coagulation. Blood. 2001;97:2314–2322.
43. Junghans U, Seitz RJ, Ritzl A, et al. Ischemic brain tissue salvaged from infarction by the GP IIb/IIIa platelet antagonist tirofiban. Neurology 2002;58:474–476.
44. Lee KY, Heo JH, Lee SI, Yoon PH. Rescue treatment with abciximab in acute ischemic stroke. Neurology 2001;56:1585–1587.
45. Houdart E, Woimant F, Chapot R, et al. Thrombolysis of extracranial and intracranial arteries after IV abciximab. Neurology 2001;56:1582–1584.
46. McDonald TC, O'Donnell J, Bemporad J, et al. The clinical utility of intravenous integrilin combined with intra-arterial tissue plasminogen activator in acute ischemic stroke: the MGH experience [abstract]. Stroke 2002;33:359.
47. Lee DH, Jo KD, Kim HG, et al. Local intraarterial urokinase thrombolysis of acute ischemic stroke with or without intravenous abciximab: a pilot study. J Vasc Interv Radiol 2002;13:769–774.

48. The Abciximab in Ischemic Stroke Investigators. Abciximab in acute ischemic stroke: a randomized, double-blind, placebo-controlled, dose-escalation study. Stroke 2000;31:601–609.
49. AbESTT Investigators. Effects of abciximab for acute ischemic stroke: final results of Abciximab in Emergent Stroke Treatment Trial (AbESTT). Stroke 2003;34:253.
50. Dahlback B. Blood coagulation. Lancet 2000;355:1627–1632.
51. Weitz JI, Hudoba M, Massel D, et al. Clot-bound thrombin is protected from inhibition by heparin-antithrombin III but is susceptible to inactivation by antithrombin III-independent inhibitors. J Clin Invest 1990;86:385–391.
52. The Global Use of Strategies to Open Occluded Coronary Arteries (GUSTO) IIb investigators. A comparison of recombinant hirudin with heparin for the treatment of acute coronary syndromes. N Engl J Med 1996;335:775–782.
53. Organisation to Assess Strategies for Ischemic Syndromes (OASIS-2) Investigators. Effects of recombinant hirudin (lepirudin) compared with heparin on death, myocardial infarction, refractory angina, and revascularisation procedures in patients with acute myocardial ischaemia without ST elevation: a randomised trial. Lancet 1999;353:429–438.
54. Thrombin inhibition in Myocardial Ischaemia (TRIM) study group. A low molecular weight, selective thrombin inhibitor, inogatran, vs heparin, in unstable coronary artery disease in 1209 patients. A double-blind, randomized, dose-finding study. Eur Heart J 1997;18:1416–1425.
55. Gold HK, Torres FW, Garabedian HD, et al. Evidence for a rebound coagulation phenomenon after cessation of a 4-hour infusion of a specific thrombin inhibitor in patients with unstable angina pectoris. J Am Coll Cardiol 1993;21:1039–1047.
56. Kong DF, Topol EJ, Bittl JA, et al. Clinical outcomes of bivalirudin for ischemic heart disease. Circulation 1999;100:2049–2053.
57. Goldhaber SZ, Ridker PM. Thrombosis and Thromboembolism. New York: Marcel Dekker; 2002.
58. Kobayashi S, Tazaki Y. Effect of the thrombin inhibitor argatroban in acute cerebral thrombosis. Semin Thromb Hemost 1997;23:531–534.
59. LaMonte M for the ARGIS-I Investigators. Results of ARGIS-I: argatroban injection in acute ischemic stroke. Stroke 2003;34:246.
60. Hossmann V, Heiss WD, Bewermeyer H, Wiedemann G. Controlled trial of ancrod in ischemic stroke. Arch Neurol 1983;40:803–808.
61. Olinger CP, Brott TG, Barsan WG, et al. Use of ancrod in acute or progressing ischemic cerebral infarction. Ann Emerg Med 1988;17:1208–1209.
62. The Ancrod Stroke Study Investigators. Ancrod for the treatment of acute ischemic brain infarction. Stroke 1994;25:1755–1759.
63. Sherman DG, Atkinson RP, Chippendale T, et al. Intravenous ancrod for treatment of acute ischemic stroke: the STAT study: a randomized controlled trial. Stroke Treatment with Ancrod Trial. JAMA 2000;283:2395–2403.
64. Orgogozo JM, Verstraete M, Kay R, et al. Outcomes of ancrod in acute ischemic stroke. Independent Data and Safety Monitoring Board for ESTAT. Steering Committee for ESTAT. European Stroke Treatment with Ancrod Trial. JAMA 2000;284:1926–1927.

15
Emerging Therapies for Ischemic Stroke

Y. Dennis Cheng, Lama Michel Al-Lhoury, and
Justin A. Zivin

Effective stroke therapy exists, but there is considerable room for further
improvement. The efficacy of recombinant tissue plasminogen activator (rt-PA)
for acute stroke is critical, because it is proof of the concept that stroke is a treatable emergency.[1] However, the 3-hour therapeutic window has significantly limited its use, with only about 2 percent of stroke patients actually treated with
rt-PA during the first year after its approval in the United States[2] and little
improvement even 7 years later. Furthermore, the risk of rt-PA, hemorrhagic
transformation of ischemic stroke, especially in patients with large infarcts and
more than 3 hours after stroke onset, has further inhibited its widespread use.[3]
Therefore searching for more specific thrombolytic agents or possibly extending
the current therapeutic window has become a priority for acute stroke therapy.

Success of rt-PA also fueled the interest in the development of supplemental
neuroprotective therapies. For the last 2 decades, neuroprotective agents have
been investigated in animal models of cerebral ischemia, and numerous agents
have been found to reduce infarct size in animal stroke models. However,
translation of neuroprotective benefits from laboratory bench to emergency
room has not been successful. According to Kidwell et al,[4] there have been more
than 100 controlled clinical trials for acute stroke therapies published in the
literature, but none has proven clinically beneficial. There are now several
questions that must be addressed: Is the whole concept of neuroprotection
fundamentally wrong? Have we just failed to optimize the conditions for
clinical trials? What were the problems that disconnected preclinical evidence
from clinical application? Most important, what we can learn from all these
failures?

The purposes of this chapter are (1) to provide clinicians and investigators
with a current summary of ongoing efforts to find safer thrombolytic agents,
(2) to review the results of some important neuroprotective agents and to
identify discrepancies between laboratory model studies and clinical trials, and
(3) to highlight emerging concepts of acute stroke therapies.

EMERGING THROMBOLYTIC THERAPIES

Newer Generation Thrombolytic Agents

Intravenous (IV) rt-PA for acute stroke treatment was approved by the Food and Drug Administration (FDA) in 1996, following the publication of National Institute of Neurological Disorders and Stroke (NINDS) study data that showed that despite an increased incidence of intracranial hemorrhages in rt-PA–treated patients versus placebo patients, there was a statistically significant improvement in clinical outcome in the rt-PA group, and comparable mortality rates between both groups. Subsequent development of mutant forms of rt-PA has changed the properties of the molecule. The most important variant or mutant form of rt-PA that has been tested in experimental stroke models and is being tested currently in clinical trials is tenecteplase (TNK), the structure of which is described in the Appendix to this chapter and shown in Figure 15.1. TNK has delayed clearance because its half-life is prolonged to 17 ± 7 minutes as compared with 3.5 ± 1.4 minutes for alteplase, when studied in acute myocardial infarction (MI) patients.[5] TNK has higher fibrin selectivity than rt-PA, and has increased resistance to plasminogen-activator inhibitor with enhanced lytic activity on the thrombus and, possibly, earlier induction of reperfusion when compared with rt-PA.

Preclinical trials have tested TNK in animal models. In 1994, Thomas et al[6] published their data on TNK versus wild type rt-PA induced clot-lysis in an embolic stroke model in rabbits. TNK was found to be more potent and more clot selective with less systemic activation of plasminogen and correspondingly lesser rates of hemorrhagic transformation of the ischemic area when compared with rt-PA. Clinical trials have tested TNK in the treatment of acute MI: the Assessment of the Safety and Efficacy of New Thrombolytic Trial, study I (ASSENT-I), evaluated the safety of TNK in 3325 patients with MI. The intracranial hemorrhage rates were 0.7 percent with the 30-milligram dose and 0.6 percent with the 40-milligram dose of TNK, rates similar to those of rt-PA in previous MI trials. Serious bleeding complications requiring transfusions were 1.4 percent with TNK compared with 7 percent with rt-PA treatment (a statistically significant difference with the lesser bleeding rates in the TNK group).[7] In the Assessment of the Safety and Efficacy of New Thrombolytic Trial, study II (ASSENT-II), the two agents TNK given as a single bolus and rt-PA given as a 30-minute infusion were compared in 16,949 patients with acute MI. All patients received heparin and aspirin as well. The intracranial hemorrhage rate (ICH) was statistically similar in both groups; however, there was a slight but statistically significant lower rate of major bleeding requiring transfusion with the TNK treatment as compared with the rt-PA treatment.[8] Therefore it was concluded that TNK is as efficacious as rt-PA and has a lower rate of major systemic bleeding. Accordingly it was approved as thrombolytic treatment for acute MI.

A phase 2, feasibility, dose-escalating trial using TNK in acute stroke treatment is ongoing. The hope is that TNK may be more efficacious and may be safer in higher doses for acute stroke treatment.

Another thrombolytic agent that had been studied experimentally is microplasmin. Microplasmin is a truncated form of recombinant plasmin. It has been shown to improve the behavioral rating scores in a small-clot embolic

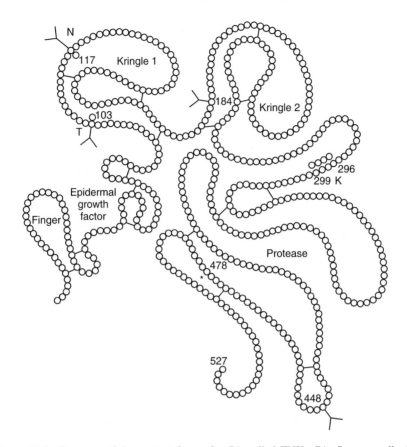

Figure 15.1 Structure of the mutant form of rt-PA called TNK-t-PA. See appendix for additional details and see reference 110. The asterisk (*) marks the serine site where plasminogen activation occurs. There are short lines that show the bridging between the different loops of the molecule. The amino acid substitutions enhance the fibrin specificity and increase the half-life of the molecule. Copyright is pending.

stroke model in rabbits and to decrease hemorrhage in the large-clot embolic stroke model, in contrast to rt-PA, which increases the hemorrhage rate in the latter model.[9] Clinical trials are needed to prove safety and efficacy of microplasmin.

Intra-Arterial Thrombolytic Treatment

Intra-arterial (IA) thrombolysis remains an unapproved procedure, but it is performed in many centers and is supported by randomized clinical trial evidence.[10,11] As with IV rt-PA, ongoing research aims to improve on this technique.[12] Arguably, it could be considered an emerging therapy, but the editors have opted to present IA thrombolysis in Chapter 13 on thrombolytic therapies.

EMERGING MECHANICAL THERAPIES

Angioplasty and Stenting for Stroke Prevention

Extracranial Internal Carotid Stenting and Angioplasty

Carotid endarterectomy (CEA), performed with a low periprocedural complication rate, is the only form of mechanical cerebral revascularization for which clinical benefit in the reduction of stroke rate has been proven. However, surgery has the disadvantage of neck incision, cranial nerve or superficial nerve injury, and wound complications, in addition to the risk of stroke, which may be fatal, and a small risk of MI. Treatment of carotid stenosis by endovascular techniques (balloon angioplasty or the use of stents) may have an advantage over CEA because they avoid the risk of surgery, but they carry a risk of stroke and restenosis.[13] We now discuss some case series and trials that shed light on the pros and cons of angioplasty and stenting of the extracranial carotid arteries.

In a meta-analysis published in 2000, Golledge et al[14] lumped together previous studies published between 1990 and 1999 that fulfilled certain inclusion and exclusion criteria that have looked at angioplasty with and without stenting of the carotid, as well as studies that looked at CEA as treatment for carotid stenosis. Thirteen studies of angioplasty with and without stenting (AS), and 20 studies of CEA were included in this meta-analysis. Carotid stents were deployed in 44 percent of angioplasty patients. Mortality within 30 days was 0.8 percent in the AS group and 1.2 percent in the CEA group (odds ratio [OR] 2.2, $p < 0.001$), and the risk of fatal or disabling stroke was 3.2 percent and 1.6 percent, respectively (OR 2.09, $p < 0.01$). The risk of stroke or death was 7.8 percent for AS and 4 percent for CEA (OR 2.02, $p < 0.001$), and disabling stroke and death was 3.9 percent and 2.2 percent, respectively (OR 1.86, $p < 0.01$). The authors concluded that the risk of stroke is significantly greater with angioplasty than with CEA.

In 2001, the results of the European, multicenter, randomized endovascular versus surgical treatment in patients with carotid stenosis in the Carotid and Vertebral Artery Transluminal Angioplasty Study (CAVATAS) were published. The authors compared endovascular treatment (angioplasty, stenting) to CEA (total patients 504). Within 30 days, the major outcome events were similar in both groups: disabling stroke and death was 6.4 percent with AS and 5.9 percent with CEA; 10 percent and 9.9 percent, respectively, for any stroke with symptoms lasting 7 days or more and death (no statistically significant difference). One year after treatment, severe ipsilateral carotid restenosis was significantly higher with the AS group (14%) compared with the CEA group (4%, $p < 0.0001$). The restenosis rate at 1 year was similar in the group who had only angioplasty and those who had angioplasty and stenting. Despite the higher restenosis rate in the AS patients, the rate of ipsilateral stroke in the survival analysis was similar in both groups up to 3 years following randomization.

Complication rates occurred as follows: cranial neuropathies in 8.7 percent after CEA, and 0 percent after AS ($p < 0.0001$); major neck or groin hematoma occurred in 6.7 percent of patients after CEA and 1.2 percent of patients after AS (also statistically different). The authors of CAVATAS concluded that endovascular treatment had similar major risks and similar effectiveness in preventing stroke during 3 years of follow-up.[13]

Carotid Revascularization Endarterectomy versus Stent Trial (CREST) is another randomized, multicenter, controlled trial that is ongoing. The patients are enrolled if they have symptomatic carotid artery stenosis greater than or equal to 50 percent. Primary outcome events of the trial will include any stroke, MI, or death during the 30-day periprocedural period.[15]

Until the results of CREST become available, the following might be considered. Based on the conclusions of a multidisciplinary panel at the recent Montefiore Vascular Symposium, subgroups of patients, including high-risk patients with significant medical co-morbidities, patients with carotid restenosis after earlier CEA, anatomically inaccessible lesions above C2, and radiation-induced stenosis should be considered for carotid artery stenting.[15]

Intracranial Cerebrovascular Stenting and Angioplasty

Intracranial angioplasty and stenting represents a challenge because of the small caliber of the cerebral vasculature. No controlled studies have been done in this domain; however, there have been many published case series that proved feasibility. For example, Gomez et al,[16] electively stented 12 patients (age 40 to 82 years) with basilar artery stenosis following events of vertebrobasilar ischemia. Stent placement was successful in all patients with a statistically significant reduction in degree of stenosis, from 71.4 percent (53% to 90%) to 10 percent (0% to 36%, $p < 0.0001$). There were no deaths, stent thromboses, perforations, ruptures, or MIs. Clinical follow-up time ranged from 0.5 to 16 months. One patient had nonspecific symptoms on his follow-up and one patient had a transient ischemic attack (TIA). The other patients remained asymptomatic. The authors concluded that basilar artery stenting is feasible and has minimal risks, although long-term impact is unknown.

Shinichi Nakano et al[17] published a Japanese study in 2002, in which 70 patients with acute middle cerebral artery (MCA) trunk occlusion were treated with IA thrombolysis or percutaneous transluminal angioplasty (PTA). Of these patients, 34 (49%) were treated with PTA in the last 5 years of the study, and subsequent thrombolytic treatment was added if necessary for distal embolization. The remaining 36 patients were treated with thrombolytic therapy alone and were used as controls mainly in the first 4 years of the study. The National Institute of Health Stroke Scale (NIHSS) and modified Rankin scale (mRS) were used as outcome measures at 90 days. There was no significant difference in the baseline NIHSS between the two groups. The rate of partial or complete recanalization in the PTA group was 91.2 percent and that of the thrombolysis group alone was 63.9 percent ($p < 0.01$). The incidence of large parenchymal hematoma with neurological deterioration in the PTA group was 2.9 percent, whereas that in the thrombolysis-alone group was 19.4 percent ($p = 0.03$). Although PTA alone did not improve the rate of favorable outcome (mRS 0–1), outcome in terms of independence (mRS ≤2) was significantly better in the PTA group (73.5%) than in the thrombolysis-alone group (50.0%, $p = 0.04$). The authors concluded that direct PTA is an effective alternative to IA thrombolysis for acute trunk MCA occlusion.

Mechanical Intra-arterial Devices

Certain IA catheter-associated devices have been developed to mechanically extract or obliterate the clot in the cerebral arteries. Case series have proven feasibility but large, controlled, randomized trials are required to prove efficacy.

The AngioJet is an IA device that uses saline jets directed back into the catheter to create a pressure zone around the catheter tip, inducing suction. The clot is pulled into the lumen and is removed from the vessel. Its safety is being evaluated in stroke patients. Another IA device called X-Sizer has small moving blades at the catheter tip that excise the thrombus and then aspirate it.

One of the simplest mechanical techniques is simple suction thrombectomy, and it has been related in a small case series. Anecdotal reports have emerged of interventional specialists employing retrieval devices such as snares and corkscrew-shaped devices for thrombectomy in acute strokes.[18]

Figure 15.2 shows a thrombus extraction device that was used in a small case series of patients with basilar artery embolism.[19] A balloon-occlusion aspiration emboli-entrapment device is another device used in conjunction with extracranial stenting. Its safety and feasibility were described in a patient series ($n = 75$) in severe internal carotid artery (ICA) stenosis. The authors reported success of the procedure in all of their patients without any major or minor stroke or death at 30 days, with visible particulate material aspirated during the procedure (fibrous plaque debris, lipid or cholesterol, and calcified plaque fragments).[20]

Hypothermia

Several experimental studies have shown that mild (34 degrees Centigrade) to moderate (30 degrees Centigrade) systemic hypothermia mitigates brain damage after cardiac arrest in dogs. A reduction in cerebral oxygen consumption and multiple chemical and physical mechanisms during and after ischemia have been postulated, including retardation of destructive enzymatic mechanisms; suppression of free-radical reactions; protection of the fluidity of the lipoprotein membranes; reduction of oxygen demand in low flow regions; reduction of intracellular acidosis; and inhibition of the biosynthesis, release, and uptake of excitatory neurotransmitters.[21]

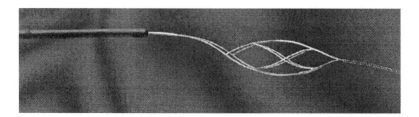

Figure 15.2   Clot retrieval device. The following parts of the device are visible, from left to right: microcatheter (0.75 millimeter), which serves as a sheath and in which the basket is advanced; microwire which is connected to the basket; and the self-expandable nitinol basket, which is released from the contracture of the microcatheter. It removes the thrombus by retraction through the vessel. Note the soft platinum coil tip. Please refer to the text and reference 19. Copyright is pending.

Several clinical studies showed that mild hypothermia after cardiac arrest improved neurological outcome without important side effects. A case-control study, published in 2002, investigated out-of-hospital cardiac-arrest patients who either were treated with mild hypothermia (33 degrees Centigrade) or were maintained normothermic. The patients were intubated, sedated, and had their shivering controlled. There was a statistically significant better neurological outcome in the hypothermia group.[22] Hyperthermia, on the other hand, had been shown to be associated with a higher mortality rate at 1 year as compared with normothermia.[23]

In 2001, Krieger et al[24] published a pilot study of 19 patients with acute major ischemic stroke (NIHSS >15). Patients were treated either with moderate hypothermia (32 degrees Centigrade) by a cooling surface blanket within 6 hours after onset of stroke or normothermia Thrombolytic therapies (IV/IA), depending on patient eligibility. Complications included bradycardia, ventricular ectopy, hypotension, melena, fever following re-warming, and infections. This study proved that induced hypothermia is feasible but that future controlled studies are needed to prove efficacy.

Ongoing multicenter trials are evaluating the safety of mild endovascular applied hypothermia in acute ischemic stroke patients with and without thrombolysis. Feasibility had been reported in few case series. For example, Georgiadis et al[25] reported six patients who had severe acute ischemic strokes and who were treated with moderate hypothermia applied through a closed-loop system entailing three balloons located near the tip of a central line that dwelled in the inferior vena cava (the minimum temperature established was 32.2 degrees Centigrade and maximum temperature 33.4 degrees Centigrade during hypothermia). Again, pulmonary infection, arterial hypotension, bradycardia, arrhythmia, and thrombocytopenia were the most common side effects.

Ultrasonication

Experimental studies in MI animal models have reported the thrombolytic effects of ultrasound (in vivo and in vitro). In stroke, the safety and feasibility of IA ultrasonication was evaluated. The ultrasound thrombolytic infusion catheter, EKOS, which combined a distal IA ultrasound transducer and IA thrombolysis using rt-PA, was demonstrated to be safe and feasible in acute stroke patients.[26]

Furthermore, ultrasound has been shown to penetrate the cranium and enhance thrombolysis in vitro. A recent paper reported that low-frequency and low-intensity transcranial ultrasound enhanced the thrombolytic activity of rt-PA in a model of artery occlusion in rabbits.[27] Future clinical trials are needed to address the safety and efficacy of transcranial ultrasonication as a thrombolytic modality in acute stroke treatment.

Endovascular Photo-Acoustic Recanalization Laser System

The safety and feasibility of Endovascular Photo-Acoustic Recanalization (EPAR) laser system in the IA treatment of stroke was reported in 2001. The device consists of a laser power source, which generates energy for the system.

The energy is delivered by fiber optics to the tip of the IA catheter. In this study, patients with acute stroke secondary to occlusion of the anterior cerebral arterial branches were treated within 6 hours and those with posterior circulation occlusion were treated within 24 hours.[28]

NEUROPROTECTIVE THERAPIES

Unlike many neurological diseases, there is no mystery about the cause of ischemic stroke. Compromised cerebral blood flow deprives brain tissue of oxygen and energy supply, and brain tissue, especially the core ischemic area, is damaged. Apart from damage resulting directly by energy depletion, injury to brain tissue, especially penumbral regions, propagates by various mechanisms. It has been well documented that cerebral ischemia leads to excessive release of glutamate and aspartate. Pathological activation of glutamate receptors on neurons and possibly glial cells, leads to cell death because of abnormal opening of ion channels, especially Na and Ca channels; activation of intracellular destructive enzymes, such as proteases, lipases, endonucleatidases, and cyclooxygenase; and initiation of programmed cell death pathways (apoptosis). Furthermore, abnormal production of toxic free radicals and recruitment of inflammatory processes also contributes to brain injury after stroke. Thus the neuroprotective therapies for stroke are designed to block these pathological cascades and minimize tissue damage in the absence of adequate blood supply. By now, drugs that have been tested in clinical trials can be classified into following categories: glutamate receptor antagonists, anti-inflammatory agents, ion channel modulators, free-radical scavengers, γ-aminobutyric acid (GABA) receptor agonists, serotonin receptor agonists, agents affecting coagulation or platelet aggregation, and agents whose functions are not yet elucidated (Table 15.1).

Glutamate Antagonists

Glutamate antagonists are probably the most studied neuroprotective agents. Glutamate is the most common excitatory neurotransmitter in the central nervous system (CNS) and is released excessively during ischemia.[29] Glutamate stimulates postsynaptic neurons by activating several types of receptors, including *N*-Methyl-D-aspartate (NMDA), α-amino-3-hydroxy-5-methyl-4-isoxazole propionate (AMPA), kainic acid (KA), and metabotropic receptors. Besides metabotropic receptors, NMDA, AMPA, and KA receptors are associated with influx of Ca^{2+}, activating Ca^{2+}-mediated enzymes that lead to cell destruction.

Selfotel (CGS19755), eliprodil, and aptiganel (Cerestat, CNS1102) are all NMDA receptor antagonists but target different sites on the receptor complex. Selfotel is a potent competitive antagonist that has shown efficacy in a number of preclinical models of stroke following systemic administration.[30] Eliprodil is a potent antagonist at the polyamine modulator site on the receptor complex and has also shown efficacy in several preclinical studies.[31-33] Cerestat, however, is a noncompetitive NMDA ion channel blocker that is characterized by a shorter

Table 15.1   Families of neuroprotective agents and their prototype drugs

Proposed Mechanism of Neuroprotection	Drug
Glutamate receptor antagonists	
NMDA antagonists	Selfotel (CGS19755)
	Eliprodil
	Aptiganel (Cerestat, CNS1102)
	Magnesium sulfate
AMPA antagonist	YM872
Ion channel modulators	
Calcium channel blockers	Nimodipine
	Flunarizine
Sodium channel blockers	Fosphenytoin
Potassium channel activator	Maxipost (BMS-204352)
Anti-inflammatory agents	Enlimomab
	LeukArrest (Hu23F2G)
	Recombinant neutrophil inhibitory factor (rNIF)
Free-radical scavengers	Tirilazad (U70046F)
	Citicoline (cytidyl diphosphocholine)
	Ebselen
GABA receptor agonists	Clomethiazole
	Diazepam
Miscellaneous	Cervene (Nalmefene)
	Lubeluzole
	Ganglioside (GMI)

AMPA = α-amino-3-hydroxy-5-methyl-4-isoxazole propionate; GABA = γ-aminobutyric acid; NMDA = N-Methyl-D-aspartate.

half-life than the other glutamate receptor antagonists introduced into clinical trials. Its efficacy was also confirmed in a numbers of stroke models.[34,35] However, a phase III trial of eliprodil was terminated prematurely when a futility analysis indicated that the drug is ineffective. The phase III trial of selfotel was also ended early because of an adverse risk/benefit ratio. The stroke trial for aptiganel was interrupted when the drug was found to be ineffective in head injury.

Although NMDA receptor antagonists produced numerous types of psychiatric and cardiovascular side effects, the hypothesis of glutamate receptor antagonism for reducing neurological damage in stroke never faded. In fact, because stroke is often a fatal disease, even serious side effects may be acceptable if counterbalanced by substantial efficacy. Furthermore, less toxic agents or existing drugs have been tested for glutamate antagonism in stroke. Magnesium has long been known to be a calcium channel blocker, especially on NMDA receptor-mediated calcium influx.[36] Currently, there are two ongoing phase III trials for accessing the possible neuroprotective effects of magnesium. Field administration of magnesium sulfate ($MgSO_4$) is targeting hyperacute stroke patients who are given $MgSO_4$ intravenously by paramedics within 2 hours of symptom onset. On the other hand, the Intravenous MAGnesium Efficacy in Stroke (IMAGES) trial includes patients within 12 hours of acute ischemic stroke.

YM872 is an AMPA receptor antagonist that has been proved to reduce brain injury in a rat MCA occlusion model.[37] Despite its initial promise, a phase III trial to assess the efficacy of YM872 in acute ischemic stroke patients who also receive rt-PA therapy was recently halted because of lack of efficacy.

Anti-Inflammatory Agents

Enlimomab was the first drug entered into clinical trials for stroke that targeted a specific step in the pathoinflammatory pathway contributing to the ischemic cascade. Enlimomab is a murine anti-intracellular adhesion module (ICAM)-1 antibody specific for the human ICAM-1 receptor. This receptor mediates neutrophil adhesion and migration through the vascular endothelium. Enlimomab was shown to inhibit these actions and demonstrated the efficacy of reducing infarct size in different stroke models.[38,39] However, the Enlimomab Acute Stroke Trial ended in failure because enlimomab-treated patients actually did worse compared with the placebo group. Although the reason for the failure is unclear, dosing schedules in the trial were different than preclinical studies. LeukArrest (Hu23F2G) is a monoclonal antibody against the neutrophil CD11/CD18 cell adhesion molecule. A phase III study of LeukArrest in patients who had an ischemic stroke was halted because interim results failed to meet predefined criteria for success.

Recombinant neutrophil inhibitory factor (rNIF) is a hookworm-derived agent that inhibits polymorphonuclear leukocyte (PMN) adhesion to the endothelium and reduces inflammatory response. Continuous treatment with a high dose of rNIF for 7 days was shown to be neuroprotective in rats up to 4 hours following MCA occlusion.[40] To select the most effective doses, the phase II trial of rNIF therapy on ischemic stroke recently conducted in Europe adapted a dose-ranging drug design, termed Adaptive Bayesian Design. The trial started with a range of doses, established an estimation of dose-response curve, and finally honed in to a possibly most effective dose and dosing schedule. The results of the trial are expected soon.

Ion Channel Modulators

Calcium Channel Blockers

Abnormal influx of calcium during ischemic episodes has been associated with pathological activation of intracellular destructive enzymes, leading to tissue damage.[41] Beside possible neuroprotective effects, nimodipine is a dihydropyridine calcium channel blocker, which has shown adequate brain penetration, dilation of intracranial vessels, and improvement in regional cerebral blood flow in the margins of cortical infarcts.[42] A multidose analysis of this drug was examined in 1064 patients treated for 21 days with treatment initiated within 48 hours of symptom onset. The result showed no overall effect.[43] However, a meta-analysis revealed a statistically significant effect of one dose when administered within 12 hours.[44] A subsequent trial, named Very Early Nimodipine Use in Stroke (VENUS) was conducted with first dose given within 6 hours after the onset of stroke. Unfortunately, the trial was terminated prematurely because futility analysis did not suggest a beneficial role of early administration of oral nimodipine. In fact, Horn et al[45] reviewed 47 trials involving calcium antagonists for stroke therapy, of which 29 were methodologically sound trials that included 7665 patients, and no beneficial effect was found.

Sodium Channel Blockers

Fosphenytoin, a disodium phosphate ester of 3-hydroxymethyl-5,5-diphenylhydantoin, was developed to overcome the poor aqueous solubility and irritant properties of IV phenytoin. It is rapidly converted to phenytoin after IV administration.[46] Phenytoin has been shown to reduce the amplitude of sodium-dependent action potentials[47] and to block voltage-dependent calcium entry into synaptosomes.[48] Although the neuroprotective effects of phenytoin may not necessarily relate to its sodium channel blockade, a phase III trial for stroke was conducted but was terminated when an interim analysis showed no differences in primary or secondary endpoints between fosphenytoin and placebo.

Potassium Channel Activation

Maxipost (BMS-204352), an activator of neuronal potassium channels, was shown to be neuroprotective by inducing neuronal hyperpolarization and decreasing the release of excitatory amino acid in an animal stroke model.[49] However, although Maxipost progressed into phase III trials for stroke, the study was halted because BMS-204352 failed to show superior efficacy compared with placebo. To our knowledge, no similar compound is currently being tested for stroke therapy.

Free-Radical Scavengers

Another class of drugs thought to have neuroprotective actions is free-radical scavengers. During ischemia, highly reactive oxygen free radicals are released from ischemic tissue because of reducing conditions and/or overexcitation of excitatory amino acid receptors.[50] Production of free radicals is potentially capable of generation of further free radicals that can destroy cell membranes. Whether this chain of events occurs to any appreciable extent during stroke has not been proven conclusively, but preclinical studies of agents with free-radical scavenging properties have shown to be effective in reducing neurological damage in some animal models.[51] In particular, tirilazad (U70046F) has been studied in a series of clinical trials in patients with ischemic stroke, subarachnoid hemorrhage, and head injury.[52] Although the drug was apparently well tolerated, a phase III acute stroke trial ended prematurely when an interim analysis revealed that results were highly unlikely to demonstrate significant treatment efficacy. Subsequently, another study using a higher dose was also terminated for the same reason.[53] Citicoline (cytidyl diphosphocholine), a phosphatidylcholine precursor, has membrane stabilization properties, but its actions are probably multiple. There are a number of preclinical studies in animal models demonstrating that citicoline administration improved either neurological outcome or infarct size.[54,55] Although phase I and II trials showed signs of neuroprotective efficacy of citicoline in acute stroke patients, subsequent phase III trials with different doses and dosing schedules failed to demonstrate its efficacy in acute stroke therapy.[56] Ebselen is a compound with antioxidant activity through a glutathione peroxidase-like action. A phase II trial was conducted in Japan and showed efficacy against acute stroke at 3 months but not at 6 months, if patients were treated within 24 hours after stroke. A phase III trial with 40 centers is currently being conducted in Japan.

GABA Receptor Antagonists

Clomethiazole is a drug derived from the thiazole moiety of thiamine that has been used clinically for years as an anticonvulsant, sedative, and hypnotic agent and for the treatment of alcohol withdrawal symptoms.[57] Receptor binding and electrophysiological studies suggest that clomethiazole appears to potentiate the effect of the neurotransmitter GABA via interaction with GABA-A receptor. According to Green,[58] the drug showed neuroprotective features on both global and focal ischemia, as assessed by various outcome measures, such as histopathology, excitatory amino acid release in vivo, and edema formation. These studies form the basis for progression of this drug into clinical trials for stroke. In a phase III trial, there was no statistically significant difference between placebo- and drug-treated groups encompassing a total of 1360 patients. However, a subgroup analysis revealed an interaction between treatment group and the severity of illness, indicating a positive effect of clomethiazole in the most severe patients.[59] Based on these findings, another phase III may be designed to confirm the subgroup of patients who seemed to benefit in the previous trial. Diazepam is another GABA antagonist currently being investigating for acute stroke therapy. A multicenter phase III trial is being conducted in Europe, targeting patients within 12 hours after stroke onset.

Serotonin Agonists

Activation of postsynaptic serotonin receptors (5-HT_{1A}) was associated with increase in potassium efflux, inhibition of cell excitability during ischemic insult, and protection of neurons from glutamate-mediated neuronal death. Repinotan (BAY X3702) is a high-affinity serotonin (5-HT_{1A}) agonist. Binding of repinotan to postsynaptic 5-HT_{1A} receptors was shown to abate excitotoxic neuronal death and protect rat brain from focal ischemic injury.[60] A phase II clinical trial involving 240 patients was completed late in 2000 and showed an improved neurological and functional outcome at 4 weeks and 3 months in those patients receiving a dose of 1.25 mg/day for 3 days within 6 hours after stroke. A phase IIb trial projected to include 680 patients is now enrolling patients in North America; however, the therapeutic window was reduced to 4.5 hours after symptom onset.

Caspase Inhibitors

As mentioned in the previous section, apoptosis was shown to extend brain injury in various animal models of stroke. One of the important elements in the apoptosis cascade is caspase activation. Caspases are a group of cysteine proteases that cleave various effectors of neuronal apoptosis including poly-adenosine diphosphate (ADP) ribose polymerase (PARP), deoxyribonucleic acid (DNA)-dependent protein kinase, U1-soluble nuclear ribonucleic acid (RNA) polymerase (U1-snRNP), spectrin, lamin A, actin, and protein kinase C. Activation of caspases has been shown in different animal ischemic models, whereas inhibition of caspase activity leads to pathological improvement of ischemic stroke.[61,62] An interesting study from Chopps' laboratory[63] indicating caspase inhibitor, Z-VAD significantly improved the survival of grafted bone marrow cells, hence improved the functional outcome of middle cerebral occlusion in a rat model. Although the protective effects of caspase inhibitors in preclinical studies are convincing, none of the caspase inhibitors has yet to progress to a clinical trial, possibly because of their hydrophobic characters.

Other Potential Neuroprotective Agents

Other drugs that have potential neuroprotective properties are also being tested in clinical trials. Nalmefene is an opioid antagonist with relative selectivity for kappa opiate receptors. It has been shown to inhibit glutamate release during global cerebral ischemia and protect neurons from ischemic damage. Nalmefene stereospecifically inhibits glutamate release during global cerebral ischemia.[64,65] However, a phase III trial completed recently showed no significant difference in 3-month functional outcome for nalmefene treatment compared with placebo.[66] Lubeluzole is a drug that may have multiple effects. Although it was shown to inhibit nitric oxide production, the neuroprotective effects of lubeluzole are currently unclear. A series of phase I to III trials have been conducted for ischemic stroke; however, they failed to show significant efficacy compared with placebo in recent phase III trials.

Gangliosides fall within a family of large-molecular-weight glycosphingolipids. A number of experiments in ischemic brain injury models have shown protection when the ganglioside G_{M1} was administered.[67,68] With regard to G_{M1}-mediated protection, a number of mechanisms have been proposed to account for this result: normalizing altered protein phosphorylation, increasing brain-derived neurotrophic factor (BDNF) expression, blocking overstimulation by excitatory amino acid, and stabilizing plasma membrane structure. In light of these results, a number of small clinical trials have subsequently examined the effect of G_{M1} administration in stroke patients. The largest trial, a collaborative effort, examined 502 patients randomly assigned to treatment with G_{M1}, G_{M1} plus hemodilution, placebo, or placebo plus hemodilution. G_{M1} was given intravenously daily starting within 12 hours after stroke onset and continuing for 15 days. However, no significant differences in Canadian Neurological Scale Scores were demonstrated among these groups at 120 days.[69]

THERAPEUTIC STRATEGIES FOR FUNCTIONAL RECOVERY

There is evidence that recovery from stroke is due, at least in part, to brain plasticity and reorganization. Methods have been proposed to augment brain reorganization, including stimulation of endogenous processes through pharmacological or molecular manipulation, gene therapy, behavioral and rehabilitation strategies, and provision of new substrates for recovery through cell transplantation. In this section, we focus on the potential therapeutic roles of neurotrophic factors and stem cell implantation in ischemic stroke.

Neurotrophic Factors

Neurotrophic factors are a group of protein peptides that affect target cells by paracrine, autocrine, or juxtacrine methods. They include epidermal growth factor (EGF); fibroblast growth factor (FGF); hepatocyte growth factor (HGF); insulin-like growth factor (IGF); transforming growth factor (TGF); platelet-derived growth factor (PDGF); glial cell line–derived neurotrophic factor (GDNF); ciliary neurotrophic factor (CNTF); and neurotrophins, which include nerve growth factor (NGF), brain-derived neurotrophic factor (BDNF), neurotrophin-3 (NT-3), and neurotrophin-4/5 (NT-4/5). In the developmental stage, neurotrophic factors are involved in cell proliferation, migration, differentiation, and production on extracellullar matrix in the nervous system. In adult CNS, neurotrophic factors are thought to play roles in normal maintenance and survival of neuronal cells after their differentiation. Although the molecular mechanisms of neurotrophic factors in adult animals are not clear, constant action of neurotrophic factors was thought to keep cell survival genes activated and suicidal genes suppressed.[70] For this reason, deprivation of neurotrophic factors in the penumbra of ischemic tissue may thus activate apoptotic signal cascades and lead to cell death.

Neurotrophic factors also play important roles in the protection and recovery of mature neurons after various type of brain injury. In preclinical studies, neurotrophic factors such as NGF, BDNF, CDNF, GDNF, VEGF, and IGF-1 have all been shown to reduced infarct size of ischemic injury in both adult[71–73] and immature animals.[74,75] However, only basic fibroblast growth factor (bFGF or FGF-2) made it to clinical trials. FGF-2 is a polypeptide that is present in high levels in the brain. It increases neuonal survival, has trophic effects on brain glial and endothelial cells, and is a potent systemic and cerebral vasodilator.[76,77] Following intraventricular injection, bFGF significantly reduced infarct size in a model of focal ischemia in rats.[78] Furthermore, IV infusion of bFGF begun after permanent[79] and transient occlusion of the MCA[80] also demonstrated anti-ischemic effects. However, the U.S. phase II trial in combination with rt-PA has been halted because the drug group did worse compared with the placebo group.

Neural Stem Cells

Neural stem cells are a group of cells that possessed the potential, such as multidirectional differentiation and self-regeneration. They were mainly found in a developing brain and their differentiation depends on both intrinsic and environmental stimuli such as nutrients, neurotrophic factors, and various sensory stimuli. For centuries, nerve cells in adult brain were considered to be fixed and nonregeneratable. The recent discovery of neural stem cells revolutionized this notion. The neural stem cells in adult brain were originally found concentrated in the subgranular zone of the hippocampal dentate gyrus or the subventricular zone,[81] but later they were also found in other brain regions including the frontal cortex.[82] A significance of these discoveries is that, in certain circumstances, these cells have the ability to regenerate and rearrange the neural network, which may restore all or part of the functions lost in injuries such as stroke. In fact, regeneration of neurons has been observed in various adult animal models in response to ischemic insults. By using a model of transient forebrain ischemia in mice, Takagi et al[83] demonstrated an increase in proliferation of neuronal precursor cells in hippocampal dentate gyrus. Furthermore, these cells were shown to proliferate in response to ischemia and subsequently migrate into the hippocampus to regenerate new neurons. Intraventricular infusion of growth factors markedly augments these responses, thereby increasing the number of newborn neurons.[84] Cell proliferation and differentiation from ependymal, subependymal, and choroid plexus cells in response to stroke were also demonstrated.[85] The therapeutic potential of stem cells is further demonstrated by increased functional recovery in an MCA occlusion model of rats even when histological recovery was not observed.[86]

To further test the possible therapeutic benefits of neuronal transplant on stroke patients, a small phase I study was conducted by Kondziolka et al.[87] LBS-Neurons, a cell line derived from human teratocarcinoma, were transplanted into the brains of 12 patients with basal ganglia stroke and fixed motor deficits. Although evaluations 12 to 18 months later showed no adverse cell-related serological or imaging-defined effects and there was a mean improvement of 2.9 points in (European Stroke Scale score) all patients ($p = 0.04$), the results must be viewed with great caution. First, LBS-Neurons are cells derived from human teratocarcinoma; a 12 to 18 month follow-up is not enough to ensure the safety of the transplants. Second, the efficacy of the study should be interpreted with caution because two of these subjects achieved improvements with p-values below the conventional 0.05, and by chance alone, 12 tests of significance of this type will result in at least one false positive approximately 50 percent of the time. Because the two positive findings reported here are strongly correlated, it is likely that the functional improvement studies did not detect anything meaningful. However, it should be emphasized that this was a phase I study that was not designed or powered to prove efficacy.

Even with all the promising evidence of neural stem cells on stroke therapy, there are two main limitations hindering the translation of laboratory studies into clinical practice. First, isolating and maintaining neural stem cells is technically difficult and the source of neural stem cells is relatively limited. Second, implantation of neural stem cells requires neurosurgical intervention, is traumatic, and may be associated with significant side effects. To approach these problems, researchers have been looking for possible alternatives. Bone marrow stromal cells were found not only to differentiate into mesodermal cells like chondrocytes, osteoblasts, and adipocytes but also to develop into neuroectodermal cells such as neurons.[88] Furthermore, bone marrow stromal cells transplanted into the ischemic boundary zone after MCA occlusion in a rat model demonstrated that animals that received bone marrow stromal cells displayed significant recovery in motor, somatosensory, and behavioral tests compared with control animals.[89,90] Interestingly, a significant recovery of motor function was observed after bone marrow stromal cells were given intravenously 1 day after stroke.[91] This suggests that their beneficial effect on recovery involves actions other than replacement of lost neurons in the infarcted region. Although the mechanisms are currently not understood, the beneficial effects were thought to derive from the increase of growth factors in the ischemic tissue, the reduction of apoptosis in the penumbral zone of the lesion, and the proliferation of endogenous cells in the subventricular zone.[91]

FROM FAILURES WE LEARN

As discussed in previous sections, many drugs have been tested in multicenter clinical trials. Although preclinical studies and some phase I and II trials suggested beneficial effects, the final results of neuroprotective therapies for acute stroke have been uniformly negative. Reasons for the failure have been subjected to intense discussion for the last several years.[92–96] In this section, we discuss potential problems that surfaced during the translation of neuroprotective agents from animal studies to clinical practice. By correcting those mistakes we may form a basis for future trials.

Problems That May Have Caused the Failure of Past Clinical Trials

The discrepancy of preclinical studies and clinical trials made it clear that current animal models (mostly rodents) may not be perfect models for the investigation of stroke therapies. There are many explanations for these divergent findings.

Animal Stroke Models May Not Reliably Predict Human Stroke

The differences between human brain and rodent brain are obvious in many aspects of anatomy, pathophysiology, and pharmacology. In rodents, more than 90 percent of brain tissue is composed of gray matter, whereas in humans, gray matter makes up about 50 percent.[97] The efficacy of neuroprotective agents in animal studies, mostly measured by reduction of infarct size, was mainly represented in gray matter protection. However, even in the most homogeneous population of cortical stroke patients, the damage to white matter will be significantly larger than in rodent models. White matter may possess completely different populations of receptors compared to gray matter, which may respond differently to neuroprotective agents. On the other hand, efficacy of neuroprotection in clinical trials is mainly measured by improvement on functional outcome. Although functional improvement was often tested in animal stroke models, the complexity of human white matter may represent different functional significance compared with animal models.

There are significant differences between the types of stroke in preclinical studies and the clinical trials. Most of the stroke models used MCA occlusion, which creates a pure cortical infarction in the animals. However, clinical trials often enroll patients with different types of stroke as long as the patient meets the inclusion criteria (mainly time window of stroke onset and severity of the stroke). In fact, only 35 percent of the trials targeted a specific stroke territory in their studies.[4] Because different types of stroke may associate with different sites of injury, response to a particular drug may also be different. Another discrepancy between preclinical studies and stroke patients is that, in stroke models, only young, healthy animals are used to create a specific focal infarct, whereas stroke patients are usually old and suffering from multiple chronic diseases such as atherosclerosis, hypertension, hyperlipidemia, hyperglycemia, and even prior stroke. Patients' pre-morbid conditions may significantly alter their functional outcome,[98] which is often the main measurement for the efficacy of neuroprotective agents.

Measurement of drug toxicity is another concern that may hinder the clinical use. Traditionally, the outcome measurement for drug toxicity is death in animal stroke studies. Other relatively mild adverse effects such as headache, myalgia, nausea, fatigue, depression, visual disturbance, cardiac arrhythmia, or asymptomatic internal hemorrhage may not be noticed. However, in clinical trials, patient tolerability becomes a most important issue. In fact, many trials were terminated because of adverse effects.

Trial Designs Do Not Represent Animal Studies

In most of the animal studies, neuroprotective drugs were given before or immediately after the onset of ischemia. In fact, most of the neuroprotective agents tested showed efficacy within 2 to 3 hours of acute artery occlusion.[99,100] However, because many pharmaceutical companies view such a short therapeutical window as a major obstacle to marketing the drugs, most of clinical trials chose the window of 6 to 12 hours after stroke. Some trials even extended the window to as long as 12 days.[4] Although animal studies indicated that neuronal death could be observed as late as 14 days after the onset of stroke,[101] the role of delayed neuronal death in human stroke is not yet clear. It is possible that most therapeutic windows chosen for clinical trials are simply too long for any meaningful neuroprotection.

Another key disagreement between animal studies and clinical trials is the drug dosing and dosing schedules. To avoid CNS complications, some of the trials chose the dose that is significantly lower than those in animal studies.[102] However, although most animal studies gave drugs for only a short period before or after ischemic insult, the dosing schedules in previous clinical trials were highly variable, ranging from one single IV infusion to multiple oral doses up to 3 months after stroke.[103] Prolonged administration of certain neuroprotective drugs may exert opposite effects because many of these drugs, especially glutamate antagonists, GABA agonists, and calcium channel blockers, are CNS suppressive and may reduce patients' efforts for rehabilitation. They can even suppress the neural plasticity during recovery.

Recommendations for Future Clinical Trials

After reviewing past unsuccessful trials on neuroprotective drugs, Stroke Therapy Academic Industry Roundtable (STAIR-II) has recently published recommendations for future trials.[104] The recommendations suggested that some key decisions must be made to ensure a good phase III acute stroke trial.

1. Dose selection should be based on preclinical studies and phase I and II trials
   Because most of the trials expect that the drugs take effect in CNS, the dose used should have reliable data proving that the drugs have good penetration into CNS at least in preclinical studies. The doses selected for the trials should achieve the plasma concentration that was projected to be therapeutic in CNS. However, the doses used in stroke animal models may not always represent the effective doses in human patients. To identify the most appropriate dose for the maximal number of patients, a 250-year-old statistical technique, Bayesian technique, has recently been given new life in advanced drug trials.[105] Patients in the trial will be randomly assigned to a range of doses initially, based on the preclinical studies and previous phase I or II trials; the outcome data from each patient will be fed back to a computer as the trial proceeds; and the optimal dose will be generated for later randomization. Bayesian technique allows statisticians to review a trial continuously, to eliminate ineffective or potentially harmful doses, and may reduce sample size in future studies.

2. Time window for initiation of drugs must reflect the preclinical studies and phase I and II trials
   The initial time window should be as short as possible after stroke onset to maximize the possibility to detect any therapeutic benefit. A follow-up trial may be needed to extend the therapeutic window if the initial trial with a shorter window proved to be effective. Although a time window for the trial is selected, researchers should be encouraged to enroll patients as soon as possible after symptom onset, and stratification by enrollment time should be considered.

3. Appropriate patient population should be selected for the trial
   As discussed in the previous section, the mechanism of injury elicited by ischemic stroke in gray matter may be different than those in white matter. If the trial is mainly targeting gray matter, then the patients with subcortical lacunar infarct that are mainly confined to the white matter should be excluded. Computed tomography (CT) scan and diffusion- and perfusion-weighted magnetic resonance imaging (MRI) may be useful tools for a timely answer if the clinical picture is not clear. By the same logic, if the drug is designed to lyse a thrombus, compromise of cerebral blood flow might be established before the patient is enrolled. CT angiogram or magnetic resonance angiography (MRA) may be good tools for confirming the diagnosis. Furthermore, although patients with mild strokes (NIHSS <6) may have a better chance for spontaneous recovery, patients with severe stroke (NIHSS >22) are less likely to have full recovery. For these reasons, patients with moderate deficit (NIHSS 7 to 22) may have a better chance to show the beneficial effects of the drugs. Thus trials enrolling only patients with NIHSS between 7 and 22 may have a better chance for success.

4. Endpoint and outcome measurement should be appropriate for the type of the drug tested

   Traditionally, 90 days after stroke was used as primary endpoint for acute stroke trials. However, some medical complications unrelated to tested drugs might alter the outcome measurement with prolonged follow-up. An earlier endpoint may help to eliminate those unwanted effects. Likewise, drugs that tested for restorative effects might need a longer follow-up period to allow beneficial effects to be shown. Another critical issue for a successful trial is what type of outcome measures should be used. Measures of impairment, disability, and handicap have been chosen in prior trials, but none was proven to be superior to others. In fact, the global statistic approach with employing multiple predefined outcome measures proved to be more effective than any single outcome measure in NINDS rt-PA stroke trial.[106] Imaging outcome measures might be included in the global outcome measures.

5. Combination therapy trials

   The proof that rt-PA is effective in stroke therapy has resulted in thrombolytic therapy becoming the standard of care in the United States and a number of foreign countries. Any acute stroke trial in the future may have to be administered in combination with rt-PA. In fact, there is preclinical evidence indicating that combinations of rt-PA and some neuroprotective agents may result in additive effects.[107,108] Administration of rt-PA might increase the perfusion to ischemic penumbra, preserve more salvageable tissue for neuroprotection, and lead to better outcomes with longer therapeutic windows.[107,108] On the other hand, co-administration of neuroprotective agents might effectively extend the therapeutic window for rt-PA.[109]

   According to their mechanisms of actions, some of the neuroprotective agents may have synergistic effects on acute ischemic stroke. Combined use of two or more neuroprotective agents from different families might increase the beneficial effects. One other potential advantage is that the dose of each drug may be reduced to limit the drug toxicity that often leads to the termination of the trials. However, combining two or more drugs in the same trial will apparently add to the complexity of trial design. No combination of neuroprotective agents was effective. Treatment window and drug-drug interactions of each drug are not known. Using two or more unknown types of drugs in the same trial is both impractical and potentially hazardous. Thus at least one neuroprotective agent must be proven effective and established as a standard of treatment before any kind of combination trial is practical.

FUTURE STROKE THERAPIES

When rt-PA became the standard treatment for selected acute stroke patients in United States, stroke became a treatable emergency. The notion that "time is brain" may extend the acute stroke therapy from emergency departments to the emergency medical service (EMS) field. Evidence from decades of stroke studies demonstrated that cerebral ischemia might elicit various pathophysiological and biochemical events that trigger intracellular cascades leading to a wide spectrum of brain damage. By interrupting the beginning of the cascades, brain tissue damage may be limited. With the possible availability of neuroprotective agents in the future, a cocktail may be developed with a combination of neuroprotective agents from different families, which may include glutamate antagonists, ion channel blockers, free-radical scavengers, and anti-inflammatory agents. By targeting the initial steps of pathological cascades leading to ischemic cell death, this cocktail may be given in the field to inhibit the propagation of ischemic injury and maximize the therapeutic window for thrombolytic therapies of the future. The EMS system should be structured to ensure that all stroke patients are taken to the hospitals that provide comprehensive stroke care, including thrombolytic therapies. On arriving in the emergency department, activities should focus on shortening the door-to-needle time, for instance, by implementation of a stroke code clinical path. In addition to treating patients within the 3-hour therapeutic window, more sophisticated diagnostic techniques, such as diffusion/perfusion CT and MRI, magnetic resonance (MR)-spectroscopy, and possible perfusion transcranial Doppler (TCD), may be used in patients who otherwise would present outside the therapeutic window, to identify salvageable brain tissue and properly select patients for thrombolytic treatments. Neuroprotective agents, especially those treating reperfusion injury, should be initiated with a thrombolytic agent. Other measures aiming at minimizing brain tissue damage, such as euglycemic, hypothermic, and normotensive therapies could be initiated. Ideally, stroke patients should be admitted to stroke units with nurses trained to take care of stroke patients. Antiapoptotic agents preventing delayed neuronal damage and restorative agents promoting neurite regeneration could be used hours after stroke to inhibit the progression of brain tissue injury and maximize functional recovery. Antiplatelet agents can also be started if hemorrhagic stroke can be ruled out. Table 15.2 is a summary of the timetable with possible main pathophysiological events and therapeutic interventions for acute stroke in the future.

CONCLUSION

This is a remarkable time in the field of acute stroke therapy. In the past, physicians had little to offer to stroke patients, and therapy for acute stroke patients appeared hopeless. However, the success of rt-PA revolutionized acute stroke therapy. Although the development of neuroprotective agents has been very difficult, what we have learned from the previous failures will certainly spur further development in this field. There is reason to expect that at least some of the drugs or combinations will be effective. Stroke remains the leading cause of adult disability and the third most common cause of death in industrialized nations. Thus there is abundant need for better methods of care.

APPENDIX: STRUCTURAL DIFFERENCES BETWEEN TNK AND RT-PA

TNK is produced by substituting the following amino acids: asparagine for threonine at position 103 (T site), glutamine for asparagine at position 117 (N site),

Table 15.2 Stroke therapies for the future: treatments targeting on possible pathophysiological events following acute ischemic stroke

Time	Time Zero	Minutes	Minutes to Hours	Hours to Days	Weeks to Months
Events	Symptoms Onset	Ambulance	Emergency Department	ICU/Inpatient Ward	Rehabilitation Center
Major pathophysiological events	Thrombosis or embolism Artery occlusion Reduce cerebral blood flow Reduce energy and O_2 supply	Release of glutamate and other excitatory amino acids Na influx Ca influx Free-radicals release Cytotoxic edema	Uncontrolled enzyme activation Apoptotic cascade activation Excitotoxic neuronal damage Inflammatory responses Reperfusion injury Tissue necrosis	Tissue necrosis and edema Apoptosis and delayed ischemic tissue injury Increase in neurotrophic factors, expression, and production Activation of regenerative pathways	Compensatory neurite regeneration Stem cell differentiation and migration Functional compensation
Possible interventions	Activation of Emergency Medical System	Neuroprotective agents such as glutamate antagonists, ion channel blockers, and free-radical scavengers	Thrombolytic therapies with patient selection for therapeutic window extension Neuroprotective agents including anti-inflammatory agents, enzyme inhibitors, free-radical scavengers, and antiapoptotic agents Hypothermic and euglycemic therapies	Continue neuroprotective agents with antiapoptotic properties Pharmacological agents to promote neurotrophic factors production and neuronal regeneration Continue hypothermic, euglycemic, and normotensive therapies Rehabilitation	Rehabilitation Stem cells implantation Gene therapy Pharmacological agents that may facilitate neurorehabilitation

and one lysine, one histidine, and two arginines for the four alanines at positions 296 through 299 (K site) of the original rt-PA structure. The main structure of both t-PA and TNK is composed of the following domains: finger domain, epidermal growth factor domain, the two-kringle structures, and the serine protease domains. Figure 15.1 demonstrates the amino acid sequence and domains of TNK. The site at which interaction and activation of plasminogen occurs is labeled by the symbol *.[110]

References

1. The NINDS t-PA Stroke Study Group. Generalized efficacy of t-PA for acute stroke. Subgroup analysis of the NINDS t-PA Stroke Trial. Stroke 1997;28:2119–2125.
2. Hademenos G. Metro stroke task force: first year experience. Stroke 1999;33:2512.
3. Clark WM, Wissman S, Albers GW, et al. Recombinant tissue-type plasminogen activator (Alteplase) for ischemic stroke 3 to 5 hours after symptom onset. The ATLANTIS Study: a randomized controlled trial. Alteplase Thrombolysis for Acute Noninterventional Therapy in Ischemic Stroke. JAMA 1999;282:2019–2026.
4. Kidwell CS, Liebeskind DS, Starkman S., Saver JL. Trends in acute ischemic stroke trial through the 20th century. Stroke 2001;32:1349–1359.
5. Verstraete M. Third generation thrombolytic drugs. Am J Med 2000;109:52–58.
6. Thomas GR, Thibodeaux H, Errett CJ, et al. A long-half-life and fibrin-specific form of tissue plasminogen activator in rabbit models of embolic stroke and peripheral bleeding. Stroke 1994;25:2072–2079.
7. Van de Werf F, Cannon C, Luyten A, et al. Safety assessment of single-bolus administration of TNK tissue-plasminogen activator in acute myocardial infarction: the ASSENT-1 trial. Am Heart J 2000;137:786–791.
8. Van de Werf F, Barron HV, Armstrong P, et al. Incidence and predictors of bleeding events after fibrinolytic therapy with fibrin-specific agents. Eur Heart J 2001;22:2253–2261.
9. Lapchak PA, Araujo DM, Pakola S, et al. Microplasm: a novel thrombolytic that improves behavioral outcome after embolic strokes in rabbits. Stroke 2002;33:2279–2284.
10. del Zoppo G, Higashida RT, Furlan AJ, et al. PROACT: a phase II randomized trial of recombinant pro-urokinase by direct arterial delivery in acute middle cerebral artery stroke. Stroke 1998;29:4–11.
11. Furlan AJ, Higashida RT, Wechsler L, et al. Intra-arterial prourokinase for acute ischemic stroke. The PROACT II study: a randomized controlled trial. JAMA 1999;282:2003–2011.
12. Lewandowski C, Frankel M, Tomsick T, et al. Combined intravenous and intra-arterial r-TPA versus intra-arterial therapy of acute ischemic stroke. Stroke 1999;30:2598–2605.
13. CAVATAS group. Endovascular versus surgical treatment in patients with carotid stenosis in the Carotid and Vertebral Artery Transluminal Angioplasty (CAVATAS). Lancet 2001;357:1729–1737.
14. Golledge J, Mitchell A, Greenhalgh RM, Davies AH. Systemic comparison of the early outcome of angioplasty and endarterectomy for symptomatic carotid artery disease. Stroke 2000;31:1439–1443.
15. Hobson RW. Update on the Carotid Revascularization Endarterectomy versus Stent Trial (CREST) protocol. J Am Coll Surg 2002;194(1 suppl):S9–14.
16. Gomez CR, Misra VK, Liu MW, et al. Elective stenting of symptomatic basilar artery stenosis. Stroke 2000;31:95–99.
17. Nakano S, Iseda T, Yoneyama T, et al. Direct percutaneous transluminal angioplasty for acute middle cerebral artery trunk occlusion: an alternative option to intra-arterial thrombolysis. Stroke 2002;33:2872–2876.
18. Lutsep H. Mechanical thrombolysis in acute stroke (www.emedicine.com/neuro/topic702.htm 2002).
19. Mayer TE, Hamann GF, Brueckmann HJ. Treatment of basilar artery embolism with a mechanical extraction device: necessity of flow reversal. Stroke 2002;33:2232–2235.
20. Whitlow PL, Lylyk P, Londero H, et al. Carotid artery stenting protected with an emboli containment system. Stroke 2002;33:1308–1314.
21. The Hypothermia After Cardiac Arrest Study Group. Mild therapeutic hypothermia to improve the neurologic outcome after cardiac arrest. New Engl J Med 2002;346:549–556.
22. Bernard SA GT, Buist MD, Jones BM, et al. Treatment of comatose survivors of out-of-hospital cardiac arrest with induced hypothermia. New Engl J Med 2002;346:557–563.

23. Wang Y, Lim L, Levi C, et al. Influence of admission body temperature on stroke mortality. Stroke 2000;31:404–409.
24. Krieger D, De Georgia M, Abou-Chebl A, et al. Cooling for acute ischemic brain damage (COOL AID). Stroke 2001;32:1847–1854.
25. Georgiadis D, Schwarz S, Kollmar R, Schwab S. Endovascular cooling for moderate hypothermia in patients with acute stroke: first results of a novel approach. Stroke 2001;32:2550–2553.
26. Mahon BR, Nesbit GM, Barnwell SL. The North American clinical experience with the EKOS ultrasound thrombolytic drug infusion catheter for treatment of embolic stroke. 1 Apr 26; 2001 (www.emedicine.com/neuro/).
27. Ishibashi T, Akiyama M, Onoue H, et al. Can transcranial ultrasonication increase recanalization flow with tissue plasminogen activator? Stroke 2002;33:1399–1404.
28. Lutsep H, Campbell M, Clark WM. EPAR therapy system for treatment of acute stroke: safety study results. Stroke 2001;32:319.
29. Guytt LL, Diaz FG, O'Regan MH, et al. Real-time measurement of glutamate release from the ischemic penumbra of the rat cerebral cortex using a focal middle cerebral artery occlusion model. Neurosci Lett 2001;299:37–40.
30. Boast CS, Gerhardt B, Pastor G, et al. The N-methyl-D-aspartate antagonist CGS19755 and CPP reduce ischemic brain damage in gerbils. Brain Res 1988;442:345–348.
31. Gotti B, Duverger D, Bertin J, et al. Ifenprodil and SL 82.0715 as cerebral anti-ischemic agents. 1. Evidence for efficacy in models of focal cerebral ischemia. J Pharmacol Exp Ther 1988;247:1211–1221.
32. O'Neill MJ, Hicks C, Ward M. Neuroprotective effects of 7-nitroindazole in gerbil model of global cerebral ischemia. Eur J Pharmacol 1996;310:115–122.
33. Patat A, Molininier P, Hergueta T, et al. Lack of amnestic, psychotomimetic or impairing effect on psychomotor performance of eliprodil, a new NMDA antagonist. Int Clin Psychopharmacol 1994;9:155–162.
34. Aronowski J, Ostrow P, Samways E, et al. Graded bioassay for demonstration of brain rescue from experimental acute ischemia in rats. Stroke 1994;25:2235–2240.
35. Cohen RA, Hasegawa Y, Fisher M. Effects of a novel NMDA receptor antagonist on experimental stroke quantitatively assessed by spectral EEG and infarct volume. Neurol Res 1994;16:443–448.
36. Muir KW. New experimental data on the efficacy of pharmacological magnesium infusions in cerebral infarcts (abstract). Magnes Res 1998;11:43–56.
37. Shimizu-Sasamata M, Kano T, Rogowska J, et al. YM872, a highly water-soluble AMPA receptor antagonist, preserves the hemodynamic penumbra and reduces brain injury after permanent focal ischemia in rats. Stroke 1998;29:2141–2148.
38. Clark WM, Madden KP, Rothlein R, Zivin JA. Reduction of central nervous system ischemic injury by monoclonal antibody to intercellular adhesion molecule. J Neurosurg 1991;75:623–627.
39. Zhang RL, Chopp M, Jiang N, et al. Anti-intercellular adhesion molecule-1 antibody reduces ischemic cell damage after transient but not permanent middle cerebral artery occlusion in the Wistar rat. Stroke 1995;26:1438–1443.
40. Jiang N, Chopp M, Chahwala S. Neutrophil inhibitory factor treatment of focal cerebral ischemia in the rat. Brain Res 1998;788:25–34.
41. Ohta K, Graf R, Rosner G, Heiss WD. Calcium ion transients in peri-infarct depolarizations may deteriorate ion homeostasis and expand infarction in focal cerebral ischemia in cats. Stroke 2001;32:535–543.
42. Steen P, Newberg LA, Milde JH, Michenfelder JD. Nimodipine improves cerebral blood flow and neurologic recovery after complete cerebral ischemia in the dog. J Cereb Blood Flow Metab 1983;3:38–43.
43. The American Nimodipine Study Group. Clinical trial of nimodipine in acute ischemic stroke. Stroke 1992;23:3–8.
44. Mohr JP, Ogogozo JM, Harrison MJG. Meta-analysis of oral nimodipine trials in acute ischemic stroke. Cerebrovasc Dis 1994;4:197–203.
45. Horn J, de Haan R, Vermeulen M, Limburg M. Very early nimodipine use in stroke (VENUS). Stroke 2001;32:461–465.
46. Bebin M, Bleck TP. New anticonvulsant drugs: Focus on flunarizine, fosphenytoin, midazolam and stiripentol. Drugs 1994;48:153–171.
47. McLean MJ, MacDonald RL. Multiple action of phenytoin on mouse spinal cord neurons in cell culture. J Pharmacol Exp Ther 1983;227:779–789.
48. Ferrendelli JA, Danials-McQueen S. Comparative actions of phenytoin and other antiepileptic drugs on potassium-and veratridine-stimulated calcium uptake in synaptosomes. J Pharmacol Exp Ther 1983;220:29–34.

49. Gribkoff VK, Starrett JE Jr, Dworetzky SI, et al. Targeting acute ischemic stroke with a calcium-sensitive opener of maxi-K potassium channels. Nat Med 2001;7:471–477.
50. Cheng Y, Sun AY. The biomechanisms of kainate-induced neurotoxicity involved in oxidative insult. Neurochemical Res 1994;19:1557–1564.
51. Lapchak PA, Chapman DF, Zivin JA. Pharmacological effects of the spin trap agents N-t-butyl-phenylnitrone (PBN) and 2,2,6, 6-tetramethylpiperidine-N-oxyl (TEMPO) in a rabbit thromboembolic stroke model: combination studies with the thrombolytic tissue plasminogen activator. Stroke 2001;32:147–153.
52. Haley EC, Kassell NF, Apperson-Hansen C, et al. A randomized, double-blind, vehicle-controlled trial of tirilazad mesylate in patients with aneurysmal subarachnoid hemorrhage: a cooperative study in North America. J Neurosurg 1997;86:467–474.
53. Haley EC Jr. High-dose tirilazad for acute stroke (RANTTAS II). RANTTAS II investigators. Stroke 1998;29:1256–1257.
54. D'Orlando KJ, Sandage BW Jr. Citicoline (CDP-choline): mechanisms of action and effects in ischemic brain injury. Neurol Res 1995;17:281–284.
55. Schabitz W, Fuhai L, Katsumi I, et al. Synergistic effects of a combination of low-dose basic fibroblast growth factor and citicoline after temporary experimental focal ischemia. Stroke 1999;30:427–432.
56. Clark WM, Warach SJ, Pettigrew LC, et al. A randomized dose-response trial of citicoline in acute ischemic stroke patients. Citicoline Stroke Study Group. Neurology 1998;49:671–678.
57. Evans JG, Feuerlein W, Glatt MM, et al. Chlomethiazole 25 years: recent developments and historical perspectives. Acta Psychiatr Scand Suppl 1986;73(suppl 329):198.
58. Green AR. Clomethiazole (Zendra®) in acute ischemic stroke: basic pharmacology and biochemistry and clinical efficacy. Pharmacol Ther 1998;80:123–147.
59. Lyden P, Jacoby M, Schim J, et al. The Clomethiazole Acute Stroke Study in tissue-type plasminogen activator-treated stroke (CLASS-T): final results. Neurology 2001;57:1199–1205.
60. Alessandri B, Tsuchida E, Bullock RM. The neuroprotective effect of a new serotonin receptor agonist, BAY X3702, upon focal ischemic brain damage caused by acute subdural hematoma in the rat. Brain Research 1999;845:232–235.
61. Cheng Y, Deshmukh M, D'Costa A, et al. Caspase inhibitor affords neuroprotection with delayed administration in a rat model of neonatal hypoxic-ischemic brain injury. J Clin Invest 1998;101:1992–1999.
62. Endres M, Namura S, Shimizu-Sasamata M, et al. Attenuation of delayed neuronal death after mild focal ischemia in mice by inhibition of the caspase family. J Cereb Blood Flow Metab 1998;18:238–247.
63. Chen J, Li Y, Wang L, et al. Caspase inhibition by Z-VAD increases the survival of grafted bone marrow cells and improves functional outcome after MCAo in rats. J Neurol Sci 2002;199:17–24.
64. Yum SW, Faden AI. Comparison of the neuroprotective effects of the N-methyl-D-aspartate antagonist MK-801 and the opiate-receptor antagonist nalmefene in experimental spinal cord ischemia. Arch Neurol 1990;47:277–281.
65. Graham SH, Shimizu H, Newman A, et al. Opioid receptor antagonist nalmefene stereospecifically inhibits glutamate release during global cerebral ischemia. Brain Res 1993;632:346–350.
66. Clark WM, Raps EC, Tong DC, Kelly RE. Cervene (Nalmefene) in acute ischemic stroke: final results of a phase III efficacy study. The Cervene Stroke Study Investigators. Stroke 2000;31:1234–1239.
67. Leon A, Lipartiti M, Seren MS, et al. Hypoxic-ischemic damage and the neuroprotective effects of GM1ganglioside. Stroke 1990;21(suppl 11):11195–11197.
68. Carolei A, Fieschi C, Bruno R, Toffano G. Monosialoganglioside GM1 in cerebral ischemia. Cerebrovasc Brain Metab Rev 1991;3:134–157.
69. Argentino C, Sacchetti ML, Toni D, et al. GM1 ganglioside therapy in acute ischemic stroke: Italian acute stroke study—hemodilution + drug. Stroke 1989;20:1143–1149.
70. Jessell TM, Sanes JR. The Generation and Survival of Nerve Cells. In ER Kandel, JH Schwartz, TM Jessell (eds), Principles of Neural Science. New York: McGraw-Hill, 2000;1041–1062.
71. Zhang Y, Pardridge WM. Neuroprotection in transient focal brain ischemia after delayed intravenous administration of brain-derived neurotrophic factor conjugated to a blood-brain barrier drug targeting system. Stroke 2001;32:1378–1384.
72. Wen TC, Matsuda S, Yoshimura T, et al. Ciliary neurotrophic factor prevents ischemic-induced learning disability and neuronal loss in gerbils. Neurosci Lett 1995;191:55–58.
73. Abe K. Therapeutic potential of neurotrophic factors and neural stem cells against ischemic brain injury. J Cereb Blood Flow Metab 2000;20:1393–1408.
74. Holtzman DM, Sheldon R, Cheng Y, et al. NGF protects the neonatal brain against hypoxic-ischemic injury. Ann Neurol 1996;39:114–122.

75. Cheng Y, Gidday JM, Yan Q, et al. Marked age-dependent neuroprotection by brain derived neurotrophic factor against neonatal hypoxic-ischemic brain injury. Ann Neurol 1997;41:521–529.
76. Rosenblatt S, Irikura K, Caday DG, et al. Basic fibroblast growth factor (bFGF) dilates rat pial arterioles. J Cereb Blood Flow Metab 1994;14:70–74.
77. Cuevas P, Carceller F, Ortega S, et al. Hypotensive activity of fibroblast growth factor. Science 1991;254:1208–1210.
78. Koketsu N, Berlove DJ, Moskowitz MA, et al. Pretreatment with intraventricular basic fibroblast growth factor (bFGF) decreases infarct size following focal ischemia in rats. Ann Neurol 1994;35:451–457.
79. Fisher M, Meadows M-E, Do T, et al. Delayed treatment with intravenous basic fibroblast growth factor reduces infarct size following permanent cerebral ischemia in rats. J Cereb Blood Flow Metab 1995;15:953–959.
80. Jiang N, Finklestein SP, Do T, et al. Delayed intravenous administration of basic fibroblast growth factor (bFGF) reduced infarction volume in a model of focal cerebral ischemia/reperfusion in the rat. J Neurol Sci 1996;139:173–179.
81. Reynolds BA, Weiss S. Generation of neurons and astrocytes from isolated cells of the adult mammalian central nervous system. Science 1992;255:1707–1710.
82. Gould E, Reeves AJ, Graziano MSA, Gross CG. Neurogenesis in the neocortex of adult primates. Science 1999;286:548–552.
83. Takagi Y, Nozaki K, Takahashi J, et al. Proliferation of neuronal precursor cells in the dentate gyrus is accelerated after transient forebrain ischemia in mice. Brain Res 1999;831:283–287.
84. Nakatomi H, Kuriu T, Okabe S, et al. Regeneration of hippocampal pyramidal neurons after ischemic brain injury by recruitment of endogenous neural progenitors. Cell 2002;110:429–441.
85. Li Y, Chen J, Chopp M. Cell proliferation and differentiation from ependymal, subependymal and choroid plexus cells in response to stroke in rats. J Neurol Sci 2002;193:137–146.
86. Modo M, Stroemer P, Tang E, et al. Effects of implantation site of stem cell grafts on behavioral recovery from stroke damage. Stroke 2002;33:2270–2278.
87. Kondziolka D, Wechsler L, Goldstein S, et al. Transplantation of cultured human neuronal cells for patients with stroke. Neurology 2000;55:565–569.
88. Woodbury D, Schwarz EJ, Prockop DJ, Black IB. Adult rat and human bone marrow stromal cells differentiate into neurons. J Neurosci Res 2000;61:364–370.
89. Chen J, Li Y, Wang L, et al. Therapeutic benefit of intracerebral transplantation of bone marrow stromal cells after cerebral ischemia in rats. J Neurol Sci 2001;189:49–57.
90. Zhao LR, Duan WM, Reyes M, et al. Human bone marrow stem cells exhibit neural phenotypes and ameliorate neurological deficits after grafting into the ischemic brain of rats. Exp Neurol 2002;174:11–20.
91. Li Y, Chen J, Chen XG, et al. Human marrow stromal cell therapy for stroke in rat: neurotrophins and functional recovery. Neurology 2002;59:514–523.
92. Zivin JA, Grotta JC. Animal stroke models: they are relevant to human disease. Stroke 1990;21:981–983.
93. Grotta J. Neuroprotection is unlikely to be effective in humans using current trial designs. Stroke 2001;33:306–307.
94. Gorelick PB. Neuroprotection in acute ischaemic stroke: a tale of for whom the bell tolls. Lancet 2000;355:1925–1926.
95. Hunter AJ, Green AR, Cross DT. Animal models of acute ischemic stroke: can they predict clinically successful neuroprotective drugs? Trends Pharmacol Sci 1995;16:123–128.
96. Morgenstern LB. What have we learned from clinical neuroprotective trials? Neurology 2001;57:S45–S47.
97. Dewar D, Yam P, McCulloch J. Drug development for stroke: importance of protecting cerebral white matter. Eur J Pharmacol 1999;375:47–50.
98. Demchuk AM, Buchan AM. Predictors of stroke outcome. Neurol Clin 2001;18:455–473.
99. Grotta JC. Acute stroke therapy at the millennium: consummating the marriage between the laboratory and bedside: the Feinberg lecture. Stroke 1999;30:1722–1728.
100. Zivin JA. Factors determining the therapeutic window for stroke. Neurology 1998;50:599–603.
101. Du C, Hu R, Csernansky CA, et al. Very delayed infarction after mild focal cerebral ischemia: a role for apoptosis? J Cereb Blood Flow Metab 1996;16:195–201.
102. Jonas A, Aiyagari V, Vieira D, Figueroa M. The failure of neuronal protective agents versus the success of thrombolysis for the treatment of ischemic stroke. The predictive value of animal models. Ann N Y Acad Sci 2001;939:257–267.
103. Dyker AG, Lees KR. Duration of neuroprotective treatment for ischemic stroke. Stroke 1998;29:535–542.

104. Stroke Therapy Academic Industry Roundtable (STAIR) II. Recommendations for clinical trial evaluation of acute stroke therapies. Stroke 2001;32:1598–1606.
105. Malakoff D. Bayes offers a "new" way to make sense of numbers. Science 1999;286:1460–1464.
106. Tilley BC, Marler J, Geller NL, et al. Use of a global test for multiple outcomes in stroke trials with application to the National Institute of Neurological Disorders and Stroke t-PA Trial. Stroke 1996;27:2136–2142.
107. Zivin JA, Mazzarella V. Tissue plasminogen activator plus glutamate antagonist improves outcome after embolic stroke. Arch Neurol 1991;48:1235–1238.
108. Bowes MP, Rothlein R, Fagan SC, Zivin JA. Monoclonal antibodies preventing leukocyte activation reduce experimental neurologic injury and enhance efficacy of thrombolytic therapy. Neurology 1995;45:815–819.
109. Lyden PD, Lonzo L, Nunez S. Combination chemotherapy extends the therapeutic window to 60 minutes after stroke. J Neurotrauma 1995;12:223–230.
110. Benedict CR, Refino CJ, Keyt BA, et al. New variant of human tissue plasminogen activator (TPA) with enhanced efficacy and a lower incidence of bleeding compared with recombinant human TPA. Circulation 1995;92:3032–3040.

16
Supportive Care of the Acute Stroke Patient

Julio A. Chalela and Jason W. Todd

Meticulous attention to the nursing and medical care provided to the patient with acute ischemic stroke (AIS) is essential in optimizing outcome. Although thrombolytic therapy may be implemented only in a select group of patients, prompt and efficient medical management applies to all stroke patients. An in-depth understanding of the type of medical complications that may afflict the stroke patient and of the impact that systemic therapies may have on stroke outcome is essential in caring for AIS patients. In addition, an understanding of the cardiac and respiratory manifestations of stroke is crucial in treating patients with cerebrovascular disease. Avoiding any potential secondary injury to the ischemic brain and avoiding common medical complications of AIS are the main goals of supportive care of the AIS patient. This chapter focuses on the general medical care of the patient with AIS. Specific management depends on the stroke type, location, cause, and coexistent systemic factors, but the general principles of medical care outlined here apply to most cases of AIS.

THE STROKE UNIT CONCEPT

In most specialized centers worldwide, stroke care has moved from general medical wards to dedicated stroke units or neurointensive care units. There is irrefutable evidence that stroke care provided in a specialized unit is associated with reduced mortality and morbidity, improved outcomes, and decreased costs.[1-4] Stroke units provide specialized care and monitoring for patients with ischemic stroke, intracranial hemorrhage, or transient ischemic attack. A stroke unit is a hospital unit that exclusively or primarily delivers care to stroke patients. The multidisciplinary team comprises neurologists, rehabilitation specialists, nurses, and other specialists who run the unit. The staff is able to monitor the effects of stroke therapies, identify complications promptly, provide patient education, direct rehabilitation efforts, and order and interpret diagnostic tests. The level of care provided varies from care similar to that provided in a general ward to full intensive care support. At a minimum, stroke units are equipped to perform cardiorespiratory monitoring and are staffed by nurses trained in neurological nursing. In some centers the stroke unit is combined with the acute rehabilitation unit; in others it functions as a neurological intensive care unit annex to a step-down unit.

Compared with general wards, stroke units reduce stroke mortality by 18 percent, death and dependence by 29 percent, and the need for institutional care by 25 percent.[5] The benefit of stroke units extends well beyond the discharge period to up to 1 year after discharge.[2] A prospective randomized trial determined that patients admitted to a stroke unit have better outcomes in the domains of energy, emotional reactions, social isolation, physical mobility, and sleep.[1] Although results of randomized trials indicate that patients of all ages and strokes of all severity benefit from stroke unit care, there is some epidemiological evidence to suggest that the benefit of stroke units is more significant in patients with nonlacunar strokes.[2] Regardless of the stroke type, when possible, patients with AIS should be admitted to a stroke unit or a neurointensive care unit.

MISCELLANEOUS ISSUES IN ACUTE STROKE CARE

Positioning

Most stroke experts recommend maintaining the head of the bed flat in the hyperacute stroke patient because this may augment cerebral perfusion. There is evidence that, in patients with unilateral middle cerebral artery occlusion, the upright position leads to a decrease in cerebral blood flow (CBF) and to an increase in the oxygen extraction ratio in the affected cortex.[6] There are no studies addressing this issue in patients with small vessel ischemic disease or in patients without a large artery occlusion. Nevertheless, at our institution we keep all patients supine until the patency of the intracranial circulation is determined and the adequacy of cerebral perfusion is documented (by magnetic resonance imaging [MRI] or computed tomography [CT]). Patients with clinical deterioration on sitting up are kept supine until the clinical condition stabilizes. In patients with orthopnea or other medical reasons that impede lying flat, we keep the patient's head of the bed at the lowest level possible.

It is not certain what the optimal position is for the patient with a large stroke and increased intracranial pressure (ICP). Elevating the head of the bed may decrease ICP but may also compromise cerebral perfusion pressure (CPP). The supine position has the opposite effects.[7] The effects of body positioning in acute neurological injury vary according to the patient's cerebral compliance and to systemic factors. Thus ideally in the patient with an ICP monitor, CPP and ICP should be measured in different positions to determine the optimal position. When ICP is not known, we favor keeping patients with the head of bed flat because the horizontal position appears to enhance CPP more than it increases ICP.[7] Frequent changes in body positioning are recommended to prevent pressure sores.

Intravenous Fluids

Stroke patients are often volume depleted as a result of nausea and vomiting, inability to access fluids, and increased insensible losses. Hypovolemia may worsen the neurological injury by compromising cerebral perfusion.[8] Elevated osmolality on admission (>296 mOsm/kg) is associated with poor outcome after AIS.[9] Mortality after acute stroke is doubled in patients with admission hypovolemia diagnosed by serum osmolality determination.[9] Diabetic patients and patients with stroke-induced hyperglycemia are more likely to have elevated plasma osmolality and volume depletion.

Volume replacement in acute stroke patients should be done using isotonic crystalloids. We use normal saline at a rate of 1 to 2 cc/kg per hour in all patients in whom normal oral fluid intake is not feasible. In patients with increased insensible losses or in patients presenting with an obvious water deficit, we provide a bolus of fluids before initiation of the maintenance infusion and increase the hourly infusion following hemodynamic parameters. In patients in whom a central venous pressure catheter is in place we titrate fluid administration to obtain a central venous pressure of 8 to 12 cm. Because of the known deleterious effects of hyperglycemia on stroke outcome, we avoid dextrose-containing solutions unless the patient has symptomatic hypoglycemia.[10] Glucose-containing solutions may induce local acidosis and worsen cerebral injury.[11] Hypo-osmolar fluids are avoided because they may worsen cerebral edema by passively diffusing into the infarcted brain.[12]

Blood Pressure Management

Preexistent hypertension is present in 30 to 50 percent of AIS patients, and acutely elevated blood pressure (BP) is noted on presentation with AIS in 70 to 80 percent.[5,13] The highest BPs are seen in patients with preexisting hypertension. BP tends to decline spontaneously to baseline levels in most patients over the first 4 to 10 days after stroke onset, with the largest drops occurring in patients with the highest initial BPs.[13,14]

Cerebral autoregulation is the homeostatic mechanism by which cerebral vascular resistance (CVR) is adjusted to accommodate variations in CPP and thus maintain relatively constant levels of CBF in normal subjects. CPP is equal to mean arterial pressure (MAP) minus venous pressure, which in the cranium is equivalent to ICP (CPP = MAP − ICP). CBF is thus governed by the following relationship: CBF = (MAP − ICP)/CVR. The BP range over which cerebral autoregulation is effective is a MAP of approximately 70 to 150 mm Hg in normal individuals and higher in chronic hypertensives.[15] In both normotensive and chronically hypertensive patients, the lower end of the effective cerebral autoregulation range is approximately 25 percent below the resting MAP. Pressures below the lower limit of effective autoregulation lead to decreased CBF, whereas MAPs exceeding the upper limit may linearly increase CBF above normal levels and result in vasogenic edema, as in hypertensive encephalopathy. In AIS, cerebral resistance vessels in the marginally perfused ischemic penumbra are maximally dilated, so that cerebral autoregulation is no longer possible, and CBF in this critical region is directly dependent on CPP.[15] Lowering BP in this setting may decrease blood flow to the ischemic penumbra, enlarge the infarction, and potentially lead to poorer outcome.[16] Markedly elevated BP in AIS could theoretically worsen endothelial injury and stroke edema and increase the risk of hemorrhagic transformation.

Acutely elevated BP in AIS is likely an adaptive brain response to increase CPP and improve blood flow to ischemic tissue. Published guidelines and recommendations on the management of AIS support the concept that elevated BP in the setting of AIS should generally not be lowered except when extreme or in special circumstances in which acute end-organ damage is documented.[5,17] Definitive data in humans to guide clinical practice are, however, lacking. The most recent Cochrane review on this subject found the existing data to be "wholly inadequate" to guide clinical practice and called for randomized controlled trials to study interventions aimed at altering BP in AIS.[18] Intentionally raising BP is beneficial in some cases but has not been studied in a controlled trial.[19,20] Intentionally lowering BP acutely has been supported, and a trial testing a nitric oxide donor with antihypertensive effects is in progress.[21] Studies correlating acutely elevated BP with poorer outcomes have been cited as rationale for such a study, but causation has not been proven.[22]

Overall, in the acute stroke patient more harm is done from overtreating elevated BP than from undertreating it. The clinical circumstances in which lowering BP promptly is warranted are summarized in Table 16.1. The preferred agents should have short half-lives and should be easily titratable (Table 16.2). Markedly elevated BP is thought to be a risk factor for intracranial hemorrhage after thrombolysis for AIS.[23] The NINDS recombinant tissue plasminogen activator (rt-PA) trial and subsequently published guidelines on thrombolytic therapy for stroke used a threshold of sustained systolic blood pressure (SBP) greater than 180 mm Hg or diastolic blood pressure (DBP) greater than 105 mm Hg for initiating antihypertensive therapy after thrombolysis.[24] In addition, nonthrombolysis patients with sustained MAP greater than 130 mm Hg should receive treatment to gently lower the BP. Our therapeutic approach to elevated BP in AIS is summarized in Table 16.2. Any worsening of the neurological symptoms related to lowering the BP should prompt the clinician to discontinue the antihypertensive medicines and to attempt to raise the BP to pretreatment levels.

In patients who do not receive rt-PA and who do not have end-organ damage, we withhold antihypertensive therapy for 5 to 7 days. It is our practice not to discontinue rate-control agents in patients with atrial fibrillation (beta blockers or calcium channel blockers) but to reduce the dose by half. Alternatively, rate-control drugs may be discontinued and the ventricular response treated as

Table 16.1   Clinical situations warranting emergent blood pressure reduction

Acute aortic dissection
Acute myocardial infarction
Acute cardiogenic pulmonary edema
Unstable angina pectoris
Eclampsia
Hypertensive encephalopathy
Subarachnoid hemorrhage
Acute renal failure

Table 16.2 Guidelines for blood pressure management in acute stroke

Mean arterial pressure ≤130 mm Hg (no end-organ damage)	Do not treat
Mean arterial pressure >130 mm Hg	Labetalol 5–20 mg IV or Enalaprilat 0.625 mg IV or Hydralazine 5–10 mg IV or Captopril 6.25–12.5 mg (PO)
End-organ damage	Sodium nitroprusside 0.5–10 μg/kg/min Labetalol 2–8 mg/minute Nicardipine 5 mg/hr (titrate up to 15 mg/hr)
Post rt-PA administration	Follow NINDS rt-PA guidelines

NINDS = National Institute of Neurological Disorders and Stroke; rt-PA = recombinant tissue plasminogen activator.

needed with intravenous (IV) beta blockers or diltiazem. If hypotension occurs, other therapeutic options include IV amiodarone, IV digoxin, or in rare circumstances, electrical cardioversion. In patients with symptomatic cervico-cranial stenosis or with symptoms worsened by the upright position we often withhold antihypertensive medicines for a prolonged period.

Temperature Management

Hyperthermia is common in AIS patients. Both infectious and neurogenic causes are thought to occur. In a prospective study, 30 of 119 (25.2%) consecutive AIS patients became febrile within 48 hours of stroke onset.[25] Eight of these (26.7%) had a history of infection during the prior week. Of infections developing after admission, pneumonia was the most common (*n* = 19), followed by bronchitis or upper respiratory infection (*n* = 7), urinary tract infection (*n* = 4), and viral infection (*n* = 3). In 5, no source of infection could be identified. Patients with severe strokes are more likely to have an increase in body temperature within the first 12 hours of onset than those with milder strokes.[26] This may be due to a higher incidence of aspiration pneumonia, or alternatively severe strokes may be more likely to cause neurogenic fever in the absence of apparent infection.[27]

In animal models, it is well established that hyperthermia increases infarct size and worsens outcomes, whereas hypothermia is neuroprotective.[27] In humans, the evidence of a similar temperature effect is suggestive but less certain. A meta-analysis of studies published up to 1998 suggested that post-stroke pyrexia is strongly associated with increased mortality and morbidity.[28] This effect seems to be independent of the presence of infection or leukocytosis. Hyperthermia has a greater impact on outcome when it occurs within the first 24 hours of stroke than when it occurs later.[29]

The impact on core body temperature of the routine administration of acetaminophen to afebrile stroke patients has been studied. In a randomized, placebo-controlled trial (RCT), a moderate dose (3900 mg/day) administered for 24 hours produced a mean temperature 0.22 degrees Centigrade lower than the control group.[30] In another RCT, a higher dose (6000 mg/day) lowered mean tympanic temperature 0.4 degrees Centigrade compared with controls.[31] Results of a three-arm trial comparing the effect on body temperature of high-dose acetaminophen, ibuprofen, and placebo in AIS patients with temperatures up to 39.0 degrees Centigrade are awaited.[32]

To date, an RCT of treatment of hyperthermia in AIS patients has not been performed, in part because of ethical concerns.[33] Lacking this data, we advise aggressive maintenance of normothermia, particularly within the first 24 to 72 hours after stroke onset. Our protocol is to use acetaminophen 650 mg every 4 hours for temperature higher than 37.2 degrees Centigrade. If hyperthermia persists, a cooling blanket is added. Nonsteroidal anti-inflammatory drugs should be avoided in patients following thrombolysis but may be used adjunctively for other patients.

The presence of hyperthermia should prompt a search for infectious causes. A detailed physical examination including inspection of venipuncture sites, lung auscultation, urinalysis, and chest x-ray should be obtained, as well as blood cultures for temperature higher than 38.3 degrees Centigrade. Documented infections should be treated with appropriate antibiotics. A lower than normal threshold should be used for instituting antibiotic therapy during fever suppression with antipyretic therapy. The potential role of induced hypothermia in AIS is currently being investigated.

Glucose Management

The relationships among diabetes mellitus (DM), acute hyperglycemia, infarct size, and outcomes in AIS are complex. Depending on the definitions and thresholds used, hyperglycemia is noted on presentation in 20 to 50 percent of AIS patients.[34] Eight to 20 percent have a previous diagnosis of DM, 5 to 28 percent have undiagnosed DM, and an additional 10 to 20 percent have hyperglycemia with a normal glycosylated hemoglobin level, possibly resulting from a stress response induced by the stroke.[34] In human studies, associations between acute hyperglycemia in AIS and increased mortality, larger final infarct size, increased inpatient costs, and poor neurological or functional outcome have been demonstrated.[35–38] These associations persist after adjusting for a history of diabetes and other factors and are more consistent in nonlacunar than in lacunar strokes. Some studies, however, have not confirmed these associations. Whether hyperglycemia has a direct detrimental effect in AIS has been controversial.

In animal models of reversible focal cerebral ischemia, a consistent relationship between hyperglycemia and greater infarct volumes has been established.[39] In models of end-arterial occlusion or irreversible ischemia, there have been mixed results.[39] These results and the inconsistent association in human lacunar stroke studies can be explained by the theory that hyperglycemia preferentially affects the ischemic penumbra. This idea is supported by a recent study which used diffusion-weighted imaging (DWI), perfusion-weighted imaging (PWI), and magnetic resonance (MR) spectroscopy to investigate the relationship between acute hyperglycemia in AIS and both imaging and clinical outcome measures.[37] In patients with a smaller DWI than PWI lesion (mismatch), acute hyperglycemia was strongly correlated with larger infarct size, decreased penumbral salvage, and higher National Institutes of Health Stroke Scale (NIHSS) and modified Rankin scores. In patients without a mismatch, acute glucose was not a significant predictor of any of these outcome variables.

The United Kingdom Glucose Insulin in Stroke Trial (GIST-UK) is an ongoing RCT to test the hypothesis that induction and maintenance of euglycemia with a 24-hour infusion of glucose, potassium, and insulin (GKI) in hyperglycemic patients with AIS improves outcomes.[40] The study seeks to include 1200 patients, and results are expected in late 2003. A prior study established the safety of GKI infusion in hyperglycemic AIS patients.[34] No other RCT data are available.

Pending the results of GIST-UK, recommendations for glucose management in AIS are empiric. Dextrose-containing IV solutions should be avoided. There is some evidence that hypoglycemia may also be harmful and should be avoided.[41] A sliding-scale insulin regimen is generally used in any AIS patient with admission hyperglycemia, even if there is no history of DM. Diabetic patients on insulin generally need to be continued on insulin, with dosages reduced by approximately 50 percent if they are receiving nil per os (NPO). Sliding-scale insulin generally begins treatment at glucose values above 200 mg/dL. Once more data become available, this practice may prove to be too conservative. Diffusion and perfusion-weighted imaging hold promise for identifying those patients most likely to benefit from aggressive glucose-lowering measures in AIS.

Prevention of Venous Thromboembolism

Deep venous thrombosis (DVT) is a preventable and potentially fatal complication of AIS. Without prophylaxis, the pooled incidence (8 studies with 346 patients) of DVT in AIS patients with a weak or paralyzed lower limb is 55 percent.[42] This figure includes asymptomatic DVTs, both distal (below knee) and proximal. Clinically apparent DVT has been reported in large clinical trials at a much lower rate—in the Trial of ORG 10172 (TOAST), DVT was reported in 1.6 percent of placebo patients.[43] Differences in reported DVT rates are largely due to differing detection methods. Older studies with higher reported rates generally screened all patients using iodine-125 (I^{125})-fibrinogen leg scanning, a highly sensitive method that is no longer available. TOAST reported clinically apparent DVT and pulmonary embolism (PE), without actively screening patients. Most DVTs occur in the paretic leg, although DVT has been reported in nonparetic limbs as well, possibly reflecting an acute or chronic hypercoagulability.[44,45] Immobility after AIS is the strongest risk factor for DVT; other high-risk conditions are listed in Table 16.3.[42,44,45] DVTs may develop as early as 48 hours after AIS, with the incidence peaking between 2 and 7 days.[44]

PE is the most serious complication of DVT and is a significant source of morbidity and mortality after stroke. Thirteen to 25 percent of deaths occurring early after AIS have been attributed to PE.[44] In autopsy studies, half of inpatients dying later than 48 hours after stroke onset have evidence of PE, suggesting a high frequency of subclinical or undiagnosed PEs after AIS.[44] Fatal PE is unusual in the first week; the incidence peaks between the second and fourth weeks. During this period, PE is the leading cause of death.[44] Fifty percent of fatal PEs present as sudden death, without preceding, clinically apparent evidence of DVT.[46] This fact underscores the importance of effective DVT prophylaxis. Distinguishing PE from aspiration pneumonia may be difficult. The two conditions may coexist, and fever is noted in up to 2/3 of patients with

Table 16.3   High risk for venous thromboembolism

Morbid obesity
Congestive heart failure
Nephrotic syndrome
Trauma (especially pelvic, hip, or leg fractures)
Major surgery
Inherited or acquired hypercoagulable state
Prior venous thromboembolism
Malignancy
Pregnancy
Inflammatory bowel disease
Acute myocardial infarction

PE.[44] The postphlebitic syndrome of persistent pain and swelling, sometimes with venous ulceration, develops in up to 90 percent of untreated symptomatic patients with DVT and is also a significant source of morbidity. Many patients presenting with this syndrome have no history of clinical DVT, implying that it can develop after asymptomatic DVT.[44]

Most studies on prophylaxis of DVT in AIS have focused on antithrombotic agents. Low-dose unfractionated heparin (LDUH), low-molecular-weight heparins (LMWH), and heparinoids have been studied. Three randomized but nonblinded trials compared LDUH (5000 U three times daily [2 trials] or 5000 U twice daily [1 trial]) to placebo. All three found statistically significant risk reduction for DVT (one trial used clinical DVT, the other two used I^{125}-fibrinogen). Several different LMWH preparations have been used for prophylaxis or treatment of thromboembolism. Two randomized placebo-controlled trials tested the LMWH Fragmin (dalteparin); one found a borderline reduction in DVT frequency, and the other found no significant difference from placebo.[47,48] At the doses tested, Fragmin has not been convincingly shown to be effective. Another LMWH, enoxaparin 40 mg daily, was compared with LDUH (5000 U three times daily) in a recently published, randomized, double-blind study of 212 patients.[49] Trends favoring enoxaparin over LDUH were noted for DVT (16.0% vs. 24.5%), PE (1.9% vs. 3.8%), death (19.8% vs. 26.4%), and hemorrhagic transformation (13.2% vs. 18.9%); these trends did not reach statistical significance. The difference in total thromboembolic events did reach statistical significance. There was only one significant bleeding event, an intracranial hemorrhage in a patient on enoxaparin (0.9%). These results are consistent with enoxaparin being at least as safe and efficacious as thrice daily LDUH; they also suggest (when contrasted with the Fragmin results) that not all LMWH preparations should be considered equivalent and that trial results favoring one should not be extrapolated to the rest of the class.[49] A heparinoid (danaparoid) has been tested both against placebo and LDUH. In the trial of danaparoid (1000 anti-factor Xa unit IV bolus, then 750 units subcutaneous [SC] twice daily) versus placebo, there were significant decreases in the rates of total DVT (4% vs. 28%) and proximal DVT (0% vs. 16%).[50] There was one major hemorrhage in the danaparoid group (2%). In one study using danaparoid (750 anti-factor Xa units SQ twice daily) against LDUH (5000 U twice daily), a significant advantage was noted in total DVT rate (9% vs. 31%) but not proximal DVT rate (4% vs. 12%, $p > 0.2$).[51] However, in a second trial of danaparoid

(1250 anti-factor Xa units SQ daily) against LDUH (5000 U twice daily) (D6), there were no significant differences between the danaparoid and heparin groups for DVT (14.6% vs. 19.8%) or death (13.5% vs. 6.7%).

Large acute stroke trials not designed specifically to test agents for efficacy in DVT prevention have reported results on rates of clinically apparent DVT or PE. In the International Stroke Trial (IST) (D2), PE was reported in 0.9 percent of control patients, 0.7 percent of aspirin-only (300 mg) patients (p = non-significant [NS]), and 0.5 percent of LDUH (5000 U twice daily) + aspirin patients ($p < 0.02$ vs. controls).[52] The Tinzaparin in Acute Ischemic Stroke Trial (TAIST) tested high (175 anti-factor Xa units SQ daily) and medium (100 anti-factor Xa units SQ daily) doses of the LMWH against aspirin 300 mg daily.[53] Rates of DVT and PE were 0 percent and 0.4 percent in the high-dose group, 0.6 percent and 0.8 percent in the medium-dose group, and 1.8 percent and 0.8 percent in the aspirin group, respectively. Only the high-dose group exhibited a significant decrease in DVT and DVT + PE. The reported event rates were low, and likely reflect under-ascertainment in both the IST and TAIST.

The efficacy of mechanical devices (pneumatic sequential compression devices [SCDs] or graded compression stockings) for DVT prevention after AIS has not been definitively evaluated.[54] In a non-randomized study, 249 consecutive AIS patients received LDUH and antithrombotic hose for DVT prophylaxis.[45] This group was compared with a group of 432 consecutive patients in whom SCDs were added to LDUH and antithrombotic hose in all nonambulatory patients. The former group had a DVT rate of 9.2 percent and a PE rate of 2.4 percent; half the PEs were fatal. All but one DVT and all PEs occurred in nonambulatory patients (odds ratio 51.9, 95% confidence interval [CI] 6.8 to 395). The latter group had DVT and PE rates of 0.23 percent and 0 percent, respectively, representing a 40-fold risk reduction with the addition of SCDs. Although a rigorous randomized controlled trial has not been completed, SCDs are generally well tolerated and carry no bleeding risk. The available data are consistent with a strong additional benefit of combining SCDs with pharmacological agents for venous thromboembolism prevention.[45]

The approach to DVT prevention in AIS requires balancing the benefit of reduction of risk of DVT and PE with the risk of bleeding, with symptomatic hemorrhagic transformation or hematoma formation in the ischemic stroke bed the most concerning and potentially dangerous. Heparin-induced thrombocytopenia (HIT) is also a significant potential adverse effect of prophylactic therapy. The risk of HIT is significantly lower with the use of LMWH (enoxaparin) than unfractionated heparin.[55] There is no universally agreed-on regimen for DVT prophylaxis after AIS. The most recent guidelines from the American College of Chest Physicians recommend LDUH or LMWH or danaparoid for nonambulatory AIS patients but specify no preferred order of use or recommended dosages.[42] The most recent American Heart Association Guidelines recommend early mobilization, and LDUH or LMWH or heparinoids, and SCDs if antithrombotic therapy is contraindicated.[17] Tables 16.3 and 16.4 summarize our approach to thromboembolism prevention and risk stratification.

The ideal length of time to continue DVT prophylaxis is also unknown. Prophylaxis has generally been administered for 10 to 14 days in clinical trials.[42] Given that the highest risk for fatal PE occurs between the second and fourth weeks after stroke, a longer course of prophylaxis for patients who remain at moderate or high risk would be logical for maximal benefit.

Table 16.4   Prevention of venous thromboembolism

Absent leg motor deficits and ambulatory within 24 hr of admission: encourage ambulation.

Fully anticoagulated patients: no further prophylaxis.

Moderate risk patients (paretic leg or nonambulatory subjects): sequential compression devices and either LDUH (5000 U bid) or enoxaparin (40 mg SC qd).

High-risk patients (paretic leg and/or nonambulatory subjects with clinical conditions listed in Table 16.3): sequential compression devices and either enoxaparin (40 mg SC qd) (preferred) or LDUH (5000 U tid). Place inferior vena cava filter in high-risk patients with anticoagulation contraindications.

bid = two times daily; LDUH = low-dose unfractionated heparin; qd = once a day; SC = subcutaneous; tid = three times daily; U = Units.

SPECIFIC CARE BY SYSTEMS

Airway and Respiratory Issues

Patients with stroke may experience airway and respiratory difficulties resulting from a variety of reasons. Stroke may disturb breathing by causing a disturbance of central rhythm generation, interrupting the descending respiratory pathways leading to a reduced respiratory drive, and by causing bulbar weakness.[56] In addition stroke may be complicated by aspiration pneumonia, atelectasis, PE, or neurogenic pulmonary edema. Acute hemiplegia resulting from stroke is associated with an increased risk of death from respiratory causes, mainly pneumonia. Aspiration pneumonia may affect up to 12 percent of AIS patients and is associated with increased risk of death.[57] PE may occur in up to 9 percent of all stroke patients but is often subclinical.[58]

As in all other medical emergencies airway control is the first priority in patients with AIS. A rapid assessment of the patient's airway and respiratory status should be performed and any signs of respiratory embarrassment should be corrected promptly. At particular risk are patients with brain stem stroke and patients with large hemispheric infarcts. Routine oxygen supplementation is not necessary, but supplemental oxygen should be provided to ensure oxygen saturation above 90 percent.[59] Management of oral and pulmonary secretions can be a difficult problem in the patient with AIS. Frequent suctioning and adequate positioning may adequately control the secretions, but, if they are copious, endotracheal intubation may be indicated. In some cases pharmacological treatment with tricyclic antidepressants or with glycopyrrolate may control the secretions. The chin-lift maneuver should be attempted if upper airway obstruction secondary to posterior displacement of the tongue is suspected. Sleep-related upper airway obstruction is common in stroke patients and is associated with supine positioning, increased neck circumference, and limb paralysis.[60]

Acute stroke patients with Glasgow coma score of less than 8, absent brain stem reflexes, or protracted vomiting should be intubated emergently.[61] Patients with evidence of hypoxemic, hypercapnic, or mixed respiratory failure should also be intubated. Endotracheal intubation should be performed expeditiously with awareness of the potential risks for worsening neurological injury.

Succinylcholine may worsen ICP and may cause fatal hyperkalemia in patients who have been bedridden because of neurogenic weakness.[62] Lidocaine may lower seizure threshold and trigger seizures. Benzodiazepines and short-acting anesthetics may lower systemic BP and compromise CPP. The combination of etomidate and a short-acting neuromuscular blocker appears to be safe and may possibly offer some neuroprotective effect.[63] Once intubated, the goal should be to keep the patient normocapnic and normoxemic. Hyperventilation should be reserved for selected cases of confirmed or suspected intracranial hypertension.[64] Although as a whole patients with AIS requiring mechanical ventilation have a poor prognosis, good outcome is possible in selected cases.[65,66]

Respiratory Patterns in Acute Stroke

Abnormal respiratory patterns may develop following acute stroke. The most common pattern is Cheyne-Stokes respiration, in which hyperventilation periodically waxes and wanes with apnea. Cheyne-Stokes respiration is due to instability of the chemoreceptor control system with hypoxemia rather than hypercapnia becoming the dominant regulator of ventilation.[62] Although Cheyne-Stokes respiration may be due to stroke, it is often caused by coexisting cardiopulmonary disease.[58] Arterial blood gases typically show hypocapnia with normal oxygenation. Cheyne-Stokes respiration does not warrant any specific treatment except in the rare case in which extreme hypocapnia is compromising cerebral perfusion; sedation and controlled mechanical ventilation will promptly correct the hypocapnia.[64,67] Ataxic breathing is an irregular, erratic breathing pattern with varying depth and rate of respiration. Its presence often indicates a lesion in the medulla in the region of the dorsal respiratory neurons that control the rhythmicity of breathing.[67] Ataxic breathing does not have any prognostic significance. Apneustic breathing is characterized by sustained deep inspiration followed by a postinspiratory pause, then rapid exhalation. It usually follows pontine infarcts and is due to dysfunction of the inspiratory cut-off mechanism.[58,67] Apneustic breathing is rarely recognized in clinical practice because patients are usually intubated and placed on mechanical ventilation on presentation. Weaning from mechanical ventilation is difficult and patients often need tracheostomy. Rapid, regular deep breaths leading to hypocapnia characterize central neurogenic hyperventilation. The diagnosis cannot be made in the presence of pulmonary edema, sepsis, or use of respiratory stimulants. The cause of central neurogenic hyperventilation is not fully understood, but the frequent association with cerebral neoplasms and the presence of acidic spinal fluid suggests that it may be triggered by alterations in pH that stimulate chemosensitive areas in the brain stem.[68]

Neurogenic Pulmonary Edema

Neurogenic pulmonary edema is a rare form of noncardiogenic pulmonary edema that may follow cerebral injuries including stroke. Following a neurological injury, the interstitium and alveoli become flooded with proteinaceous, hemorrhagic fluid leading to impaired gas exchange and hypoxemia. The pathogenesis of neurogenic pulmonary edema is not fully understood, but most putative mechanisms involve an acute exaggerated sympathetic discharge related to solitary tract and nucleus dysfunction.[62] Pulmonary vascular constriction induces a dramatic leakage of fluid into the interstitium and the alveoli. Neurogenic pulmonary edema has a mixed cause with both increased permeability and increased hydrostatic pressure playing a role in its genesis.[69] Radiographically, neurogenic pulmonary edema is indistinguishable from cardiogenic pulmonary edema. The heart size may be normal, a feature atypical for cardiogenic pulmonary edema but not specific enough to differentiate the two conditions. The rapid development of pulmonary edema, minutes to hours after the neurological injury, is the most characteristic clinical feature of neurogenic pulmonary edema. The differential diagnosis includes cardiogenic pulmonary edema and aspiration pneumonia. Treatment involves controlling the underlying cause and providing mechanical ventilatory support with positive expiratory pressure.[62] Dobutamine and alpha antagonists have been used empirically with variable results.

Cardiac Care in Acute Stroke

The relation between the heart and the brain in acute stroke is twofold; cardiac disorders may be the cause of the stroke and stroke can cause a variety of cardiac disturbances. Most neurogenically induced cardiac conditions are transient and require either no therapy or brief supportive therapy. On the other hand, cardiac conditions that have caused stroke may require specific acute therapy. Cardiac abnormalities after stroke can be classified into repolarization and electrocardiographic (ECG) abnormalities, cardiac arrhythmias, and myocardial injury.

ECG Alterations in Acute Stroke

ST-segment alterations, T-wave changes, U waves, and QT prolongations are the most common ECG abnormalities in AIS. In most patients the ECG abnormalities do not reflect underlying coronary disease, because they are known to occur in young patients with normal coronary vessels.[70] The ST changes may closely mimic myocardial ischemia. ECG features that allow differentiation from myocardial ischemia include T-wave asymmetry, absence of reciprocal changes, and preferential involvement of the anterior leads with sparing of the limb leads.[70] Stroke-related T-wave abnormalities include upright, peaked T waves and inverted T waves. Laboratory evaluation should be performed to rule electrolyte disturbances and myocardial ischemia before attributing the T-wave changes to the stroke. Prolongation of the QT interval may precede cardiac arrhythmias and sudden death after stroke. If hypokalemia is absent and the QT prolongation is associated with U waves, it is likely secondary to the stroke.[71] QT prolongation occurs more commonly with right hemispheric infarctions as a result of lateralization of autonomic function.[72] Transient aberrant Q waves may follow evolutionary changes similar to those seen in acute transmural infarction but myocardial enzymes are usually normal and echocardiography does not reveal areas of segmental hypokinesis. With the exception of prolongation of the QT interval, the above-mentioned ECG findings do not appear to have prognostic significance.[70,71]

Cardiac Arrhythmias in Acute Stroke

Cardiac arrhythmias may follow stroke or may be the inciting event that caused the stroke. The most common type of arrhythmia is ventricular extrasystoles, followed by atrial extrasystoles, supraventricular tachycardia, and atrial fibrillation.[73] The acute stroke may be the inciting event causing the cardiac arrhythmia, but not all cardiac phenomena after cerebral ischemia should be regarded as secondary because there is often coincident myocardial ischemia with acute cerebrovascular disease.[5,71] In most patients with acute stroke, atrial fibrillation is chronic and precedes the stroke; in 10 percent of patients with atrial fibrillation after stroke it is transient and will not recur.[74] There is an increased incidence of fatal ventricular arrhythmias among patients with right hemisphere stroke likely related to the frequent occurrence of QT-interval prolongation.[75]

Cardiac Injury in Acute Stroke

Neurogenic cardiac damage can follow any acute cerebral injury including stroke. Evidence of subendocardial infarction or anterolateral ischemia is common after stroke, particularly after subarachnoid hemorrhage. In most patients, the ECG abnormalities and enzyme elevation do not reflect underlying coronary disease but more likely reflect a nonischemic cardiac injury. The injury is distinct from classic cardiac necrosis because it occurs in the vicinity of epicardial nerves, occurs within minutes of the neurological injury, and leads to cell death in a hypercontracted state with early calcifications.[71] Troponin-I elevation occurs in up to 6 percent of stroke patients and is associated with stroke severity.[76] In most patients with troponin-I elevation, there is no clinical or other laboratory evidence of myocardial necrosis. Treatment is supportive; beta blocker use may be indicated to ameliorate the exaggerated sympathetic response that mediates neurogenically induced cardiac damage.

Cardiac Function in Acute Stroke

Optimization of cardiac output and maintenance of a high normal BP and a normal heart rate is essential in acute stroke care. BP measurement and jugular venous pressure are useful bedside estimates of the patient's volume status. When available, a central line can be used to assess central venous pressure and optimize volume status with a goal of euvolemia. If hypotension does not correct with volume administration, inotropic support with dobutamine, dopamine, or phenylephrine should be attempted. Dopamine may be particularly useful in patients with renal insufficiency or persistent hypotension not secondary to cardiac pump failure. Restoration of normal cardiac rhythm using pharmacological agents, cardioversion, or pacemaker should be performed when there is evidence of compromised cerebral or systemic perfusion. Controlling the heart rate in the patient with rapid atrial fibrillation and acute stroke is a challenging task because the agents used (beta blockers and calcium channel blockers) may cause hypotension and a decline in CPP. In such a situation, ensuring adequate volume status, using inotropic agents, and reversing the action of the drugs used are useful therapeutic options. IV digoxin is a useful therapeutic alternative, although it is not as effective in controlling the heart rate.[77]

Nutritional and Gastrointestinal Issues

Gastrointestinal and nutritional issues are often neglected in the patient with AIS. Nevertheless, there is clear evidence that malnutrition is common after stroke and that it may have a negative impact on stroke outcome.[78] Gastrointestinal disturbances after stroke may increase morbidity and mortality, delay discharge, and interfere with rehabilitation.[79,80]

Nutritional Issues in Acute Stroke

Chronic protein-caloric malnutrition is a risk factor for poor outcome after AIS.[78] Acute malnutrition occurring in the first week after stroke onset also worsens stroke prognosis. Malnutrition after stroke results from dysphagia and possibly from the catabolic state that follows acute neurological injury.[78] Malnutrition in the stroke patient leads to increased risk of infection, impaired immunological function, impaired functional capacity, increased risk of bedsores, and increased mortality.[78] A nutritional evaluation should be performed in all stroke patients receiving tube feedings or parenteral nutrition and in patients receiving enteral nutrition in whom the risk of protein-caloric malnutrition is evident. A calorie count is a reasonable way to gauge whether the patient is consuming enough calories. In patients receiving tube feedings or parenteral nutrition we determine nitrogen balance and adjust intake accordingly. In intubated patients, indirect calorimetry allows determination of energy expenditure and adjustment of enteral or parenteral feeding.

Dysphagia is very common after acute stroke, affecting up to 47 percent of all stroke victims.[81] Dysphagia is particularly common in patients with bilateral strokes and in patients with brain stem strokes.[82] Dysphagia may lead to aspiration pneumonia, dehydration, and malnutrition. Dysphagia is an independent marker of poor outcome after stroke. Dysphagic patients tend to have poor functional outcome, increased length of hospital stay, and increased mortality.[81] Although in some patients aspiration is easily recognized, in many stroke patients aspiration is silent and evident only after performing videofluoroscopy.

A swallowing evaluation performed by a speech pathologist should be obtained in all patients with moderate to severe stroke, and in all other patients in whom the clinical examination indicates that the patient is at risk for aspiration. Useful bedside parameters that help determine that the patient is at risk for aspiration include cough on swallowing, changes in the voice after swallowing, and difficulty swallowing water. The so-called 3-ounce water test is performed by asking the patient to drink 3 ounces of water from a cup without interruption. Coughing for up to a minute after completing the test or the presence of a postswallow wet or hoarse voice is abnormal and predicts aspiration risk.[83] In such patients either a modified diet with aspiration precautions should be instituted or an alternate feeding route should be considered. In our institution we favor placing a temporary small-bore nasogastric or postpyloric feeding tube in patients at high risk for aspiration. When prolonged tube feeding is necessary, percutaneous endoscopic gastrostomy is the preferred option.

Gastrointestinal Issues in Acute Stroke

The most common gastrointestinal disorders in patients with acute stroke are disorders of gastric motility (diarrhea, constipation, and gastroparesis) and gastrointestinal bleeding. Constipation affects up to 16 percent of stroke patients and is multifactorial in origin.[79] Immobility following stroke, medications, dehydration, hypokalemia, and changes in diet are the principal culprits in stroke-related constipation. Treatment involves early mobilization; hydration; avoidance of drugs with anticholinergic properties; and the use of stool softeners, bulk-forming agents, and laxatives. Gastroparesis may complicate any acute neurological injury but is more common among diabetics and among patients receiving agents that interfere with gastric emptying (e.g., tricyclic antidepressants and barbiturates). Treatment includes control of hyperglycemia, avoidance of high-fat foods, and the use of prokinetic agents like metoclopramide or erythromycin.[84]

In a clinical study of the medical complications occurring in acute stroke, diarrhea occurred in 3 percent of all patients.[79] Causes include drugs, infections, enteral nutrition, and changes in gastrointestinal flora. Multiple adverse effects ensue from diarrhea in the stroke patient. In conscious patients, embarrassment and discomfort add to the distress of suffering a stroke, and in unconscious or incontinent patients, diarrhea complicates skin care and allows bowel organisms to contaminate the skin and surrounding areas, increasing the risk of urinary tract infection. Treatment depends on the cause, often withdrawing an offending drug or supporting the patient with supplemental intravenous fluids is all that is required.

Gastrointestinal hemorrhage occurs in approximately 5 percent of all stroke patients.[79] Risk factors for hemorrhage include tetraplegia, respiratory failure, sepsis, hypotension, renal failure, hepatic failure, and intracranial hypertension.[85] We do not use stress ulcer prophylaxis in all stroke patients but limit it to patients with the above-mentioned risk factors or with history of peptic ulcer disease or gastrointestinal bleeding. The agent used for stress ulcer prophylaxis depends on the availability of the enteral route for drug administration. If administering drugs via the enteral route is not feasible, intravenous histamine-2 (H_2) or proton pump antagonists are the drugs of choice. If the enteral route is available sucralfate, H_2 antagonists, or proton pump antagonists can be used.

Neuropsychiatric Issues

Psychomotor agitation, anxiety, and delirium are not unusual complications in AIS. The unfamiliar environment and the use of psychotropic medications make the elderly particularly vulnerable to acute confusional states. Delirium affects between 28 to 40 percent of all stroke patients. Delirium in acute stroke is more common among older patients, patients with left-sided lesions, patients with extensive motor impairment, patients with preexisting cognitive decline, patients with apnea-related hypoxemia, and patients with low body mass.[86,87] Functional outcome at 6 months is worse in patients that have in-hospital delirium than in those that have no delirium.[87] Although delirium may occur in patients with diverse stroke locations, it appears to be particularly common in patients with bilateral thalamic lesions, bilateral frontal lesions, and posterior cerebral artery lesions.[86]

The management of delirium after stroke does not differ much from the management of delirium resulting from other causes. A careful investigation must be done to exclude any medical factors that could explain the delirium (e.g., infections, drugs, hypoxemia, substance withdrawal). The patient should be reassured and placed in a comfortable, well-lit environment. Nonpharmacological measures should be the therapy of first resort except in the patient with hyperkinetic delirium who is at great risk for self-injury and in whom pharmacological treatment may be warranted upfront. Haloperidol may be used to control agitation, although there is some evidence that dopamine-blocking drugs may interfere with recovery after stroke.[88] Benzodiazepines are a useful therapeutic alternative. In the intubated agitated patient we favor using a propofol infusion. Care must be taken when using any sedatives as hypotension and respiratory depression may worsen the cerebral injury.

References

1. Indredavik B, Bakke F, Slordahl SA, et al. Stroke unit treatment improves long-term quality of life: a randomized controlled trial. Stroke 1998;29:895–899.
2. Evans A, Harraf F, Donaldson N, et al. Randomized controlled study of stroke unit care versus stroke team care in different stroke subtypes. Stroke 2002;33:449–455.
3. Diringer MN, Edwards D. Admission to a neurologic/neurosurgical intensive care unit is associated with reduced mortality rate after intracerebral hemorrhage. Crit Care Med 2001;29:635–640.
4. Mamoli A, Censori B, Casto L, et al. An analysis of the costs of ischemic stroke in an Italian Stroke Unit. Neurology 1999;53:112–116.
5. Hacke W, Kaste M, Skyhoj Olsen T, et al. European Stroke Initiative (EUSI) recommendations for stroke management. The European Stroke Initiative Writing Committee. Eur J Neurol 2000;7: 607–623.
6. Ouchi Y, Nobezawa S, Yoshikawa E, et al. Postural effects on brain hemodynamics in unilateral cerebral artery occlusive disease: a positron emission tomographic study. J Cereb Blood Flow Metab 2001;9:1058–1066.
7. Schwarz S, Georgiadis D, Aschoff A, Schwab S. Effects of body position on intracranial pressure and cerebral perfusion in patients with large hemispheric stroke. Stroke 2002;33:497–501.
8. Yamaguchi T, Minematsu K, Hasegawa Y. General care in acute stroke. Cerebrovasc Dis 1997;7: 12–17.
9. Bhalla A, Sankaralingam S, Dundas R, et al. Influence of raised plasma osmolality on clinical outcome after acute stroke. Stroke 2000;31:2043–2048.
10. Bruno A, Biller J, Adams HP, et al. Acute blood glucose level and outcome from ischemic stroke. Trial of ORG 10172 in Acute Stroke Treatment (TOAST) Investigators. Neurology 1999;52: 280–284.
11. Li P-A, Siesjo BK. Role of hyperglycaemia-related acidosis in ischemic brain damage. Acta Physiol Scand 1997;161:567–580.
12. Berger L, Hakim AM. The association of hyperglycemia with cerebral edema in stroke. Stroke 1986;17:865–871.
13. Wallace JD, Levy LL. Blood pressure after stroke. JAMA 1981;246:2177–2180.
14. Britton M, Carlsson A, de Faire U. Blood pressure course in patients with acute stroke and matched controls. Stroke 1986;17:861–864.

15. Powers WJ. Acute hypertension after stroke. Neurology 1993;43:461–467.
16. Britton M, de Faire U, Helmers C. Hazards of therapy for excessive hypertension after stroke. Acta Med Scand 1980;207:253–257.
17. Adams HP Jr, Brott TG, Crowell RM, et al. Guidelines for the management of patients with acute ischemic stroke. A statement for healthcare professionals from a special writing group of the Stroke Council, American Heart Association. Stroke 1994;25:1901–1914.
18. The Cochrane Library. Blood pressure in acute stroke collaboration (BASC). Cochrane Review 2002(3).
19. Rordorf G, Koroshetz WJ, Ezzeddine MA, et al. A pilot study of drug-induced hypertension for treatment of acute stroke. Neurology 2001;56:1210–1213.
20. Hillis AE, Barker PB, Beauchamp NJ, et al. Restoring blood pressure reperfused Wernicke's area and improved language. Neurology 2001;56:670–672.
21. Bath P. Efficacy of nitric oxide in stroke (ENOS) trial. Stroke 2002;33:2529.
22. Bath PMW, Weaver C, Iddenden R, Bath FJ. A trial of blood pressure reduction in acute stroke. Age Aging 2001;30:554–555.
23. Levy DE, Brott TG, Haley EC Jr, et al. Factors related to intracranial hematoma formation in patients receiving tissue-type plasminogen activator for acute stroke. Stroke 1994;25:291–297.
24. Special Writing Group of the Stroke Council. Guidelines for thrombolytic therapy for acute stroke: a supplement to the guidelines for the management of patients with acute ischemic stroke. Stroke 1996;27:1711–1718.
25. Grau A, Buggle F, Schnitzler P, et al. Fever and infection early after ischemic stroke. J Neurol Sci 1999;171:115–120.
26. Boysen G, Christensen H. Stroke severity determines body temperature in acute stroke. Stroke 2001;32:413–417.
27. Ginsberg MD, Busto R. Combating hyperthermia in acute stroke: a significant clinical concern. Stroke 1998;29:529–534.
28. Hajat C, Hajat S, Sharma P. Effects of poststroke pyrexia on stroke outcome: a meta-analysis of studies in patients. Stroke 2000;31:410–414.
29. Castillo J, Davalos A, Marrugat J, Noya M. Timing for fever-related brain damage in acute ischemic stroke. Stroke 1998;29:2455–2460.
30. Kasner SE, Wein T, Piriyawat P, et al. Acetaminophen for altering body temperature in acute stroke: a randomized clinical trial. Stroke 2002;33:130–134.
31. Dippel DW, van Breda EJ, van Gemert HM, et al. Effect of paracetamol (acetaminophen) on body temperature in acute ischemic stroke: a double-blind, randomized phase II clinical trial. Stroke 2001;32:1607–1612.
32. Breda EJ, van der Worp B, Gemert M, et al. PISA. The effect of paracetamol (acetaminophen) and ibuprofen on body temperature in acute stroke: protocol for a phase II double-blind randomised placebo-controlled trial. BMC Cardiovasc Disord 2002;2:1–7.
33. De Keyser J. Antipyretics in acute ischaemic stroke. Lancet 1998;352:6–7.
34. Scott JF, Robinson GM, French JM, et al. Glucose potassium insulin infusions in the treatment of acute stroke patients with mild to moderate hyperglycemia: the Glucose Insulin in Stroke Trial (GIST). Stroke 1999;30:793–799.
35. Williams LS, Rotich J, Fineberg N, et al. Effects of admission hyperglycemia on mortality and costs in acute ischemic stroke. Neurology 2002;59:67–71.
36. Capes SE, Hunt D, Malmberg K, et al. Stress hyperglycemia and prognosis of stroke in nondiabetic and diabetic patients: a systematic overview. Stroke 2001;32:2426–2432.
37. Parsons MW, Barber PA, Desmond PM, et al. Acute hyperglycemia adversely affects stroke outcome: a magnetic imaging and spectroscopy study. Ann Neurol 2002;52:20–28.
38. Els T, Klisch J, Orszagh M, et al. Hyperglycemia in patients with focal cerebral ischemia after intravenous thrombolysis: influence on clinical outcome and infarct size. Cerebrovasc Dis 2002;13:89–94.
39. Kagansky N, Levy S, Knobler H. The role of acute hyperglycemia in acute stroke. Arch Neurol 2001;58:1209–1212.
40. Gray CS. The United Kingdom glucose insulin in stroke trial (GIST-UK). Stroke 2002;33:1736.
41. de Courten-Myers GM, Kleinholz M, Wagner KR, Meyers RE. Normoglycemia (not hypoglycemia) optimizes outcome from middle cerebral artery occlusion. J Cereb Blood Flow Metab 1994;14:227–236.
42. Geerts WH, Heit JA, Clagett GP, et al. Prevention of venous thromboembolism. Chest 2001;119:132S–175S.
43. The Publications Committee for the Trial of ORG 10172 in Acute Stroke Treatment (TOAST) Investigators. Low molecular weight heparinoid ORG 10172 (danaparoid), and outcome after acute ischemic stroke. JAMA 1998;279:1265–1272.

44. Kelly J, Rudd A, Lewis R, Hunt BJ. Venous thromboembolism after acute stroke. Stroke 2001;32:262–267.
45. Kamran SI, Downey D, Ruff RL. Pneumatic sequential compression reduces the risk of deep vein thrombosis in stroke patients. Neurology 1998;50:1683–1688.
46. Wijdicks EF, Scott JP. Pulmonary embolism associated with acute stroke. Mayo Clin Proc 1997;72:297–300.
47. Prins MH, Gelsema R, Sing AK, et al. Prophylaxis of deep venous thrombosis with a low-molecular-weight heparin (Kabi 2165/Fragmin) in stroke patients. Haemostasis 1989;5:245–250.
48. Sandset PM, Dahl T, Stiris M, et al. A double-blind and randomized placebo-controlled trial of low molecular-weight heparin once daily to prevent deep-vein thrombosis in acute ischemic stroke. Semin Thromb Hemost 1990;16:S25–S33.
49. Hillbom M, Erila T, Sotaniemi K, et al. Enoxaparin vs heparin for prevention of deep-vein thrombosis in acute ischemic stroke: a randomized, double-blind study. Acta Neurol Scand 2002;106:84–92.
50. Turpie AG, Levine MN, Hirsh J, et al. Double-blind randomised trial of Org 10172 low-molecular-weight heparinoid in prevention of deep-vein thrombosis in thrombotic stroke. Lancet 1987;8352:523–526.
51. Turpie AG, Gent M, Cote R, et al. A low-molecular-weight heparinoid compared with unfractionated heparin in the prevention of deep vein thrombosis in patients with acute ischemic stroke. A randomized, double-blind study. Ann Intern Med 1992;117:353–357.
52. International Stroke Trial Collaborative Group. The International Stroke Trial (IST): a randomised trial of aspirin, subcutaneous heparin, both, or neither among 19435 patients with acute ischemic stroke. Lancet 1997;349:1569–1581.
53. Bath PM, Lindenstrom E, Boysen G, et al. Tinzaparin in Acute Ischaemic Stroke (TAIST): a randomized aspirin-controlled trial. Lancet 2001;358:702–710.
54. Mazzone C, Chiodo GF, Sandercock P, et al. Physical methods for preventing deep vein thrombosis in stroke. Cochrane Library 2002(3).
55. Warkentin TE, Levine MN, Hirsh J, et al. Heparin-induced thrombocytopenia in patients treated with low-molecular-weight heparin or unfractionated heparin. N Engl J Med 1995;332:1330–1335.
56. Howard RS, Rudd AG, Wolfe CD, Williams AJ. Pathophysiological and clinical aspects of breathing after stroke. Postgrad Med J 2001;77:700–702.
57. Davenport R, Dennis M, Wellwood I, Warlow CP. Complications after acute stroke. Stroke 1996;27:415–420.
58. Polkey MI, Lyall RA, Moxham J, Leigh PN. Respiratory aspects of neurological disease. J Neurol Neurosurg Psychiatry 1999;66:5–15.
59. Ronning OM, Guldvog B. Should stroke victims routinely receive supplemental oxygen? A quasi-randomized controlled trial. Stroke 1999;30:2033–2037.
60. Turkington PM, Bamford J, Wanklyn P, Elliot MW. Prevalence and predictors of upper airway obstruction in the first 24 hours after acute stroke. Stroke 2002;33:2037–2042.
61. Wijdicks EF, Borel CO. Respiratory management in acute neurologic illness. Neurology 1998;50:11–20.
62. Nardin RA, Drislane FW. Neurologic causes of acute respiratory dysfunction. J Intensive Care Med 2000;15:29–47.
63. Cheng MA, Theard A, Tempelhoff R. Intravenous agents and intraoperative neuroprotection. Beyond barbiturates. Crit Care Clin 1997;13:185–199.
64. Borel CO, Guy J. Ventilatory management in critical neurologic illness. Neurol Clin 1995;13:627–644.
65. Steiner T, Mendoza G, De Georgia M, et al. Prognosis of stroke patients requiring mechanical ventilation in a neurological critical care unit. Stroke 1997;28:711–715.
66. Gujjar AR, Deibert E, Manno EM, et al. Mechanical ventilation for ischemic stroke and intracerebral hemorrhage: indications, timing, and outcome. Neurology 1998;51:447–451.
67. North JB, Jennet S. Abnormal breathing patterns associated with acute brain damage. Arch Neurol 1974;31:338–344.
68. Plum F. Mechanisms of central hyperventilation. Ann Neurol 1982;11:636–638.
69. Smith WS, Matthay MA. Evidence for a hydrostatic mechanism in human neurogenic pulmonary edema. Chest 1997;111:1326–1333.
70. Perron AD, Brady W. Electrocardiographic manifestations of CNS events. Am J Emerg Med 2000;18:715–720.
71. Oppenheimer S, Hachinski VC. The cardiac consequences of stroke. Neurol Clin 1992;10:167–176.
72. Hachinski VC, Oppenheimer SM, Wilson JX, et al. Asymmetry of sympathetic consequences of experimental stroke. Stroke 1992;49:497–502.

73. Rem JA, Hachinski VC, Boughner MD, et al. Value of cardiac monitoring and echocardiography in TIA and stroke patients. Stroke 1995;16:950–956.
74. Lin H-J, Wolf PA, Benjamin EJ, et al. Newly diagnosed atrial fibrillation and acute stroke. The Framington Study. Stroke 1995;26:1527–1530.
75. Tokgozoglu SL, Batur MK, Topcuoglu MA, et al. Effects of stroke localization on cardiac autonomic balance and sudden death. Stroke 1999;30:1307–1311.
76. Chalela JA, Ezeddine MA, Davis LA, et al. Myocardial ischemia in acute stroke patients: a troponin I study. Stroke 2002;33:383.
77. Marik PE, Zaloga GP. The management of atrial fibrillation in the ICU. J Intensive Care Med 2000;15:181–190.
78. Davalos A, Ricart W, Gonzalez-Huix F, et al. Effect of malnutrition after acute stroke on clinical outcome. Stroke 1996;27:1028–1032.
79. Johnston KC, Li JY, Lyden PD, et al. Medical and neurologic complications of ischemic stroke: experience from the RANTTAS trial. Stroke 1998;29:447–453.
80. Roth EJ, Lovell L, Harvey RL, et al. Stroke rehabilitation: indwelling urinary catheters, enteral feeding tubes, and tracheostomies are associated with resource use and functional outcomes. Stroke 2002;33:1845–1850.
81. Smithard DG, O'Neill PA, Park SC, Morris J. Complications and outcome after acute stroke. Does dysphagia matter? Stroke 1996;27:1200–1204.
82. Smith Hammond CA, Goldstein LB, Zajac DJ, et al. Assessment of aspiration risk in stroke patients with quantification of voluntary cough. Neurology 2001;56:502–506.
83. Mari F, Matei M, Ceravolo MG, et al. Predictive value of clinical indices in detecting aspiration in patients with neurological disorders. J Neurol Neurosurg Psychiatry 1997;63:456–460.
84. Añel RL, Pingleton SK, Dellinger RP. Respiratory and Nonrespiratory Complications of Critical Illness. In JE Parrillo, RP Dellinger (eds), Critical Care Medicine: Principles of Diagnosis and Management in the Aduct. St. Louis: Mosby, 2001;846–880.
85. Mutlu GM, Mutlu EA, Factor P. GI complications in patients receiving mechanical ventilation. Chest 2001;119:1222–1241.
86. Ferro JM, Caerio L, Verdelho A. Delirium in acute stroke. Curr Opin Neurol 2002;15:51–55.
87. Henon H, Lebert F, Durieu I, et al. Confusional state in stroke: relation to preexisting dementia, patient characteristics, and outcome. Stroke 1999;30:773–779.
88. Goldstein LB. Common drugs may influence motor recovery after stroke. The Sygen in Acute Stroke Study Investigators. Neurology 1995;45:865–871.

17
Medical Complications of Stroke

Devin L. Brown, Teresa L. Smith, and Karen C. Johnston

Medical complications of acute ischemic stroke are common and are related to clinical outcome. The frequency of medical complications must be recognized by physicians involved in the care of stroke patients to allow for the proper implementation of preventive and treatment strategies. In this chapter we review some of the major medical complications known to be associated with stroke.

GENERAL CONSIDERATIONS

When data collection and reporting of complications are performed rigorously, the rates of reported medical complications of ischemic stroke are quite high (Table 17.1) (Figure 17.1). In a recent prospective study, 95 percent of patients were reported to have had at least one medical complication and 32 percent had at least one serious complication, defined as a complication that is prolonged, immediately life threatening, or resulting in hospitalization or death.[1] Patients who sustain a serious medical complication have an increased risk of poorer outcomes, with an odds ratio of 6:1 for poor outcome, including death or disability (as measured by the Barthel index).[1] The most common serious medical complications are pneumonia (5%), gastrointestinal (GI) bleeding (3%), congestive heart failure (CHF) (3%), and cardiac arrest (2%) (Table 17.2).[1] Prospectively collected data suggest that direct effects of ischemic stroke account for most deaths within the first week after stroke, but mortality resulting from medical complications predominate thereafter.[1,2] Approximately 50 percent of deaths after stroke are attributed to medical complications.[1,2] An autopsy series confirmed these findings, demonstrating that the most common cause of death after ischemic and hemorrhagic strokes in the first week is cerebrovascular disease; the second through fourth weeks, pulmonary embolism (PE); the second and third months, bronchopneumonia; and after 3 months, cardiac disease.[3]

Table 17.1 Common complications after acute stroke[a]

Falls	25%
Urinary tract infection	24%
Chest infection	22%
Pressure sores	21%
Depression	16%
Shoulder pain	9%
Deep venous thrombosis	2%
Pulmonary embolism	1%

Data derived from Langhorne P, Stott DJ, Robertson L, et al. Medical complications after stroke: a multicenter study. Stroke 2000;31:1223–1229.
[a]Data from a prospective multicentered study with patients followed up to 30 months. Of those patients, 89 percent had ischemic strokes and 11 percent had primary intracerebral hemorrhages.

SYSTEMIC THROMBOTIC COMPLICATIONS

Deep Venous Thrombosis/Pulmonary Embolism

Deep venous thrombosis (DVT) is a serious problem for stroke patients. Patients with leg paresis are predisposed to developing DVTs, and the degree of paresis confers a graded risk of DVT.[4] Because isolated DVTs on the nonparetic side are uncommon, finding a DVT on the nonparetic side suggests a DVT on the paretic side.[4,5] The risk of DVT may be as high as 75 percent in the paretic side and 7 percent on the nonparetic side.[6] DVTs may develop as early as the second day but have a peak incidence at 2 to 7 days.[7] It has been suggested that the risk of death from untreated proximal DVT in stroke patients is 15 percent.[7] The most widely used screening test for DVT is duplex scanning. If a DVT is found, the risks of anticoagulation, especially in the setting of a large stroke,

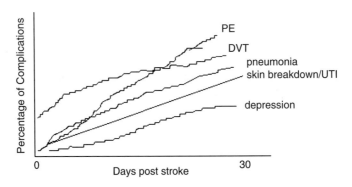

Figure 17.1   Timing of stroke complications in the first 30 days poststroke.
Adapted from Langhorne P, Stott DJ, Robertson L, et al. Medical complications after stroke: a multicenter study. Stroke 2000;31:1223–1229.

Table 17.2 Serious medical complications after stroke

All pneumonias	5%
Aspiration pneumonia alone	3%
Congestive heart failure	3%
Gastrointestinal bleeding	3%
Cardiac arrest	2%
Angina/MI/cardiac ischemia	1%
Deep venous thrombosis	1%
Pulmonary embolism	1%
Hypoxia	1%
Urinary tract infection	1%

From Johnston KC, Li JY, Lyden PD, et al. Medical and neurological complications of ischemic stroke: experience from the RANTTAS trial. RANTTAS Investigators. Stroke 1998;29:447–453.
MI = myocardial infarction.

should be weighed against the risks of DVT propagation or recurrence, or development of PE. DVT prevention strategies are discussed in Chapter 16.

PE represents 13 to 25 percent of early deaths after stroke and is the most common cause of death at its peak occurrence, 2 to 4 weeks.[7] Some recent studies have shown a low incidence of PE in the first few months after stroke.[1,8]

Heparin has been shown to decrease the risk of recurrence and mortality after PE.[9] Thrombolytic therapy compared with heparin for the treatment of PE has been shown to hasten resolution of the thrombus by angiography and lung scan and the sequelae of PE as measured by pulmonary artery pressure and echocardiography in the first 24 hours, but there appears to be no difference 7 or 30 days after the PE.[10] In assessing the major trials of thrombolysis for PE, which excluded acute stroke patients, intracranial hemorrhage (ICH) occurs in approximately 2 percent, with fatal ICH in 1.6 percent.[10] Higher diastolic blood pressure and advanced age appear to increase risk of ICH.[11] Overall, in adults, the risk of any bleeding complications from thrombolysis for PE increases with age at a rate of 4 percent per year.[12] Although the absolute increase in risk of ICH with the use of a thrombolytic for PE in an acute stroke patient is unknown, it stands to reason that it is substantially higher than 2 percent. Embolectomy in patients with large central emboli may have better survival results than previously suggested.[13] This represents another treatment option for those with life-threatening PE. Although heparin is administered during the procedure, the theoretical risks of ICH are lower with embolectomy than with systemic thrombolytic administration.

PULMONARY COMPLICATIONS

Aspiration

When videofluoroscopy rather than clinical assessment is used to assess swallowing in poststroke patients, rates of pathology may exceed 50 percent.[14] On initial presentation, male gender, age greater than 70, disabling stroke, impaired pharyngeal response, incomplete oral clearance, and palatal weakness or asymmetry are independent predictors of dysphagia.[15] Bedside tests to screen for swallowing dysfunction are important but, of course, are not completely accurate. The best bedside predictors of aspiration to thin liquid have been shown to be spontaneous cough during test swallows and the overall sense of the presence of aspiration by the examiner.[16] The absence of a gag reflex is not a helpful finding in predicting aspiration.[16] In healthy elderly subjects, gag reflex may be absent bilaterally in 43 percent.[17]

Dysphagia is a risk factor for developing aspiration pneumonia. The relative risk of developing pneumonia is greater for aspirating thick liquids or solids than for thin liquids.[18] One series showed a chest infection rate of 33 percent in those with an unsafe swallow and 16 percent in those with a safe swallow.[19] In another series, 92 percent of those stroke patients who developed chest infections had demonstrated dysphagia on initial videofluoroscopy. In this same group, although at 6 months 87 percent had returned to their prestroke diet, 50 percent had evidence of a swallowing abnormality on clinical assessment.[14] Interestingly, the presence of dysphagia, but not aspiration as detected on videofluoroscopy, was shown in one study to be related to increased mortality.[19] Prevention of aspiration in patients with dysphagia includes initial nil per os (NPO) status for those who may be at risk for aspiration.

Pneumonia is the most common medical complication 2 to 4 weeks after a supratentorial ischemic infarction.[2] It has been shown to represent a serious medical complication in 5 percent of stroke patients; 66 percent of cases are caused by aspiration.[1] Pneumonia is the most common cause of fever in stroke patients within the first 48 hours.[20]

Aspiration pneumonia occurs because of aspiration of colonized oropharyngeal material, not typically from aspiration of sterile gastric contents. The most common sites of involvement are the posterior segments of the upper lobes or apical segments of the lower lobes if aspiration occurs while recumbent, and the basal segments of the lower lobes if the patient aspirates while upright or semi-upright.[21] The most likely organisms are *Streptococcus pneumoniae, Staphylococcus aureus, Haemophilus influenzae,* and *Enterobacteriaceae* in community-acquired aspiration pneumonias, and gram-negative organisms (including *Pseudomonas*) in hospital-acquired aspiration pneumonias. Anaerobic organisms are uncommon.[21] Antibiotic coverage for anaerobes should be considered in patients with putrid sputum, severe periodontal disease, alcoholism, or evidence of a necrotizing process on chest films, whereas gram-negative organism coverage, such as a third-generation cephalosporin or fluoroquinolone, is routine.[21]

Oxygen Desaturation

The occurrence of oxygen desaturation, as detected by continuous pulse oximetry in acute hemiparetic ischemic and hemorrhagic stroke patients, is associated with increased age, higher National Institutes of Health Stroke Scale (NIHSS), and the presence of dysphagia.[22] Even stroke patients deemed safe to eat have a greater likelihood of desaturation after completion of a meal than do elderly controls.[23] Patients with a history of cardiac and pulmonary diseases are also at higher risk for desaturation.[22] In most cases, the patients are asymptomatic during periods of desaturation, suggesting that silent desaturation may be more common than previously recognized.[22]

Oxygen desaturation is a common problem in sleep apnea, which itself is not uncommon in stroke patients. One polysomnographic study showed signs of sleep apnea during the first night of sleep in 62 percent of patients after first hemispheric ischemic stroke.[24] Although this prevalence exceeds that of the general population, it is likely that in these cases sleep apnea was not caused by the stroke but rather the existence of co-occurring stroke and sleep apnea is common perhaps because of shared risk factors.[24]

Mechanical Ventilation

Most ischemic stroke patients who require intubation do so because of neurological deterioration. The morbidity and mortality are very high in this group. Fortunately, intubation is infrequently required; one retrospective study demonstrated that only 6 percent of 1275 patients with stroke required intubation.[25] In a group of 74 ischemic stroke patients receiving mechanical ventilation, 76 percent were dead or had severe enough disability to require nursing home placement at discharge.[25]

In a series of 24 patients, Wijdicks and Scott[26] found three major reasons for stroke patients to require mechanical ventilation: pulmonary edema (10 patients), brain swelling (8 patients), and seizures (6 patients). Of these 24 patients, 17 died. It is tempting to invoke neurogenic pulmonary edema as the cause of pulmonary edema in stroke patients; however, the data are lacking. In the 10 aforementioned patients with pulmonary edema, 6 had echocardiograms, all of which demonstrated a depressed ejection fraction thereby accounting for the pulmonary edema on the basis of congestive failure.[26] Stroke patients should be intubated and mechanically ventilated if they are not protecting their airway or require ventilatory support from partial airway obstruction, hypoventilation, aspiration pneumonia, or decreased level of consciousness. The use of mechanical ventilation and hyperventilation in the setting of elevated intracranial pressures is addressed in Chapter 18.

CARDIAC COMPLICATIONS

Arrhythmias

Through effects of the autonomic nervous system, likely via a combination of humorally mediated and direct effects, electrocardiographic (ECG) changes often occur in the setting of stroke.[27] Of 68 patients with cerebral thrombosis or embolism, Table 17.3 shows the rates of abnormal ECG findings.[28]

Given the concurrence of coronary disease with cerebrovascular disease, it is likely that some of these findings represent previous ECG changes rather than changes associated with acute stroke. However, based on electrocardiograms performed three times within the first week of cerebral thrombosis or cerebral embolism in those without any history of preexisting heart disease, only

Table 17.3   Cardiac arrhythmia after stroke[a]

Goldstein[28]		Ramani et al[29]	
Prolonged QT	37%	QTc prolonged	28%
U waves	25%	Tall U waves	9%
ST depression	25%	ST changes	25%
T-wave inversion	24%	T-wave changes	34%
Tachycardia	22%	Sinus tachycardia	15%
LVH	22%	LVH	4%
Q waves	22%	Q waves	9%
AF	13%	AF	0%
VPCs	13%	VPCs	0%
Decreased HR	9%	Sinus bradycardia	11%
RBBB	7%		NR
1st degree HB	6%	1st degree HB	2%
PACs	6%		NR
LAE	3%	LAH	2%
ST elevation	3%		NR
LBBB	0%		NR

AF = atrial fibrillation; HB = heart block; HR = heart rate; LAE = left atrial enlargement; LAH = left atrial hypertrophy; LBBB = left bundle branch block; LVH = left ventricular hypertrophy; NR = not reported; PAC = premature atrial contracture; RBBB = right bundle branch block; VPC = ventricular premature contraction.

[a]Comparison of rates of arrhythmias in two different studies. The left columns detail arrhythmias detected in the study by Goldstein[28] of stroke patients including those with a history of heart disease. In comparison, the right columns outline the arrhythmias detected in stroke patients without a known history of cardiac disease as documented by Ramani et al.[29]

23 percent had normal tracings.[29] The abnormalities detected in this group are found in Table 17.3.

In another series using controls matched for age and previous history of heart disease, two factors known to be associated with an increased risk of cardiac arrhythmias, the presence of heart disease did not appear to confer an increased risk of arrhythmia poststroke, again suggesting a causative association between stroke and arrhythmias.[30] Occurrence of potentially lethal arrhythmias may be more common than anticipated. In one series, 6 of 30 patients had asystole, complete atrioventricular block, or ventricular tachycardia.[31] Hemispheric infarcts have a higher degree of association with serious arrhythmias than brain stem infarcts.[30] The literature also supports a differential effect of hemisphere laterality on cardiac function. For instance, right hemisphere strokes are associated with more severe supraventricular tachycardias, whereas left hemisphere strokes have been proposed to be associated with ventricular arrhythmias.[32]

Sudden cardiac death occurs in 1 percent of supratentorial ischemic infarction within the first 30 days.[2] This may be due to the high prevalence of comorbid cardiac disease in this population. However, because cardiac arrhythmias and elevated catecholamine levels have been shown to be more frequent in stroke patients, cerebral ischemia per se may account for sudden death in this population. In those with first ischemic infarcts within the middle cerebral distribution, the sympathovagal balance, as assessed by heart rate variability parameters, appears to be shifted toward a sympathetic predominance.[33]

Although postulated to have significant input into autonomic function, involvement of the right insula was not statistically significantly associated with cases of sudden death, despite a trend.[33] Insular lesions have been found to be associated with prolonged QTc intervals, however, which may theoretically predispose to sudden cardiac death.[34]

Elevated Cardiac Enzymes

In a study of patients with first-ever acute large hemispheric ischemic infarctions, creatine kinase (CK)-MB, myoglobin, and total CK rose over 3 days (above the normal threshold values) and then decreased on day 4, whereas troponin T, a more sensitive and specific marker of myocytolysis, remained within the normal range.[35] Seventeen percent of a large group of patients admitted with acute ischemic stroke who had a history, but not active symptoms, of ischemic heart disease were shown to have an elevated troponin T level.[36] Forty percent of those with an elevated troponin T, but only 13 percent of those with a normal troponin T level, died while in the hospital, suggesting that elevated troponin T is a poor prognostic sign. Troponin levels can be useful in attempting to differentiate neurogenic left ventricular dysfunction associated with subarachnoid hemorrhage and dysfunction associated with myocardial infarction (MI).[37] Similarly, there may be a lower level of troponin elevation accompanying the reversible myocardial dysfunction associated with a stroke than with an MI.

Myocardial Infarction

Coincident stroke and MI are not uncommon. Literature from the pre–computed tomography (CT) era when cardiac markers were less sensitive support a concurrence rate of 12.7 percent in patients older than 60 years presenting within 72 hours of stroke symptom onset.[38] In most cases, the MI was asymptomatic underscoring the need for screening tests in this population. Excluding initial presentation, angina, MI, and cardiac ischemia complicate 6 percent of acute stroke patients, but only 1 percent have been considered to have a serious medical event secondary to cardiac ischemia.[1] Treatment options for acute MI are more limited in the setting of acute ischemic stroke. Not only is MI a contraindication to thrombolysis in acute stroke but also the converse is true.[39] Primary angioplasty may be an option for coronary revascularization in the acute stroke setting. Commonly, medical therapy concurrently administered with angioplasty and stenting include aspirin, clopidogrel, and heparin (or a low-molecular-weight heparinoid), in combination with a glycoprotein IIB/IIIA receptor inhibitor.[40] This combination is untested in acute stroke patients but likely increases the risk of symptomatic intracerebral hemorrhage. Risks and benefits must be weighed together with the cardiologists. Recommendations for treatment of acute coronary ischemia include aspirin, beta blockers (first dose given intravenously), nitrates, and angiotensin-converting enzyme (ACE) inhibitors (for those with persistent hypertension with CHF, systolic dysfunction, or diabetes) in typical cases.[40] In stroke patients, agents that affect blood pressure must be used cautiously, given the risks associated with abrupt lowering of blood pressure.[41]

GENITOURINARY COMPLICATIONS

Urological Complications

Urinary incontinence is a common problem after stroke. Between 32 percent and 79 percent of stroke patients on admission and 25 to 28 percent on discharge experience incontinence.[42] The most common urodynamic finding is detrusor hyperreflexia.[43] The loss of inhibitory input from higher neurological centers is thought to cause this hyperreflexia leading to urinary urgency, frequency, and urge incontinence. The characteristics of urological dysfunction are irrespective of laterality of hemisphere involvement. Although frontoparietal and internal capsule infarcts are most often associated with detrusor hyperreflexia, some lesions in the temporal and occipital lobes, thalamus, and basal ganglia despite urological symptoms may be unassociated with urodynamic abnormalities.[43] The presence of incontinence in ischemic stroke patients studied around 21 days poststroke has been associated with large infarcts (cortical plus subcortical area involvement), although this finding has not been consistent throughout studies.[44,45]

Detrusor hyporeflexia or areflexia may also occur leading to overflow incontinence. Although this may be a more common finding in hemorrhages, only 10 percent of patients with ischemic strokes have been demonstrated to have detrusor areflexia within 72 hours of stroke symptom onset.[43] Infarcts in the cerebellum, internal capsule, basal ganglia, thalamus, pons, and frontoparietal regions have been associated with this type of incontinence.[43] Other contributions to urinary retention also include the use of anticholinergic drugs, diabetic cystopathy, and bladder outlet obstruction. Unlike other neurological disorders associated with incontinence, in the stroke population detrusor-sphincter dyssynergia is an uncommon phenomenon.

The prevalence of incontinence post stroke decreases with time. Of a group of 95 patients with incontinence 7 to 10 days after stroke, 20 percent were still incontinent at 3 months, 8 percent at 1 year, and 3 percent at 2 years.[46] Urinary incontinence is a poor prognostic sign after stroke. In one study that assessed outcome 1 year after a first-time stroke in patients younger than age 75, initial incontinence was the best single predictor of moderate to severe disability with a sensitivity of 62 percent and specificity of 82 percent.[47] At 6 months, those who initially had complete urinary incontinence have a mortality of 60 percent; partial urinary incontinence of 25 percent; and no urinary incontinence of 7 percent.[48] Urinary incontinence is associated with an increased death rate at 5 years, perhaps as a marker of stroke severity.[49]

Physicians can easily overlook the diagnosis of urinary incontinence if patients or nursing staff are not directly queried. Diagnosis of the type of incontinence and appropriate treatment can be coordinated with a urologist. Detrusor hyperreflexia can be treated with scheduled voiding, tailored fluid restriction, and anticholinergic drugs. When possible, Foley catheter placement should be avoided to decrease the risks of nosocomial infections.

Urinary Tract Infections

Urinary tract infections (UTIs) occur in 11 percent of stroke patients followed for 3 months but are only considered a serious medical complication in

1 percent.[1] UTIs not only are a frequent complication directly after strokes but also remain a common complication when patients are followed for up to 30 months.[8]

Indwelling Foley catheters are often placed in stroke patients because of immobility, incontinence, urinary retention, or convenience. It is recommended that the placement of urinary catheters be avoided to reduce the incidence of UTIs if possible.[41] The duration of catheterization is directly related to risk of UTI.[50] In short-term catheterization, the bacteriuria is typically caused by a single organism rather than a polymicrobial infection. The most common organism is *Escherichia coli*; although other intestinal flora such as the enterococci are not uncommon.[50] Most patients with catheter-related UTIs are asymptomatic and do not have peripheral white blood cell counts different from other catheterized hospitalized patients without UTIs.[51] Although the presence of pyuria is considered necessary for the diagnosis of a non–catheter-related UTI, the sensitivity, related to a catheter-related UTI, of a urinary white blood cell count greater than 10 is only 37 percent, with a specificity of 90 percent.[51] The degree of pyuria does not correlate with the absolute level of bacteriuria with the exception of very high levels of microbial counts.[51] Urine cultures are therefore important in diagnosing catheter-related UTIs. After the diagnosis is made, using a threshold of 10^5 bacteria on culture, treatment options should be tailored to the culture results and regional organism sensitivities.

Sexual Dysfunction

Changes in sexual function after stroke may be related to a variety of factors including fear of stroke recurrence, physical disability, medication effects, and sensory deficits. Two months after stroke, 40 percent of patients express moderate or complete dissatisfaction with their sex lives.[52] In men, the most commonly sited aspect of sexual dysfunction is libido; next, ejaculatory dysfunction; and last, impotence. In women, decreased vaginal lubrication is somewhat more common than orgasmic failure.[52] In men, incontinence should be treated before tackling treatment of sexual dysfunction. In those with decreased libido, there should be an evaluation for depression or hormonal deficiencies. Options for treatment of erectile dysfunction in the setting of stroke are not different from those associated with other causes; however, a cardiac evaluation and recognition of possible risks in stroke patients should be considered before using sildenafil. Treatment of sexual dysfunction in women is more limited. Oral or vaginal estrogen replacement and sexual counseling are options.[52]

GASTROINTESTINAL COMPLICATIONS

Gastrointestinal Bleeding

Although rates of GI hemorrhage associated with acute stroke are often not reported as part of medical complications, we know from a recent study that it is one of the more common complications, being designated a serious medical complication in 3 percent and an additional nonserious complication in 2 percent of patients.[1] These statistics are in keeping with other reports.[53] Older patients, those with more significant impairment from the stroke, and those with more disability predating the incident stroke appear to be at higher risk for GI hemorrhage, whereas the use of antiplatelet and anticoagulation may not be related.[53] Those acute stroke patients with GI hemorrhage have higher mortality rates, but in most cases this does not appear to be directly related to the hemorrhage.[53]

GI prophylaxis is recommended for intensive care unit (ICU) patients with a central nervous system (CNS) process but not as routine therapy for all stroke patients.[54] However, given that patients not receiving enteral feeds are at higher risk for GI bleeding than those receiving feeds, the use of GI prophylaxis in stroke patients who are NPO may be reasonable.[55] Withholding of antiplatelet or anticoagulant therapy in the setting of GI bleeding should be individualized.

MISCELLANEOUS COMPLICATIONS

Falls

Falls have been sited as the most common complication of acute stroke.[56] Hip fractures are two to four times more common in the stroke population in comparison with an age-matched reference population and represent 45 percent of poststroke fractures.[57] Hospitalized stroke patients not only have skeletal "unloading" secondary to bed rest but also have disuse of the paretic limbs. These factors predispose patients to bone resorption. Patients who are able to ambulate early poststroke appear to lose bone density only on the paretic side (hemiosteoporosis), whereas those who are not ambulatory lose bone mineral density on both sides. Relearning to walk by 2 months predicts less bone density loss.[58]

Most fractures after stroke occur on the paretic side and are secondary to accidental falls.[57] Patients tend to fall toward the paretic side and without ample protective responses, such as outstretching an arm, these patients are at higher risk for fractures. Both lower bone mineral density and ipsilateral triceps weakness are associated with higher risk of postfall fractures.[59] Direction of the fall also helps determine fracture risk. Falls forward are associated with decreased wrist fractures, whereas falls backward are associated with an increased risk of wrist fractures but a decreased rate of hip fractures.[59] As would be expected, outstretching an arm during the fall increases the risk of wrist fractures and decreases the risk of hip fractures.[59] Risk of hip fractures may also be increased in the setting of serum 25-hydroxyvitamin D deficiency.[60] Diagnostic x-rays should be obtained in fall patients in the appropriate clinical setting. Although fall precautions should be considered in all stroke patients, those with cognitive impairment, neglect, and anosognosia may be at especially high risk. The role of bisphosphonates and other osteoporosis preventive therapies in the acute stroke patient have not yet been determined.

Skin Breakdown

Skin breaks and pressure sores are a common complication in stroke patients occurring in approximately 20 percent of patients.[8,56] Their frequency increases within the first month but decreases by 6 months post stroke.[8,56] As would be expected, skin breakdown is more common in those who are less independent.[8] Early mobilization, frequent turning, and use of specialized alternating pressure mattresses help prevent the development of decubitus ulcers.[41] Close surveillance is also an important measure for prevention. When pressure sores do develop, the principles of treatment include reducing pressure and friction, removing necrotic debris, managing bacterial contamination, and optimizing nutritional status.

Depression

Poststroke depression is difficult to quantify because of methodological differences in studies, but the incidence appears to range from 18 to 61 percent.[61] Both left and right hemispheric infarcts have both been related to poststroke depression, without an apparent predominance of one side.[62] Similar to the lack of laterality, there also does not appear to be an anterior to posterior hemispheric gradient in poststroke depression.[62] Higher disability scores, female gender, and most notably a prior history of depression are risk factors for poststroke depression.[63] There are many depression scales that can be used to assess depression. Recently, the single question "Do you often feel sad or depressed?" was found to have a sensitivity of 86 percent and a specificity of 78 percent when used against the Montgomery Asberg depression rating in screening for depression in poststroke patients.[64]

Depression at 3 months is correlated with a poor outcome at 1 year, although causation cannot be inferred from this.[63] Nonetheless, when matched for initial functional outcome, patients whose depression remits have a better functional outcome at 3 and 6 months.[65]

Selective serotonin reuptake inhibitors are effective and safe in treating early poststroke depression.[66,67] Although the data are controversial, treatment of depression may positively affect functional outcome; this effect does not appear robust, and often does not meet statistical significance.[67–69] Those patients whose mood responds to treatment also have a benefit in Mini-Mental status scores; although, placebo treated patients whose mood disorder remits also have a positive cognitive effect.[70] There appears to be a relationship between depression and 12- and 24-month mortality, but confounders likely exist.[71]

CONCLUSION

Medical complications are common and influence outcome after ischemic stroke. Recognition of risk for developing DVT, aspiration, and falls, among other medical complications, can affect the care of stroke patients. Implementation of preventive strategies and recognition of complications as they arise are essential in the proper treatment of stroke patients.

References

1. Johnston KC, Li JY, Lyden PD, et al. Medical and neurological complications of ischemic stroke: experience from the RANTTAS trial. RANTTAS Investigators. Stroke 1998;29:447–453.
2. Silver FL, Norris JW, Lewis AJ, Hachinski VC. Early mortality following stroke: a prospective review. Stroke 1984;15:492–496.
3. Viitanen M, Winblad B, Asplund K. Autopsy-verified causes of death after stroke. Acta Med Scand 1987;222:401–408.
4. Landi G, D'Angelo A, Boccardi E, et al. Venous thromboembolism in acute stroke: prognostic importance of hypercoagulability. Arch Neurol 1992;49:279–283.
5. Warlow C, Ogston D, Douglas AS. Deep venous thrombosis of the legs after strokes: part I— incidence and predisposing factors. BMJ 1976;1:1178–1183.
6. Consensus Conference. Prevention of venous thrombosis and pulmonary embolism. JAMA 1986;256:744–749.
7. Kelly J, Rudd A, Lewis R, Hunt BJ. Venous thromboembolism after acute stroke. Stroke 2001; 32:262–267.
8. Langhorne P, Stott DJ, Robertson L, et al. Medical complications after stroke: a multicenter study. Stroke 2000;31:1223–1229.
9. Barritt DW, Jordan SC. Anticoagulant drugs in the treatment of pulmonary embolism: a controlled trial. Lancet 1960;1:1309–1312.
10. Dalen JE, Alpert JS, Hirsch J. Thrombolytic therapy for pulmonary embolism: is it effective? Is it safe? When is it indicated? Arch Intern Med 1997;157:2550–2556.
11. Kanter DS, Mikkola KM, Patel SR, et al. Thrombolytic therapy for pulmonary embolism: frequency of intracranial hemorrhage and associated risk factors. Chest 1997;111:1241–1255.
12. Mikkola KM, Patel SR, Parker JA, et al. Increasing age is a major risk factor for hemorrhagic complications after pulmonary embolism thrombolysis. Am Heart J 1997;134:69–72.
13. Aklog L, Williams CS, Byrne JG, Goldhaber SZ. Acute pulmonary embolectomy: a contemporary approach. Circulation 2002;105:1416–1419.
14. Mann G, Hankey GJ, Cameron D. Swallowing function after stroke: prognosis and prognostic factors at 6 months. Stroke 1999;30:744–748.
15. Mann G, Hankey GJ. Initial clinical and demographic predictors of swallowing impairment following acute stroke. Dysphagia 2001;16:208–215.
16. McCullough GH, Wertz RT, Rosenbek JC. Sensitivity and specificity of clinical/bedside examination signs for detecting aspiration in adults subsequent to stroke. J Commun Disord 2001;34:55–72.
17. Davies AE, Kidd D, Stone SP, MacMahon J. Pharyngeal sensation and gag reflex in healthy subjects. Lancet 1995;345:487–488.
18. Holas MA, DePippo KL, Reding MJ. Aspiration and relative risk of medical complications following stroke. Arch Neurol 1994;51:1051–1053.
19. Smithard DG, O'Neill PA, Parks C, Morris J. Complications and outcome after acute stroke: does dysphagia matter? Stroke 1996;27:1200–1204.
20. Grau AJ, Buggle F, Schnitzler P, et al. Fever and infection early after ischemic stroke. J Neurol Sci 1999;171:115–120.
21. Marik PE. Aspiration pneumonitis and aspiration pneumonia. N Engl J Med 2001;344:665–671.
22. Sulter G, Elting JW, Stewart R, et al. Continuous pulse oximetry in acute hemiparetic stroke. J Neurol Sci 2000;179:65–69.
23. Rowat AM, Wardlaw JM, Dennis MS, Warlow CP. Does feeding alter arterial oxygen saturation in patients with acute stroke? Stroke 2000;31:2134–2140.
24. Iranzo A, Santamaría J, Berenguer J, et al. Prevalence and clinical importance of sleep apnea in the first night after cerebral infarction. Neurology 2002;58:911–916.
25. Gujjar AR, Deibert E, Manno EM, et al. Mechanical ventilation for ischemic stroke and intracerebral hemorrhage: indications, timing, and outcome. Neurology 1998;51:447–451.
26. Wijdicks EF, Scott JP. Causes and outcome of mechanical ventilation in patients with hemispheric ischemic stroke. Mayo Clin Proc 1997;72:210–213.
27. Davis TP, Alexander J, Lesch M. Electrocardiographic changes associated with acute cerebrovascular disease: a clinical review. Prog Cardiovasc Dis 1993;36:245–260.
28. Goldstein DS. The electrocardiogram in stroke: relationship to pathophysiologic type and comparison with prior tracings. Stroke 1979;10:253–259.
29. Ramani A, Shetty U, Kundaje GN. Electrocardiographic abnormalities in cerebrovascular accidents. Angiology 1990;41:681–686.
30. Myers MG, Norris JW, Hachinski VC, et al. Cardiac sequelae of acute stroke. Stroke 1982;13:838–842.

31. Mikolich JR, Jacobs WC, Fletcher GF. Cardiac arrhythmias in patients with acute cerebrovascular accidents. JAMA 1981;246:1314–1317.
32. Lane RD, Wallace JD, Petrosky PP, et al. Supraventricular tachycardia in patients with right hemisphere strokes. Stroke 1992;23:362–366.
33. Tokgozoglu SL, Batur MK, Topcuoglu MA, et al. Effects of stroke localization on cardiac autonomic balance and sudden death. Stroke 1999;30:1307–1311.
34. Eckardt M, Gerlach L, Welter FL. Prolongation of the frequency-corrected QT dispersion following cerebral strokes with involvement of the insula of Reil.Eur Neurol 1999;42:190–193.
35. Ay H, Arsava EM, Saribas O. Creatine kinase-MB elevation after stroke is not cardiac in origin: comparison with troponin T levels. Stroke 2002;33:286–289.
36. James P, Ellis CJ, Whitlock RM, et al. Relation between troponin T concentration and mortality in patients presenting with an acute stroke: observational study. BMJ 2000;320:1502–1504.
37. McGirt MJ, Bulsara KR, Lynch JR, et al. Troponin trend differentiates myocardial infarction from reversible neurogenic cardiac ventricular dysfunction following SAH (abstract). Stroke 2002; 33: 379.
38. Chin PL, Kaminski J, Rout M. Myocardial infarction coincident with cerebrovascular accidents in the elderly. Age Ageing 1977;6:29–37.
39. Wong CK, White HD. Medical treatment for acute coronary syndromes. Curr Opin Cardiol 2000;15:441–462.
40. Braunwald E, Antman EM, Beasley JW, et al. ACC/AHH 2002 Guideline update for the management of patients with unstable angina and non-ST-segment elevation myocardial infarction: a report of the American College of Cardiology/American Heart Association Task Force on Practice Guidelines (Committee on the Management of Patients with Unstable Angina). ACC/AHA Practice Guidelines. J Am Coll Cardiol 2002;40:1366–1374.
41. Adams HP Jr, Brott TG, Crowell RM, et al. Guidelines for the management of patients with acute ischemic stroke. A statement for healthcare professionals from a special writing group of the Stroke Council, American Heart Association. Circulation 1994;90:1588–1601.
42. Brittain KR, Peet SM, Castleden CM. Stroke and incontinence. Stroke 1998;29:524–528.
43. Burney TL, Senapti M, Desai S, et al. Acute cerebrovascular accident and lower urinary tract dysfunction: a prospective correlation of the site of brain injury with urodynamic findings. J Urol 1996;156:1748–1750.
44. Gelber DA, Good DC, Laven LJ, Verhulst SJ. Causes of urinary incontinence after acute hemispheric stroke. Stroke 1993;24:378–382.
45. Reding MJ, Winter SW, Hochrein SA, et al. Urinary incontinence after unilateral hemispheric stroke: a neurologic-epidemiologic perspective. J Neurol Rehabil 1987;1:25–30.
46. Patel M, Coshall C, Rudd AG, Wolfe CD. Natural history and effects on 2-year outcomes of urinary incontinence after stroke. Stroke 2001;32:122–127.
47. Taub NA, Wolfe CD, Richardson E, Burney PG. Predicting the disability of first-time stroke sufferers at 1 year: 12–month follow-up of a population-based cohort in southeast England. Stroke 1994;25:352–357.
48. Nakayama H, Jørgensen HS, Pedersen PM, et al. Prevalence and risk factors of incontinence after stroke: the Copenhagen Stroke Study. Stroke 1997;28:58–62.
49. Hankey GJ, Jamrozik K, Broadhurst RJ, et al. Five-year survival after first-ever stroke and related prognostic factors in the Perth Community Stroke Study. Stroke 2000;31:2080–2086.
50. Sedor J, Mulholland SG. Hospital-acquired urinary tract infections associated with the indwelling catheter. Urol Clin North Am 1999;26:821–828.
51. Tambyah PA, Maki DG. The relationship between pyuria and infection in patients with indwelling urinary catheters: a prospective study of 761 patients. Arch Intern Med 2000;160: 673–677.
52. Marinkovic S, Badlani G. Voiding and sexual dysfunction after cerebrovascular accidents. J Urol 2001;165:359–370.
53. Davenport RJ, Dennis MS, Warlow CP. Gastrointestinal hemorrhage after acute stroke. Stroke 1996;27:421–424.
54. Navab F, Steingrub S. Stress ulcer: is routine prophylaxis necessary? Am J Gastroenterol 1995; 90:708–712.
55. Cook D, Heyland D, Griffith L. Risk factors for clinically important upper gastrointestinal bleeding in patients requiring mechanical ventilation: Canadian Critical Care Trials Group. Crit Care Med 1999;27:2812–2817.
56. Davenport RJ, Dennis MS, Wellwood I, Warlow CP. Complications after acute stroke. Stroke 1996; 27:415–420.
57. Ramnemark A, Nyberg L, Borssén B, et al. Fractures after stroke. Osteoporos Int 1998;8:92–95.

58. Jørgensen L, Jacobsen BK, Wilsgaard T, Magnus JH. Walking after stroke: does it matter? Changes in bone mineral density within the first 12 months after stroke. A longitudinal study. Osteoporos Int 2000;11:381–387.
59. Nevitt MC, Cummings SR. The Study of Osteoporotic Fractures Research Group. Type of fall and risk of hip and wrist fractures: the study of osteoporotic fractures. J Am Geriatr Soc 1993;41:1226–1234.
60. Sato Y, Asoh T, Kondo I, Satoh K. Vitamin D deficiency and risk of hip fractures among disabled elderly stroke patients. Stroke 2001;32:1673–1677.
61. Gainotti G, Marra C. Determinants and consequences of post-stroke depression. Curr Opin Neurol 2002;15:85–89.
62. Carson AJ, MacHale S, Allen K, et al. Depression after stroke and lesion location: a systematic review. Lancet 2000;356:122–126.
63. Herrmann N, Black SE, Lawrence J, et al. The Sunnybrook Stroke Study. A prospective study of depressive symptoms and functional outcome. Stroke 1998;29:618–624.
64. Watkins C, Daniels L, Jack C, et al. Accuracy of a single question in screening for depression in a cohort of patients after stroke: comparative study. BMJ 2001;323:1159.
65. Chemerinski E, Robinson RG, Kosier JT. Improved recovery in activities of daily living associated with remission of poststroke depression. Stroke 2001;32:113–117.
66. Andersen G, Vestergaard K, Lauritzen L. Effective treatment of poststroke depression with the selective serotonin reuptake inhibitor citalopram. Stroke 1994;25:1099–1104.
67. Wiart L, Petit H, Joseph PA, et al. Fluoxetine in early poststroke depression. A double-blind placebo-controlled study. Stroke 2000;31:1829–1832.
68. Gainotti G, Antonucci G, Marra C, Paolucci S. The relation between depression after stroke, antidepressant therapy, and functional recovery. J Neurol Neurosurg Psychiatry 2001;71:258–261.
69. Robinson RG, Schultz SK, Castillo C, et al. Nortriptyline versus fluoxetine in the treatment of depression and in short-term recovery after stroke: a placebo-controlled, double-blind study. Am J Psychiatry 2000;157:351–359.
70. Kimura M, Robinson RG, Kosier JT. Treatment of cognitive impairment after poststroke depression; a double-blind treatment trial. Stroke 2000;31:1482–1486.
71. House A, Knapp P, Bamford J, Vail A. Mortality at 12 and 24 months after stroke may be associated with depressive symptoms at 1 month. Stroke 2001;32:696–701.

18
Neurological Deterioration in Acute Stroke

Devin L. Brown, Teresa L. Smith, and Karen C. Johnston

Worsening of stroke symptoms is a frustrating problem for those physicians involved in the care of stroke patients. In some patients, the initial clinical presentation is marked by fluctuations or an early clinical decline, whereas in others the worsening is delayed by hours or days. This variable time course suggests that different pathophysiological mechanisms may play a role in neurological deterioration after stroke. An understanding of the possible causes and pathophysiology of neurological worsening is helpful in determining the appropriate evaluation and treatment of stroke patients. This chapter addresses the major causes of neurological worsening in acute stroke and attempts to identify methods of differentiating among them and treating them.

OVERVIEW

The variability in terms often used interchangeably, including stroke in evolution, progressing stroke, stroke extension, stuttering stroke, and others, suggests confusion regarding clinical worsening after stroke. However, it remains a common problem with prognostic import. Deterioration is related to both poorer neurological outcome and higher mortality rates,[1] with impairment in level of consciousness appearing to confer a poorer prognosis than deterioration in other realms. Again, this suggests that different mechanisms play a role in symptom worsening after stroke.

Deterioration in neurological condition after stroke can be due to a variety of factors, including cerebral edema, hemorrhagic conversion of the infarct, recurrent stroke, concurrent infection, metabolic disturbance, and other less well understood contributors. Because the definition of neurological deterioration differs dramatically among studies, comparisons are difficult. One determinant of the variability in reported deterioration is the timing of presentation. Higher

363

rates of observed deteriorations are seen in patients who present earlier. This suggests that early deteriorations may be under-reported in patients presenting for medical care later. Patients with higher National Institutes of Health Stroke Scale (NIHSS) scores are more likely to have progression of neurological dysfunction; deterioration is seen in approximately 66 percent of those with an NIHSS greater than 7 and only approximately 15 percent in those with an NIHSS less than or equal to 7.[2] This, however, may be confounded by the fact that more severe strokes tend to present to a medical care facility earlier. When deterioration in level of consciousness is excluded and only motor progression assessed, lacunar infarctions are the most common stroke subtype found.[3]

RECURRENT STROKE

Recurrent stroke is a relatively uncommon occurrence in the acute setting but obviously can lead to cumulative neurological deficits. Data from one large randomized controlled trial showed a recurrence rate of 2.8 percent in those treated with aspirin and 3.9 percent in those not receiving aspirin in the first 14 days[4] (Table 18.1). The 7-day recurrence rate in another trial was 1.2 percent with no significant difference between the heparinoid-treated group and the placebo group.[5] Both of these trials (International Stroke Trial [IST] and the Trial of ORG 10172 in Acute Stroke Treatment [TOAST]) had longer enrollment windows and thus could have underestimated recurrences. In the study reported by Johnston et al,[6] the enrollment window was 6 hours from original stroke symptom onset and patients were followed for 3 months. In this study, new infarct or extension was found to have occurred in 18 percent of patients and designated a serious complication in 5 percent.[6] Another 1 percent had a transient ischemic attack. In this study, however, 3-month disability was primarily due to direct stroke effect, 10 percent of disabled patients had a new stroke or extension of stroke as at least a contributing cause of disability.

Even in a high-risk population such as those with atrial fibrillation, the recurrence risk in the acute setting is low, with recent data showing less than 1 percent per day for the first 14 days.[7,8] Although the use of high-dose subcutaneous heparin was shown to decrease the risk of recurrence, it was offset by the increased rate of hemorrhagic stroke in the IST.[7] Low-dose aspirin, begun

Table 18.1   Outcomes at 14 days in the different treatment groups stratified by the presence of aspirin or heparin treatment

	Aspirin (%)	No Aspirin (%)	Heparin (%)	No Heparin (%)
Recurrent ischemic stroke	2.8	3.9	2.9	3.8
Hemorrhagic stroke	0.9	0.8	1.2	0.4
Death or nonfatal stroke	11.3	12.4	11.7	12

Adapted from the International Stroke Trial (IST): a randomised trial of aspirin, subcutaneous heparin, both, or neither among 19435 patients with acute ischemic stroke. International Stroke Trial Collaborative Group. Lancet 1997;349:1569–1581.

within the first 48 hours after stroke, is recommended to decrease the risk of early ischemic stroke recurrence based on two large studies showing a modest but statistically significant effect.[4,9] (See also Chapter 14.)

HEMORRHAGE

Hemorrhagic transformation of an ischemic infarct can be symptomatic or asymptomatic. In patients with symptomatic transformation, headache, worsening of the underlying focal deficit, or decreased level of consciousness can occur. In a prospective study assessing 65 patients with acute supratentorial infarcts who had serial computed tomography (CT) scans at various points throughout the subsequent 4 weeks, 28 (43%) were found to have hemorrhagic transformation.[10] Although asymptomatic hemorrhagic conversion was common, only three (5%) of the 65 patients, or 10 percent of those with hemorrhagic transformation, had deterioration of neurological status associated with the hemorrhagic conversion.[10] None of the patients had an abnormal partial thromboplastin time (PTT). In this study, there was a positive correlation between size of infarction and the presence of hemorrhagic transformation.

Toni et al,[11] in a series of 150 first-ever supratentorial strokes, determined that hemorrhagic transformation was not an independent predictor of early neurological deterioration or 30-day outcome but that large infarcts and mass effect were predictors. The only early (within 5 hours) CT characteristic to predict hemorrhagic transformation was a focal hypodensity, with hemorrhage occurring predominantly in those with medium- or large-sized infarctions and those with mass effect.[11]

Thrombolysis is known to increase the risk of symptomatic intracerebral hemorrhage. In the placebo arm of the National Institutes of Neurological Disorders and Stroke (NINDS) recombinant tissue plasminogen activator (rt-PA) trial, 0.6 percent of the patients had symptomatic intracerebral hemorrhage within the first 36 hours, although substantially higher rates (6.4%) were seen in the rt-PA–treated group.[12] Restricted to patients with middle cerebral artery (MCA) occlusions, Prolyse in Acute Cerebral Thromboembolism II (PROACT II) showed a 2 percent symptomatic hemorrhage rate at 24 hours in its placebo group (heparin treated but no prourokinase) and 10 percent in the treated group (prourokinase plus heparin).[13] In addition to the increased risk associated with thrombolytics, it is known that rates of symptomatic intracerebral hemorrhage are increased by the use of high-dose subcutaneous heparin and heparinoids.[4,5] In IST, symptomatic hemorrhagic stroke was increased from 0.4 percent in the no heparin group to 1.2 percent in the subcutaneous heparin-treated group (Table 18.1). Rates of symptomatic hemorrhagic transformation of infarction in the TOAST study were 0.6 percent in the placebo group and 1.7 percent in the danaparoid group.

In analysis of the European Cooperative Acute Stroke Study (ECASS) I and II data, a 6-hour window thrombolysis trial, types of hemorrhagic conversion were subdivided into four categories: (1) small petechial hemorrhage, (2) confluent petechial hemorrhage, (3) hematoma less than or equal to 30 percent of the infarcted area with some mild space-occupying effect, and (4) larger hematoma with greater than 30 percent of the infarcted area with significant space-occupying effect, or a clot remote from the original infarct site. Retrospective analysis of ECASS I and II showed that in both the placebo group and the rt-PA–treated group, petechial hemorrhage (Figure 18.1) was not associated with a negative outcome.[14,15] In both studies, only development of the large parenchymal hematoma was associated with both deterioration at 24 hours and increased mortality at 3 months in the placebo and rt-PA–treated groups.[14] Large parenchymal hematoma formation was not, however, associated with disability at 3 months in ECASS I but was in ECASS II. Only in ECASS II were small parenchymal hematomas (Figure 18.2) associated with clinical deterioration at 24 hours in the combined placebo and rt-PA–treated groups.[15]

In patients treated with rt-PA, high NIHSS scores and edema or mass effect on baseline CT scan predict symptomatic intracerebral hemorrhage.[16] Three percent of those rt-PA–treated patients with an NIHSS score less than 10 and 17 percent of those with an NIHSS score greater than or equal to 20 developed symptomatic intracerebral hemorrhage.[16] In the subgroup of patients with a severe neurological deficit or edema or mass effect on CT scan, however, 3-month outcomes were still superior in those who were treated with rt-PA in comparison with those given placebo.

In cases of suspected intracerebral hemorrhage associated with thrombolytics, if the infusion has not already been completed, it should be held while emergent imaging is obtained.[17] Blood should be sent for fibrinogen, prothrombin time (PT)/PTT, platelets, hemoglobin, and hematocrit. Cryoprecipitate, packed red blood cells, and platelets can be administered if necessary.

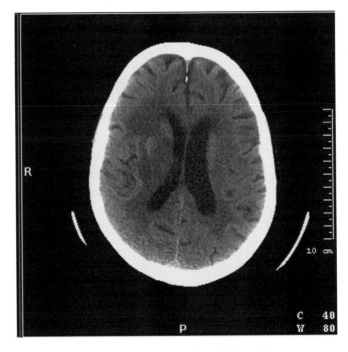

Figure 18.1   Petechial hemorrhage can be seen in the right hemisphere.

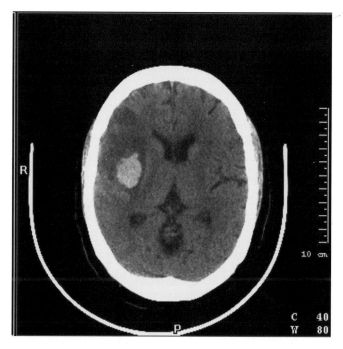

Figure 18.2 A small parenchymal hematoma is seen in the right hemisphere within a right middle cerebral artery (MCA) infarction.

Neurosurgical options may exist for select patients. In cases of intracranial hemorrhage (ICH) in the nonthrombolysis patients, supportive care and neurosurgical consultation are appropriate. Secondary stroke prevention may need to be reconsidered in the setting of a large ICH. Treatment recommendations for ICH are listed[18] (Table 18.2).

CEREBRAL EDEMA

Symptomatic cerebral edema is typically related to larger infarcts and tends to have a delayed clinical presentation. Globally elevated intracranial pressure (ICP) is not a common cause of deterioration even in large hemispheric infarctions.[19] The correlation between initial CT hypodensity and mass effect and progressing neurological deficits, however, suggests an important role of cerebral edema in early deterioration after stroke.[1] Although maximal edema of infarcted tissue occurs between days 2 and 5, brain herniation can occur as early as 20 hours.[20] Clinically, drowsiness is often accompanied by pupillary asymmetry, an extensor plantar response contralateral to the hemiparesis, or periodic breathing.

Brain edema was found to complicate 8 percent of acute strokes, with 4 percent considered a serious complication in one study.[6] Brain herniation, reported separately, was found in 3 percent of patients. In a series of 55 patients admitted

Table 18.2   Treatment of intracerebral hemorrhage

Blood pressure (BP)	Mean arterial pressure <130 mm Hg in those with a history of hypertension
	Avoid mean arterial pressure >110 mm Hg if patient is postoperative
	Give pressors for systolic BP <90 mm Hg
Intracranial pressure (ICP)	Defined as >20 mm Hg for >5 min
	Maintain cerebral perfusion pressure (CPP) >70 mm Hg
	Osmotherapy–mannitol 20% 0.25–0.5 g/kg every 4 hr with serum osmolality goal of ≤310 mOsm/dL
	Hyperventilation—pCO_2 30–35
	No steroids
	Muscle relaxants
	Nondepolarizing neuromuscular blockade (with appropriate sedation)
Volume	Maintain euvolemia
Temperature	Treat temperatures >38.5° C
Surgery	For cerebellar hemorrhage >3 cm who are deteriorating or have brain stem compression and hydrocephalus from ventricular compression
	Consider if hemorrhage >10 cc, Glasgow
	Coma Scale (GCS) >4, young patient with a moderate or large hemorrhage with clinical deterioration

Adapted from Broderick JP, Adams HP, Barsan W. Guidelines for the management of spontaneous intracerebral hemorrhage: a statement for healthcare professionals from a Special Writing Group of the Stroke Council, American Heart Association. Stroke 1999;30:905–915.

to an intensive care setting because of a complete MCA infarction, the mortality rate was 78 percent owing to cerebral herniation.[20] Poor prognostic findings include necessity for artificial ventilation, pupillary asymmetry, history of hypertension or heart failure, early hypodensity on CT scan involving greater than half of the MCA territory, baseline white blood cell count, nausea and vomiting during the first day, and degree of ICP elevation.[20–22] ICP monitoring demonstrating a level greater than 35 mm Hg at any point during the clinical course is predictive of death.[23] Although ICP monitoring can be helpful in guiding therapy, its ability to positively effect outcome is questioned.[23]

In one series, patients who died from brain edema tended to have high initial NIHSS scores, confined to scores greater than 15 for a right hemispheric infarct and 20 for a left hemispheric infarct.[21] Perhaps because of higher initial brain volumes, younger patients appear to be at higher risk of fatal edema from stroke.[21]

Treatment of elevated ICP in stroke patients is complex because most treatments have the capacity to simultaneously decrease cerebral perfusion while decreasing ICP. Both mechanical/physical and pharmacological methods can be used. The simplest physical method to reduce ICP is to elevate the head of the bed by 15 to 30 degrees. Morraine et al[24] reported that elevations of 30 to 45 degrees may worsen ICP. A recent transcranial Doppler (TCD) study of patients with large hemispheric infarcts (excluding those with ICP >20 mm Hg or pupillary abnormalities) showed that both ICP and cerebral perfusion pressure (CPP) are highest when supine, whereas CPP and ICP are lowest when the head is elevated by 30 degrees.[25] The uncertainty of the effect of decreasing

CPP for the sake of decreasing ICP underscores the complexity inherent in treating elevated ICP.

Another mechanical intervention, hyperventilation, acts almost immediately to lower ICP by leading to vasoconstriction secondary to alkalosis of cerebrospinal fluid (CSF). The effects of hyperventilation are short lived and should be reserved for emergency situations while a more definitive intervention is planned.[26] Hyperventilation below a pCO$_2$ of 30 mm Hg can likely further ischemia via vasoconstriction and should be avoided.[27]

Pharmacological treatment can also be used to treat elevated ICP. The administration of mannitol causes an almost immediate decrease in whole blood viscosity thereby leading to vasoconstriction and resultant decrease in ICP.[28,29] Studies have shown that the effects of mannitol in brain volume reduction preferentially involve the noninfarcted brain[30] (Figure 18.3). Although there is a theoretical concern that this may actually exacerbate midline shift, this has not been demonstrated.[31] The maximal duration of effect on ICP ranges from 20 to 360 minutes with a mean of 88 minutes.[32]

Mannitol can be given at a dosage of 0.25 to 0.5 g/kg over 20 minutes and repeated every 6 hours,[26] while matching input and output and monitoring the serum osmolality. The typical maximum daily dose is 2 g/kg.[26] Smaller doses of mannitol such as 0.25 and 0.5 g/kg have been shown to be just as effective as 1 g/kg with fewer side effects.[33]

Surgical interventions can be undertaken in specific circumstances to treat elevated ICP in acute stroke patients. Hemicraniectomy can be used as a definitive procedure to reduce ICP in space-occupying hemispheric infarcts (Figure 18.4). Of 32 patients who received large craniotomies with dural patch enlargement for

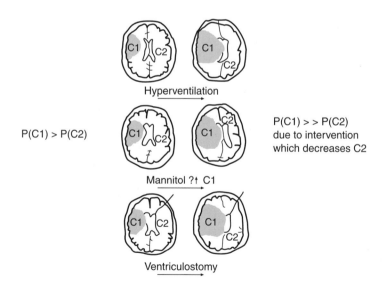

Figure 18.3 This figure shows two compartments: C1 the area of infarction, and C2 the area of normal brain. Initially, the pressure in C1 (P[C1]) is greater than the pressure of C2 (P[C2]). Hyperventilation, mannitol, and hemicraniectomy decrease the volume of C2 thereby decreasing intracranial pressure (ICP). As the volume of C2 decreases, the pressure gradient between C1 and C2 increases (P[C1] >> P[C2]) thereby theoretically worsening midline shift.

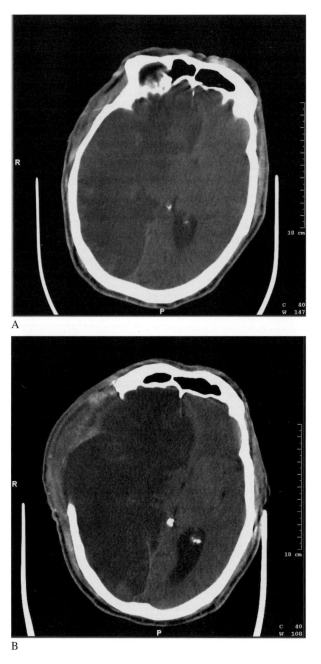

Figure 18.4 (A) This noncontrast head computed tomography (CT) demonstrates a malignant right middle cerebral artery (MCA) infarction with significant mass effect and edema. Note the obliteration of the right lateral ventricle. (B) This follow-up study demonstrates the appearance after right hemicraniectomy.

malignant hemispheric infarctions associated with decreased level of consciousness, midline shift, and requirement for mechanical ventilation, 21 survived.[34] In this small series, most were severely but not completely disabled, a few were disabled but independent, and one had minimal deficits on discharge from the intensive care unit (ICU). In another series of 31 patients with early hemicraniectomy, the mortality rate was only 16 percent with a mean Barthel index of 70, suggesting that earlier intervention may lead to improved outcomes.[35]

Another group, in addition to malignant middle cerebral infarct patients, for whom there are surgical options are those with large cerebellar infarcts and depressed level of consciousness. Of 34 patients with large cerebellar infarcts treated with craniotomy, 19 of whom were comatose, 65 percent had a good outcome.[36] In another series of 11 patients who received suboccipital craniectomies for cerebellar infarcts with signs of brain stem compression, most were at minimum living independently by 3 months.[37] It appears that decompressive surgery for cerebellar infarcts is not likely valuable for those whose level of consciousness is superior to coma.[36]

SEIZURES AND EPILEPSY

Seizure and its accompanying postictal state can lead to depressed level of consciousness and worsening of focal neurological deficits. The incidence of seizures in patients after ischemic stroke has been found to be 8.6 percent in a large prospective study.[38] In the same study, early-onset seizures (within 2 weeks) occurred in 4.8 percent of stroke patients. Many (40%) occurred within the first 24 hours. Late-onset seizures (after 2 weeks) occurred in 3.8 percent. Late-onset seizures were a predictor of recurrent seizures; 55 percent of patient with late-onset seizures developed epilepsy. Both cortical infarcts (hazard ratio 2.09) and stroke disability (hazard ratio 2.10) were risk factors for seizure occurrence.

Although mortality in some studies is higher in stroke patients with seizures, this appears to be related to stroke severity rather than the occurrence of seizures. Supporting this concept is the lack of association between patients with subcortical infarcts and poststroke seizures and mortality rates.[38] Status epilepticus is uncommon in stroke patients, occurring in 9 percent of those with poststroke seizure, although it has been said to account for 22 percent of all cases of status epilepticus in adults.[39] The presence of status epilepticus does not appear to be related to location or size of infarction; it also does not predict a higher mortality rate.[40]

Anticonvulsant therapy is recommended for patients who have seizures in the acute stroke setting; however, long-term therapy may not be necessary for all patients. Traditional antiepileptic drugs (AEDs) used for partial epilepsies, such as carbamazepine and phenytoin, are appropriate for prophylaxis in poststroke epilepsies, although some of the newer AEDs have a more favorable side-effect profile. Treatment of status epilepticus in the acute stroke setting should be managed similarly to its management in other clinical venues. Our preferred sequence of drugs is as follows: lorazepam 0.1 mg/kg; if this fails, phenytoin 20 mg/kg; if this fails, midazolam 0.2 mg/kg bolus followed by 0.1 to 2 mg/kg per hour with electroencephalographic (EEG) monitoring.

UNKNOWN CAUSES OF DETERIORATION IN SMALL-VESSEL AND LARGE-VESSEL INFARCTS

Although one typically thinks of stroke symptoms as maximal at onset, this is not always the case. Some strokes begin with a fluctuating course, which can be stepwise or gradually progressive. Overall, early deterioration (within 7 days of symptom onset) occurs in approximately 25 percent of patients.[41] When deterioration in level of consciousness is excluded and only progression in motor deficits included, lacunar stroke is the most common cause of progressive stroke[3] (Table 18.3). Of those with lacunar infarctions, the presence of diabetes and more significant motor dysfunction at hospital admission are predictive of progression of motor deficits, whereas infarct size is not statistically significantly related.[42]

The mechanism of deterioration in lacunar infarctions is not well understood. Previous emphasis was placed on the hypothesis of thrombus propagation despite limited evidence.[43] The relevance of large-artery parent disease remains undetermined. In one study of Korean patients, those who presented with a classic lacunar syndrome and had small deep striatocapsular infarcts had a high (36%) incidence of MCA disease by magnetic resonance angiography (MRA) or angiography.[44] Clinical worsening or a fluctuating presentation were more common in those with imaging suggestive of MCA stenosis and were more common with a larger degree of stenosis. Although microemboli or low perfusion could be inferred, this may represent the co-occurrence of two separate processes.

More recently, in lacunar infarctions, elevations in serum glutamate and depression in serum γ-aminobutyric acid (GABA) have been found in association with motor deterioration within the first 48 hours.[45] These changes may prove to be of prognostic significance even if a pathophysiological role of excitotoxicity is not borne out.[45] A secondary analysis of these data showed elevations in certain inflammatory markers, including interleukin-6 (IL-6), tumor necrosis factor-α (TNF-α), and intercellular adhesion molecule–1 (ICAM) in those with early neurological deterioration raising the possibility of an inflammatory contribution.[46]

Other hypotheses of the causes of early neurological deterioration include hypoperfusion. Suggesting against this as a common mechanism are data showing that a decrease in mean arterial pressure by 20 mm Hg from baseline during

Table 18.3 Determined stroke pathogenesis in those with and without a progressive motor deficit

	Patients with Progressive Motor Deficit (%)	*Patients Without a Progressive Motor Deficit (%)*
Small vessel stroke	63.6	21.4
Embolic from arterial, cardiac, or undetermined source	27.3	61.4
Low-flow in cortical or subcortical junctional zone	0	2.9

Adapted from Steinke W, Ley SC. Lacunar stroke is the major cause of progressive motor deficits. Stroke 2002;33:1510–1516.

the first 24 hours is not related to deterioration following initial improvement.[47] In another large study, maximum decrease in systolic blood pressures in the first 24 hours was not related to early progressing stroke either.[48] The data from two large thrombolysis trials do not demonstrate a difference in placebo versus thrombolysis groups in rates of early progression or early deterioration following improvement, thus suggesting against re-occlusion following early recanalization as a common mechanism for progressing stroke.[47,48]

Some studies have found deterioration to be common in large-vessel strokes. In 80 consecutive patients presenting within 5 hours of stroke onset who were studied with angiography, 91 percent of those with a progressive course, and 71 percent of those with a nonprogressive course had extracranial and/or intracranial arterial occlusions.[1] The finding of more frequent collateral supply (63% vs. 35%) in those without neurological deterioration underscores the significance of alternative sources of perfusion in arterial occlusions. In this study, the highest rate of neurological deterioration was observed in those with carotid siphon occlusions.

MR imaging has provided some insight into the pathophysiology of deterioration in large infarcts. Those patients with lower cerebral blood flow, as measured indirectly by bolus-tracking magnetic resonance imaging (MRI), have larger diffusion-weighted imaging volumes, larger perfusion defects, and higher NIHSS scores suggesting that decreased perfusion is correlated with poorer outcomes.[49]

Unfortunately, no effective treatment has been proven to halt neurological deterioration. Heparin cannot be recommended for routine treatment because it has not been shown to be effective.[50] In one study, half of the patients continued to progress despite immediate initiation of continuous intravenous (IV) heparin.[51] Induced hypertension may be another consideration in treating neurological progression in some cases. Some patients have a blood pressure threshold below which symptoms worsen and above which they improve. Those with such a threshold are more likely to be those with stenotic or occluded large vessels (internal carotid artery [ICA], MCA, basilar, and vertebral arteries).[52] As in the treatment of vasospasm associated with subarachnoid hemorrhage, it is believed that drug-induced hypertension improves leptomeningeal collateral blood flow and cerebral blood flow in maximally dilated vascular beds. This would theoretically lead to improved perfusion of the ischemic penumbra, a region with impaired autoregulatory function.[53] In patients with large MCA strokes, a 10 mm Hg elevation in blood pressure has been shown by TCD to increase peak mean flow velocities of the MCA, a surrogate for perfusion.[54] A small pilot study suggested that the use of phenylephrine to increase systolic pressures by 20 percent up to 200 mm Hg may be safe in the acute stroke setting.[55] More studies are needed to select the appropriate treatment population and prove efficacy.

SYSTEMIC CONDITIONS

Systemic processes may affect neurological status in stroke patients by furthering cerebral ischemia or by leading to presumed neuronal dysfunction. Those processes that further ischemia can lead to worsening of original symptoms, whereas those processes that work through other means may only cause transient worsening of baseline symptoms or recurrence of original symptoms. An example of a systemic process that can affect cerebral ischemia is fever. Pyrexia has been shown to be associated with increased morbidity and mortality in stroke patients.[56] Potential mechanisms by which ischemia may be furthered include release of excitatory amino acids and hydroxyl radicals.[57,58]

Worsening of focal symptoms in the face of sedative medications is not unusual. Two small series of patients with either previous stroke or mass lesion showed reemergence of previous focal neurological symptoms or exacerbation of an existing deficit in some patients after receiving either midazolam or fentanyl.[59,60] This type of stroke symptom recurrence, an anamnestic response, is a reversible phenomenon. Other systemic conditions such as infection, hypoglycemia, or hyperglycemia can have a similar response. These systemic and metabolic derangements must be considered in the setting of neurological worsening, after major neurological events have been ruled out.

CONCLUSION

Neurological worsening after stroke is a not uncommon phenomenon influencing both morbidity and mortality. Deterioration in neurological status can be very early, with a fluctuating initial course associated with a not-well-understood pathophysiology, or can be related to secondary phenomena such as cerebral edema, hemorrhagic transformation, recurrent stroke, or systemic derangements. Aspirin is recommended for prevention of early recurrence, but further studies are needed to determine a proven strategy for preventing and treating primary progression of symptoms.

References

1. Toni D, Fiorelli M, Gentile M, et al. Progressing neurological deficit secondary to acute ischemic stroke: a study on predictability, pathogenesis, and prognosis. Arch Neurol 1995;52:670–675.
2. DeGraba TJ, Hallenbeck JM, Pettigrew KD, et al. Progression in acute stroke: value of the initial NIH stroke scale score on patient stratification in future trials. Stroke 1999;30:1208–1212.
3. Steinke W, Ley SC. Lacunar stroke is the major cause of progressive motor deficits. Stroke 2002;33:1510–1516.
4. The International Stroke Trial (IST): a randomised trial of aspirin, subcutaneous heparin, both, or neither among 19435 patients with acute ischaemic stroke. International Stroke Trial Collaborative Group. Lancet 1997;349:1569–1581.
5. The Publications Committee for the Trial of ORG 10172 in Acute Stroke Treatment (TOAST) Investigators. Low molecular weight heparinoid, ORG 10172 (danaparoid), and outcome after acute ischemic stroke: a randomized controlled trial. JAMA 1998;279:1265–1272.
6. Johnston KC, Li JY, Lyden PD, et al. Medical and neurological complications of ischemic stroke: experience from the RANTTAS trial. RANTTAS Investigators. Stroke 1998;29:447–453.
7. Saxena R, Lewis S, Berge E, et al. Risk of early death and recurrent stroke and effect of heparin in 3169 patients with acute ischemic stroke and atrial fibrillation in the International Stroke Trial. Stroke 2001;32:2333–2337.
8. Berge E, Abdelnoor M, Nakstad PH, Sandset PM. Low molecular-weight heparin versus aspirin in patients with acute ischaemic stroke and atrial fibrillation: a double-blind randomized study. Lancet 2000;355:1205–1210.
9. CAST (Chinese Acute Stroke Trial) Collaborative Group. CAST: randomised placebo-controlled trial of early aspirin use in 20,000 patients with acute ischaemic stroke. Lancet 1997;349:1641–1649.

10. Hornig CR, Dorndorf W, Agnoli AL. Hemorrhagic cerebral infarction—a prospective study. Stroke 1986;17:179–185.
11. Toni D, Fiorelli M, Bastianello S, et al. Hemorrhagic transformation of brain infarct: predictability in the first 5 hours from stroke onset and influence on clinical outcome. Neurology 1996;46:341–345.
12. The National Institute of Neurological Disorders and Stroke rt-PA Stroke Study Group. Tissue plasminogen activator for acute ischemic stroke. N Engl J Med 1995;333:1581–1587.
13. Furlan A, Higashida R, Wechsler L, et al. Intra-arterial prourokinase for acute ischemic stroke. The PROACT II study: a randomized controlled trial. Prolyse in Acute Cerebral Thromboembolism. JAMA 1999;282:2003–2011.
14. Fiorelli M, Bastianello S, von Kummer R, et al. Hemorrhagic transformation within 36 hours of a cerebral infarct: relationships with early clinical deterioration and 3-month outcome in the European Cooperative Acute Stroke Study I (ECASS I) cohort. Stroke 1999;30:2280–2284.
15. Berger C, Fiorelli M, Steiner T, et al. Hemorrhagic transformation of ischemic brain tissue: asymptomatic or symptomatic? Stroke 2001;32:1330–1335.
16. The NINDS t-PA Stroke Study Group. Intracerebral hemorrhage after intravenous t-PA therapy for ischemic stroke. Stroke 1997;28:2109–2118.
17. Adams HP Jr, Brott TG, Furlan AJ, et al. Guidelines thrombolytic therapy for acute stroke: a supplement to the guidelines for the management of patients with acute ischemic stroke. A statement for healthcare professionals from a special writing group of the Stroke Council, American Heart Association. Stroke 1996;27:1711–1718.
18. Broderick JP, Adams HP Jr, Barsan W. Guidelines for the management of spontaneous intracerebral hemorrhage: a statement for healthcare professionals from a special writing group of the Stroke Council, American Heart Association. Stroke 1999;30:905–915.
19. Frank JI. Large hemispheric infarction, deterioration, and intracranial pressure. Neurology 1995;45:1286–1290.
20. Hacke W, Schwab S, Horn M, et al. 'Malignant' middle cerebral artery territory infarction. Clinical course and prognostic signs. Arch Neurol 1996;53:309–315.
21. Krieger DW, Demchuk AM, Kasner SE, et al. Early clinical and radiological predictors of fatal brain swelling in ischemic stroke. Stroke 1999;30:287–292.
22. Kasner SE, Demchuk AM, Berrouschot J, et al. Predictors of fatal brain edema in massive hemispheric ischemic stroke. Stroke 2001;32:2117–2123.
23. Schwab S, Aschoff A, Spranger M, et al. The value of intracranial pressure monitoring in acute hemispheric stroke. Neurology 1996;47:393–398.
24. Moraine JJ, Berre J, Melot C. Is cerebral perfusion pressure a major determinant of cerebral blood flow during head elevation in comatose patients with severe intracranial lesions? J Neurosurg 2000;92:606–614.
25. Schwarz S, Georgiadis D, Aschoff A, Schwab S. Effects of body position on intracranial pressure and cerebral perfusion in patients with large hemispheric stroke. Stroke 2002;33:497–501.
26. Adams HP Jr, Brott TG, Crowell RM, et al. Guidelines for the management of patients with acute ischemic stroke. A statement for healthcare professionals from a special writing group of the Stroke Council, American Heart Association. Circulation 1994;90:1588–1601.
27. Muizelaar JP, Marmarou A, Ward JD, et al. Adverse effects of prolonged hyperventilation in patients with severe head injury: a randomized clinical trial. J Neurosurg 1991;75:731–739.
28. Burke AM, Quest DO, Chien S, Cerri C. The effects of mannitol on blood viscosity. J Neurosurg 1981;55:550–553.
29. Muizelaar JP, Wei EP, Kontos HA, Becker DP. Mannitol causes compensatory cerebral vasoconstriction and vasodilation in response to blood viscosity changes. J Neurosurg 1983;59:822–828.
30. Videen TO, Zazulia AR, Manno EM, et al. Mannitol bolus preferentially shrinks non-infarcted brain in patients with ischemic stroke. Neurology 2001;57:2120–2102.
31. Manno EM, Adams RE, Derdeyn CP, et al. The effects of mannitol on cerebral edema after large hemispheric cerebral infarct. Neurology 1999;52:583–587.
32. James HE, Langfitt TW, Kumar VS, Ghostine SY. Treatment of intracranial hypertension. Analysis of 105 consecutive, continuous recordings of intracranial pressure. Acta Neurochir 1977;36:189–200.
33. Marshall LF, Smith RW, Rauscher LA, Shapiro HM. Mannitol dose requirements in brain-injured patients. J Neurosurg 1978;48:169–172.
34. Rieke K, Schwab S, Krieger D, et al. Decompressive surgery in space-occupying hemispheric infarction: results of an open, prospective trial. Crit Care Med 1995;23:1576–1587.
35. Schwab S, Steiner T, Aschoff A, et al. Early hemicraniectomy in patients with complete middle cerebral artery infarction. Stroke 1998;29:1888–1893.

36. Jauss M, Krieger D, Hornig C, et al. Surgical and medical management of patients with massive cerebellar infarctions: results of the German-Austrian Cerebellar Infarction Study. J Neurol 1999;246:257–264.
37. Chen HJ, Lee TC, Wei CP. Treatment of cerebellar infarction by decompressive suboccipital craniectomy. Stroke 1992;23:957–961.
38. Bladin CF, Alexandrov AV, Bellavance A, et al. Seizures after stroke: a prospective multicenter study. Arch Neurol 2000;57:1617–1622.
39. DeLorenzo RJ, Hauser WA, Towne AR, et al. A prospective, population-based epidemiologic study of status epilepticus in Richmond, Virginia. Neurology 1996;46:1029–1035.
40. Velioglu SK, Özmenoglu M, Boz C, Alioglu Z. Status epilepticus after stroke. Stroke 2001;32:1169–1172.
41. Tei H, Uchiyama S, Ohara K, et al. Deteriorating ischemic stroke in 4 clinical categories classified by the Oxfordshire Community Stroke Project. Stroke 2000;31:2049–2054.
42. Nakamura K, Saku Y, Ibayashi S, Fujishima M. Progressive motor deficits in lacunar infarction. Neurology 1999;52:29–33.
43. Fisher M, Garcia JH. Evolving stroke and the ischemic penumbra. Neurology 1996;47:884–888.
44. Bang OY, Heo JH, Kim JY, et al. Middle cerebral artery stenosis is a major clinical determinant in striatocapsular small, deep infarction. Arch Neurol 2002;59:259–263.
45. Serena J, Leira R, Castillo J, et al. Neurological deterioration in acute lacunar infarctions: the role of excitatory and inhibitory neurotransmitters. Stroke 2001;32:1154–1161.
46. Castellanos M, Castillo J, Garcia MM, et al. Inflammation-mediated damage in progressing lacunar infarctions: a potential therapeutic target. Stroke 2002;33:982–987.
47. Grotta JC, Welch KM, Fagan SC, et al. Clinical deterioration following improvement in the NINDS rt-PA stroke trial. Stroke 2001;32:661–668.
48. Dávalos A, Toni D, Iweins F, et al. Neurological deterioration in acute ischemic stroke: potential predictors and associated factors in the European Cooperative Acute Stroke Study (ECASS) I. Stroke 1999;30:2631–2636.
49. Thijs VN, Adami A, Neumann-Haefelin T, et al. Clinical and radiological correlates of reduced cerebral blood flow measured using magnetic resonance imaging. Arch Neurol 2002;59:233–238.
50. Coull BM, Williams LS, Goldstein LB, et al. Anticoagulants and antiplatelet agents in acute ischemic stroke: report of the Joint Stroke Guideline Development Committee of the American Academy of Neurology and the American Stroke Association (a division of the American Heart Association). Stroke 2002;33:1934–1942.
51. Haley EC Jr, Kassell NF, Torner JC. Failure of heparin to prevent progression in progressing ischemic infarction. Stroke 1988;19:10–14.
52. Rordorf G, Cramer SC, Efird JT, et al. Pharmacological elevation of blood pressure in acute stroke: clinical effects and safety. Stroke 1997;28:2133–2138.
53. Fieschi C, Agnoli A, Battistini N, et al. Derangement of regional cerebral blood flow and of its regulatory mechanisms in acute cerebrovascular lesions. Neurology 1968;18:1166–1179.
54. Schwarz S, Georgiadis D, Aschoff A, Schwab S. Effects of induced hypertension on intracranial pressure and flow velocities of the middle cerebral arteries in patients with large hemispheric stroke. Stroke 2002;33:998–1004.
55. Rordorf G, Koroshetz WJ, Ezzeddine MA, et al. A pilot study of drug-induced hypertension for treatment of acute stroke. Neurology 2001;56:1210–1213.
56. Hajat C, Hajat S, Sharma P. Effects of poststroke pyrexia on stroke outcome: a meta-analysis of studies in patients. Stroke 2000;31:410–414.
57. Globus MY, Busto R, Lin B, et al. Detection of free radical activity during transient global ischemia and recirculation: effects of intraischemic brain temperature modulation. J Neurochem 1995;65:1250–1256.
58. Monda M, Viggiano A, Sullo A, De Luca V. Aspartic and glutamic acids increase in the frontal cortex during prostaglandin E1 hyperthermia. Neuroscience 1998;83:1239–1243.
59. Thal GD, Szabo MD, Lopez-Bresnahan M, Crosby G. Exacerbation or unmasking of focal neurologic deficits by sedatives. Anesthesiology 1996;85:21–25.
60. Lazar RM, Fitzsimmons BF, Marshall RS, et al. Reemergence of stroke deficits with midazolam challenge. Stroke 2002;33:283–285.

19
Rehabilitation After Stroke

Alexander W. Dromerick

REHABILITATION OVERVIEW

Large numbers of stroke survivors have less than full recovery, even with the best of early medical management. In the United States, about one quarter will be discharged from the acute hospital to an inpatient rehabilitation setting. In most of Europe and elsewhere, most stroke patients receive inpatient rehabilitation where they were initially admitted for stroke care. In less-developed countries, little or no organized rehabilitation may be available, and patients are discharged directly to the care of their family within a few days. No data are available to compare these different systems of care, but within the European model, patients admitted to specialized stroke units have less long-term disability than those admitted to general geriatric units.[1-5] In the United States, two retrospective studies suggest that the intensive "acute" level rehabilitation programs are more effective than less aggressive "subacute" programs.[6,7]

In considering how rehabilitation interventions might improve the status of an individual with stroke, it is useful to organize one's thinking around the World Health Organization International Classification of Impairments, Disabilities, and Handicaps.[8] In the context of stroke, pathology refers to characteristics of the stroke lesion, such as the cause, size, and location of the injury. Impairment encompasses the neurological deficits associated with the stroke, such as hemiparesis, aphasia, and neglect. Disability refers to the loss of ability to do specific tasks; basic activities of daily living (ADLs) include walking, eating, and grooming, whereas instrumental ADLs are more complex and include cooking, medication management, driving, and using a telephone. At the highest level, handicap (now called participation) refers to the ability of the person to function in the roles and activities normally expected for that individual and includes the ability to be a worker, a parent or grandparent, or a member of the community.

Rehabilitation can target any of these levels, and examples of interventions at the impairment level include strengthening the affected side with motor therapies or reducing cardiovascular deconditioning by aerobic training. Interventions

377

at the disability level can include teaching the person with hemiparesis to dress with one arm, teaching the use of a cane or brace to improve walking, or teaching the use of gestures or devices to improve communication in the presence of language impairment such as a nonfluent aphasia. Participation might be increased by changing the physical environment (curb cuts, elevators, and transportation) or the social milieu with the use of vocational rehabilitation interventions at the workplace. Thus there are many opportunities to improve the status of persons with stroke sequelae that do not involve reducing lesion size. Often, the most effective intervention to increase independence and quality of life of a stroke survivor may not be a medication or a therapy. Instead, simply persuading the individual to move to a more enabling setting with elevators, public transportation, and social activities may yield the greatest gains in community and activity participation.

RECOVERY PATTERNS

Some useful rules of thumb are available to answer the questions of patients and families. Patients without voluntary movement in the arm within 2 weeks of stroke rarely recover fully, and those without voluntary movement at 3 weeks rarely regain any functional use of the arm.[9] Walking with some degree of assistance occurs in a remarkably large proportion of patients, as high as 85 percent in the inpatient rehabilitation population. Up to 50 percent of stroke rehabilitation inpatients will be discharged as independent ambulators.[10] Mortality is high in those who initially present with leg paralysis, but about 20 percent of these survivors will ambulate independently.[11] Urinary incontinence persists at 6 months in 10 to 20 percent of patients and may be single largest detriment to quality of life at 6 months after stroke.[12]

Some overall statements can be made about patterns of recovery after stroke. Most data come from large cohort studies in Denmark, the United Kingdom, and the United States.[13–15] In all these studies, care was the usual and customary care; few studies can inform us of the untreated natural history of stroke. For the group of all stroke survivors, recovery was completed in 95 percent of patients at 12.5 weeks.[16] Recovery plateaus sooner for those with relatively mild deficits and later (4 to 6 months) for patients with larger hemispheric injuries.[17] These statements must be tempered by the understanding that the studies were done using simple scales that are sensitive only to relatively large changes.[18] Patients universally report changes months and years later that they value as clinically significant, and these late improvements in impairment should be viewed as opportunities to reduce disability. It is the most severely affected patients that improve over the longest period, and these patients should be monitored regularly for improvement that can be exploited to increase independence. No large-scale studies exist to allow the physician to predict recovery based on lesion size or location,[19] although a few studies that focus on specific brain regions have found some differences.[20,21]

Motor recovery is generally fastest and most complete in the proximal antigravity muscles. Twitchell[22] described a sequence of recovery stages in his landmark study, beginning with the flaccid cerebral shock stage and the subsequent return of some tone and deep tendon reflexes. This is followed by the development of some voluntary movement, followed by "synergy" patterns, in which many surrounding muscles are activated indiscriminately during attempted muscle activation. An example of synergy is the flexion of the wrist and elbow that occurs when the hemiparetic patient attempts to make a fist. As synergy in flexion improves, voluntary extension appears, at first also in a synergy pattern. Finally, the patient begins to activate individual muscles in a discriminate fashion, and progresses to full recovery. Those who recover fully often report some residual easy fatigability, and hyperreflexia often is present on examination. Twitchell observed that the difference between patients who recover well and those who recover poorly is the number of stages through which they progress.

REHABILITATION IMMEDIATELY AFTER STROKE

If one defines rehabilitation as the care intended to maximize recovery from stroke, then rehabilitation begins at the time of hospital admission. For most U.S. stroke patients, who will be on the acute medicine or neurological floor for only a few days, the major rehabilitation issues revolve around prevention of complications and assessment of rehabilitation needs. The Stroke Rehabilitation Clinical Practice Guidelines published by the Agency for Health Research and Quality[23] outline the appropriate rehabilitation assessment. This assessment should include evaluation for physical and cognitive impairment as well as the need for assistance or supervision with ADLs. Key rehabilitation interventions during this period include a swallowing evaluation to reduce the likelihood of aspiration pneumonia, mobilizing the patient out of bed into a chair or into ambulation to prevent deconditioning, and preventing falls.

SELECTING THE REHABILITATION SETTING

Choosing the appropriate rehabilitation setting, intervention, and duration of treatment for an individual stroke patient is an art rather than a science. Pragmatically, the need for inpatient rehabilitation depends on the patient's medical complexity, degree of disability, the availability of support at home, and access to sophisticated therapy services. There is nothing magical about the delivery of rehabilitation treatment in the inpatient setting, and some large-scale forays into home-based rehabilitation programs are underway. However, a well-run inpatient program will immerse the patient in a medical, nursing, and therapy environment that allows for the efficient delivery and integration of rehabilitation interventions. It can also provide a physically and emotionally supportive setting for the newly impaired person to adjust to a life-changing event with profound impact on self-image, economic status, and lifestyle. Inpatient rehabilitation also allows the family time to adjust and to plan.

In the United States, there are two levels of inpatient rehabilitation, and a stay in one setting does not preclude a stay in the other. Both require medical and neurological stability and that the patient be willing and able to participate in treatment. There should also be a clinically significant goal for the rehabilitation intervention. However, such a goal does not require a discharge to the community; even for the person likely to go to a nursing home, improving the independence can lead to important gains in quality of life and survival. The traditional "acute" or "intensive" rehabilitation program consists of 3 to 6 hours per day of therapies in a setting of nursing care focused on incorporating therapy procedures in the patient's daily life. Patients must demonstrate their ability to tolerate this level of activity and must show clinically significant progress from week to week. The "subacute" or "skilled" setting provides 0 to 3 hours of daily therapy, typically within a population of patients with a broad array of physical and cognitive conditions. The amount and sophistication of therapy and nursing care varies greatly from center to center and is for all practical purposes unregulated. Although progress in rehabilitation must also be demonstrated in this setting, standards and time pressures are generally more forgiving. Thus this setting may be particularly helpful for persons with severe impairments or for those with other conditions such as fractures, wounds, or congestive heart failure that prevent more intense participation.

The use of subacute settings for persons who can tolerate 3 hours a day of therapy cannot be condoned. At least two U.S. studies suggest that outcomes are inferior for stroke patients in subacute settings,[6,7] even when controlled for stroke severity. Subacute rehabilitation should not be considered an acceptable substitute for acute rehabilitation for patients who can tolerate the latter.

TIMING AND DURATION

Little is known about the optimal timing or dose of rehabilitation after stroke. Most rehabilitation authorities advocate as much treatment as possible, as soon as possible, and for as long as possible; but there are few randomized controlled trials to support this recommendation. Circumstantial evidence for early rehabilitation does exist; most case series have found that subjects who received rehabilitation earlier made better recoveries. Clinical judgment would suggest that early mobilization would minimize complications such as aspiration pneumonia, deep venous thrombosis (DVT), and pressure ulcers.

At the other end of the spectrum, rehabilitation interventions months, years, or even decades after stroke can be appropriate and valuable. These interventions usually involve 5 to 20 sessions of outpatient physical, occupational, or speech therapy or may involve evaluation and treatment by a recreational or vocational therapist. Late recovery does happen, and brief courses of therapy may help the patient learn to use that recovery to improve independence and participation. Also, late complications do occur; often a short course of therapy can help patients who develop late musculoskeletal injuries, increases in tone, deconditioning, or contracture.

In those with mild impairments (discharged home within a few days), the case is often made for deferring therapies until it is clear that those impairments will not resolve spontaneously. This may lead to the most parsimonious use of rehabilitation resources, but it can lead to unnecessarily prolonged disability. There are also at least two theoretical reasons not to defer treatment. One is that it permits the development of suboptimal compensatory behaviors on the part of the untutored patient; these can be difficult and time-consuming to unlearn. The other is that it may miss a window of opportunity to shape the recovering brain. Increasingly, animal evidence suggests that there is a burst of synapse formation and pruning within a few days or weeks of injury[24]; there are also data suggesting that the types of activities that the animal engages in may modify these processes. Although sooner is probably better than later, decisions about how soon and how much must be left up to the judgment of the clinician.

MEDICAL MANAGEMENT DURING THE INPATIENT REHABILITATION PHASE

The goals of medical management in the first few weeks after stroke are to provide an optimal physiological environment for brain recovery, to prevent complications, and to refine and extend the stroke evaluation and prophylaxis plan initiated at stroke onset. There are several medical management issues that are unique to the rehabilitation phase of stroke care, and death rates during inpatient stroke rehabilitation are 2 to 4 percent. The rate of transfer back to the general hospital has been reported at 13 to 20 percent, most commonly for cardiopulmonary complications. Although pain syndromes, urinary tract infection (UTI), and depression are frequent, the stereotypical complications of pneumonia, recurrent stroke, and pressure sores are actually rather uncommon.[25,26]

Just as in the first few days after stroke, little is specifically known about the optimal physiological management during the first several weeks. With data accumulating regarding the deleterious effects of fever after stroke, timely management of any febrile illness seems in order. For patients with diabetes, euglycemia is the obvious long-term goal. However, many patients with new stroke may have difficulty perceiving the symptoms of hypoglycemia or may have difficulty communicating these symptoms to caregivers. Although hyperglycemia is not desirable, hypoglycemia can have immediate and catastrophic effects; loose glucose control is often desirable in the first few weeks after stroke. Afterward, diabetic management can become more exacting. Regarding hypertension, many experts recommend allowing systolic blood pressures to rise to somewhere between 140 and 220 mm Hg after ischemic stroke; tighter blood pressure management can be achieved a few weeks after stroke. Of course, cardiovascular stability must have first priority; in cases in which there is unstable angina or active congestive heart failure, the cardiac status must be aggressively addressed.

Several other complications are often encountered. Depression is common after stroke, but mimics such as neglect, sleep apnea, dysprosody, and impaired initiation should be ruled out before counseling and antidepressant therapy is begun. Only a handful of antidepressants have been tested for effectiveness specifically in poststroke depression; these include nortriptyline, citalopram, fluoxetine, and trazodone. DVT is a widely feared but relatively uncommon complication during inpatient rehabilitation, and prophylaxis practice should follow standard guidelines. In some studies, DVT incidence peaks between 2 and 7 days after stroke, with fatal pulmonary emboli peaking between weeks 2 and 4 after stroke. Diagnosis of DVT is the same in stroke rehabilitation setting as in other settings, but the physician must be more alert because sensory or cognitive impairments may delay the discovery of DVT. A vexing issue is when to discontinue DVT prophylaxis; some experts suggest discontinuation when the patient is able to reliably walk 150 feet at a time. Falls occur in about 25 percent of patients undergoing inpatient rehabilitation; fortunately, fracture or other serious injury is uncommon. The goal of rehabilitation is to maximize independence, but there is a natural tension with a second important goal, to maximize safety. Rehabilitation programs with an undue number of fall-related serious injuries may be unsafe; programs with few or no falls risk sacrificing effectiveness to safety.

SPECIFIC REHABILITATION ISSUES

Deconditioning is the constellation of the consequences of prolonged immobility or bed rest. Deconditioning affects virtually every organ system, and deconditioning-related impairments can be just as disabling as those related to stroke. Reversal of deconditioning is often the most effective strategy to improve the status of the stroke patient, particularly when the neurological impairments themselves cannot be lessened. Although most studies of immobility and bed rest were performed on healthy young males, the data seem relevant to the care of persons with stroke.

The most obvious manifestations of deconditioning are cardiovascular. As many of 75 percent of stroke patients have coexisting heart disease, and they can ill afford the doubling of cardiac demand that hemiparesis imposes on gait.[27] Effects of immobility include increased resting heart rate, elevated pulse during submaximal exercise, decreased stroke volume, and reduction in cardiac size. Symptomatic exertional cardiac ischemia can be precipitated in persons with no previous history of angina because the increased heart rate causes reduction in the diastolic filling time and reduced cardiac perfusion. The return to resting heart rate after exercise is prolonged, and aerobic capacity (VO_2 max) is reduced. Postural reflexes are also affected, and symptomatic orthostasis can present within 3 days of bed rest.

The musculoskeletal system is also profoundly affected by immobility. In healthy young males at strict bed rest, muscle strength loss averages about 1 percent per day. Similar results are found in the limbs of persons immobilized by casting, with generated torque reduced by about 15 percent after 2 weeks of casting. Weight-bearing muscles in the proximal limbs and trunk are disproportionately affected. Distal muscles are relatively spared, and simply testing grip strength alone will not demonstrate the finding of reduced ability to sustain that grip described after bed rest.

The treatment of deconditioning is straightforward in concept but is time consuming and incomplete in practice.[28] The clinical rule of thumb is that 3 days of treatment are required to reverse the effects of each day of bed rest. The most efficient approach is to eliminate deconditioning altogether by incorporating preventative measures in the first 48 hours of stroke care. For most stroke patients whose neurological impairments are stable regardless of position, time out of bed can begin within 24 hours of stroke onset. A seating schedule consists of at least two sessions per day up in an upright (not reclining) chair; the duration and frequency of these sessions should be aggressively increased to the patient's tolerance. Exercises in the supine position will improve strength and VO_2 max but do not address the positional reflexes. For patients with severe hemiparesis who have difficulty in maintaining an upright position, seating with trunk supports is essential. For patients who have undergone lengthy bed rest in the intensive care unit (ICU) or other settings, even the upright seated position may be intolerable. In such cases, the use of a "tilt in space" wheelchair followed by a tilt table is usually effective.

Pain syndromes are commonly found in stroke patients. Knee pain on the affected side, caused by repeated hyperextension seen in hemiplegic gait, is discussed later. A substantial number of patients develop flexor spasms, particularly during sleep onset, and these can be treated with low doses of an anti-spasticity medication. Central pain is well known but uncommon. It is classically associated with thalamic injuries and typically follows a "cortical" pattern, involving hand and mouth areas most severely. Clinically, central pain can be difficult to distinguish from musculoskeletal causes of pain. Brachial plexus injuries can also occur, although these are also infrequent.

Much more common is hemiplegic shoulder pain, which is probably a syndrome with several different causes. The incidence has been reported as high as 84 percent of stroke patients, and onset is usually within days to weeks after stroke. Patients report pain both at rest and on active or passive range of motion exercises. The cause of pain is poorly understood, but many cases are caused by local musculoskeletal causes such as biceps tendonitis, subacromial bursitis, and adhesive capsulitis. Although the downward subluxation of the humeral head out of the glenoid fossa in patients with flaccid hemiparesis would seem to be an obvious cause for shoulder pain, most studies have been unable to establish a relationship between pain and subluxation. Thus the aggressive treatment of subluxation in absence of pain is not warranted. Dependent edema in the hand and forearm are common, and are often a source of arm and hand pain. There is also a regional pain syndrome, the "shoulder-hand syndrome," which is said to be autonomically mediated. However, the findings of skin reddening, distal edema, and trophic changes can also be seen in simple disuse, and clear diagnostic criteria have not been established.

In the absence of much useful data regarding treatment, a symptom-based approach is useful. Several approaches may reduce the frequency and severity of pain. First, training of staff and family caregivers regarding transfer techniques can prevent mechanical trauma to the flaccid shoulder joint. There is a natural tendency to assist the hemiplegic individual by grabbing them under the affected shoulder, but this can cause trauma. Training in the use of a gait belt and stand-pivot transfer techniques can prevent this trauma. Second, mechanical support of the elbow to prevent downward traction on the shoulder should be provided. In the seated position, the use of an arm board or pillows under the elbow and forearm can unload the shoulder joint and provide elevation to minimize dependent edema. In the standing position, a sling can be used during ambulation and transfers. The constant use of slings is controversial because they discourage the voluntary use of the arm, and they place the arm in a position that may encourage shoulder contracture. Use of slings for short periods is unlikely to cause contracture but can keep the paretic arm out of harm's way and assist ambulation by moving the arm closer to the center of gravity. The third aspect of management is stretching to reduce spastic hypertonia and maintain shoulder range of motion. Exercises should be performed under the guidance of a therapist to ensure that unintended shoulder trauma does not occur. Simple analgesia with scheduled (not "as needed") acetaminophen will usually provide adequate pain relief; narcotics are rarely needed. Corticosteroid injections are often used, and at least one case series has found it useful. In the unusual case of severe intractable pain and physical findings consistent with a regional pain syndrome, an oral corticosteroid course or stellate ganglion blocks are sometimes used.

Driving requires the coordinated high-level activity of the motor, sensory, and cognitive systems, and one would intuitively expect that most people with persistent stroke impairments would have at least some difficulty with driving. At least 40 percent of those who were driving before stroke resume driving after stroke.[29] The available data do not document an increase in accident rates after stroke,[30] but stroke patients do report modification of driving activities and greater reliance on others for transportation,[31] and this may mask decreased driving safety.

Because driving can be essential to independence in many settings, it is a high priority for patients. Determining who is a safe driver after stroke is not trivial. Most studies have focused on populations of stroke patients who were referred for driving evaluations, and evaluated mostly neuropsychological impairment.[31–33] These studies used performance on an on the road driving evaluation as the endpoint and not driving performance in the community as measured accident rate or frequency of moving violations.

Faced with the impaired individual who requests clearance for driving, clinicians have little on which to base a judgment. The data available suggest persons with hemianopia, hemineglect, and other subtle visuoperceptual problems are at high risk for poor performance. The degree of impairment in persons with pure motor hemiparesis that raises the accident rate is unknown. Executive function in the form of attention and impulsivity must play some role in driving safety. An on-the-road driving evaluation with an experienced instructor is probably the best available predictor for driving safety and should be considered in any individual with a question of visual or perceptual impairment. The value of simple reaction time and color perception evaluations done at many institutions is questionable. Detailed neuropsychological evaluations may be more helpful, but they are expensive and of uncertain relevance. Useful driving simulators are on the horizon and may prove to be a convenient and inexpensive method of safety determination.

Spasticity management should be attempted only when the patient and physician agree on the goals of treatment. Available spasticity treatments are of limited benefit and are often quite costly. Although most patients present requesting improvement in the negative symptoms of the upper motor neuron syndrome (weakness and clumsiness), the available treatments are best at addressing the positive symptoms such as flexor spasms, posturing, and resistance to passive movement. Thus the patient who presents requesting that stiffness be reduced so that movement can be improved will be disappointed. Available data indicate that the difficulty in movement encountered in spastic hemiparesis is due to poor activation of motor units; simply reducing the passive resistance to stretch does not address the underlying pathophysiology.

Some goals of spasticity management are clearly achievable. For example, painful muscle spasms respond to almost any antispasticity medication. Spasticity often interferes with the range of motion exercises that are necessary to prevent joint contracture. Frustration and pain often limit stretching; antispasticity treatment can reduce the passive resistance to stretch, and thus facilitate preservation of joint function. Another achievable goal is cosmetic; many patients object to the appearance of the flexed and adducted arm posture that worsens with walking and are grateful for the reduction in spastic posturing that takes place with treatment.

Treatment should be approached in a stepwise fashion. The first step is to eliminate exacerbations of spastic hypertonia. These can include infection, intraabdominal processes, bladder distension, and bowel obstipation. Other sources of pain, such as joint injury, skin wounds, and neuropathy should be addressed. Next is the addition of physical medicine techniques such as stretching, active exercise regimens, and splinting.

If hypertonia is still troublesome, then pharmacological intervention is indicated. Oral medications are usually the first choice. Many stroke patients are highly sensitive to the central side effects of these medicines, and initial doses should be very low. Each of the major oral antispasticity agents has advantages and weaknesses.[34] Baclofen is probably the most widely used, but can cause drowsiness at therapeutic doses. Dantrolene is the traditional first choice in patients with "cerebral" (as opposed to "spinal") spasticity, and causes relatively little sedation. However, it can cause weakness, and there are reports of hepatic dysfunction.[35] Tizanidine was shown in an open label trial to reduce resistance to passive range of motion without increasing weakness, but was poorly tolerated by a large proportion of subjects.[36] Second-line agents include benzodiazepines, clonidine, and mexiletine.

Botulinum toxin is a widely publicized spasticity treatment, and it is a lucrative intervention for practitioners and pharmaceutical companies. Intramuscular injections every few months cause focal weakness, and the treatment is effective in reducing flexor spasm, resistance to passive movement, and tonic posturing. For such symptoms, it can be considered when less invasive treatments are insufficient; it is particularly useful in patients who have dystonic features. Advocates also contend that botulinum toxin treatment actually increases use of the upper extremity, but this is much more controversial. Most studies have showed no such effect,[34] and one would predict no significant improvement based on the underlying physiology of spasticity. A recent, large randomized trial of botulinum toxin did report improvements in arm function,[37] but this result has been questioned[38,39] because of potential unblinding of the raters. A persuasive, double-blinded randomized controlled clinical trial has yet to be done. In clinical experience, most patients without painful spasms lose enthusiasm for botulinum toxin after a few treatments.

Other treatments are less widely used. Acupuncture[40] has been reported helpful in some case series. Intrathecal baclofen[41] can effective when oral medication and botulinum toxin fail to control pain and posturing and is very useful for patients with severe spastic dystonia. The use of phenol to focally ablate peripheral nerves has been largely replaced by botulinum toxin.

ADDRESSING THE NEEDS OF THE CHRONIC OR DEBILITATED STROKE PATIENT

With 4.7 million stroke survivors in the United States alone, the clinician is often challenged by the individual who had a stroke months or years before, who has persistent impairments or disabilities, and who comes seeking an improvement in functional status. Rather than simply reassess the patient's stroke prophylaxis and remind him or her of the lack of impairment improvement after the first few months, the stroke physician can take a proactive and productive approach to substantively increase the quality of life of the patient. Questioning will usually reveal specific and achievable goals that can increase independence or lead to more participation in the community. Such patients should be viewed as long-term projects, in whom the treatment plan will be executed over 2 or 3 years.

Improving walking months or years after stroke typically requires increases in gait speed and endurance and requires a patient who is willing and able to engage in a daily training regimen indefinitely. Physical medicine techniques, strength training, and endurance training are the relevant approaches. Optimizing management of coexisting conditions such as congestive heart failure or depression can also make important contributions. Collaboration with a physical therapist is essential, but simple referral for a handful of therapy sessions rarely makes much difference. In those patients for whom an increase in the safety or speed of walking is the issue, reduction of cardiac deconditioning with endurance training will usually be part of the answer. Stroke patients typically reduce their walking speed to maintain the same perceived level of exertion that they experienced before stroke[27]; improved aerobic conditioning will allow a higher gait speed. Contracture of the knee or ankle reduces gait efficiency because the patient must compensate for the lost function; treatment will involve stretching and sometimes the pharmacological management of spastic hypertonia. Most people with decreased mobility resulting from stroke will have bilateral weakening and atrophy of muscles due to disuse that can be addressed by resistance training. Improvements in skeletal muscle strength, independent of any changes in neurological impairment, will typically improve gait mechanics, walking speed, and endurance. Musculoskeletal pain syndromes also impair walking. The most common is genu recurvatum, a traumatic arthropathy of the knee. This condition is due to the vigorous knee hyperextension that takes place each time that the patient puts weight on the affected side. The treatment for this condition is to improve gait mechanics via retraining with a physical therapist, strengthening of the quadriceps and hamstrings, and adjustment of the ankle brace to allow more dorsiflexion of the ankle. Corticosteroid injections of the knee bring short-term relief, but the pain will return after a few weeks if gait biomechanics are not improved. When these conventional approaches have been exhausted, an emerging treatment such as body-weight supported treadmill training should be considered. As a last resort, powered wheelchairs can offer the physically impaired person the opportunity to participate in community activities such as shopping, theater attendance, and family events.

Transition from gastrostomy tube to oral feedings typically takes place in the first few weeks to 3 months after stroke. Permanent tube feeding is rare in the aware person with unilateral hemispheric stroke. An enteral feeding tube should be viewed as temporary in all but those with impaired consciousness or persistent profound neglect. Patients with lower brain stem injury may take the longest to become oral feeders, but even those with large bilateral pontine or medullary injuries typically become oral feeders within 6 to 24 months. In such cases, there may be a transitional period where the patient's needs are partially met by oral feeding and partly met by tube feeding. In most cases, withdrawal of tube feedings is generally done by first reducing daytime feeds. This will facilitate oral feeding by increasing appetite during the day and will encourage activity because the patient is no longer attached to a feeding pump and can move about freely.

Urinary incontinence may cause more patients to be homebound than any other neurological impairment and is an important contributor to quality of life. Although the notion of "upper motor neuron" and "lower motor neuron" bladder dysfunction may be useful in understanding basic neurophysiology, the clinical reality is much different. Although it would seem obvious that stroke patients universally have upper motor neuron disturbance, incontinent stroke patients are equally likely to have upper, lower, or mixed disturbances of bladder function.[42] Preexisting stress incontinence and prostatism are frequent contributors. There are few data regarding optimal evaluation and treatment of urinary incontinence. Like other impairments, there are rapid changes in the first few weeks, and a pragmatic, symptom-oriented approach is reasonable. Incontinence management begins with treatment of UTIs. Discontinuation of diuretics is obvious but often overlooked; in most cases, drugs other than diuretics can be chosen to manage hypertension or congestive heart failure. Timed voiding, in which the patient is on the toilet at specific times, is the mainstay of incontinence management. Simply put, the patient attempts to void on the toilet or bedside commode every 2 to 4 hours while awake, whether there is a perceived need to void or not. Besides the obvious goal of regularly draining the bladder before incontinence episodes occur, this technique also helps the patient relearn sensory cues for a bladder that is filled near capacity. Timed voids may also promote a bladder emptying rhythm. Because incontinence is often most common at night, eliminating fluid intake after dinner, except to take medications, can also be an effective maneuver.

Medications can be a useful adjunct to the basic techniques mentioned previously, but simply writing a prescription will likely be unsuccessful. Urodynamic studies are often performed to further understand the underlying pathophysiology of bladder dysfunction, and this is the most rational approach to the pharmacological treatment of incontinence in individual patients. Because urodynamic studies are invasive and expensive, they are typically deferred until a few months after stroke. During the interim, postvoid residual (PVR) determinations can be useful to determine whether urinary retention is occurring, but available data suggest that any single PVR reading may be misleading and that three determinations may be more informative.[43] Rather than attempt to globally restore continence, a more realistic goal is to achieve continence during certain key points during the day or to reduce the frequency of urinary loss. The easiest syndrome to address is the individual who is continent during the day but who has multiple episodes of nighttime incontinence or nocturia. In this case, evening fluid restriction and a small amount of a short acting anticholinergic such as oxybutynin will often provide relief. Nighttime condom catheters for men can help, although most men who can tolerate this will prefer to use a bedside urinal. For more severely affected patients, timed voids and elimination of diuretics may be the best available choices for improving continence status. For patients with preexisting prostatism or pelvic floor dysfunction, careful anatomical and physiological evaluation by a urologist or gynecologist is essential.

Improving the status of the institutionalized stoke patient requires patience but can be very rewarding. Many of these patients will have been discharged from therapies months or years before, but, in the interim, there has been slow improvement in impairments that can now be exploited to reduce disability. Most of these patients will have deconditioning and contracture that can be addressed as described previously. A seating schedule to address neurovascular deconditioning is often the first order of business because little else can be achieved if the patient cannot sit up for at least an hour or two. Once this level of endurance is achieved, the use of a standing frame can allow the development of the standing endurance necessary to engage in useful transfer or gait training. Incontinence is typically addressed via timed voiding schedules and discontinuation of diuretics.

EMERGING TREATMENTS

Recently, the scientific attention directed toward fundamental mechanisms of brain recovery and means of enhancing those mechanisms has yielded an array of clinical treatments that are based on those laboratory and animal findings. The best studied of these involve motor restoration. None of these has been subjected to large-scale randomized controlled trials, but because no regulatory approval is required for patient use, many of them are being applied in ongoing patient care. These treatments have not been standardized, but many centers and clinicians are using them. Given the lack of data, it is impossible to state with confidence when, how, or whether such treatments should be applied. Advocates of some of these treatments state the need for specific aspects of the treatment to be executed in specific ways, but little or no data are available. Nonetheless, the risk of these treatments seems low, and decisions about whether or when to use them is left to the judgment of the clinician. Certainly, until more data are available, these treatments should not be considered until treatments that are more traditional are exhausted.

Body weight-supported treadmill training (BWSTT) has the most extensive data supporting its use. The technique is derived from the motorized treadmill-training paradigm applied to cats with surgical spinal cord transsections. In the laboratory, animals are made paraplegic and then given motorized treadmill sessions. These animals often begin to display gait patterns in the hind limbs, and in certain cases, these walking motions will occur in overground walking, not just on the treadmill. The mechanism by which this takes place has been shown to be a pool of motor neurons in the lumbosacral spinal cord that apparently have been trained to elaborate the hind limb walking pattern in the absence of influence from higher motor centers. In humans, work has proceeded along two lines. The first is an explicit attempt to replicate the laboratory work to improve gait endurance, gait velocity, and balance. There have been reports of some success in stroke patients,[44,45] and a multicenter study in spinal cord injury is underway. The second approach is to view the intervention as a means of addressing cardiovascular deconditioning in patients with motor impairment. The primary goal is to reduce disability by improving aerobic capacity for physical activity, especially walking.[46] The data are limited but promising.

Constraint-induced therapy (CIT) or forced use therapy has received a great deal of attention, although at the time of this writing there is only modest, randomized clinical trial evidence for effectiveness. Nonetheless, there is a significant basic literature regarding this technique that extends back into the 19th century. The treatment consists of two components: constraint of the unaffected arm for several hours per day and shaping. Shaping is the stepwise approach toward a desired behavior; the concept is from the experimental psychology literature.[47] Clinically, the patient engages in highly repetitive exercises that are directed toward the execution of some valued tasks; the difficulty of the exercises is gradually increased as progress is made. Three potential mechanisms are cited. One is the overcoming of learned nonuse, in which the use of compensation techniques (such as learning how to dress one-handed) masks latent motor function because the individual does not attempt to exploit these abilities. The second mechanism invoked is massed practice; large numbers of repetitions are more an effective means of learning than other motor learning paradigms. Third is that cortical reorganization is driven by CIT and that shifting of function to neighboring or functionally related cortical areas accounts for a (presumed) response to CIT.[48] Two randomized, controlled studies that use another motor treatment as a control have been performed, and both show a small but clinically significant superiority of CIT over conventional motor treatment.[49,50] Other studies have not been of a randomized design or use the pretreatment baseline of each subject as the control.[51]

Dextroamphetamine also has a significant basic science literature to support potential efficacy and is the best-known candidate for a pharmacological enhancer of recovery or rehabilitation. Animal data demonstrates that amphetamine can modulate spinal reflexes, and Feeney and Gonzalez[52] have found that amphetamine can speed motor recovery in rodent models of recovery from experimentally induced stroke. In Feeney's model, amphetamine alone had no effect, but when amphetamine dosing was followed by motor activity, motor recovery was accelerated. The data in humans have been mixed. The original report[53] and studies by Walker-Batson in motor recovery[54] and aphasia[55] were positive. Other studies showed no treatment effect[56,57]; advocates of the treatment suggest that the dosing must be accompanied shortly after by motor therapy, just as in the laboratory model. Simple administration without paired motor therapy within a few days of stroke has not been effective. Other drugs that have been reported in small studies to enhance recovery include piracetam, levodopa[58], and methylphenidate.[59] There are no multicenter, randomized controlled trial data to confirm these findings.

References

1. Indredavik B, Bakke F, Solberg R, et al. Benefits of a stroke unit: a randomized controlled trial. Stroke 1991;22:1026–1031.
2. Indredavik B, Bakke F, Slordahl SA, et al. Stroke unit treatment. 10-year follow-up. Stroke 1999; 30:1524–1527.
3. Jorgensen HS, Krammersgaard LP, Nokayama H, et al. Treatment and rehabilitation on a stroke unit improves 5-year survival. Stroke 1999;30:930–933.
4. Ronning OM, Guldvog B. Outcome of subacute stroke rehabilitation. A randomized controlled trial. Stroke 1998;29:779–784.
5. Kalra L. The influence of stroke unit rehabilitation on functional recovery from stroke. Stroke 1994;25:821–825.

6. Duncan PW, Horner RD, Reker DM, et al. Adherence to postacute rehabilitation guidelines is associated with functional recovery in stroke. Stroke 2002;33:167–178.
7. Kramer AM, Steiner JF, Schlenker PE, et al. Outcomes and costs after hip fracture and stroke. A comparison of rehabilitation settings. JAMA 1997;277:396–404.
8. World Health Organization. The International Classification of Impairments, Disabilities, and Handicaps Geneva: World Health Organization, 1980.
9. Heller A, Wade DT, Wood VA, et al. Arm function after stroke: measurement and recovery over the first three months. JNNP 1987;50:714–719.
10. Jorgensen HS, Nakayama H, Raaschou HO, et al. Recovery of walking function in stroke patients: the Copenhagen Stroke Study. Arch Phys Med Rehabil 1995;76:27–32.
11. Wandel A, Jorgensen HS, Nakayama H, et al. Prediction of walking function in stroke patients with initial lower extremity paralysis: the Copenhagen Stroke Study. Arch Phys Med Rehabil 2000;81:736–738.
12. Dromerick AW, Hahn MG, Klein A, et al. Urinary incontinence predicts quality of life and participation after stroke. Stroke 2003;34:313.
13. Gresham GE, Phillips TF, Wolf PA, et al. Epidemiologic profile of long-term stroke disability: the Framingham study. Arch Phys Med Rehabil 1979;60:487–491.
14. Wade DT, Hewer R. Functional abilities after stroke: measurement, natural history, and prognosis. JNNP 1987;50:177–182.
15. Jorgensen HS, Nakayama H, Raaschou HO, et al. Outcome and time course of recovery in stroke. Part I: outcome. The Copenhagen Stroke Study. Arch Phys Med Rehabil 1995;76:399–405.
16. Jorgensen HS, Nakayama H, Raaschou HO, et al. Outcome and time course of recovery in stroke. Part II: time course of recovery. The Copenhagen Stroke Study. Arch Phys Med Rehabil 1995;76:406–412.
17. Reding MJ, Potes E. Rehabilitation outcome following initial unilateral hemispheric stroke: life table analysis approach. Stroke 1988;19:1354–1358.
18. Dromerick AW, Edwards DF, Diringer MN. Sensitivity to changes in disability after stroke: a comparison of four scales used in clinical trials. J Rehabil Res Dev 2003;40:1–8.
19. Dromerick AW, Reding MJ. Functional outcome for patients with hemiparesis, hemihypesthesia, and hemianopsia: does lesion location matter? Stroke 1995;26:2023–2026.
20. de NAP, Shelton F, Reding MJ. Effect of lesion location on upper limb motor recovery after stroke. Stroke 2001;32:107–112.
21. Binkofski F, Seitz RJ, Arnold S, et al. Thalamic metabolism and corticospinal tract integrity determine motor recovery in stroke. Ann Neurol 2000;39:460–470.
22. Twitchell TE. The restoration of motor function following hemiplegia in man. Brain 1951;54:443–480.
23. Gresham Glenn E, Duncan PW, Stason WB. Post-Stroke Rehabilitation Clinical Practice Guideline, No. 16. Rockville, Maryland: Department of Health and Human Services. Public Heath Service, Agency for Health Care Policy Research, 1995.
24. Kozlowski DA, Schallert T. Relationship between dendritic pruning and behavioral recovery following sensorimotor cortex lesions. Behav Brain Res 1998;97:89–98.
25. Davenport RJ, Dennis MS, Warlow CP. Complications after acute stroke. Stroke 1996;27:425–420.
26. Dromerick A, Reding MJ. Medical and neurological complications during stroke rehabilitation. Stroke 1994;25:358–361.
27. Corcoran PJ, Jebson RH, Brengleman GL, et al. Effects of plastic and metal braces on speed and energy cost of hemiparetic ambulation. Arch Phys Med Rehabil 1970;51:69–77.
28. Greenleaf JE. Intensive exercise training during bed rest attenuates deconditioning. Med Sci Sports Exerc 1997;29:207–215.
29. Leigh-Smith J, Wade DT, Langton-Hewer R. Driving after stroke. J Royal Soc Med 1986; 79:200–203.
30. Haselkorn JK, Mueller BA, Rivara FA. Characteristics of drivers and driving record after traumatic and non-traumatic brain injury. Arch Phys Med Rehabil 1998;79:738–742.
31. Fisk GD, Owsley C, Mennemeier M. Vision, attention, and self-reported driving behaviors in community-dwelling stroke survivors. Arch Phys Med Rehabil 2002;83:469–477.
32. Akinwuntan AE, Feys H, DeWeerdt W, et al. Determinants of driving after stroke. Arch Phys Med Rehabil 2002;83:334–341.
33. Korner-Bitensky NA, Mazer BL, Sofer S, et al. Visual testing for readiness to drive after stroke: a multicenter study. Am J Phys Med Rehabil 2000;79:253–259.
34. Deibert EM, Dromerick AW. Motor restoration and spasticity management after stroke. Curr Treat Options Neurol 2002;4:427–433.
35. Schmidt RT, Lee RH, Spehlman R. Comparison of dantrolene sodium and diazepam in the treatment of spasticity. J Neurol Neurosurg Psychiatry 1976;39:350–356.

36. Gelber DA, Good DC, Dromerick AW, et al. Open-label dose-titration study of tizanidine hydrochloride in the treatment of spasticity associated with chronic stroke. Stroke 2001;32:1841–1846.
37. Brashear A, Gordon MF, Elovic E, et al. Intramuscular injection of botulinum toxin for the treatment of wrist and finger spasticity after a stroke. N Engl J Med 2002;347:395–400.
38. Landau WM. Botulinum toxin for spasticity after stroke (correspondence). N Engl J Med 2003; 348:258–259.
39. Dobkin BH. Botulinum toxin for spasticity after stroke (correspondence). N Engl J Med 2003; 348:258–259.
40. Sze FK, Wong E, Or KK, et al. Does acupuncture improve motor recovery after stroke? A meta-analysis of randomized controlled trials. Stroke 2002;33:2604–2619.
41. Meyerthaler JM, Guin-Renfroe S, Brunner RC, et al. Intrathecal baclofen for spastic hypertonia after stroke. Stroke 2001;32:2099–2109.
42. Gelber DA, Good DC, Laven LJ, et al. Causes of urinary incontinence after acute hemispheric stroke. Stroke 1993;24:378–382.
43. Dromerick AW, Edwards DF. Relationship of post-void residual to urinary tract infection during stroke rehabilitation. Arch Phys Med Rehabil. 2003 (in press).
44. Hesse S, Bertelt C, Jahnke MT, et al. Treadmill training with partial body weight support compared with physiotherapy in nonambulatory hemiparetic stroke patients. Stroke 1995;26:976–981.
45. Visintin M, Barbeau H, Korner-Bitensky N, et al. A new approach to retrain gait in stroke patients through body weight support and treadmill stimulation. Stroke 1998;29:1122–1128.
46. Macko RF, Smith GV, Dobrovolny CL, et al. Treadmill training improves fitness reserve in chronic stroke patients. Arch Phys Med Rehabil 2002;82:879–884.
47. Taub E, Uswatte G. Constraint-induced movement therapy based on behavioral neuroscience. In R Frank, T Elliott (eds), Handbook of Rehabilitation Psychology. Washington DC: American Psychological Association, 2000:475–496.
48. Liepert J, Bauder H, Miltner WHR, et al. Treatment-induced cortical reorganization after stroke in humans. Stroke 2000;31:1210–1216.
49. Dromerick A, Edwards DA, Hahn M. Does the application of constraint-induced movement therapy during acute rehabilitation reduce hemiparesis after ischemic stroke? Stroke 2000;31:2984–2988.
50. van der Lee JH, Wagenaar RC, Lankhorst GJ, et al. Forced use of the upper extremity in chronic stroke patients. Stroke 1999;30:2369–2375.
51. Taub E, Miller NE, Novack TA, et al. Technique to improve chronic motor deficit after stroke. Arch Phys Med Rehabil 1993;74:347–354.
52. Feeney DM, Gonzalez ALWA. Amphetamine, haloperidol, and experience interact to affect rate of recovery after motor cortex injury. Science 1980;217:855–857.
53. Crisistomo EA, Duncan PW, Propst M, et al. Evidence that amphetamine paired with physical therapy promotes recovery of motor function in stroke patients. Ann Neurol 1988;23:94–97.
54. Walker-Batson D, Smith P, Curtis S, et al. Amphetamine paired with physical activity accelerates motor recovery after stroke. Stroke 1995;26:2254–2259.
55. Walker-Batson D, Curtis S, Natarajan R, et al. A double-blind, placebo-controlled study of the use of amphetamine in the treatment of aphasia. Stroke 2001;32:2093–2098.
56. Sonde L, Nordstrom M, Nilsson C-G, et al. A double-blind placebo-controlled study of the effects of amphetamine and physiotherapy after stroke. Cerebrovasc Dis 2001;12:253–257.
57. Reding MJ, Solomon B, Borucki S. Effect of dextroamphetamine on motor recovery after stroke. Neurology 1995;45:A222.
58. Scheidtmann K, Fries W, Muller K, et al. Effect of levodopa in combination with physiotherapy on functional motor recovery after stroke: a prospective, randomized, controlled study. Lancet 2001;358:787–790.
59. Grade C, Redford B, Chrostowski J, et al. Methylphenidate in early poststroke recovery: a double-blind, placebo-controlled study. Arch Phys Med Rehabil 1998;79:1047–1050.

Index

A

AAASPS. *See* African-American
    Antiplatelet Stroke Prevention
    Study
Abciximab, 296–297
Abciximab in Emergency Stroke Treatment
    Trial, 297
Abdominal obesity, 28
AbESTT. *See* Abciximab in Emergency
    Stroke Treatment Trial
Absorption, of dipyridamole, 191
Abuse, alcohol, 8t, 23–24, 25f
Accidents Ischémiques Cérébraux À
    L'athérosclérose
  on aspirin, 133
  on dipyridamole, 191–192
  endpoint in, 183t
ACE. *See* Aspirin and Carotid
    Endarterectomy Trial
Acetaminophen
  for fever, 333–334
  for pain, 383–384
Acupuncture, 385
Acute Noninterventional Therapy in
    Ischemic Stroke, 268, 268t, 269
Acute posterior multifocal placoid pigment
    epitheliopathy, 149
Adenosine diphosphate receptor,
    187–188
Adenosine diphosphate receptor blocker,
    287

AFCAPS/TexCAPS. *See also* Air
    Force/Texas Coronary Atherosclerosis
    Prevention Study
  trial, 38
African-American Antiplatelet Stroke
    Prevention Study, 188
African-American patient
  atherosclerosis in, 103
  lacunar stroke in, 123
  lisinopril less effective in, 14
  stroke risk for, 1–2, 6t
Age
  antihypertensive treatment and, 15
  atrial fibrillation and, 80–81
  hyperlipidemia and, 17–18
  hypertension and, 7, 11t, 12
  risk of stroke and, 1–2
AICLA. *See also* Accidents Ischémiques
    Cérébraux À L'athérosclérose
  aspirin trial of, 133
Air Force/Texas Coronary Atherosclerosis
    Prevention Study, 19
Airway management, 338–339
Alaska native, 6t
Alberta Stroke Program Early CT Score,
    239, 241f
Alcohol
  primary prevention and, 8t, 23–24,
    25f
  secondary prevention and, 204–205
Aldosterone, 199

Algorithm
    for ischemic stroke, 64f
    for transient ischemic attack, 68–78
ALLHAT. *See also* Antihypertensive and
    Lipid-Lowering Treatment to
    Prevention Heart Attack
    trial, 13–14, 21
Alteplase Thrombolysis for Acute
    Noninterventional Therapy in
    Ischemic Stroke, 268, 268t, 269
American Academy of Emergency
    Medicine, 273
American-Canadian Cooperative Study,
    192
American College of Chest Physicians, 89
American Indian, 6t
American Stroke Association, 212
α-Amino-3-hydroxy-5-methyl-4-isoxazole
    propionate, 310
Amino acid, homoocyst(e)ine and, 30–34
Amphetamine, 389
Analgesia, 383–384
Anastomosis, primitive artery and,
    153–154
Ancrod, 298
Aneurysm
    atrial septal, 88
    cerebral, 154
    mycotic, 91
    in Von Recklinghausen disease, 165
Angiography
    computed tomography, 244–245
    conventional, 258
    in Ehlers-Danlos syndrome, 161–162
    in fibromuscular dysplasia, 152, 152f
    magnetic resonance. *See* Magnetic
        resonance angiography
    for rapid diagnostic evaluation, 258
    in transient ischemic attack, 76
AngioJet, 308
Angiokeratoma corporis diffusum,
    162–163, 162f
Angioma
    facial, 159–160, 160f
    in Sturge-Weber syndrome, 160, 161f
Angiomatosis
    encephalo-facial, 159–161, 160f, 161f
    and leukoencephalopathy, 144–145
Angiopathy
    arterial dissection and, 150–151
    cerebral aneurysm, 154
    of cervical arteries, 155–156
    congenital, 159–166
        Ehlers-Danlos syndrome, 161–162
        Fabry disease, 162–163, 162f

Angiopathy *(Continued)*
    Grönblad-Strandberg syndrome, 163,
        164f, 165
    hereditary hemorrhagic telangiectasia,
        163
    Marfan syndrome, 165–166
    Sturge-Weber syndrome, 159–161,
        160f, 161f
    Von Recklinghausen disease with, 165
    endovascular lymphoma causing, 157
    fibromuscular dysplasia and, 151–153,
        152f, 153f
    moyamoya syndrome causing, 157–159
    primitive arteries and, 153–154
    radiation-induced, 154–155
    reversible vasoconstriction and, 156–157
Angioplasty
    for extracranial disease, 113–114
    in fibromuscular dysplasia, 153
    percutaneous transluminal coronary, 84
    stenting with, 306–307
Angiotensin, 199
Angiotensin-converting enzyme inhibitor
    effects of, 199t
    hypertension and, 16
    in secondary prevention, 199
    stroke risk and, 13
Animal stroke model, 318–319
Annulus calcification, mitral, 88–89
Anterior carotid circulation, 108–112,
    110f, 111f
Anterior cerebral artery, 230t
Anterior choroidal artery, 230t
Anterior inferior cerebellar artery, 230t
Anterior watershed, 231t
Antiatherosclerotic drug, 20t
Antibiotic for infective endocarditis, 90
Antibody
    antiphospholipid, 179
    in Sneddon syndrome, 144
Anticoagulant
    for atrial fibrillation, 81–82
    in congestive heart failure, 86
    in coronary artery disease, 83–84
    coumarins as, 177–179
    heparin as, 288–296. *See also* Heparin
    for large vessel atherosclerosis, 106–107
    in malignant atrophic papulosis, 142
    in moyamoya, 159
    in patent foramen ovale, 87–88
    prosthetic heart valve and, 89
    in valvular disease, 88
Anticonvulsant
    as emergency therapy, 314
    for seizure, 371

Antiepileptic drug, 371
Antihypertensive agent
    as secondary prevention, 107–108
    studies of, 13–17
Antihypertensive and Lipid-Lowering
    Treatment to Prevention Heart Attack,
    13–14, 21
Antiinflammatory agent, 312
Antiphospholipid antibody, 179
Antiplatelet therapy
    aspirin for. *See* Aspirin
    in congestive heart failure, 86
    currently available, 284t
    dipyridamole as, 191–193. *See also*
        Dipyridamole
    IIb/IIIA receptor antagonists as,
        180–181
    in infective endocarditis, 90
    for lacunar stroke, 132–133
    for large vessel atherosclerosis, 106
    in malignant atrophic papulosis, 142
    in moyamoya, 159
    in patent foramen ovale, 87
    prosthetic heart valve and, 89, 90
    in Sneddon syndrome, 144
    thienopyridines as, 187–191
        aspirin with, 190–191
        clopidogrel, 187, 189–190
        ticlopidine, 187–189
    triflusal as, 187
Antiplatelet Trialists Collaboration,
    181, 182
Antithrombotic therapy
    for acute stroke, 283–299
        ancrod for, 298
        antiplatelet. *See* Antiplatelet therapy
        in congestive heart failure, 85–86
        direct thrombin inhibitor for,
            297–298
        glycoprotein IIb/IIIa antagonist for,
            296–297
        heparin for, 288–296. *See also*
            Heparin
        for large vessel atherosclerosis, 106
    as secondary prevention, 175–193
        antiplatelet agents as, 180–193. *See
            also* Antiplatelet therapy
        direct thrombin inhibitors as, 179–180
        oral anticoagulants as, 177–179, 178t
        thrombus formation and, 175–177,
            176f
Apneustic breathing, 339
Apoptosis, 315
Apparent diffusion coefficient, 70, 252,
    253

APTC. *See* Antiplatelet Trialists
    Collaboration
Aptiganel, 310–311
Areflexia, detrusor, 356
Argatroban, 297–298
Arrhythmia
    as complication, 353–355, 354t
    supportive care for, 341
Arterial dissection, 150–151
    heparin for, 293
Arterial stroke
    disorders causing, 56t
    mechanism of, 55–58, 56t
Arteriolopathy, retinocochleocerebral,
    149–150
Arteriopathy, 55–56, 56t
Arteriovenous angioma, 160, 161f
Artery
    anterior inferior cerebellar, 230t
    coronary, 82f, 83f
        atrial fibrillation and, 82–85
    distal basilar, 231t
    lateral medullary circumferential, 230t
    lateral pontine circumferential, 230t
    middle cerebral. *See* Middle cerebral
        artery
    primitive, 153–154
    superior cerebellar, 231t
    vertebral, 104
    in Von Recklinghausen disease, 165
Artery-to-artery embolization, 55–56
Artifact in magnetic resonance imaging,
    248–249
ASA. *See* Atrial septal aneurysm
Asian patient, 6t
ASPECTS. *See* Alberta Stroke Program
    Early CT Score
Aspiration, 351–352
Aspiration pneumonia, 352
Aspirin
    clopidogrel and, 189–191
    in congestive heart failure, 86
    effectiveness of, 181–185, 182t–184t,
        286
    effects of, 288t
    failure of, 185–186
    in infective endocarditis, 90
    in intracranial atherosclerosis, 107
    for lacunar stroke, 133
    mechanism of, 181
    prosthetic heart valve and, 89, 90
    safety of, 186, 286–287
    in sinus rhythm, 106–107
    ticlopidine with, 190–191
    time to treatment with, 285–286

Aspirin *(Conitnued)*
 trials of, 284–285
 warfarin *vs.,* 179
Aspirin and Carotid Endarterectomy
  (ACE) Trial, 185
Asymptomatic Carotid Artery Study,
  111–112
Asymptomatic small artery disease,
  lacunar stroke and, 132
Ataxic hemiparesis, 127
Atenolol, losartan *vs.,* 14
Atheroma, 99, 100f
Atherosclerosis
 C-reactive protein and, 36–37
 infection and, 38–39
 insulin resistance in, 26–27
 intracranial, anticoagulation for, 107
 large-vessel, 99–117
  drugs to prevent, 105–108
  endovascular treatment of, 113–115,
   114f
  examples of, 105f
  future treatments of, 115–116
  mechanism of stroke in, 103–104
  pathology of, 99–103, 100f–102f
  prevention of, 104–115
  strategies for prevention of, 104–105
  surgery to prevent, 108–113, 110f,
   111f
 stroke caused by, 56–57
ATLANTIS. *See* Alteplase Thrombolysis
  for Acute Noninterventional Therapy
  in Ischemic Stroke
Atorvastatin, mechanism of, 20t
Atrial fibrillation, 80–82
 in cardioembolic stroke, 58–59
 treatment of, 332–333
Atrial myxoma-lentiginosis, 146
Atrial septal aneurysm, 88
Atrophic papulosis, malignant, 139–142,
  140f, 141f
Australian Streptokinase Trial, 267, 268t
Autoimmune disorder, 142
Autoregulation, cerebral, 331

B

Baltimore-Washington Cooperative Young
  Stroke Study, 7
Basilar artery
 atherosclerosis of, 102f
 distal, 231t
 occlusion of, 106
BAY X3702, 314
Bed rest, 382

Behavioral Risk Factor Surveillance
  System, 28
Bezafibrate Infarction Prevention
  Study, 37
Beta blocker, stroke risk and, 13
Bjork-Shiley heart valve, 89
Black patient. *See* African-American
Bleeding
 gastrointestinal, 357–358
 intracranial, 238–239
 warfarin and, 179
Blood disorder, 60, 60t
Blood flow, cerebral, 331
Blood pressure
 hypertension categories and, 198t
 induced hypertension and, 373
 intracranial hemorrhage and, 368t
 management of, 331–333, 332t, 333t
 in primary prevention, 7, 8t, 10t, 12–17,
  12t, 14f–16f
 in secondary prevention, 198–200,
  198t–200t
BMS-204352, 313
Body mass index, 28, 29t, 30
Body weight-supported treadmill training,
  388
Botulinum toxin, 385
Brain
 in cardioembolic stroke, 79
 cerebral edema and, 367–371, 369f, 370f
 imaging of, 63f
  computed tomography of, 2f, 4f–6f,
   238–243
  magnetic resonance, 249–250
 laboratory evaluation of, 260
Brain stem, 229f
Breathing pattern, 339

C

C-reactive protein, 36–37
Calcification
 mitral annulus, 88–89
 in Sturge-Weber syndrome, 160
Calcium channel blocker, 312–313
 hypertension and, 17
 stroke risk and, 13
cAMP, dipyridamole and, 191
Canadian Activase for Stroke Effectiveness
  Study, 273, 274t
Canadian American Ticlopidine Study,
  133, 188
CAPRIE. *See* Clopidogrel and Aspirin
  Prevention in Recurrent Ischemic
  Events

Cardiac care, 340–342
Cardiac damage in stroke, 341
Cardiac enzyme, 355
Cardiac output, 341–342
    cardioembolic stroke and, 85–86
Cardiac study, 63f
Cardioembolic stroke, 58–60, 59t, 79–95
    atrial fibrillation causing, 80–82
    atrial septal aneurysm causing, 88
    cardiomyopathy causing, 86–87
    causes of, 56t, 57
    congestive heart failure causing, 85–86
    coronary artery disease causing, 82–85,
        82f, 83f
    disease associated with, 80t
    echocardiography in, 92–93, 93f
    endocarditis causing
        infective, 90–91
        noninfective thrombotic, 91–92
    management of, 93–95
    mechanism of, 79–80
    neoplasm causing, 92
    patent foramen ovale causing, 87–88,
        87f
    valvular heart disease causing, 88–90
Cardioembolism
    heparin for, 292–293
    lacunar stroke with, 130
Cardiomyopathy, 86–87
Cardiovascular disorder in Marfan
    syndrome, 165
Cardioversion of atrial fibrillation, 81
CARE trial. *See* Cholesterol and Recurrent
    Events trial
Carotid and Vertebral Artery Transluminal
    Angioplasty Study, 306–307
Carotid artery
    atherosclerosis of, 101, 101f, 102f
    neurovascular examination of, 225
Carotid artery disease, 84–85
    surgery for
        for nonsymptomatic disease, 111–112
        for symptomatic disease, 108–112,
            110f, 111f
Carotid Atherosclerosis Progression
    Study, 38
Carotid dissection, heparin for, 293
Carotid endarterectomy
    for lacunar stroke, 134
    stenting and angioplasty and, 306–307
Carotid imaging
    duplex, 74f, 75
    in lacunar stroke, 130
Carotid Revascularization Endarterectomy
    versus Stent Trial, 307

Cascade, coagulation, in atrial fibrillation,
    81
CASES. *See* Canadian Activase for Stroke
    Effectiveness Study
Caspase inhibitor, 315
CAST. *See* Chinese Acute Stroke Trial
Cationic protein, eosinophil, 146
CATS. *See* Canadian American Ticlopidine
    Study
CAVATAS. *See* Carotid and Vertebral
    Artery Transluminal Angioplasty
    Study
Cell, neural, stem, 316–318
Cell death, 314, 315
Cellular disorder, 60t
Central nervous system
    in Eales disease, 148–149
    in malignant atrophic papulosis, 140,
        141
    neuroprotective therapy and, 310–312
    vasculitis of, 58
Central pain, 383
Cerebellar artery
    anterior inferior, stroke symptoms of,
        230t
    superior, stroke symptoms of, 231t
Cerebellar infarct, 371
Cerebellum, stroke symptoms and, 229f
Cerebral aneurysm, 154
Cerebral angiopathy, 150–166. *See also*
    Angiopathy
Cerebral artery
    atherosclerosis of, 101
    middle
        atherosclerosis of, 101
        bypass procedure and, 112
        computed tomography of, 239
        deterioration of, 372
        hyperdense, 243–244
        stenting and, 307
        thrombolytic therapy and, 277
    stroke symptoms of, 230t
    in Von Recklinghausen disease, 165
Cerebral autoregulation, 331
Cerebral blood flow management, 331–332
Cerebral edema, 367–371, 369f, 370f
Cerebral Embolism Study Group, 289
Cerebral infarction, eosinophil-induced,
    146–147, 146t
Cerebral ischemia, markers of, 260
Cerebral perfusion pressure
    cerebral edema and, 368–369
    positioning and, 330
Cerebral vascular resistance, 331
Cerestat, 310–311

Cerivastatin, 20t
Cervical artery, 155–156
Cessation, smoking, 204
CHAD2 index in atrial fibrillation, 82
Cheyne-Stokes respiration, 339
Child, Kawasaki syndrome in, 148
Chinese Acute Stroke Trial, 285–287
  on lacunar stroke, 133
Chlamydia pneumoniae, 38
Cholesterol, 17–22, 21f
Cholesterol-lowering drug. *See also* Statin
  in large-vessel atherosclerosis, 107–108
  in secondary prevention, 201–203, 202t
Cholesterol and Recurrent Events trial, 18,
  201–202
Cigarette smoking
  primary prevention and, 8t, 10t, 22–23
  secondary prevention and, 204
Cilostazole Stroke Prevention Study, 133
Cincinnati Prehospital Stroke Screen,
  218, 219f
Circumferential artery
  lateral medullary, 230t
  lateral pontine, 230t
Citicoline, 314
Clinical evaluation, rapid, 211–233. *See
  also* Evaluation, rapid
Clomethiazole, 314
Clopidogrel, 187, 189–190
  aspirin with, 287
Clopidogrel and Aspirin Prevention in
  Recurrent Ischemic Events, 189–190
  trial, 189–190
Clopidogrel for the Reduction of Events
  During Observation, 190
Clopidogrel in High-Risk Patients trial,
  191
Clopidogrel in Unstable Angina to Prevent
  Recurrent Events Trial, 190, 287
Clot formation, 176–177, 176f
Clot retrieval device, 308, 308f
Clumsy-hand syndrome, 127
Coagulation
  cascade of, in atrial fibrillation, 81
  diffuse, 91
  thrombus formation and, 177
Cocaine abuse, 9t, 39, 41
Coiling of cervical artery, 155
Collagen in Ehlers-Danlos syndrome, 161
Combination therapy trial, 321
Complications, 349–359
  cardiac, 353–355, 354t
  depression as, 359
  falls as, 358
  general considerations in, 349, 350t

Complications *(Continued)*
  genitourinary, 356–357
  skin breakdown as, 359
  thrombotic, 350–351
  timing of, 350f
Compression device, pneumatic sequential,
  337
Computed tomography
  of brain, 2f, 4f–6f, 238–243
  in cerebral edema, 370f
  in emergency department, 223
  in moyamoya, 158
  physiologic, 247
  practical considerations in, 237–238
  single-photon emission
    in moyamoya, 158
    in rapid diagnosis, 258–259
  in Sturge-Weber syndrome, 160
  thrombolytic therapy and, 272
  in transient ischemic attack, 69–70, 70f,
    72, 76
  vascular, 243–246, 243f–246f
Computed tomography angiography,
  244–245
Computed tomography perfusion, 247
Congenital disorder
  diffuse meningocerebral angiomatosis,
    144–145
  Ehlers-Danlos syndrome, 161–162
  Fabry disease, 162–163, 162f
  Grönblad-Strandberg syndrome, 163,
    164f, 165
  hereditary hemorrhagic telangiectasia,
    163
  Marfan syndrome, 165–166
  moyamoya, 158
  Sturge-Weber syndrome, 159–161, 160f,
    161f
  Von Recklinghausen disease with, 165
Congestive heart failure, 85–86
Connective tissue disease, 57–58
  in Grönblad-Strandberg syndrome, 163
  in Marfan syndrome, 166
Constipation, 363
Constraint-induced therapy, 389
Continuum of care, 3, 3f
Contrast, intravenous, in CT scan of brain,
  242–243
Contrast-enhanced magnetic resonance
  angiography, 255
Coronary angioplasty, percutaneous
  transluminal, 84
Coronary artery bypass graft, 84–85
Coronary artery disease, 82–85, 82f, 83f
Coronary reperfusion, 86

Coumarin
  effectiveness of, 178
  mechanism of action of, 177
Creatinine kinase, 355
Crescendo transient ischemic attack, 294
CREST. *See* Carotid Revascularization Endarterectomy *versus* Stent Trial
Crystalloid, 331
CURE. *See* Clopidogrel in Unstable Angina to Prevent Recurrent Events Trial
Cutaneous lesion. *See* Skin disorder
Cyclic adenosine monophosphate, 191
Cytokine, 35–36

D

Dalteparin, 292
Danaparoid, 336
Death
  lacunar stroke and, 130
  neuron, 314, 315
  risk of, 1–2
  seizure and, 371
  on stroke unit, 330
  sudden cardiac, 354
Debilitated patient, 385–388
Deconditioning, 382–383
Deep venous thrombosis
  as complication, 350–351
  prevention of, 335–337, 338t
  in rehabilitation phase, 381–382
Delirium, 343–344
Dementia, vascular, 131–132
Depression, 359
Desaturation, oxygen, 352–363
Deterioration, neurological. *See* Neurological disorder
Detrusor hyporeflexia, 356
Dextroamphetamine, 389
Diabetes
  hyperglycemia and, 334
  primary prevention and, 9t, 25–28
  secondary prevention and, 200
Diagnosis, differential, 229, 231, 232t
Diagnostic evaluation, rapid, 237–261. *See also* Evaluation, rapid
Diarrhea, 363
Diastolic hypertension, 7, 12–17
Diazepam, 314
Diet
  nutritional issues and, 342–343
  primary prevention and, 34
Differential diagnosis, 229, 231, 232t

Diffuse intravascular coagulation, endocarditis and, 91
Diffuse meningocerebral angiomatosis, 145
Diffuse meningocerebral angiomatosis and leukoencephalopathy, 144–145
Diffusion tensor imaging, 260
Diffusion-weighted imaging, 248
  of brain, 251, 252–253
  in hyperglycemia, 334
  in lacunar stroke, 129
Digital subtraction angiography, 76
Dipyridamole
  effectiveness of, 191–192
  for lacunar stroke, 133
  mechanism of, 191
  safety of, 192–193
  in sinus rhythm, 107
Direct thrombin inhibitor, 179–180, 297–298
  currently available, 284t
  as emerging therapy, 297–298
Dissection, 57–58
  arterial, 150–151
  carotid, heparin for, 293
  vertebral, heparin for, 293
Distal basilar artery, 231t
Diuretic, hypertension and, 16
Divry-Van Bogaert syndrome, 144–145
Dolichoectasia
  of cervical artery, 156
  of vertebral and basilar arteries, 103
Doppler ultrasonography, transcranial, 256–257
  in cerebral edema, 368
  for large-vessel atherosclerosis, 115–116
  thrombolytic therapy and, 279
  in transient ischemic attack, 72–73, 75f, 76
Dot sign, 243–244
Driving, 384
Drug abuse, 9t, 39, 40t, 41
Duplex ultrasonography, 257–258
Dutch TIA trial. *See* Dutch TIA trial
Dutch Transient Ischemic Stroke trial, 185
Dysarthria clumsy-hand syndrome, 127
Dysphagia, 352, 362–363
Dysplasia
  in epidermal nevus syndrome, 145
  fibromuscular, 151–153, 152f, 153f

E

Eales disease, 148–149
Ear disorder, 149–150

ECASS. *See* European Cooperative Acute
    Stroke Study
Echo-planar hemorrhagic susceptibility
    weighted image, 248
Echocardiography
    in cardioembolic stroke, 92–93, 93f
    in patent foramen ovale, 87, 87f
    in transient ischemic attack, 72–73
Edema
    cerebral, 367–371, 369f, 370f
    neurogenic pulmonary, 339–340
Ehlers-Danlos syndrome, 57–58,
    161–162
Elastic lumina in moyamoya, 158–159
Elderly, antihypertensive treatment in,
    15
Electrocardiography, 340–341
    arrhythmias and, 354–355, 354t
Electron microscopy in malignant atrophic
    papulosis, 142
Eligibility criteria for thrombolytic therapy,
    270–271, 270t
Eliprodil, 310–311
Embolism
    cardiac, 58–60, 59t
    in cardioembolic stroke, 79–80
    pulmonary, 335–336, 350–351
Embolization, artery-to-artery, 55–56
Embolus, septic, 91
Emergency department, 221–224, 222f
Emergency Management of Stroke, 276
    trial, 276–277
Emergency Management of Stroke
    Bridging Trial, 276–277
Emergency medical services, 213–214
Emerging therapy, 303–328
    direct thrombin inhibitor as, 297–298
    failure of, 318–319
    in future, 321–322, 323t
    glycoprotein IIb/IIIa inhibitor as,
        296–297. *See also* Glycoprotein
        IIb/IIIa inhibitor
    mechanical
        angioplasty and stenting, 306–307
        endovascular photo-acoustic
            recanalization laser system,
            309–310
        hypothermia, 308–309
        intra-arterial, 308, 308t
        ultrasonication, 309
    neural stem cells as, 316–318
    neuroprotective, 310–315, 311t
        antiinflammatory agents for, 312
        caspase inhibitor for, 315
        GABA receptor antagonists for, 314

Emerging therapy *(Continued)*
        glutamate antagonist, 310–312
        ion channel blocker for, 312–314
        potential, 315
        serotonin agonists for, 314
    neurotrophic factors as, 316
    recommendations for, 319–321
    rehabilitation and, 388–389
    tenecteplase *vs.* tissue plasminogen
        activator, 322, 324
    thrombolytic
        intra-arterial, 305
        newer generation, 304–305
EMS. *See* Emergency Management of
    Stroke
Enalapril, 14
Encephalo-facial angiomatosis, 159–161,
    160f, 161f
Encephalopathy
    retinocochleocerebral arteriolopathy,
        149–150
    vasculitis and, 58
Endarterectomy
    carotid
        for lacunar stroke, 134
        for nonsymptomatic disease,
            111–112
        for symptomatic disease, 108–111,
            110f, 111f
    in fibromuscular dysplasia, 153
    vertebral artery, 113
Endocarditis
    infective, 90–91
    noninfective thrombotic, 91–92
Endocardium, 79
Endothelial injury, 176
Endotoxin receptor CD14, 38
Endotracheal intubation, 338–339
Endovascular lymphoma, 157
Endovascular Photo-Acoustic
    Recanalization, 309
    laser system, 309–310
Endovascular treatment of large-vessel
    atherosclerosis, 113–115, 114f
Enlimomab, 312
Enoxaparin, 336
Enzyme, cardiac, 355
Eosinophil-induced neurotoxicity,
    146–147, 146t
EPAR. *See* Endovascular Photo-Acoustic
    Recanalization
Epidemiology of stroke, 1–2
Epidermal nevus syndrome, 145–146
Epilepsy, 371
Epitheliopathy, placoid pigment, 149

ESPS-2. *See* European Stroke Prevention Study-II
ESTAT. *See* European Stroke Treatment with Ancrod Trial
Estrogen replacement, 203–204
Ethnicity, risk of stroke and, 1–2
European Carotid Surgery Trial, 108–109
European Cooperative Acute Stroke Study, 268–269, 268t
  on hemorrhage, 365, 366
  thrombolytic therapy and, 268, 268t, 277
European Stroke Prevention Study-II, 182–183, 192–193
European Stroke Treatment with Ancrod Trial, 298
Evaluation, rapid
  clinical, 211–233
    data needed for, 224–233, 226f–227f, 228t, 229t
    detection of symptoms and, 212–214, 213f
    in emergency department, 221–224, 222f
    emergency dispatch and, 214–215
    identification of stroke and, 215–216, 217f–218f, 219–221, 219f, 220f
    knowledge of stroke and, 215
    stroke chain of survival and recovery in, 211, 212f
  diagnostic, 237–261
    angiography for, 258
    computed tomography for, 237–247. *See also* Computed tomography
    in future, 260–261
    laboratory, 259–260, 259t
    magnetic resonance imaging in, 247–256. *See also* Magnetic resonance imaging
    nuclear medicine for, 258–259
    ultrasonography for, 256–258, 257f
Exclusion criteria for thrombolytic therapy, 270–271, 270t
Exercise
  in rehabilitation, 382–383
  secondary prevention and, 206
Extended-release dipyridamole, side effects of, 192–193
Extracranial atherosclerosis, 99–100, 100f
Extracranial carotid stenting, 306–307
Extracranial disease, endovascular treatment of, 113–114

Extracranial vertebral artery disease, 104
Extraction device, thrombus, 308
Eye disorder, 148–150
  in Eales disease, 148–149
  in Grönblad-Strandberg syndrome, 163, 164f
  in malignant atrophic papulosis, 141–142
  in Marfan syndrome, 165–166

F
Fabry disease, 162–163, 162f
Face Arm Speech Test, 218
Facial angioma, 159–160, 160f
Fall, 358
FAST. *See* Face Arm Speech Test
FDA. *See* Food and Drug Administration
Fever, 333–334
Fibrillation, atrial, 80–82
  in cardioembolic stroke, 58–59
  treatment of, 332–333
Fibrinogen, 177
Fibroelastoma, papillary, 59
Fibromuscular dysplasia, 57–58, 151–153, 152f, 153f
Field, recognition and treatment in, 219–221, 220f
Filament in mitral valvular strand, 92–93, 93f
Fish oil, 34
FISS. *See* Fraxaparine in Ischemic Stroke Study
FISS-bis, 292
FLAIR imaging. *See* Fluid-attenuated inversion-recovery imaging
Fluid-attenuated inversion-recovery imaging
  of brain, 251
  in lacunar stroke, 125f
  in rapid diagnosis, 248–249
  vascular, 253–254
Fluid therapy, 331
Fluvastatin, 20t
Focal neurological deficit, 69–71, 70f, 71f
Food and Drug Administration, 185
Forced use therapy, 389
Fosphenytoin, 313
Fracture, 358
Framingham Study, 7
Fraxaparine in Ischemic Stroke Study, 291–292, 292t
Free-radical scavenger, 313–314
Fruits in diet, 34
Functional recovery, 316–318
Funduscopic examination, 225

G

GABA receptor antagonist, 310, 311t, 314
Gadolinium imaging, 251
Gamma-aminobutyric acid, 372
Gamma-aminobutyric acid receptor antagonist, 310, 311t, 314
Ganglioside, 315
Gastric motility, 363
Gastrointestinal disorder
  bleeding as, 357–358
  care for, 343
  dipyridamole causing, 192
  in malignant atrophic papulosis, 140–141
Gastroparesis, 363
Gastrostomy tube, 386–387
Gender
  atherosclerosis and, 99
  hyperlipidemia and, 17
  risk of stroke and, 6t
Generic prevention of stroke, 2
Genitourinary complications, 356–357
Genotype, MTHFR, 30, 32
GIST-UK. *See* Glucose Insulin in Stroke Trial, United Kingdom
Glasgow coma score, 338
Glucose
  insulin resistance and, 25–28
  management of, 334–335
  stroke risk and, 200
Glucose Insulin in Stroke Trial, United Kingdom, 335
Glutamate antagonist, 310–312
Glycoprotein IIb/IIIa inhibitor
  characteristics of, 180–181
  currently available, 284t
  as emerging therapy, 296–297
Gradient-recalled echo, 248
  of brain, 251
Grönblad-Strandberg syndrome, 163, 164f, 165
Growth factor, neurotrophic, 316

H

HAEST. *See* Heparin in Acute Embolic Stroke Trial
Heart and Estrogen/Progestin Replacement Study, 203
Heart disorder in Marfan syndrome, 165
Heart failure, congestive, 85–86
Heart Outcomes Prevention Evaluation, 199
Heart rate, 341–342
Helicobacter pylori, 38
Hematological stroke, 56t, 60, 60t
Hemichorea-hemiballismus syndrome, 128
Hemiparesis
  ataxic, 127
  motor, 124, 126, 129f
Hemispherectomy in Sturge-Weber syndrome, 160–161
Hemodynamics in cardioembolic stroke, 80
Hemiplegic shoulder pain, 383
Hemorrhage
  anticoagulation contraindicated in, 82
  antithrombotic therapy for, 283–299.
    See also Antithrombotic therapy
  aspirin in, 286–287
  as complication, 365–367, 366f, 367f, 368t
  computed tomography and, 238
  in Fabry disease, 162–163
  gastrointestinal, 343
  pulmonary embolism and, 351
  subarachnoid
    cerebral aneurysm and, 154
    endocarditis and, 91
  symptoms of, 229f
  thrombolytic therapy for, 267–280.
    See also Thrombolytic therapy
Hemorrhagic Stroke Project, 41
Hemorrhagic telangiectasia, hereditary, 163
Hemorrhagic transformation, 365–367, 366f, 367f, 368t
Hemostasis, thrombus formation and, 175–176
Heparin, 288–296, 288t
  in coronary artery disease, 83–84
  currently available, 284t
  in deep venous thrombosis, 336
  early trials of, 288–291
  effects of, 288t
  for large-vessel disease, 293
  low-molecular-weight, 291–293, 291t
    in deep venous thrombosis, 336
    for large-vessel occlusion, 293
    trials with, 291–293, 291t
    unfractionated heparin *vs.,* 288
  in neurological deterioration, 373
  for pulmonary embolism, 351
  thrombocytopenia induced by, 337
  for transient ischemic attack, 293
  for vertebral or carotid dissection, 293
Heparin in Acute Embolic Stroke Trial, 291t, 292
Hepatocyte growth factor, 316

Hereditary disorder
  diffuse meningocerebral angiomatosis,
    144–145
  Fabry disease as, 162–163, 162f
  hemorrhagic telangiectasia as, 163
  Marfan syndrome, 165–166
  moyamoya as, 158
  Von Recklinghausen disease, 165
HERS II. *See* Heart and Estrogen/
    Progestin Replacement Study
High-density lipoprotein, stroke risk and,
    17–18
Hispanic patient
  atherosclerosis in, 103
  lacunar stroke in, 123
  risk of stroke in, 1–2, 6t
History, patient, 224–225
HMG Co-A reductase inhibitor
  in coronary artery disease, 84
  in primary prevention, 18–19, 20t,
    21–22
  in secondary prevention, 201–203, 202t
Homocyst(e)inemia, 30–34, 31f, 33f
Homocystinuria, 30, 32
HOPE. *See* Heart Outcomes Prevention
    Evaluation
Hormone replacement therapy, 203–204
Hospital notification, 221
Housefield density measurement, 238–239
Hydrochlorothiazide, 14
Hyperdense middle cerebral artery, 243–244
Hypereosinophilia, 146–147
Hyperhomocysteinemia
  primary prevention and, 30–34, 31f, 33f
  secondary prevention and, 205
Hyperlipidemia
  primary prevention and, 8t, 10t, 17–19,
    19f, 20t, 21f, 22
  secondary prevention and, 201–203,
    202t
Hypertension
  categories of, 198t
  induced, 373
  primary prevention and, 7, 8t, 10t,
    12–17, 12f, 14f–16f
  secondary prevention and, 198–200,
    198t–200t
Hyperthermia, 333–334
Hypertonia, spastic, 384–385
Hyperventilation, 369
Hyperviscosity, causes of, 60t
Hypodensity
  in computed tomography, of brain,
    238–240, 242
  on CT scan of brain, 240

Hypoperfusion
  in arterial stroke, 55
  systemic, 60
Hypoplasia of cervical artery, 155–156
Hyporeflexia, detrusor, 356
Hypotension, postmyocardial infarction,
    83
Hypothermia, 308–309
Hypovolemia, 331

I

ICAM-1. *See* Intercellular adhesion
    molecule-1
Identification of stroke, 214–219, 217f
IIb/IIIa antagonist. *See* Glycoprotein
    IIb/IIIa inhibitor
Illicit drug use, 9t, 39, 40t, 41
Imaging. *See also* Computed tomography;
    Magnetic resonance imaging;
    Ultrasonography
  carotid
    duplex, 74f, 75
    in lacunar stroke, 130
  diffusion tensor, 260
  diffusion-weighted, 248
    of brain, 251, 252–253
    in hyperglycemia, 334
    in lacunar stroke, 129
  fluid-attenuated inversion-recovery
    of brain, 251
    in lacunar stroke, 125f
    in rapid diagnosis, 248–249
    vascular, 253–254
  gadolinium, 251
  in lacunar stroke, 129–130, 129f
Immune complex, in vasculitis, 58
Impotence, 357
Inclusion criteria for thrombolytic therapy,
    270–271, 270t
Incontinence, 356
  treatment of, 387
Index, body mass, 28, 29t, 30
Induced hypertension, 373
Infarct
  cerebellar, 371
  computed tomography and, 239
  lacunar, 123. *See also* Lacunar stroke
Infarction
  eosinophil-induced neurotoxicity and,
    146–147, 146t
  epidermal nevus syndrome and,
    145
  in malignant atrophic papulosis, 140
  myocardial, as complication, 355

Infection
  aspiration pneumonia and, 352
  atherosclerosis and, 38–39
  hyperthermia with, 333–334
  primary prevention and, 35–39, 36f
  urinary tract, 356–357
  vasculitis caused by, 57
Infective endocarditis, 90–91
Inferior cerebellar artery, anterior, 230t
Infiltration, lymphocytic, 143, 144f
Inflammation, 35–39, 36f
Inpatient rehabilitation, 379–380
Insulin resistance, 9t, 25–28
Intercellular adhesion molecule-1, 35
Interleukin, 35–36
Internal carotid artery, 108–112, 110f,
  111f
International normalized ratio
  in atrial fibrillation, 81
  coumarins and, 178
  mechanical heart valve and, 89
International Stroke Trial
  recurrence and, 364
  thrombolytic therapy and, 284–287,
    290–291
Intoxication, 24
Intra-arterial mechanical therapy, 308,
  308t
Intra-arterial thrombolytic therapy,
  275–279
  intravenous therapy with, 276–278,
    277t
  newer, 305
  primary, 275
  rescue with, 278–279, 278f, 279t
Intra-arterial ultrasonication, 309
Intracardiac neoplasm, 92
Intracerebral angioma, 160
Intracerebral hemorrhage, endocarditis
  and, 91
Intracranial atherosclerosis, 100, 100f
  anticoagulation for, 107
Intracranial carotid artery, 112
Intracranial disease, transluminal
  angioplasty for, 114–115
Intracranial hemorrhage
  antithrombotic therapy for, 283–299.
    See also Antithrombotic
    therapy
  aspirin in, 286–287
  computed tomography in, 238
  pulmonary embolism and, 351
  symptoms of, 229f
  thrombolytic therapy for, 267–280. *See
    also* Thrombolytic therapy

Intracranial pressure
  blood pressure and, 331
  cerebral edema and, 367–369
  hemorrhage and, 368t
  positioning and, 330
Intracranial stenting, 307
Intravascular coagulation, diffuse, 91
Intravenous contrast, in CT scan of brain,
  242–243
Intravenous fluids therapy, 331
Intravenous thrombolytic therapy,
  267–275, 268t
  in clinical practice, 272–273
  correct dose of, 271
  criteria for, 271–272, 271t
  newer, 304–305, 305f
  outcomes for, 273, 274t, 275, 275t
  time window for, 270
Intubation, endotracheal, 338–339
Ion channel blocker, 312–314
Iovastatin, 38
Ischemia marker, 260
Ischemic heart disease, 128–129

J
JNC. *See* Joint National Committee
Joint National Committee on hypertension,
  198
Joint National Committee on the
  Prevention, Detection, Evaluation,
  and Treatment of High Blood
  Pressure, 13

K
Kawasaki syndrome, 147–148
Kinking of cervical artery, 155
Kohlmeier-Degos disease, 139–142, 140f,
  141f
Kuopio Ischaemic Heart Disease Risk
  Factor Study, 28

L
Laboratory evaluation
  in rapid clinical evaluation, 228–229, 232t
  in rapid diagnostic evaluation, 259–260,
    259t
Lacunar stroke, 123–134
  antiplatelet therapy for, 132–133
  ataxic hemiparesis in, 127
  carotid endarterectomy for, 134
  causes of, 57
  characteristics of, 123–124, 125f
  deterioration of, 372–373

Lacunar stroke *(Continued)*
  dysarthria clumsy-hand syndrome in, 127
  hemichorea-hemiballismus in, 128
  imaging of, 129–130, 129f
  incidence of, 124t
  lesion sites of, 126t
  prognosis for, 130–132, 131t
  pure motor hemiparesis in, 124
  pure sensory, 126–127
  risk factors for, 128–129
  sensorimotor, 127
  symptoms of, 229f, 231t
Large-vessel disease
  atherosclerotic, 99–117. *See also*
    Atherosclerosis, large vessel
  heparin for, 293
Large-vessel stroke, deterioration after, 373
Laser system, endovascular photo-acoustic recanalization, 309–310
Lateral medullary circumferential artery, 230t
Lateral pontine circumferential artery, 230t
LBS-Neurons, 317
Left hemisphere, 229f
Left ventricle
  congestive heart failure and, 85
  thrombus of, 83, 83f
Lentiginosis, facial, 146
Leptomeningeal angioma, 160
Leukoencephalopathy, 144–145
Libido, 357
LIPID trial, 18–19
Lipohyalinosis, 123
Lipoprotein
  statins and, 202
  stroke risk and, 17–18
Livedo racemosa, 143–144, 143f, 144f
Livedo reticularis, 145
Los Angeles Motor Scale, 220, 220f
Los Angeles Prehospital Stroke Screen, 216–218, 217f
Losartan, 14
Lovastatin, 20t
Low cardiac output state, 85–86
Low-density lipoprotein
  diet and, 34
  statins and, 202
  stroke risk and, 1718
Low-dose unfractionated heparin, in deep venous thrombosis, 336
Low-molecular-weight heparin, 291–293, 291t
  in deep venous thrombosis, 336
  for large-vessel occlusion, 293

Low-molecular-weight heparin *(Continued)*
  trials with, 291–293, 291t
  unfractionated heparin *vs.,* 288
Lubeluzole, 315
Lumina, 158–159
Lymph node syndrome, mucocutaneous, 147–148
Lymphocytic infiltration, 143, 144f
Lymphoma, endovascular, 157

M

Macrophage, statins and, 202
Magnesium sulfate, 311–312
Magnetic resonance angiography
  contrast-enhanced, 255
  CT angiography and, 244–246, 245f, 246f
  in rapid diagnosis, 254–255
  in Sturge-Weber syndrome, 160
  in transient ischemic attack, 72, 76
Magnetic resonance imaging
  of brain, 249–253, 250f, 251t–253t
  future of, 260
  in hyperglycemia, 334
  in lacunar stroke, 129
  of lacunar stroke, 125f
  perfusion, 255–256
  physiological, 255–256
  practical considerations for, 247–249, 249t
  in Sturge-Weber syndrome, 160
  in transient ischemic attack, 69–70, 70f, 72, 76
  vascular, 253–255, 254f, 255f
Magnetic resonance spectroscopy, 260
Magnetic resonance venography, 254–255
Malformation, vascular, 160
Malignancy
  cardioembolic stroke caused by, 92
  endovascular lymphoma, 157
Malignant atrophic papulosis, 139–142, 140f, 141f
Malnutrition, 362
Management of Atherothrombosis with Clopidogrel in High-Risk Patients, 191
Mannitol in cerebral edema, 369
MAP. *See* Malignant atrophic papulosis
Marantic endocarditis, 91–92
Marfan syndrome, 165–166
Marker
  for cerebral ischemia, 260
  inflammatory, 36–37

MATCH. *See* Management of Atherothrombosis with Clopidogrel in High-Risk Patients
Maxipost, 313
Mean arterial pressure, 331
Mechanical heart valve, 89
Mechanical therapy
    angioplasty and stenting, 306–307
    endovascular photo-acoustic recanalization laser system, 309–310
    hypothermia, 308–309
    intra-arterial, 308, 308t
    ultrasonication, 309
Mechanical ventilation, 339, 353
Medial medullary penetrator, 230t
Medial pontine penetrator, 230t
Medical Research Council and British Heart Foundation Heart Protection Study, 201–202
Medullary circumferential artery, lateral, 230t
Medullary penetrator, medial, 230t
Meningocerebral angiomatosis and leukoencephalopathy, 144–145
Metabolism of homocyst(e)ine, 31f
Methionine, 30
Methylene tetrahydrofolate reductase, 30
Mexican-American patient, 6t
Microatheroma, 123
Microscopy in malignant atrophic papulosis, 142
Microvascular disorder, 26
Midazolam
    for seizure, 371
    worsening of symptoms after, 374
Midbrain penetrator, 230t
Middle cerebral artery
    atherosclerosis of, 101
    bypass procedure and, 112
    computed tomography of, 239
    deterioration of, 372
    hyperdense, 243–244
    stenting and, 307
    stroke symptoms of, 230t
    thrombolytic therapy and, 277
Mitral stenosis, 88–89
Mitral valve prosthesis, 59–60
Mitral valvular strand, 92–93
Mobile telemedicine, 219
Mobility, improvement of, 386
Model, animal, 318–319
Mortality
    lacunar stroke and, 130
    neuron, 314, 315

Mortality *(Continued)*
    risk of, 1–2
    seizure and, 371
    on stroke unit, 330
    sudden cardiac, 354
Motor deficit, progressive, 372, 372t
Motor hemiparesis, 129f
    lacunar stroke causing, 124, 126
Motor recovery, 378–379
Moyamoya, 57–58, 157–159
MRC/BHF Heart Protection Study, 19
MTHFR genotype, 30, 32
Mucocutaneous lymph node syndrome, 147–148
Multicenter Acute Stroke Trial-Europe Study Group, 267, 268t
Multicenter Acute Stroke Trial-Italy
    on aspirin, 285–286
    on thrombolytic therapy, 267, 268t
Multifocal placoid pigment epitheliopathy, 149
Multimodal Computed tomography, 247
Multiple metabolic syndrome, 26
Multiple Risk Factor Intervention Trial, 17
Mycotic aneurysm, 91
Myocardial infarction
    aspirin in, 286
    as complication, 355
    ischemic stroke after, 83
Myocardium, 86
Myoglobin, 355
Myxoma, 59
Myxoma-lentiginosis, atrial, 146

N

N-Methyl-D-asparate, 310–311
Nalmefene, 315
NASCET. *See* North American Symptomatic Carotid Endarterectomy Trial
National American Stroke Association 212
National Cholesterol Education Program, 27t
National Cholesterol Education Program Adult Treatment Panel, 203
National Health and Nutrition Examination Survey
    on diabetes, 200
    on homoocyst(e)ine, 30
    on hyperlipidemia, 201
    on hypertension, 13, 198

National Institute of Neurological
    Disorders and Stroke trial, 268,
    268t, 277
  blood pressure and, 332
  on education program, 213
  hemorrhage and, 365
  on thrombolytic therapy, 268, 268t
National Institutes of Health Stroke Scale,
    226f–227f, 227
  hyperglycemia and, 334
  neurological deterioration and, 364
  oxygen desaturation and, 352–353
  post-stroke hemorrhage and, 366
  stenting and angioplasty and, 307
  thrombolytic therapy and, 269t, 277,
    279–280
National Registry of Myocardial
    Infarction, 22
NCEP ATP III. *See* National Cholesterol
    Education Program Adult Treatment
    Panel
Neoplasm, cardiac, 92
Nerve growth factor, 316
Neural stem cell, 316–318
Neurofibromatosis, 165
Neurogenic pulmonary edema, 339–340
Neuroimaging in lacunar stroke, 129–130,
    129f
Neurological disorder, 364t
  cerebral edema causing, 367–371, 369f,
    370f
  in diffuse meningocerebral angiomatosis,
    145
  hemorrhagic transformation as,
    365–367, 366f, 367f, 368t
  in Kawasaki syndrome, 148
  in malignant atrophic papulosis, 140,
    141
  overview of, 363–364
  recurrent stroke and, 364–365
  seizure as, 371
  systemic, 373–374
  of unknown cause, 372–373, 372t
Neurological examination, 225, 227
Neuron death, 314, 315
Neuroprotective therapy, 310–315,
    311t
  antiinflammatory agents for, 312
  caspase inhibitor for, 315
  GABA receptor antagonists for, 314
  glutamate antagonist as, 310–312
  ion channel blocker for, 312–314
  potential, 315
  serotonin agonists for, 314
Neuropsychiatric care, 343–344

Neurotoxicity, eosinophil-induced,
    146–147, 146t
Neurotrophic factor, 316
Neurotrophin-4/5r, 316
Neurovascular examination, 225, 227
Neutrophil inhibitory factor, recombinant,
    312
Nevus syndrome, epidermal, 145–146
NHANES III. *See* Third National Health
    and Nutrition Examination Survey
NIHSS. *See* National Institutes of Health
    Stroke Scale
Nimodipine, 312–313
NINDS. *See* National Institute of
    Neurological Disorders and Stroke
    trial
911 emergency system, 213, 214
Node, lymph, mucocutaneous, 147–148
Noninfective thrombotic endocarditis,
    91–92
Noninflammatory vasculopathy, 57–58
North American Symptomatic Carotid
    Endarterectomy Trial, 108–109, 185
Northern Manhattan Stroke Study, 7
Nuclear medicine, 258–259
Nutritional issues, 342–343

O
Obesity, 9t, 28, 30
Occlusion of primitive artery, 153–154
Occlusive stroke, small-vessel, 123–134.
    See also Lacunar stroke
Ocular disorder, 148–150
  Eales disease, 148–149
  in Grönblad-Strandberg syndrome, 163,
    164f
  in malignant atrophic papulosis,
    141–142
  in Marfan syndrome, 165–166
  placoid pigment epitheliopathy, 149
  retinocochleocerebral arteriolopathy,
    149–150
Oil, fish, 34
Ontario Regional Acute Stroke Protocol,
    223–224
Ophthalmological disorder. *See* Eye
    disorder
Oral feeding, 386–387
Oral platelet antagonist. *See* Antiplatelet
    therapy
Organ damage in hypertension, 199–200,
    200t
Osler-Weber-Rendu disease, 163
Overweight, 9t, 28, 30

Oxidized low-density lipoprotein, 202
Oxygen, supplemental, 338
Oxygen desaturation, 352–363
Oxygen free radical, 313–314

P

Pacific Islander, 6t
Pain syndrome, 383
Papillary fibroelastoma, 59
Papule in Fabry disease, 162, 162f
Papulosis, malignant atrophic, 139–142,
    140f, 141f
Paradoxical embolism, 80
Paraneoplastic endocarditis, 91–92
Partial thromboplastin time, 296
Patent foramen ovale
    cardioembolic stroke and, 87–88, 87f
    warfarin and, 179
Patient history, 224–225
Pattern
    recovery, 378–379
    respiratory, 339
Percutaneous transluminal angioplasty
    intracranial, 307
    for large-vessel atherosclerosis, 115
Percutaneous transluminal coronary
    angioplasty, 84
Perfusion computed tomography, 247
Perfusion magnetic resonance imaging,
    255–256
Perfusion pressure, cerebral, 330, 331–332
    cerebral edema and, 368–369
Perfusion-weighted imaging, 334
Perindopril pROtection aGainst REcurrent
    Stroke Study, 107–108, 199
Perivascular disorder, retinal, 148–149
Petechial hemorrhage, 366f
Phase contrast magnetic resonance
    venography, 254–255
Photo-acoustic recanalization laser system,
    endovascular, 309–310
Physical examination, 225, 227
Physical inactivity, secondary prevention
    and, 206
Physical therapy, 386
Physiological imaging
    computed tomographic, 247
    magnetic resonance, 255–256
Pigment epitheliopathy, placoid, 149
Placoid pigment epitheliopathy, 149
Plaque, 105f
    composition of, 202
    extracranial, 99–100
    thrombus formation and, 176, 176f

Plasma, inflammation and, 35
Plateau, recovery, 378
Platelet antagonist. *See* Antiplatelet
    therapy
Platelet-derived growth factor, 316
Platelet in thrombus formation, 176–177
Pneumatic sequential compression
    device, 337
Pneumonia, aspiration, 352
Pontine circumferential artery, lateral,
    230t
Port wine angioma, 160, 161f
Positioning, 330
Positron emission tomography
    in moyamoya, 158
    in rapid diagnosis, 258–259
Posterior carotid circulation, 112
Posterior cerebral artery, 113
Posterior inferior cerebellar artery, 113
Posterior multifocal placoid pigment
    epitheliopathy, 149
Posterior watershed, 231t
Postmenopausal woman, 203
Postmyocardial infarction hypotension,
    83
Postvoid residual, 387
Potassium channel activation, 313
Pravastatin
    in elderly, 21
    in elderly persons at risk of vascular
        disease trial, 21
    mechanism of, 20t
Pravastatin Inflammation/CRP Evaluation
    study, 38
Pressure
    blood. *See* Blood pressure
    cerebral perfusion, 330
        cerebral edema and, 368–369
    intracranial. *See* Intracranial pressure
Prevention of stroke
    generic, 2
    large-vessel atherosclerosis and,
        104–115. *See also* Atherosclerosis,
        large vessel
    risk factors and, 5–42, 197–206. *See
        also* Risk factor modification
Primary prevention of stroke, 2
Primitive artery, 153–154
PRINCE study. *See* Pravastatin
    Inflammation/CRP Evaluation study
PROACT I. *See* Prolyse in Acute Cerebral
    Thromboembolism I
PROACT II. *See* Prolyse in Acute Cerebral
    Thromboembolism II
Procoagulant, inflammation and, 35–36

Procoagulant state, 60t
PROGRESS. *See* Perindopril pROtection aGainst REcurrent Stroke Study
Progressive motor deficit, 372, 372t
Progressive stroke, heparin and, 295
Prolapse, mitral valve, 88–89
Prolyse in Acute Cerebral Thromboembolism I, 276
Prolyse in Acute Cerebral Thromboembolism II, 276, 365
Prophylaxis
  deep venous thrombosis, 335–337, 338t
  gastrointestinal, 358
PROSPER trial. *See* Pravastatin in elderly persons at risk of vascular disease trial
Prosthetic heart valve, 89
  mitral, 59–60
Protein, eosinophil, 146
Protein-caloric malnutrition, 362
Proximal vertebral artery disease, surgery for, 113
Pseudoxanthoma elasticum, 163, 164f, 165
Psychiatric disorder, 343–344
Pulmonary complications, 351–353
Pulmonary edema, neurogenic, 339–340
Pulmonary embolism
  as complication, 350–351
  treatment of, 335–336
Pure motor hemiparesis, 129f
  lacunar stroke causing, 124, 126
Pure sensory stroke, 126–127
Purpura, thrombotic thrombocytopenic, 189
PWI imaging, 255–256

Q

QT interval, 340–341

R

Race
  atherosclerosis and, 99, 103
  lacunar stroke and, 123
  lisinopril effectiveness and, 14
  stroke risk and, 1–2, 6t
Radiation-induced angiopathy, 154–155
Rapid evaluation. *See* Evaluation, rapid
Rapid recognition of stroke, 228
Rating, stroke, 219–220, 220f
Ratio, international normalized
  in atrial fibrillation, 81
  mechanical heart valve and, 89

Recanalization laser system, endovascular photo-acoustic, 309–310
Recombinant neutrophil inhibitory factor, 312
Recombinant tissue plasminogen activator, 267–280. *See also* Tissue plasminogen activator, recombinant
Recovery, functional, 316–318
Recovery pattern, 378–379
Recurrence
  as complication, 364–365
  of lacunar stroke, 131, 131t
  neurological disorder and, 364–365
  of transient ischemic attack, 294
Regional Acute Stroke Protocol, 223–224
Rehabilitation, 377–389
  of debilitated patient, 385–388
  duration of, 380–381
  emerging treatment and, 388–389
  immediate, 379
  issues in, 382–385
  medical management during, 381–382
  overview of, 377–378
  recovery patterns in, 378–379
  setting for, 379–380
Renin-angiotensin-aldosterone system, hypertension and, 199
Reperfusion in congestive heart failure, 86
Repinotan, 314
Residual, postvoid, 387
Resistance
  to aspirin, 185–186
  cerebral vascular, 331
  insulin, 9t, 25–28
Respiratory complications, 351–353
Respiratory pattern, 339
Respiratory system, 338–339
Retinal perivascular disorder, 148–149
  in Eales disease, 148–149
Retinocochleocerebral arteriolopathy, 149–150
Reversible vasoconstriction, 156–157
Right hemisphere stroke, 229f
  arrhythmia and, 354
Risk factor. *See also* Risk factor modification
  for lacunar stroke, 128–129
  by race and gender, 6t
Risk factor modification
  for primary prevention
    alcohol and, 8t, 11t, 23–24, 25f
    cocaine abuse and, 9t
    diabetes and, 9t, 25–28, 128

Risk factor modification *(Continued)*
  hyperhomocyst(e)inemia and, 30–34,
    31f, 33f
  hyperlipidemia and, 8t, 10t, 17–19,
    19f, 20t, 21f, 22
  hypertension and, 7, 8t, 10t, 12–17,
    12f, 14f–16f, 128
  inflammation/infection and, 35–39,
    36f
  insulin resistance and, 9t, 25–28
  obesity and, 9t, 28, 30
  recommendations about, 41–42
  smoking and, 8t, 10t, 22–23
  for secondary prevention, 197–206
    alcohol and, 204–205
    diabetes, 200
    hormone replacement therapy and,
      203–204
    hyperhomocyteinemia and, 205
    hyperlipidemia and, 201–203, 202t
    hypertension and, 198–200,
      198t–200t
    physical inactivity and, 206
    smoking and, 204
rt-PA. *See* Tissue plasminogen activator,
    recombinant
Rupture, arterial dissection, 150–151

S
Safety
  of aspirin, 186, 286–287
  of clopidogrel, 189–190
  driving, 384
  of ticlopidine, 188
  of ximelagatran, 180
Scale
  Alberta Stroke Program Early CT Score,
    239, 241f
  Los Angeles Motor Scale, 220, 220f
  National Institutes of Health Stroke
    Scale. *See* National Institutes of
    Health Stroke Scale
  Thrombolysis in Brain Ischemia score,
    257
Scandinavian Simvastatin Survival Study,
    18, 201
Scavenger, free-radical, 313–314
Score. *See* Scale
Screen, stroke, 216–219, 217f, 219f
Secondary prevention of stroke, 2
Secretion, pulmonary, 338
Seizure
  neurological deterioration and, 371
  in Sturge-Weber syndrome, 160–161

Selfotel, 310–311
Sensorimotor stroke, 127
Sensory stroke, 126–127
Septal aneurysm, atrial, 88
Septic embolus, 91
Sequential compression device, pneumatic,
    337
Serotonin agonist, 314
Setting, rehabilitation, 379–380
Sexual dysfunction, 357
Shoulder pain, 383
Shunt in patent foramen ovale, 87, 87f
Simvastatin
  for hyperlipidemia, 18
  mechanism of, 20t
Single-photon emission computed
    tomography
  in moyamoya, 158
  in rapid diagnosis, 258–259
Sinus rhythm, anticoagulation therapy in,
    106
Skin disorder, 139–148
  atrial myxoma-lentiginosis as, 146
  as complication, 359
  in Divry-Van Bogaert syndrome,
    144–145
  in eosinophil-induced neurotoxicity and
    cerebral infarction, 146–147, 146t
  epidermal nevus syndrome as, 145–146
  in Kawasaki syndrome, 147–148
  malignant atrophic papulosis as,
    139–142, 140f, 141f
  in Sneddon syndrome, 143–144, 143f,
    144f
Small-vessel deterioration, 372–373
Small-vessel occlusive disease, 37
Small-vessel stroke, 57, 123–134. *See also*
    Lacunar stroke
Smoking
  primary prevention and, 8t, 10t, 22–23
  secondary prevention and, 204
Sneddon syndrome, 143–144, 143f, 144f
Sodium channel blocker, 313
Spasticity, 384–385
Spectroscopy, magnetic resonance, 260
SPIRIT. *See* Stroke Prevention in
    Reversible Ischemia Trial
Standard Treatment with Alteplase to
    Reverse Stroke, 273, 274t
Standardization of stroke subtype
    determination, 62
STARS. *See* Standard Treatment with
    Alteplase to Reverse Stroke
STAT. *See* Stroke Treatment with Ancrod
    Trial

Statin
  C-reactive protein and, 38
  in coronary artery disease, 84
  in primary prevention, 18–19, 20t,
    21–22
  in secondary prevention, 201–203,
    202t
Steal, subclavian, 113
Stem cell, neural, 316–318
Stenosis
  in arterial stroke, 55
  atherosclerotic, 100–101, 101f, 102f
  carotid artery, 84–85
    surgery for, 108–112, 110f, 111f
  intracranial, 107
  of middle cerebral artery, 372
  mitral, 88–89
  in moyamoya, 158–159
Stenting, angioplasty with, 306–307
STOP-Hypertension. *See* Swedish Trial of
    Old Patients with Hypertension
Strand, mitral valvular, 92–93, 93f
Stroke
  continuum of care for, 3, 3f
  definition of, 1
  diagnosis of, 2–3
  epidemiology of, 1–2
  prevention of, 2
  territorial symptoms of, 230t–231t
Stroke chain of survival and recovery,
    211–233
  data in, 224–233, 226f–227f, 228t, 229t
  delivery in, 215–216, 217f–219f,
    219–221, 220f
  detection in, 212–214, 213f
  dispatch in, 214–215
  "door" in, 221–224, 222f
Stroke model, animal, 318–319
Stroke Prevention by Oral Thrombin
    Inhibitor in Atrial Fibrillation, 180
Stroke Prevention in Atrial Fibrillation
    trial, 178
Stroke Prevention in Reversible Ischemia
    Trial, 178
Stroke syndrome, 229f
Stroke Treatment with Ancrod Trial, 298
Stroke unit, 329–330
Study
  Abciximab in Emergency Stroke
    Treatment Trial, 297
  Acute Noninternventional Therapy in
    Ischemic Stroke, 268, 268t, 269
  AFCAPS/TexCAPS. *See* Air
    Force/Texas Coronary
    Atherosclerosis Prevention Study

Study *(Continued)*
  AICLA. *See also* Accidents Ischémiques
    Cérébraux À L'athérosclérose
    aspirin trial, 133
  Air Force/Texas Coronary Atherosclerosis
    Prevention Study, 19
  ALLHAT. *See also* Antihypertensive
    and Lipid-Lowering Treatment to
    Prevention Heart Attack
    trial, 13–14, 21
  animal, 319
  Antihypertensive and Lipid-Lowering
    Treatment to Prevention Heart
    Attack, 13–14, 21
  on antiplatelet agents, 181–184,
    182t–184t
  Asymptomatic Carotid Artery Study,
    111–112
  Australian Streptokinase Trial, 267, 268t
  Baltimore-Washington Cooperative
    Young Stroke Study, 7
  Bezafibrate Infarction Prevention Study,
    37
  Canadian Activase for Stroke
    Effectiveness Study, 273, 274t
  CARE trial. *See* Cholesterol and
    Recurrent Events trial
  Carotid and Vertebral Artery Transluminal
    Angioplasty Study, 306–307
  Carotid Atherosclerosis Progression
    Study, 38
  Carotid Revascularization Endarterectomy
    versus Stent Trial, 307
  Cerebral Embolism Study Group, 289
  Chinese Acute Stroke Trial, 133
  Clopidogrel for the Reduction of Events
    During Observation, 190
  Clopidogrel in High-Risk Patients trial,
    191
  Clopidogrel in Unstable Angina to
    Prevent Recurrent Events Trial, 190
  Dutch TIA trial, 185
  Emergency Management of Stroke
    Bridging Trial, 276–277
  European Carotid Surgery Trial, 108–109
  European Cooperative Acute Stroke
    Study, 268–269, 268t, 365
  European Stroke Prevention Study-II,
    182–183
  Framingham Study, 7
  Fraxaparine in Ischemic Stroke Study,
    291–292
  Glucose Insulin in Stroke Trial, 335
  Heart and Estrogen/Progestin
    Replacement Study, 203

Study *(Continued)*
  Heart Outcomes Prevention Evaluation, 199
  Heparin in Acute Embolic Stroke Trial, 292
  International Stroke Trial, 284–287, 290–291, 364
  Kuopio Ischaemic Heart Disease Risk Factor Study, 28
  Medical Research Council and British Heart Foundation Heart Protection Study, 19, 201–202
  MRC/BHF Heart Protection Study. *See* Medical Research Council and British Heart Foundation Heart Protection Study
  Multicenter Acute Stroke Trial-Europe Study Group, 267, 268t
  Multicenter Acute Stroke Trial-Italy, 267, 268t
  National Institute of Neurological Disorders and Stroke, 268, 268t, 277
  Neurological Disorders and Stroke Trial, 268, 268t
  NHANES III trial. *See* Third National Health and Nutrition Examination Survey
  North American Symptomatic Carotid Endarterectomy Trial, 108–109, 185
  Northern Manhattan Stroke Study, 7
  Perindopril Protection Against Recurrent Stroke Study, 107–108, 199
  Pravastatin Inflammation/CRP Evaluation study, 38
  Prolyse in Acute Cerebral Thromboembolism I and II, 276
  PROSPER trial. *See* Pravastatin in elderly persons at risk of vascular disease trial
  recommendations for, 320–321
  Scandinavian Simvastatin Survival Study, 18, 201
  Standard Treatment with Alteplase to Reverse, 273, 274t
  Stroke Prevention by Oral Thrombin Inhibitor in Atrial Fibrillation, 180
  Stroke Prevention in Atrial Fibrillation trial, 178
  Stroke Prevention in Reversible Ischemia Trial, 178
  Swedish Trial of Old Patients with Hypertension, 15
  Systolic Hypertension in Europe, 15

Study *(Continued)*
  Systolic Hypertension in the Elderly Program, 15
  Therapy of Patients with Acute Stroke, 292
  Thrombolysis in Myocardial Ischemia, 277
  Ticlopidine Aspirin Stroke Study, 188
  Tinzaparin in Acute Ischemic Stroke, 292–293
  Trial of ORG 10172 in Acute Stroke Treatment, 61–62, 64f
    on recurrence, 364
  Triflusal *versus* Aspirin in Cerebral Infarction Prevention, 187
  Very Early Nimodipine Use in Stroke, 313
  Veteran Affairs HDL Intervention Trial, 21
  Vitamin Intervention for Stroke Prevention, 205
  Vitamins to Prevent Stroke, 205
  Warfarin-Aspirin Recurrent Stroke Study, 133
  Warfarin Versus Aspirin in Reduced Cardiac Ejection Fraction Study, 86
Sturge-Weber syndrome, 159–161, 160f, 161f
Subacute rehabilitation setting, 380
Subarachnoid hemorrhage
  cerebral aneurysm and, 154
  endocarditis and, 91
  symptoms of, 229f
Subclavian steal, 113
Subcortical stroke, 123. *See also* Lacunar stroke
  vascular dementia with, 131–132
Subcutaneous heparin, 295–296
Subluxation, shoulder, 383
Subtraction angiography, 76
Subtype of stroke
  determination of, 63–64
  future of, 65
  importance of, 61–62
  pitfalls in diagnosis of, 64–65
  standardization of, 62–63, 62t
Suction thrombectomy, 308
Suctioning, 338
Sudden cardiac death, 354
Superior cerebellar artery, 231t
Supplemental oxygen, 338
Supportive care, 329–344
  airway management in, 338–339
  blood pressure management of in, 331–333, 332t, 333t

Supportive care *(Continued)*
cardiac, 340–342
of gastrointestinal disorder, 343
glucose management in, 334–335
intravenous fluids and, 331
neuropsychiatric, 343–344
nutritional, 342–343
positioning in, 330
pulmonary edema and, 339–340
respiratory patterns and, 339
stroke unit and, 329–330
temperature regulation in, 333–334
thromboembolism prevention in,
335–337, 338t
Surgery. *See also* Endarterectomy
for cerebral edema, 369, 371
in moyamoya, 159
Swallowing evaluation, 362–363
Swedish Trial of Old Patients with
Hypertension, 15
Symptoms of stroke, 212–213, 213t
Syndrome X, 26
Systemic disorder
cerebral angiopathy, 150–166. *See also*
Angiopathy
dermatologic
atrial myxoma-lentiginosis, 146
Divry-Van Bogaert syndrome,
144–145
eosinophil-induced neurotoxicity and
cerebral infarction, 146–147,
146t
epidermal nevus syndrome, 145–146
Kawasaki syndrome, 147–148
Sneddon syndrome, 143–144, 143f,
144f
neurological deterioration caused by,
373–374
ocular, 148–150
Eales disease, 148–149
placoid pigment epitheliopathy, 149
Systemic disorder causing stroke,
139–175
dermatologic, 139–148. *See also* Skin
disorder
Systemic hypoperfusion, 60
Systolic hypertension, 7, 12–17
Systolic Hypertension in Europe study, 15
Systolic Hypertension in the Elderly
Program, 15

T

T lymphocyte, statins and, 202
T wave, 340

T1-weighted imaging of brain, 249–250
T2-weighted imaging of brain, 250
Tachycardia, 354
TACIP. *See* Triflusal *versus* Aspirin in
Cerebrak Infarction Prevention
Study
TAIST. *See* Tinzaparin in Acute Ischemic
Stroke Trial
Target organ damage in hypertension,
199–200, 200t
TASS. *See* Ticlopidine Aspirin Stroke
Study
Telangiectasia, hereditary hemorrhagic,
163
Temperature regulation, 308–309,
333–334
Tenecteplase
tissue plasminogen activator *versus,* 322,
324
trials with, 304–305
Terminal endocarditis, 91–92
Territorial ischemic stroke symptoms,
230t–231t
Therapy of Patients with Acute Stroke,
292
Thiazide diuretic, stroke risk and, 13
Thienopyridine, 187–191
Third National Health and Nutrition
Examination Survey
homoocyst(e)ine and, 30
on hypertension, 13
Three-hour window for thrombolytic
therapy, 270
Thrombin inhibitor, direct, 179–180,
297–298
currently available, 284t
as emerging therapy, 297–298
Thrombocytopenia, heparin-induced,
337
Thromboembolic stroke
hormone replacement and, 203
prosthetic heart valve and, 89
Thromboembolism prevention, 335–337,
338t
Thrombolysis in Brain Ischemia score,
257
Thrombolysis in Myocardial Ischemia,
277
Thrombolytic therapy, 267–280
in coronary artery disease, 84
emerging, intra-arterial, 305
intra-arterial, 275–279
intravenous therapy with, 276–278,
277t
primary, 275

Thrombolytic therapy *(Continued)*
    rescue therapy, 278–279, 278f,
        279t
    intravenous, 267–275, 268t
        3-hour time window for, 270
        in clinical practice, 272–273
        correct dose of, 271
        criteria for, 271–272, 271t
        outcomes for, 273, 274t, 275, 275t
    risk of hemorrhage and, 365
Thrombosis, deep venous
    as complication, 350–351
    prevention of, 335–337, 338t
    in rehabilitation phase, 381–382
Thrombotic complications of stroke,
    350–351
Thrombotic endocarditis, noninfective,
    91–92
Thrombus
    in cardioembolic stroke, 58–59,
        79–80
    formation of, 175–177, 176f, 177f
    left ventricular, 83, 83f
TIBI score. *See* Thrombolysis in Brain
    Ischemia score
Ticlopidine, 187–189
    for lacunar stroke, 133
Ticlopidine Aspirin Stroke Study, 188
Timing
    of complications, 350f
    of rehabilitation, 380–381
    of thrombolytic therapy, 270
Tinzaparin in Acute Ischemic Stroke Trial,
    292–293
Tirilazad, 313–314
Tissue plasminogen activator, recombinant,
    267–280
    blood pressure management and,
        332
    intra-arterial, 275–279
        glycoprotein IIb/IIIa inhibitor and,
            296–297
        intravenous therapy with, 276–278,
            277t
        primary, 275
        as rescue therapy with, 278–279,
            278f, 279t
    intravenous, 267–275, 268t
        3-hour time window for, 270
        in clinical practice, 272–273
        correct dose of, 271
        criteria for, 271–272, 271t
        outcomes for, 273, 274t, 275,
            275t
    tenecteplase *vs.,* 322, 324

Tissue replacement heart valve,
    90
TOAST. *See* Trial of ORG 10172 in
    Acute Stroke Treatment
Tobacco smoking. *See* Smoking
Top-of-the-basilar syndrome, 153
TOPAS, 292
Toxin, botulinum, 385
Training, treadmill, 388
Transcranial Doppler ultrasonography,
    256
    in cerebral edema, 368
    for large-vessel atherosclerosis,
        115–116
    thrombolytic therapy and, 279
    in transient ischemic attack, 72–73,
        75f, 76
Transesophageal echocardiography,
    72–73
Transformation, hemorrhagic, 365–367,
    366f, 367f, 368t
Transforming growth factor, 316
Transient ischemic attack, 67–77
    atherosclerosis and, 104
    common symptoms of, 69t
    coumarins for, 178
    heparin for, 293
    large-vessel atherosclerosis and,
        104
    mechanism of, 72–73, 74f–76f
    origin of, 69–71, 70f, 71f
    risk of stroke after, 197
    stroke *vs.,* 71–72
Transluminal angioplasty
    for extracranial disease, 113–114
    percutaneous, intracranial, 307
Transluminal coronary angioplasty,
    percutaneous, 84
Transport of patient, 221
Treadmill training, 388
Trial of ORG 10172 in Acute Stroke
    Treatment
    on antiplatelet therapy, 292, 293
    on recurrence, 364
Triflusal, 187
Triflusal *versus* Aspirin in Cerebral
    Infarction Prevention study,
    87
Trousseau syndrome, 91
Tube, gastrostomy, 386–387
Tumor, cardiac, 59
    cardioembolic stroke caused by,
        92
Turbulence, atherosclerosis and,
    99

U

U70046F, 313–314
UK-TIA trial. *See* United Kingdom
    Transient Ischemic Attack trial
Ultrasonication, 309
Ultrasonography, 256–258, 257
    transcranial Doppler, 256
    in cerebral edema, 368
    for large-vessel atherosclerosis,
        115–116
    thrombolytic therapy and, 279
    in transient ischemic attack, 72–73,
        75f, 76
Unfractionated heparin
    in deep venous thrombosis, 336
    trials using, 288–291
United Kingdom Glucose Insulin in Stroke
    Trial, 335
United Kingdom Transient Ischemic
    Attack trial, 107, 185
Unknown cause of neurological
    deterioration, 372–373, 372t
Urinary incontinence, 356
    treatment of, 387
Urinary tract infection, 356–357
Urokinase, 296–297
Urological complications, 356

V

VA-HIT. *See* Veteran Affairs HDL
    Intervention Trial
Valve prosthesis, 59–60
Valvular heart disease
    cardioembolic stroke caused by, 88–90
    mitral valvular strand, 92–93, 93f
Vascular dementia, 131–132
Vascular disorder in transient ischemic
    attack, 69–71, 70f, 71f
Vascular dysplasia, 145
Vascular imaging, 63f
    computed tomography, 243–246,
        243f–246f
    magnetic resonance, 253–255, 254f,
        255f
Vascular malformation in Sturge-Weber
    syndrome, 160
Vascular resistance, cerebral, 331
Vascular system, homocyst(e)ine affecting,
    33f
Vasculitis, 57
Vasculopathy. *See also* Angiopathy
    Kawasaki syndrome in, 148
    in malignant atrophic papulosis, 140
    noninflammatory, 57–58

Vasoconstriction, reversible, 156–157
Vegetables in diet, 34
Vegetation, valve, 59–60
Venography, magnetic resonance,
    254–255
Venous thrombosis
    as complication, 350–351
    prevention of, 335–337, 338t
    in rehabilitation phase, 381–382
Ventilation, mechanical, 339, 353
Ventricle, thrombus of, 83, 83f
VENUS. *See* Very Early Nimodipine
    Use in Stroke
Verrucous endocarditis, 91–92
Vertebral artery disease, 104, 113
Vertebral dissection, heparin for, 293
Very Early Nimodipine Use in Stroke,
    313
Veteran Affairs HDL Intervention Trial,
    21
Viral infection, 38
VISP. *See* Vitamin Intervention for Stroke
    Prevention
Vitamin, 34
Vitamin Intervention for Stroke Prevention,
    205
Vitamin K, 177
Vitamins to Prevent Stroke, 205
VITATOPS. *See* Vitamins to Prevent
    Stroke
Volume replacement, 331
Von Recklinghausen disease, 165

W

Walking, improving, 386
Warfarin
    for atrial fibrillation, 81
    in congestive heart failure, 86
    in intracranial atherosclerosis, 107
    for lacunar stroke, 133
    in patent foramen ovale, 87
    in sinus rhythm, 106–107
Warfarin-Aspirin Recurrent Stroke Study,
    133, 179
Warfarin Versus Aspirin in Reduced
    Cardiac Ejection Fraction Study,
    86
Warfarin *versus* aspirin study, 107,
    116–117
Warning signs of stroke, 212–213, 213t
WARSS. *See* Warfarin-Aspirin Recurrent
    Stroke Study
WASID. *See* Warfarin *versus* aspirin
    study

Watershed, anterior and posterior,
    231t
White matter in lacunar stroke,
    123–124
Window, time, for thrombolytic therapy,
    270
Women's Estrogen for Stroke Trial, 203
Women's Health Initiative
    on exercise, 206
    on hormone replacement, 203
World Health Organization, on metabolic
    syndrome, 27t

X

X-linked disorder, Fabry disease as, 162
XeCT. *See* Xenon-CT
Xenon computed tomography, 247
Xenon-CT, 247
Ximelagatran
    for atrial fibrillation, 81
    effectiveness of, 180

Z

Z-VAD, 315